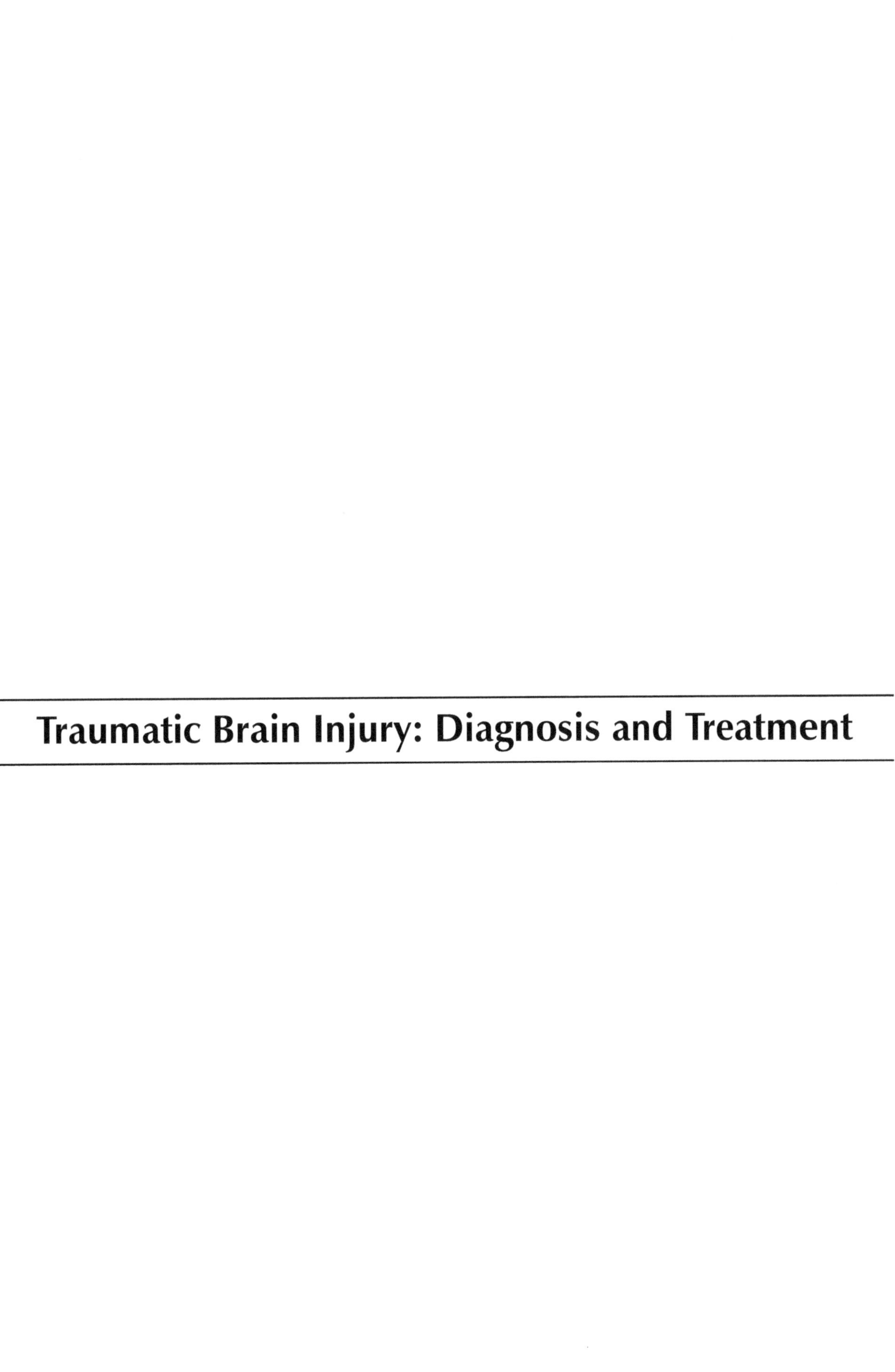

Traumatic Brain Injury: Diagnosis and Treatment

Traumatic Brain Injury: Diagnosis and Treatment

Editor: Analise Phelps

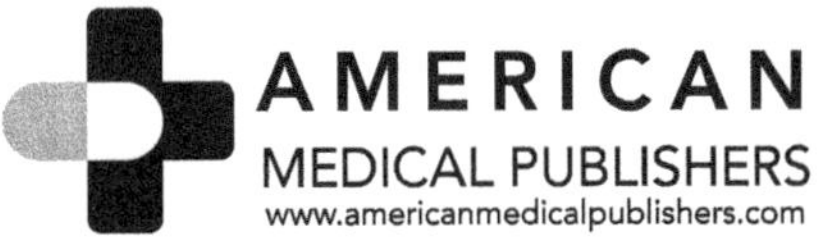

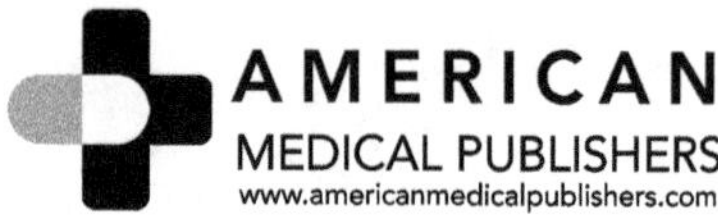

Cataloging-in-Publication Data

Traumatic brain injury : diagnosis and treatment / edited by Analise Phelps.
p. cm.
Includes bibliographical references and index.
ISBN 978-1-63927-333-1
1. Brain--Wounds and injuries. 2. Brain--Wounds and injuries--Diagnosis.
3. Brain--Wounds and injuries--Treatment. I. Phelps, Analise.
RD594 .T73 2022
617.481--dc23

American Medical Publishers,
41 Flatbush Avenue,
1st Floor, New York,
NY 11217, USA

ISBN 978-1-63927-333-1 (Hardback)

Contents

Preface

Traumatic brain injury (TBI) refers to the occurrence of brain injuries caused by an external force. It is also known as intracranial injury. TBI can cause physical, cognitive and behavioral symptoms. These symptoms include headache, vomiting, nausea, blurred vision, fatigue, etc. Their outcomes can range from complete recovery to permanent disability or sometimes fatal. It can be diagnosed using many techniques of neurological examination such as computed tomography, magnetic resonance imaging, electroencephalography, etc. The major cause of TBI is vehicle accidents. The two stages of TBI are acute stage and chronic stage. The treatment of acute stage includes use of sedatives, analgesics and paralytic agents. Chronic stage can be managed through rehabilitation, physiotherapy and occupational therapy. The topics included in this book on traumatic brain injury are of utmost significance and bound to provide incredible insights to readers. It contains some path-breaking studies in the diagnosis and treatment of traumatic brain injury. This book will serve as a valuable source of reference for graduate and postgraduate students.

The researches compiled throughout the book are authentic and of high quality, combining several disciplines and from very diverse regions from around the world. Drawing on the contributions of many researchers from diverse countries, the book's objective is to provide the readers with the latest achievements in the area of research. This book will surely be a source of knowledge to all interested and researching the field.

In the end, I would like to express my deep sense of gratitude to all the authors for meeting the set deadlines in completing and submitting their research chapters. I would also like to thank the publisher for the support offered to us throughout the course of the book. Finally, I extend my sincere thanks to my family for being a constant source of inspiration and encouragement.

Editor

1

Transiently lowering tumor necrosis factor-α synthesis ameliorates neuronal cell loss and cognitive impairments induced by minimal traumatic brain injury in mice

Renana Baratz[1], David Tweedie[2], Jia-Yi Wang[3], Vardit Rubovitch[1], Weiming Luo[2], Barry J Hoffer[4], Nigel H Greig[2*†] and Chaim G Pick[1†]

Abstract

Background: The treatment of traumatic brain injury (TBI) represents an unmet medical need, as no effective pharmacological treatment currently exists. The development of such a treatment requires a fundamental understanding of the pathophysiological mechanisms that underpin the sequelae resulting from TBI, particularly the ensuing neuronal cell death and cognitive impairments. Tumor necrosis factor-alpha (TNF-α) is a cytokine that is a master regulator of systemic and neuroinflammatory processes. TNF-α levels are reported to become rapidly elevated post TBI and, potentially, can lead to secondary neuronal damage.

Methods: To elucidate the role of TNF-α in TBI, particularly as a drug target, the present study evaluated (i) time-dependent TNF-α levels and (ii) markers of apoptosis and gliosis within the brain and related these to behavioral measures of 'well being' and cognition in a mouse closed head 50 g weight drop mild TBI (mTBI) model in the presence and absence of post-treatment with an experimental TNF-α synthesis inhibitor, 3,6'-dithiothalidomide.

Results: mTBI elevated brain TNF-α levels, which peaked at 12 h post injury and returned to baseline by 18 h. This was accompanied by a neuronal loss and an increase in astrocyte number (evaluated by neuronal nuclei (NeuN) and glial fibrillary acidic protein (GFAP) immunostaining), as well as an elevation in the apoptotic death marker BH3-interacting domain death agonist (BID) at 72 h. Selective impairments in measures of cognition, evaluated by novel object recognition and passive avoidance paradigms - without changes in well being, were evident at 7 days after injury. A single systemic treatment with the TNF-α synthesis inhibitor 3,6'-dithiothalidomide 1 h post injury prevented the mTBI-induced TNF-α elevation and fully ameliorated the neuronal loss (NeuN), elevations in astrocyte number (GFAP) and BID, and cognitive impairments. Cognitive impairments evident at 7 days after injury were prevented by treatment as late as 12 h post mTBI but were not reversed when treatment was delayed until 18 h.

Conclusions: These results implicate that TNF-α in mTBI induced secondary brain damage and indicate that pharmacologically limiting the generation of TNF-α post mTBI may mitigate such damage, defining a time-dependent window of up to 12 h to achieve this reversal.

* Correspondence: greign@grc.nia.nih.gov
†Equal contributors
[2]Drug Design and Development Section, Translational Gerontology Branch, Intramural Research Program, National Institute on Aging, National Institutes of Health, BRC Room 05C220, 251 Bayview Blvd., Baltimore, MD 21224, USA
Full list of author information is available at the end of the article

Introduction

Traumatic brain injury (TBI) is a common cause of morbidity and mortality across both the civilian and military populations, with a reported worldwide annual incidence of some ten million cases [1]. Indeed, within the US alone, TBI accounts for some 1.7 million emergency department visits - a number that likely underestimates its true incidence [2] - and is credited with some 30% of all injury-related deaths [3]. In essence, TBI is elicited following the unexpected application of an external force to the head. Patients who survive such injury often present with persistent long-term disabilities that require rehabilitation - a costly 52 billion dollars annual expense in the US alone [4-6]. The severity of ensuing disabilities varies and often may be associated with the severity of the injury itself [7]. Mild TBI (mTBI) accounts for some 80% to 90% of cases, and arising common disabilities include sensory-motor problems, learning and memory deficits, anxiety, and depression [8,9]. Of significant additional concern, mTBI may predispose long-term survivors to age-related neurodegenerative disorders by providing a risk factor for the development of Alzheimer's disease, Parkinson's disease, and post-traumatic dementia [10-14], with the older people being most vulnerable [15,16]. Despite significant ongoing research and advancements in our understanding of the molecular and cellular changes that occur after TBI, no effective pharmacological treatment is currently available [17,18].

mTBI-associated brain damage can be subdivided into two phases: an initial primary phase that is immediate and results from the mechanical force(s) applied to the skull and brain at the time of impact, potentially inducing shearing and compression of neuronal and vascular tissue that results in brain contusion, axonal injury, blood vessel rupture, and hemorrhage. This is followed by an extended second phase that involves cascades of biological processes initiated at the time of injury that may persist over subsequent days, weeks, and possibly months, consequent to ischemia, neuroinflammation, glutamate toxicity, altered blood-brain barrier permeability, oxidative stress, astrocyte reactivity, cellular dysfunction, and apoptosis [19-22]. As secondary brain injury may be reversible, in order to develop an effective treatment, it is imperative to understand the biological cascades that drive the delayed secondary phase that occurs following TBI [23-25].

It is widely recognized that inflammatory cytokines, chemokines, and growth factors play significant roles in the pathophysiology of TBI. Albeit that initiation of an inflammatory response can be essential to promote neuroreparative mechanisms in response to a physiological insult [26-28], if this is excessive or unregulated, it can augment neuronal dysfunction and degeneration by inducing a self-propagating pathological cascade of neuroinflammation [29-31]. Shortly following TBI, substantial synthesis and release of proinflammatory cytokines occur from astrocytes and microglia, particularly tumor necrosis factor-α (TNF-α) with mRNA and protein levels becoming acutely elevated within as little as 17 min after injury seen in post-mortem brains from patients who died shortly after TBI [32]. A parallel rapid sequence has been described in rodent TBI animal models in which a TNF-α rise precedes the appearance of ensuing cytokines [33-35]. Depending on its signaling pathway, TNF-α can exacerbate trauma and oxidative stress within the brain and contribute to glutamate release and blood-brain barrier dysfunction that can lead to further influx of inflammatory factors from blood to brain [36].

Inhibiting the generation of TNF-α may thus reinforce its role in mTBI and define its value as a potential treatment target, as it is considered a master regulator of the inflammatory response. Sudden and substantial rises in TNF-α can induce a diverse array of cell death processes, including NF-kB activation, apoptosis, and necrosis [37]. In addition, an increase in TNF-α levels trigger glutamate release from astrocytes, which can lead to glutamate excitotoxicity [38]. Although the elevation of TNF-α levels in the early hours post TBI can be harmful [39-41], cytokine balance has been reported as essential for long-term recovery from injury [40-42]. In this current study, rather than utilizing a TNF-α antibody approach to capture and clear it before it can potentially reach its target, as is effectively achieved in the treatment of rheumatoid arthritis, the experimental drug 3,6′-dithiothalidomide was employed to reduce TNF-α synthesis [43] and thereby maintain but dramatically lower its physiological release pattern. In our previous studies, we effectively used 3,6′-dithiothalidomide to ameliorate cognitive deficit following mTBI [44]. However, our previous work did not define the therapeutic window for 3,6′-dithiothalidomide, the extended time course of TNF-α overproduction, and the histochemical changes in neurons and glia correlated with injury. We extend our previous finding in the present study, correlating the potential role of mTBI-induced TNF-α release with neuronal loss, apoptosis, and astrocyte elevation, and defining a window of opportunity for potential treatment.

Materials and methods

Animals

Male ICR mice (30 to 40 g of weight and 6 to 8 weeks of age) were bred and raised within the vivarium of Tel Aviv University, Israel, originally derived from breeding pairs purchased from HSD Jerusalem, Israel. They were housed four to six per cage, maintained at a constant 22 ± 1°C, had *ad libitum* access to food and water, and kept on a 12:12 h light/dark cycle. Lighting during the light phase remained constant, and all experimental manipulations were undertaken during this light phase of the cycle. A minimum number of animals were included into studies, and all efforts were made to minimize potential suffering. Each animal was used for only a single experiment, and all experimental procedures and housing conditions were approved by the Institutional Animal Care and Use Committee of Tel Aviv University (M-10-006).

Mild traumatic brain injury

Mice were subjected to mTBI using a weight drop device that has previously been described [44-46]. Mice were anesthetized with isoflurane (Merck & Co., Inc., Whitehouse Station, NJ, USA) and then placed under the device. The weight drop apparatus comprised of a cylindrical-shaped 50-g piece of metal with a rounded spherical tip, which was dropped through a vertical metal guide tube (diameter 13 mm × length 80 cm). Anesthetized mice were carefully positioned with their head supported and immobilized by a sponge so that the right temporal side of the head, between the corner of the eye and the ear, was directly below the guide tube opening. The sponge allowed anterior/posterior motion of the head without rotational movement at the moment of impact following weight drop [44-46]. Sham mice were submitted to the same procedure as described for mTBI, but without release of the weight.

Drug administration

Synthesis of 3,6′-dithiothalidomide (Merck & Co., Inc., Whitehouse Station, NJ, USA) was achieved by a published synthetic route [43], and chemical characterization confirmed the structure of the final product with a chemical purity of 99.8%. The agent was prepared as a suspension in 1% carboxymethyl cellulose (formulated in isotonic saline; Merck & Co., Inc., Whitehouse Station, NJ, USA) immediately prior to daily use in each study to provide a final dose of 28 mg/kg (0.1 ml/10 g) body weight. Either 3,6′-dithiothalidomide or similarly prepared vehicle was administered by the intraperitoneal (i.p.) route from 1 to 18 h post injury or sham procedure, depending on the measures evaluated (whether for ELISA, immunohistochemistry, or behavioral studies).

TNF-α analysis by ELISA

To verify the occurrence of TNF-α elevation in our mTBI model and define its time dependence, mice were subjected to mTBI and brains were removed at specific times thereafter (1 to 18 h; $n = 4$ to 5 per time). The right cortex was immediately frozen in liquid nitrogen and homogenized with appropriate protease inhibitors (Halt Protease Inhibitor Cocktail; Sigma-Aldrich, St. Louis, MO, USA). The samples were then quantified for TNF-α levels by ELISA assay (BioLegend, San Diego, CA, USA).

Physiological parameters of well-being

Rectal temperature was recorded with a mouse thermometer. Baseline values (°C) were evaluated 30 min before 3,6′-dithiothalidomide administration and at 1 and 4 h following mTBI or sham procedure.

Anxiety-like behavior and motor activity were evaluated by elevated plus maze. The maze was elevated 60 cm above the floor level and comprised of 4 arms (30 × 5 × 15 cm) along which mice could walk that formed a '+' shape [47]. Two conjoined arms were open (without walls) and the other two were closed (with walls but no ceiling). On evaluation days, mice were placed at the center of the plus-maze, facing one of the open arms and their time spent within the open arms was recorded over a 5-min period. The maze was cleansed with 70% ethanol (ETOH; *v*/*v*) between animals.

Cognitive behavioral tests

Two behavioral paradigms were evaluated: Y-maze and novel object recognition (NOR).

Y-maze test

Spatial memory was evaluated by Y-maze, as initially described by Dellu and colleagues [48], and is a task that takes advantage of a preference of rodents to explore novel rather than familiar places. The Y-maze was erected from black Plexiglas and comprised of three alike arms (30 × 8 × 15 cm length, set at an angle of 120° from one another). Evaluation comprised of two trials separated by a 2-min interval (during which the mouse was returned to its home cage). The initial 'familiarization' trial was of 5-min duration with only two arms open (one termed the 'start' arm and the other the 'old' arm), with the third ('novel') arm blocked by a door. The second trial was of 2-min duration, and all three arms were open. The time spent in each of the arms was recorded, and discrimination of spatial novelty was determined as a preference index [49] calculated as (time in the novel – time in the old arm)/(time in the novel + time in the old arm). The apparatus was cleansed between trials with 70% ETOH (*v*/*v*).

NOR test

An object recognition test to evaluate short-term recognition memory [50] was undertaken within an open field that comprised a black Plexiglas arena (59 × 59 cm size) surrounded by 20-cm black walls. The task takes advantage of a predisposition for rodents to explore new objects and included three trials of 5-min duration separated by a 24-h interval. On the initial day of evaluation, mice were individually placed within the empty arena for habituation. The following day, mice were placed into the same arena that had two identical objects, A and B, positioned 40 cm from one another and 10 cm from the walls. On the third day, mice were again placed into the arena; however, object A remained the same as the preceding day and new object C replaced prior object B. The arena and objects were thoroughly cleansed (70% ETOH *v/v*) between each trial. Object exploration (defined as rearing on the object or sniffing it at a distance of less than 2 cm and/or nose touching it) was recorded and discrimination of recognition novelty was determined as a preference index [49]: (time exploring the new object – time exploring the old object)/(total time exploring an object). Mice that explored objects for less than 10% of the total available time were excluded from analyses.

Immunohistochemistry/immunofluorescence brain slice studies

A cohort of mTBI and sham mice were anesthetized at 72 h following the procedure by excess ketamine + xylazine administration and were immediately perfused transcardially with PBS followed by 4% paraformaldehyde ((PFA) in 0.1 M phosphate buffer, pH 7.4). Their brains were removed, fixed overnight (4% PFA in 0.1 M phosphate buffer, pH 7.4), and then placed in 30% sucrose for 48 h. Coronal sections (30 μm) were cut on a cryostat, placed in cryoprotectant, and stored at −20°C until use. Thereafter, 5 sections of cortex and 5 of hippocampus were blocked by incubation with 0.1% Triton X-100 in phosphate-buffered saline (PBST) and 10% normal horse serum for 1 h at 25°C. The primary antibodies, mouse anti-neuronal nuclei (NeuN; 1:50, Millipore, Danvers, MA, USA, Cat#MAB3377), mouse anti-glial fibrillary acidic protein (GFAP; 1:10,000, Millipore, Cat#MAB3402), and rabbit anti-BH3-interacting domain death agonist (BID; 1:50, Cell Signaling, Danvers, MA, USA, Cat#9942), were then dissolved in PBST and 2% normal horse serum and incubated with the sections for 48 h at 4°C. Following rinsing in PBST, sections were incubated for 1 h at 25°C with DyLight™ 594-conjugated AffinityPure Donkey Anti-rabbit IgG and DyLight™ 488-conjugated AffinityPure Donkey Anti-mouse IgG (1:300; Jackson Laboratories, Bar Harbor, ME, USA). After rinses in PBST, sections were mounted on dry gelatin-coated slides and evaluated for fluorescence with a Zeiss LSM 510 confocal microscope with × 20 and × 63 lens (Carl Zeiss, Jena, Germany). For each brain, three to five sections were taken and the average numbers of cells within the hippocampus and the temporal cortex were calculated within defined fields of either 140^2 or 440^2 μM. Evaluation of immunohistochemical slides for immunofluorescence was undertaken in a blinded manner, and the omission of primary antibodies was routinely undertaken in the generation of negative control sections. Analyses were performed by Imaris program for color quantification (Bitplane AG, Zurich, Switzerland).

Data analyses

Results throughout are presented as mean ± SEM values and were analyzed by SPSS 18 software (Genius Systems, Petah Tikva, Israel). One-way ANOVAs were performed to compare between all groups, followed by least significant difference (LSD) *post hoc* tests. ANOVA-repeated measures were performed to compare rectal temperatures.

Results

Evaluation of well-being

'Basic well-being,' a concept that underlies the combined health and wellness of an animal [51], was evaluated across all mice groups and combined subjective measures, such as the grooming and appearance, righting skills, ambulation, and blinking reflex, with objective ones that included the parameters of weight, body temperature, anxiety-like behavior, and motor skills.

Subjectively and in accord with prior studies [45], mice subjected to this type of mTBI were indistinguishable from those subjected to the sham procedure when evaluated at 1 or 24 h later, irrespective of 3,6′-dithiothalidomide or vehicle administration. Rectal temperature measurements were used to monitor potential core temperature changes induced by either brain injury or 3,6′-dithiothalidomide administration, and no significant difference (NS) was found either between animal groups [$F(2,12) = 0.084$, NS] or across measurement times (30 min before injury and 1 and 4 h post-mTBI/injection) [$F(2,12) = 3.630$, NS] (data not shown).

The elevated plus maze was used to examine anxiety-like behavior and motor activity. No differences were found between any groups in anxiety-like behavior at 72 h and 7 days post-injury [$F(5,56) = 0.791$, NS] [$F(5,47) = 0.765$, NS], respectively (data not shown). Likewise, no differences were evident between any groups in relation to motor skills evaluated at 72 h and 7 days post-injury [$F(5,56) = 1.13$ NS] [$F(5,47) = 0.798$, NS], respectively (data not shown). Together these result indicate that mice were healthy and that neither mTBI nor 3,6′-dithiothalidomide impacted their well-being.

Time-dependent changes in TNF-α levels in brain tissue

As illustrated in Figure 1, mice challenged with mTBI demonstrated a time-dependent rise in brain protein levels of TNF-α that were increased by 2.5-fold, peaked at 12 h post injury, and returned to baseline by 18 h [$F(3,13) = 30.529$, $p < 0.0001$]. LSD *post hoc* analyses confirmed that the 12-h mTBI group was significantly different from all other groups ($p < 0.0001$). Levels were elevated to 132.9 pg/ml at 12 h versus a baseline value of 53.4 pg/ml. In animals subjected to mTBI and administered 3,6′-dithiothalidomide 1 h post injury, the elevated TNF-α 12 h post injury response was ameliorated. Specifically, mice treated with 3,6′-dithiothalidomide post

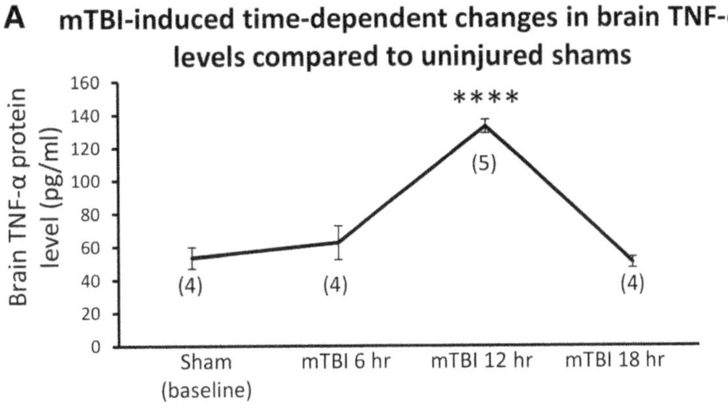

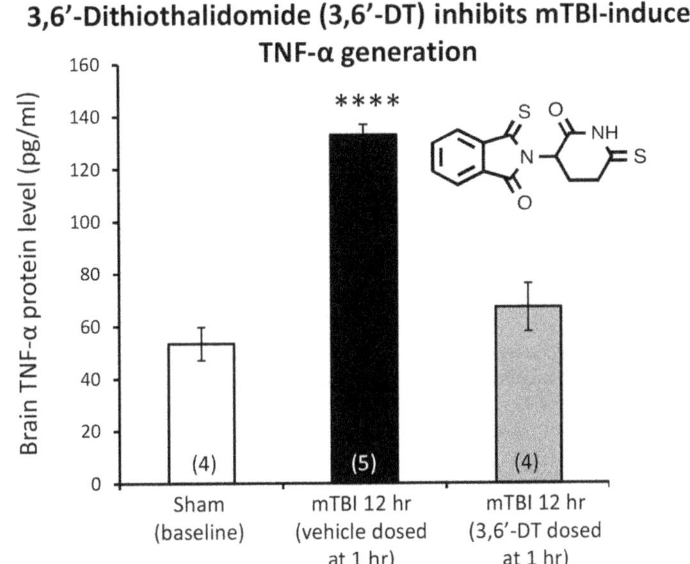

Figure 1 mTBI induces a time-dependent rise in brain TNF-α levels. Right (ipsilateral to mTBI) cerebral cortex protein extracts were prepared from sham or mTBI mice at the indicated time points post injury. **(A)** Time-dependent brain levels of TNF-α at baseline (sham) and post injury. At 12 h post mTBI, TNF-α levels peaked (132.8 vs. 53.4 (sham) pg/ml, $p < 0.0001$). By 18 h post injury, TNF-α levels returned to baseline (50.5 pg/ml). **(B)** Treatment with 3,6'-dithiothalidomide (3,6-DT) at 1 h after mTBI prevented the TNF-α elevation evident at 12 h post mTBI (3,6'-DT + mTBI 67.1 pg/ml vs. mTBI 132.8 pg/ml, $p < 0.0001$). In both **(A)** and **(B)**, **** was significantly different from all other groups ($p < 0.0001$).

injury had similar brain TNF-α levels as the sham group, 67.0 and 53.4 pg/ml, respectively, $F(4,17) = 14.579$, $p < 0.0001$, Figure 1B. LSD *post hoc* analyses confirmed that the mTBI 12-h group was significantly different from all other groups ($p < 0.0001$).

mTBI- and treatment-induced changes in cognitive function

When evaluated by Y-maze at 7 days post procedure, vehicle-treated mTBI-challenged mice demonstrated a significant impairment in spatial memory, as compared to sham control animals. This mTBI-induced deficit was ameliorated by a single dose of 3,6′-dithiothalidomide administered either 1 or 12 h post injury. However, when 3,6′-dithiothalidomide administration was withheld until 18 h, mice displayed impairment and, together with the mTBI vehicle group, their preference index was significantly reduced compared to sham controls [$F(4,57) = 6.462$, $p < 0.01$] (Figure 2A). LSD *post hoc* analyses confirmed that the mTBI + vehicle and the mTBI + 18 h 3,6′-dithiothalidomide groups were significantly different from all other groups ($p < 0.05$).

As illustrated in Figure 2B, the spatial deficit evident in vehicle-treated mTBI mice in the Y-maze was also seen with the NOR paradigm. Here too, the administration of a single dose of 3,6′-dithiothalidomide to mTBI mice 1 or 12 h following injury fully mitigated the deficit, but delaying administration to 18 h post injury did not. Specifically, the mTBI vehicle and mTBI + 18 h 3,6′-dithiothalidomide groups displayed a significantly reduced index preference versus sham controls [$F(4,57) = 8.975$, $p < 0.001$]. LSD *post hoc* analyses established that the mTBI + vehicle and the

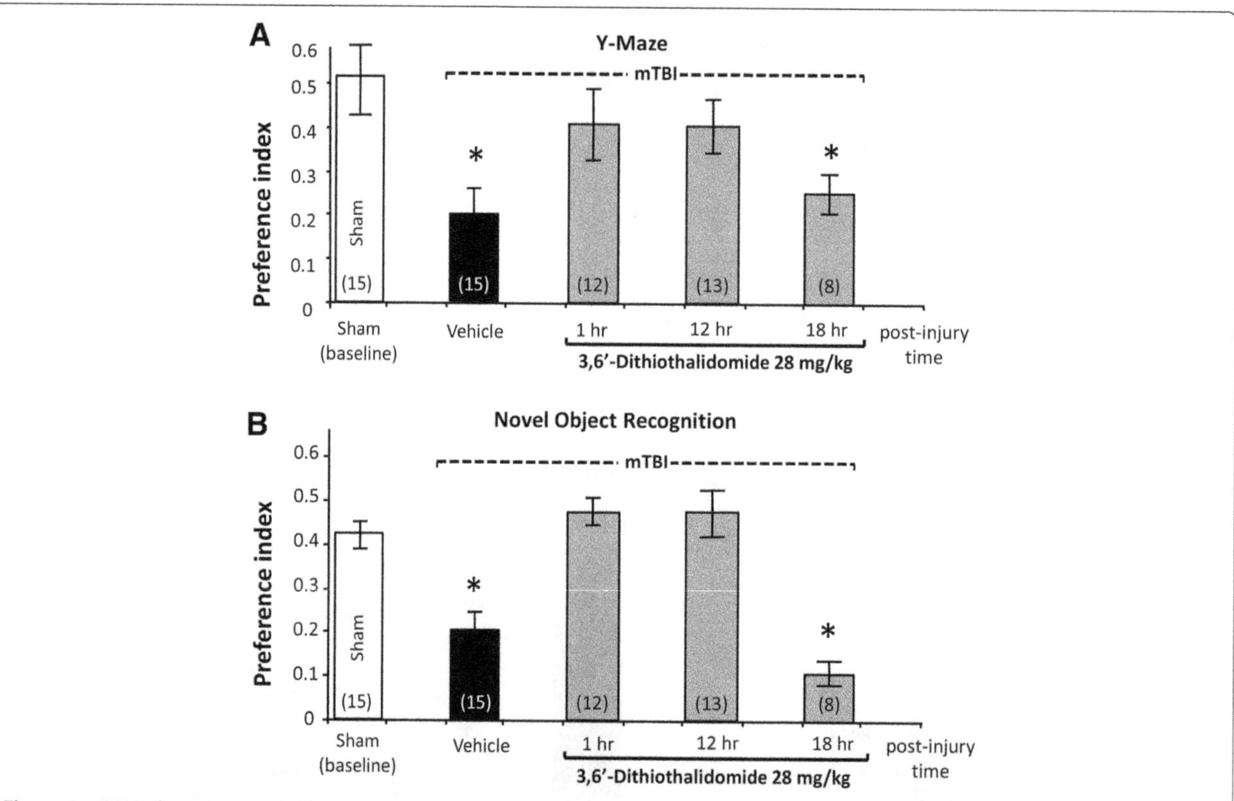

Figure 2 mTBI induces impairments in performance in both a Y-maze and novel object recognition (NOR) preference index paradigms that are ameliorated by 3,6′-dithiothalidomide when administered up to 12 but not 18 h post injury. (A) Performance of mice was quantitatively assessed in a Y-maze and **(B)** in a NOR paradigm at 7 days following mTBI as a preference index that was calculated as (time associated with the novel – time with the old arm or object)/(time with the novel + time with the old arm or object). Values are mean ± SEM values; a one-way ANOVA indicates that mTBI animals had a deficit in spatial (Y-maze) and visual (NOR) memory performance compared with all the other groups (*$p < 0.05$) with the exception of animals dosed with 3,6′-dithiothalidomide at 18 h post injury. No differences were found between any of the other groups (control (sham) 1 and 12 h 3,6′-dithiothalidomide dosing), suggesting complete amelioration by 3,6′-dithiothalidomide when administered within 12 h of injury.

mTBI + 18 h 3,6′-dithiothalidomide groups were significantly different from all other groups ($p < 0.05$).

Together these results extend the work of Baratz and colleagues [44] and define a therapeutic window of up to 12 h post mTBI to mitigate cognitive deficits by lowering TNF-α generation, as well as documenting the time course of TNF-α elevation.

Immunofluorescence

To evaluate the impact of mTBI at the cellular level, particularly in relation to the described amelioration of cognitive deficits imparted by lowering TNF-α generation, immunohistochemical analyses were undertaken at 72 h post injury. These focused on two key brain areas ipsilateral to injury: the cerebral cortex, as the area closest to impact, and the dentate gyrus, a region of the hippocampal formation considered to contribute to the formation of new episodic memory [52,53], the spontaneous exploration of novel environments, and other mnemonic functions [53,54].

Illustrated in Figures 3A and 4A are brain regions (cerebral cortex and dentate gyrus, respectively) displaying immunofluorescence associated with (i) NeuN, a neuronal nuclear protein that is widely used as a marker of adult neurons, and with (ii) BID, a proapoptotic Bcl-2 protein. Quantification of NeuN staining revealed a neuronal loss in both the cortex [$F(3,13) = 7.198$, $p < 0.005$, Figure 3B] and dentate gyrus [$F(3,15) = 5.641$, $p < 0.05$, Figure 4B]. *Post hoc* analyses revealed that the mTBI alone group was different from all other groups ($p < 0.05$) in both brain regions and was reduced by 42.5% and 22.3% versus sham values in cortex and dentate gyrus, respectively. Correlated with this was an elevation in apoptotic cell number, as revealed from BID staining in the cortex [$F(3,13) = 23.067$, $p < 0.0001$, Figure 3C] and in dentate gyrus [$F(3,13) = 6.301$, $p < 0.05$, Figure 4C]. Likewise, *post hoc* analyses demonstrated that the mTBI group was different from all other groups ($p < 0.0001$, $p < 0.05$, respectively; and 2.76- and 1.91-fold compared to their respective sham values). In addition and illustrated in Figures 5A and 6A, mTBI-challenged mice had an elevation in astrocyte number (3.37- and 1.39-fold, respectively), as revealed by GFAP staining, within the cortex [$F(3,13) = 37.641$, $p < 0.0001$, Figure 5B] and dentate

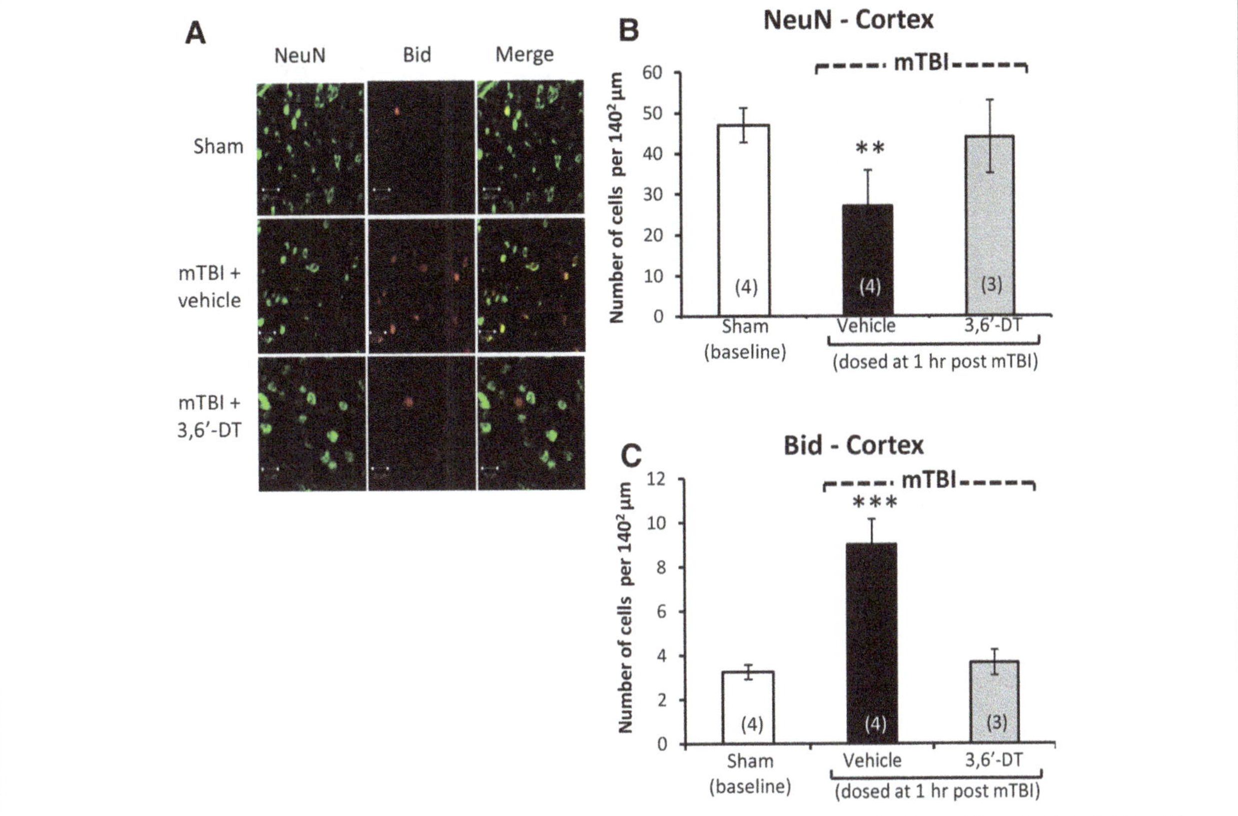

Figure 3 Neuronal loss and apoptosis is induced by mTBI in cerebral cortex ipsilateral to injury and mitigated by 3,6′-dithiothalidomide. At 72 h post injury, cerebral cortex ipsilateral to mTBI was assessed for cellular changes. **(A)** and **(B)** A decline in neuronal number indicative of neuronal loss (NeuN - green) was evident post mTBI ($p < 0.01$). Treatment with 3,6′-dithiothalidomide at 1 h post-injury prevented such a change. **(A)** and **(C)** An elevation in BID (a marker for apoptosis - red) was evident within mTBI brains ($p < 0.001$). No changes in apoptotic cell death were found in animals that were treated with 3,6′-dithiothalidomide (as compared to sham animals). Within **(A)** (representative sections within the cerebral cortex), the bar is equal to 20 μm in length.

gyrus [$F(3,13) = 13.284$, $p < 0.001$, Figure 6B]. The administration of 3,6′-dithiothalidomide 1 h post injury ameliorated all mTBI-induced changes in neuron, BID, and astrocyte number as, notably, no differences were found between the mTBI + 3,6′-dithiothalidomide and the sham groups. Finally, no changes were evident between any groups (sham, mTBI, and mTBI + drug) in the total cell numbers, as revealed from DAPI staining, within the cortex and dentate gyrus [$F(3,15) = 1.009$, NS, Figure 5C; $F(3,15) = 2.251$, NS, Figure 6C].

In conclusion, the early administration (1 h post injury) of a single dose of the TNF-α synthesis inhibitor 3,6′-dithiothalidomide inhibited cellular changes induced by mTBI in two key brain regions evaluated, cerebral cortex and dentate gyrus.

Discussion

TNF-α has been implicated in the pathogenesis of a wide number of neurological disorders that develop both acutely, as in TBI and stroke, and chronically, as in Alzheimer's disease and Parkinson's disease [29-36,40-42,55,56]. The current study confirms the rapid generation and release of TNF-α in a mouse closed head 50 g weight drop mTBI model, emulating a concussive head injury in humans, which led to neuronal loss and specific cognitive deficits. The inhibition of TNF-α synthesis blocked the mTBI-induced rise in brain TNF-α and protected against neuronal loss and cognitive deficits with a therapeutic window of 12 h. These results underline a role for TNF-α as a key regulator of cascades leading to neuronal loss and cognitive impairment in mTBI and highlights TNF-α as an amenable drug target for future mTBI treatment.

In light of (i) the high incidence of mTBI (approximately 600 per 100,000 people); (ii) the increased risk of dementia resulting from mTBI, particularly in the older people [15]; (iii) the upregulation of pathways leading to chronic neurodegenerative disorders induced by mTBI [12,20,57,58]; (iv) the long-term care, suffering, and economic debt associated with mTBI patients [59]; and (v) the lack of any available therapeutic [60], it is important to understand the mechanisms that underlie head injury.

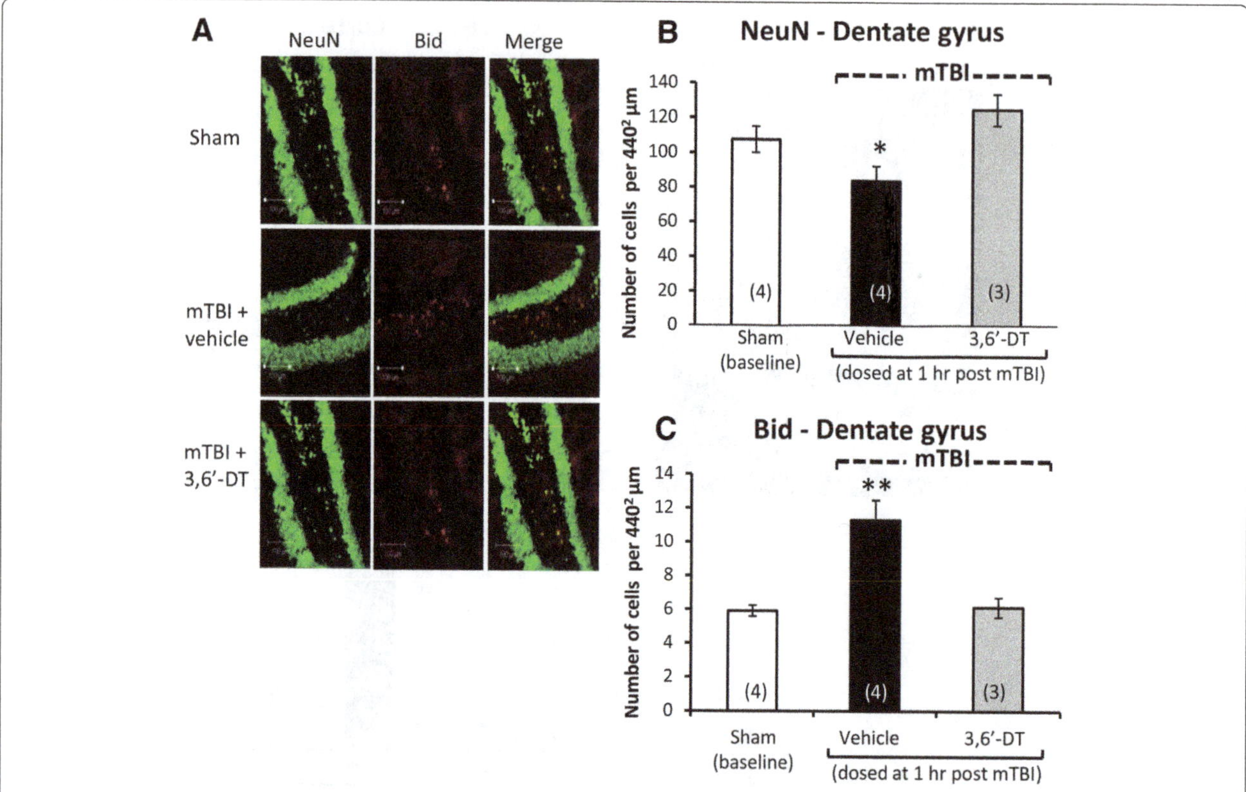

Figure 4 Neuronal loss and apoptosis is induced by mTBI in the dentate gyrus ipsilateral to injury and mitigated by 3,6′-dithiothalidomide. At 72 h post injury, the dentate gyrus of the hippocampus ipsilateral to mTBI was evaluated for cellular changes. **(A)** and **(B)** Neuronal loss (NeuN - green) was found post mTBI ($p < 0.05$). Treatment with the 3,6′-dithiothalidomide at 1 h post-injury prevented this loss. **(A)** and **(C)** An increase in BID (a marker for apoptosis in red) was evident in the mTBI brains ($p < 0.01$). No change in apoptotic cell death was apparent in animals treated with 3,6′-dithiothalidomide (as compared to sham animals). Within **(A)** (representative sections within the dentate gyrus), the bar is equal to 100 μm in length.

TNF-α is a well-characterized protein that regulates numerous cellular processes, including inflammation and cell death as well as cellular differentiation and survival, by binding to and activation of two cognate receptors: TNF-α receptor 1 (TNFR1) (p55) and TNFR2 (p75) [29-31,61].

TNFR1 is expressed ubiquitously, including neurons, astrocytes, and microglia throughout the brain. With its intracellular death domain, it contributes to neuronal dysfunction and death and primarily is activated by soluble TNF-α [62]. TNFR2, on the other hand, is principally expressed on hematopoietic cells but also is present on other cell types, including neurons, has been associated with cell survival [61,63-65] and chiefly responds to membrane-bound TNF-α [66,67]. The engagement of homotrimeric TNF-α (either soluble or membrane bound) to either receptor can activate three major signaling pathways: an apoptotic cascade initiated via the TNF-α receptor-associated death domain, a nuclear factor kappa B (NFκB) signaling a pro-survival pathway implemented via NFκB-mediated gene transcriptional actions, and a c-Jun N-terminal kinase (JNK) cascade involved in cellular differentiation and proliferation that is generally proapoptotic [38,68]. In large part, the contrasting pro-survival versus death-induced actions of TNF-α plausibly rely on which TNF-α receptor subtype is activated, the target cell types involved and their expression ratio of TNFR1/2 and associated coupling proteins, and the temporal concentrations of available soluble and membrane-bound TNF-α [64]. However, cross talk between the different signaling pathways and the degree and duration of neuroinflammation combine in determining the eventual physiological consequences of TNF-α receptor activation [69]. Consequent to the diverse actions of TNF-α and the influence of the brain microenvironment in which they occur, it is not always clear under which conditions TNF-α promotes beneficial versus deleterious neuronal effects. This explains the sometimes contradictory literature in the TNF-α neuroscience field [29-31,36,38,55,69] and its involvement in cascades promoting neuronal dysfunction and loss in both acute and long-term neurodegenerative disorders. In the present study, no differences were evident across the sham and mTBI groups in relation to the broad measure of 'well being' or in the evaluation of body temperature, anxiety-related behavior, and motor activity,

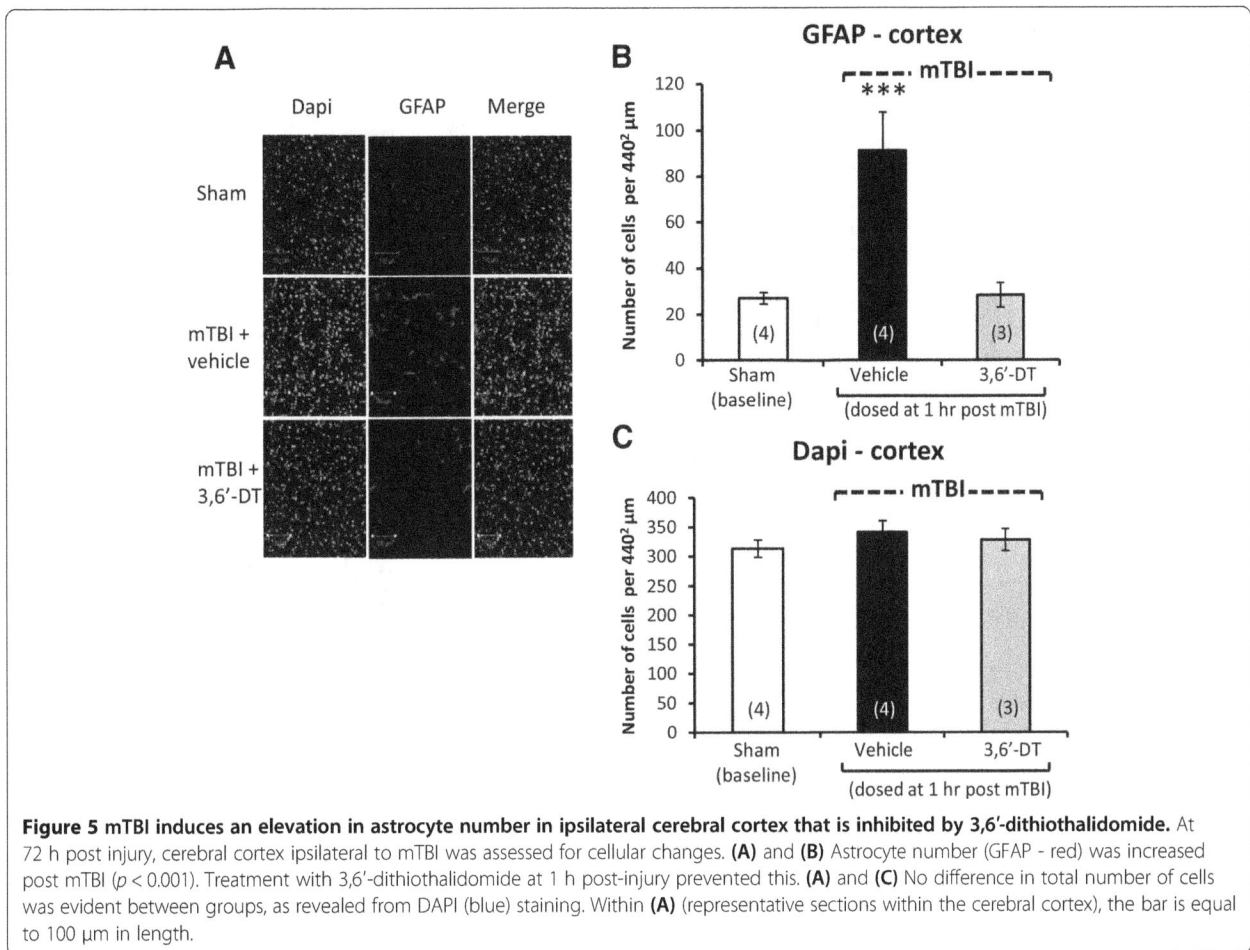

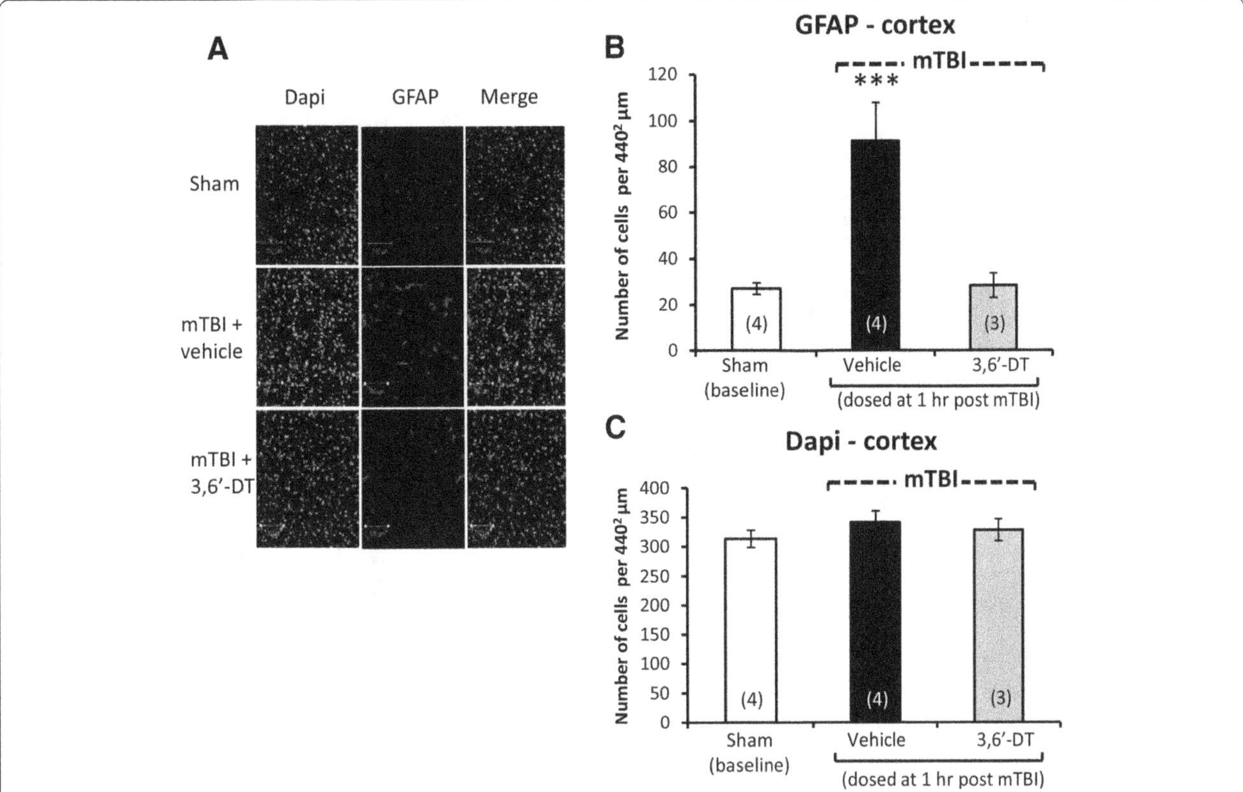

Figure 5 mTBI induces an elevation in astrocyte number in ipsilateral cerebral cortex that is inhibited by 3,6'-dithiothalidomide. At 72 h post injury, cerebral cortex ipsilateral to mTBI was assessed for cellular changes. **(A)** and **(B)** Astrocyte number (GFAP - red) was increased post mTBI ($p < 0.001$). Treatment with 3,6'-dithiothalidomide at 1 h post-injury prevented this. **(A)** and **(C)** No difference in total number of cells was evident between groups, as revealed from DAPI (blue) staining. Within **(A)** (representative sections within the cerebral cortex), the bar is equal to 100 μm in length.

which is in accord with previous results in rodents [51] and humans [70]. Although indistinguishable across a wide number of measures, importantly, deficits in cognitive performance were apparent in mTBI mice in accordance with past studies in mice [24,44-46] and humans [71]. In evaluating potential mechanisms responsible for these cognitive changes, a mTBI-triggered inflammatory cascade mediated by the generation of proinflammatory cytokines appears likely [72]. In this regard, the proinflammatory cytokine TNF-α is considered essential for both initiating and regulating an inflammatory response to trauma, and early transient elevations in brain mRNA expression of TNF-α as well as rises in IL-1β and IL-6 have been described in rodent closed head TBI, and associated adverse events [33,35,73]. In the current study, a time-dependent elevation in brain TNF-α protein levels was apparent in mTBI-challenged mice that peaked at 12 h and declined to baseline by 18 h. In line with this, elevated brain protein levels of TNF-α, IL-1β, and IL-6 have been reported in rodent mTBI models as well as within human CSF within hours of injury [74-78], as they have in other neurological disorders [79-81]. Inhibiting such an elevation in brain TNF-α in this model allowed the evaluation of the role of this transient TNF-α rise in neuronal cell loss, neuroinflammation, and cognitive deficits known to accompany mTBI.

To define the relationship between the mTBI-induced elevation in TNF-α and cognitive impairment evident 7 days later, 3,6'-dithiothalidomide was administered 1, 12, and 18 h following mTBI, extending our initial concentration-dependent studies of the compound in this same mTBI model [44]. Notably, mTBI-induced impairments in both the Y-maze and NOR paradigms were blocked by a single drug dose either at 1 or 12 h post injury, the peak of TNF-α generation in brain, but were not mitigated when administration was delayed to 18 h, thereby defining a treatment window of opportunity.

To evaluate the basis of the mTBI-induced cognitive impairment, brain regions ipsilateral to the side of injury were evaluated at 72 h, as this time coincides with the substantial occurrence of markers of neuronal apoptosis [24,82]. Assessment of the cerebral cortex, the area closest to the site of impact, and dentate gyrus of the hippocampus was performed, as dysfunction in the former and latter might explain the decline in performance in visual memory evaluated by NOR [83] and in spatial learning as assessed by the Y-maze [48], respectively. Neuronal loss (NeuN), an

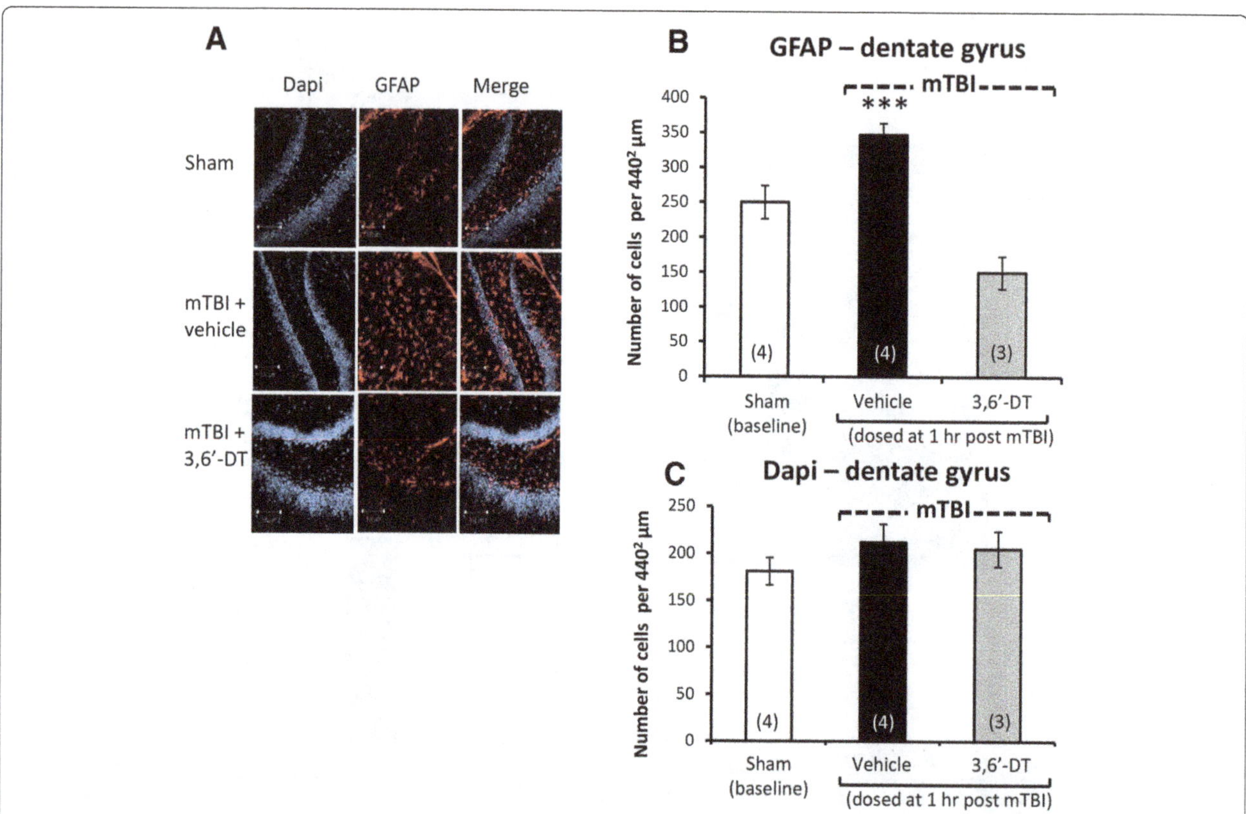

Figure 6 mTBI induces an elevation in astrocyte number in ipsilateral dentate gyrus that is inhibited by 3,6′-dithiothalidomide. At 72 h post injury, dentate gyrus ipsilateral injury was assessed for cellular changes. **(A)** and **(B)** Astrocyte number (GFAP - red) was elevated post mTBI ($p < 0.001$). Treatment with 3,6′-dithiothalidomide at 1 h post-injury inhibited this. **(A)** and **(C)** No difference in total number of cells was apparent between groups, as evaluated by DAPI (blue) staining. Within **(A)** (representative sections within the dentate gyrus), the bar is equal to 100 µm in length.

increase neuronal apoptosis (BID), and an elevation in astrocyte number (GFAP) were evident in both brain regions, which is in accord with prior studies in this mTBI model describing elevations in apoptotic proteins (p53, c-Jun, and Bcl-2) as well as TUNEL-positive and silver stain-impregnated degenerating neurons [82,84], as well as other animal models of brain injury [20,60,85,86]. Importantly, early post injury treatment with 3,6′-dithiothalidomide fully prevented these changes. In line with this, this same agent has recently been reported to ameliorate neuroinflammation and alleviate cognitive deficits arising from intracerebral administration of LPS or amyloid-β peptide [79,87,88]. 3,6′-Dithiothalidomide is also reported to attenuate inflammatory markers, Alzheimer's disease pathology, and behavioral deficits evident in aged Alzheimer transgenic mice [79,80], as well as mitigate neuroinflammation and apoptosis within the penumbra of focal ischemic stroke in mice [81]. Additionally, 3,6′-dithiothalidomide has recently been described to lower TNF-α and cerebral aneurysm formation and progression to rupture in mice [89,90].

Taken together, these studies support an important role for TNF-α in neuroinflammation and the modulation of neuronal function and viability across a broad range of neurological disorders. Consequent to the availability of both biological and small molecular weight TNF-α inhibitors in preclinical and clinical research, there is growing evidence that whereas physiological TNF-α levels are critical in normal brain physiology [37,38,55], excess TNF-α plays a key role in brain dysfunction [29-31,69]. In relation to the former, among a host of functions in brain, TNF-α serves as a gliotransmitter that, when secreted from glial cells surrounding synapses, can regulate synaptic communication between neurons as well as neuronal networks [36-38]. With respect to the latter, TNF-α reductions achieved with the clinical TNF-α binding protein etanercept, when administered i.p. following fluid percussion injury-induced TBI, attenuated TBI-induced contusion, ischemia, and resulting motor and cognitive deficits [91]. As in our studies, this brain TNF-α lowering approach also mitigated TBI-induced elevations in [91]. Albeit that these animal studies utilized a far higher etanercept dose than achievable in humans [91], in an open-label analysis of 12 TBI patients given perispinal etanercept up to more than 10 years following injury, motor impairment and spasticity were reported significantly reduced [55], supporting both clinical and translational relevance. Additionally, in rat studies using a TBI weight drop paradigm with some parallels to our studies in mice, immediate i.v. administration of a TNF-α binding protein or the competitive nonselective phosphodiesterase inhibitor, pentoxifylline, that lowers TNF-α at a transcriptional level, has been reported to mitigate mTBI-induced brain edema at 24 h and neurological dysfunction evaluated up to 14 days [75]. Finally, in other animal models that include ischemic and spinal cord injury, thalidomide has been reported to effectively reduce inflammation and improve the injury outcome when administered either before [92], immediately after [93], or within an hour of injury [94] in doses that varied between 20 and 300 mg/kg.

The single dose of 3,6′-dithiothalidomide used in the current study (28 mg/kg in mouse) compares favorably with former studies of thalidomide (20 to 300 mg/kg) and equates to a dose of 150 mg in a 65 kg human (2.3 mg/kg), following normalization of body surface area in accord with FDA guidelines [95]. Prior cellular [43,79] and animal studies [80,81] indicate that 3,6′-dithiothalidomide (albeit administered systemically by the i.p. route, as in the current study) is more potent in reducing TNF-α elevations than thalidomide and that it enters the brain but does not appear to be soporific [44,79,80]. In light of recent studies suggesting that thalidomide analogues can express more potent anti-inflammatory action with less neurotoxicity than the parent compound [96,97], the development of new and well-tolerated small molecular weight TNF-α inhibitors that can be administered orally may be of great clinical potential. Past studies evaluating genetically engineered mice that either lack TNF-α or its receptors have suggested a 'Jekyll and Hyde' scenario in which elevated TNF-α is detrimental during the acute phase after a TBI incident, but a part of the regenerative processes during the later chronic post-injury phase [42,98,99]. More recent studies in which the two individual receptors, TNFR1 (p55) and TNFR2 (p75), have been separately deleted suggest that each may have a distinct time-dependent function in TBI [40,41]. TNFR1 knockout mice possessed a smaller contusion volume and a clearly improved neurobehavioral performance for up to 4 weeks following a controlled cortical impact TBI, as compared with wild-type mice, whereas TNFR2 knockout mice demonstrated significant worsening post injury [42]. This implicates TNFR1 involvement in the immediate deleterious actions associated with acute TNF-α release following an injury and an involvement of TNFR2 in later tissue repair.

In summary, our studies suggest that the administration of a TNF-α synthesis inhibitor, 3,6′-dithiothalidomide, within the initial 12-h window of a mTBi event, may be therapeutically valuable at a time when elevated TNF-α interacts with TNFR1 to drive the development of neuro-inflammation, neuronal dysfunction, and apoptosis. But such a therapeutic strategy should best be acute to allow later potentially beneficial actions of TNF-α mediated via TNFR2. Our results, together with other studies [33,36,39-41,44,56,74-78,97], underscore the potential of TNF-α as a potential therapeutic target in TBI and other neurological disorders.

Conclusion

This study implicates TNF-α in the delayed neuronal cell death and gliosis that occurs within the brain following mTBI, which leads to cognitive deficits. It additionally indicates that pharmacologically limiting the elevation of TNF-α within 12 h of the mTBI event markedly reduces such secondary damage and leads to improved cognitive outcome measures. Such a window provides an opportunity for translational studies in mTBI that is more difficult to define for other neurological disorders [100]. Building on the growing literature on the role of TNF-α in the initiation and perpetuation of the neuroinflammation that can drive the progression of acute and chronic neurological disorders [29-31,36,55,56,68,69,101,102], the present study underscores the value of targeting of TNF-α as a treatment strategy for TBI and the development of new and well-tolerated oral small molecular weight TNF-α inhibitors and related approaches as clinical treatment options.

Competing interests

The small molecule TNF-α synthesis inhibitor 3,6′-dithiothalidomide was originally synthesized within the laboratory of NHG and colleagues within the Intramural Research Program of NIA, NIH. Whereas NHG is a co-inventor of the agent, neither he nor any of the authors hold any rights to the agent. All authors declare that they are without any financial and non-financial competing interests (political, personal, religious, ideological, academic, intellectual, commercial, or any other) in relation to this article.

Authors' contributions

RB, DT, VR, and WL undertook 'hands-on' experimental studies generating data used within the manuscript, preliminary data on which studies were then optimized, and synthetic chemistry to provide compounds used within the studies. RD, DT, JYW, VR, WL, BJH, NHG, and CGP analyzed immunohistochemical, ELISA, behavioral, or chemical characterization data essential to the studies within the manuscript. CGP, BJH, and NHG conceived and planned the studies. RB, DT, JYW, BJH, CGP, and NHG prepared the manuscript. All authors have read the manuscript in full and are in agreement with the data and its interpretation.

Acknowledgements

This study was supported in part by the Intramural Research Program, National Institute on Aging, NIH, Baltimore, USA; by Tel-Aviv University, Tel-Aviv, Israel; and by a grant from the Ministry of Science and Technology, Taiwan (MOST103-2321-B-038-002 to JY Wang). None of the authors have any competing interests in the manuscript.

Author details

[1]Department of Anatomy and Anthropology, Sackler School of Medicine, Tel-Aviv University, Tel-Aviv, Israel. [2]Drug Design and Development Section, Translational Gerontology Branch, Intramural Research Program, National Institute on Aging, National Institutes of Health, BRC Room 05C220, 251 Bayview Blvd., Baltimore, MD 21224, USA. [3]Graduate Institute of Medical Sciences, College of Medicine, Taipei Medical University, Taipei, Taiwan.

[4]Department of Neurosurgery, Case Western Reserve University School of Medicine, Cleveland, OH, USA.

References

1. Hyder AA, Wunderlich CA, Puvanachandra P, Gururaj G, Kobusingye OC. The impact of traumatic brain injuries: a global perspective. NeuroRehabilitation. 2007;22:341–53.
2. Setnik L, Bazarian JJ. The characteristics of patients who do not seek medical treatment for traumatic brain injury. Brain Inj. 2007;21(1):1–9.
3. Faul M, Xu L, Wald M, Coronado VG. Traumatic Brain Injury in the United States: Emergency Department Visits, Hospitalizations and Deaths 2002–2006. Atlanta (GA): Centers for Disease Control and Prevention, National Center for Injury Prevention and Control; 2010.
4. McGarry LJ, Thompson D, Millham FH, Cowell L, Snyder PJ, Lenderking WR, et al. Outcomes and costs of acute treatment of traumatic brain injury. J Trauma. 2002;53(6):1152–9.
5. McAllister TW. Neurobehavioral sequelae of traumatic brain injury: evaluation and management. World Psychiatry. 2008;7(1):3–10.
6. Coronado VG, Xu L, Basavaraju SV, McGuire LC, Wald MM, Faul MD, et al. Centers for Disease Control and Prevention (CDC). Surveillance for traumatic brain injury-related deaths–United States, 1997–2007. MMWR Surveill Summ. 2011;60(5):1–32.
7. Yu S, Kaneko Y, Bae E, Stahl CE, Wang Y, van Loveren H, et al. Severity of controlled cortical impact traumatic brain injury in rats and mice dictates degree of behavioral deficits. Brain Res. 2009;1287:157–63.
8. Iverson GL. Outcome from mild traumatic brain injury. Curr Opinion Psychiatry. 2005;18:301–7.
9. Schreiber S, Barkai G, Gur-Hartman T, Peles E, Tov N, Dolberg OT, et al. Long-lasting sleep patterns of adult patients with minor traumatic brain injury (mTBI) and non-mTBI subjects. Sleep Med. 2008;9:481–7.
10. Mortimer JA, van Duijn CM, Chandra V, Fratiglioni L, Graves AB, Heyman A, et al. Head trauma as a risk factor for Alzheimer's disease: a collaborative re-analysis of case–control studies, EURODEM Risk Factors Research Group. Int J Epidemiol. 1991;20 Suppl 2:S28–35.
11. Mayeux R, Ottman R, Maestre G, Ngai C, Tang MX, Ginsberg H, et al. Synergistic effects of traumatic head-injury and apolipoprotein-epsilon-4 in patients with Alzheimers-disease. Neurology. 1995;45:555–7.
12. Tweedie D, Rachmany L, Rubovitch V, Zhang Y, Becker KG, Perez E, et al. Changes in mouse cognition and hippocampal gene expression observed in a mild physical- and blast-traumatic brain injury. Neurobiol Dis. 2013;54:1–11.
13. Goldstein LE, Fisher AM, Tagge CA, Zhang XL, Velisek L, Sullivan JA, et al. Chronic traumatic encephalopathy in blast-exposed military veterans and a blast neurotrauma mouse model. Sci Transl Med. 2012;4(134):134ra60.
14. Barnes DE, Kaup A, Kirby KA, Byers AL, Diaz-Arrastia R, Yaffe K. Traumatic brain injury and risk of dementia in older veterans. Neurology. 2014;83(4):312–9.
15. Gardner RC, Burke JF, Nettiksimmons J, Kaup A, Barnes DE, Yaffe K. Dementia risk after traumatic brain injury vs nonbrain trauma: the role of age and severity. JAMA Neurol. 2014 [Epub ahead of print].
16. Kumar A, Stoica BA, Sabirzhanov B, Burns MP, Faden AI, Loane DJ. Traumatic brain injury in aged animals increases lesion size and chronically alters microglial/macrophage classical and alternative activation states. Neurobiol Aging. 2013;34(5):1397–411.
17. Loane DJ, Faden AI. Neuroprotection for traumatic brain injury: translational challenges and emerging therapeutic strategies. Trends Pharmacol Sci. 2010;31(12):596–604.
18. Diaz-Arrastia R, Kochanek PM, Bergold P, Kenney K, Marx CE, Grimes CJ, et al. Pharmacotherapy of traumatic brain injury: state of the science and the road forward: report of the Department of Defense Neurotrauma Pharmacology Workgroup. J Neurotrauma. 2014;31(2):135–58.
19. Finnie JW, Blumbergs PC, Manavis J, Vink R. Pattern of cerebrospinal immediate early gene c-fos expression in an ovine model of non-accidental head injury. J Clin Neurosci. 2013;20:1759–61.
20. Greig NH, Tweedie D, Rachmany L, Li Y, Rubovitch V, Schreiber S, et al. Incretin mimetics as pharmacologic tools to elucidate and as a new drug strategy to treat traumatic brain injury. Alzheimers Dement. 2014;10(1 Suppl):S62–75.
21. Barkhoudarian G, Hovda DA, Giza C. The molecular pathophysiology of concussive brain injury. Clin Sports Med. 2011;30:33–48.
22. Greve MW, Zink BJ. Pathophysiology of traumatic brain injury. Mt Sinai J Med. 2009;76:97–104.
23. Finnie JW, Blumbergs PC. Traumatic brain injury. Vet Pathol. 2002;39(6):679–89.
24. Tweedie D, Milman A, Holloway HW, Li YZ, Harvey BK, Shen H, et al. Apoptotic and behavioral sequelae of mild brain trauma in mice. J Neurosci Res. 2007;85:805–15.
25. Stoica BA, Byrnes KR, Faden AI. Cell cycle activation and CNS injury. Neurotox Res. 2009;16:221–37.
26. Morganti-Kossmann MC, Rancan M, Stahel PF, Kossmann T. Inflammatory response in acute traumatic brain injury: a double-edged sword. Curr Opinion Crit Care. 2002;8:101–5.
27. Stoll G, Jander S, Schroeter M. Detrimental and beneficial effects of injury-induced inflammation and cytokine expression in the nervous system. Adv Exp Med Biol. 2002;513:87–113.
28. Schmidt OI, Heyde CE, Ertel W, Stahel PF. Closed head injury - an inflammatory disease? Brain Res Rev. 2005;48:388–99.
29. McCoy MK, Tansey MG. TNF signaling inhibition in the CNS: implications for normal brain function and neurodegenerative disease. J Neuroinflammation. 2008;5:45.
30. Frankola KA, Greig NH, Luo W, Tweedie D. Targeting TNF-α to elucidate and ameliorate neuroinflammation in neurodegenerative diseases. CNS Neurol Disord Drug Targets. 2011;10(3):391–403.
31. Clark IA, Alleva LM, Vissel B. The roles of TNF in brain dysfunction and disease. Pharmacol Ther. 2010;128(3):519–48.
32. Frugier T, Morganti-Kossmann MC, O'Reilly D, McLean CA. In situ detection of inflammatory mediators in post mortem human brain tissue after traumatic injury. J Neurotrauma. 2010;27:497–507.
33. Shohami E, Gallily R, Mechoulam R, Bass R, Ben-Hur T. Cytokine production in the brain following closed head injury: dexanabinol (HU-211) is a novel TNF-α inhibitor and an effective neuroprotectant. J Neuroimmunol. 1997;72:169–77.
34. Lu J, Goh SJ, Tng PY, Deng YY, Ling EA, Moochhala S. Systemic inflammatory response following acute traumatic brain injury. Front Biosci. 2009;14:3795–813.
35. Yang J, You Z, Kim HH, Hwang SK, Khuman J, Guo S, et al. Genetic analysis of the role of tumor necrosis factor receptors in functional outcome after traumatic brain injury in mice. J Neurotrauma. 2010;27:1037–46.
36. Tuttolomondo A, Pecoraro R, Pinto A. Studies of selective TNF inhibitors in the treatment of brain injury from stroke and trauma: a review of the evidence to date. Drug Des Devel Ther. 2014;8:2221–38.
37. Li J, Yin Q, Wu H. Structural basis of signal transduction in the TNF receptor superfamily. Adv Immunol. 2013;119:135–53.
38. Santello M, Volterra A. TNFα in synaptic function: switching gears. Trends Neurosci. 2012;35(10):638–47.
39. Bermpohl D, You Z, Lo EH, Kim HH, Whalen MJ. TNF alpha and Fas mediate tissue damage and functional outcome after traumatic brain injury in mice. J Cerebral Blood Flow Metabol. 2007;27:1806–18.
40. Longhi L, Ortolano F, Zanier ER, Perego C, Stocchetti N, De Simoni MG. Effect of traumatic brain injury on cognitive function in mice lacking p55 and p75 tumor necrosis factor receptors. Acta Neurochir Suppl. 2008;102:409–13.
41. Longhi L, Perego C, Ortolano F, Aresi S, Fumagalli S, Zanier ER, et al. Tumor necrosis factor in traumatic brain injury: effects of genetic deletion of p55 or p75 receptor. J Cereb Blood Flow Metab. 2013;33(8):1182–9.
42. Scherbel U, Raghupathi R, Nakamura M, Saatman KE, Trojanowski JQ, Neugebauer E, et al. Differential acute and chronic responses of tumor necrosis factor-deficient mice to experimental brain injury. Proc Natl Acad Sci U S A. 1999;96:8721–6.
43. Zhu X, Giordano T, Yu QS, Holloway HW, Perry T, Lahiri DK, et al. Thiothalidomides: novel isosteric analogues of thalidomide with enhanced TNF-alpha inhibitory activity. J Med Chem. 2003;46:5222–9.
44. Baratz R, Tweedie D, Rubovitch V, Luo W, Yoon JS, Hoffer BJ, et al. Tumor necrosis factor-alpha synthesis inhibitor, 3,6′-dithiothalidomide, reverses behavioral impairments induced by minimal traumatic brain injury in mice. J Neurochem. 2011;118:1032–42.
45. Zohar O, Schreiber S, Getslev V, Schwartz JP, Mullins PG, Pick CG. Closed-head minimal traumatic brain injury produces long-term cognitive deficits in mice. Neuroscience. 2003;118:949–55.
46. Milman A, Rosenberg A, Weizman R, Pick CG. Mild traumatic brain injury induces persistent cognitive deficits and behavioral disturbances in mice. J Neurotrauma. 2005;22:1003–10.
47. Hogg S. A review of the validity and variability of the elevated plus-maze as an animal model of anxiety. Pharmacol Biochem Behav. 1996;54:21–30.
48. Dellu F, Mayo W, Cherkaoui J, Lemoal M, Simon H. A 2-trial memory task with automated recording - study in young and aged rats. Brain Res. 1992;588:132–9.

49. Dix SL, Aggleton JP. Extending the spontaneous preference test of recognition: evidence of object-location and object-context recognition. Behav Brain Res. 1999;99:191–200.
50. Meisser C. Object recognition in mice: improvement of memory by glucose. Neurobiol Learning Memory. 1997;67:172–5.
51. Edut S, Rubovitch V, Schreiber S, Pick CG. The intriguing effects of ecstasy (MDMA) on cognitive function in mice subjected to a minimal traumatic brain injury (mTBI). Psychopharmacol. 2011;214:877–89.
52. Amaral D, Scharfman H, Lavenex P. The dentate gyrus: fundamental neuroanatomical organization (dentate gyrus for dummies). Prog Brain Res. 2007;163:3–22. 788–790.
53. Saab BJ, Georgiou J, Nath A, Lee FJ, Wang M, Michalon A, et al. NCS-1 in the dentate gyrus promotes exploration, synaptic plasticity, and rapid acquisition of spatial memory. Neuron. 2009;63(5):643–56.
54. Perederiy JV, Westbrook GL. Structural plasticity in the dentate gyrus- revisiting a classic injury model. Front Neural Circuits. 2013;7:17.
55. Tobinick E, Kim NM, Reyzin G, Rodriguez-Romanacce H, DePuy V. Selective TNF inhibition for chronic stroke and traumatic brain injury: an observational study involving 629 consecutive patients treated with perispinal etanercept. CNS Drugs. 2012;26(12):1051–70.
56. Tuttolomondo A, Di Raimondo D, di Sciacca R, Pinto A, Licata G. Inflammatory cytokines in acute ischemic stroke. Curr Pharm Des. 2008;14:3574–89.
57. Tweedie D, Rachmany L, Rubovitch V, Lehrmann E, Zhang Y, Becker KG, et al. Exendin-4, a glucagon-like peptide-1 receptor agonist prevents mTBI-induced changes in hippocampus gene expression and memory deficits in mice. Exp Neurol. 2013;239:170–82.
58. Sharp DJ, Scott G, Leech R. Network dysfunction after traumatic brain injury. Nat Rev Neurol. 2014;10(3):156–66.
59. Ryu WH, Feinstein A, Colantonio A, Streiner DL, Dawson DR. Early identification and incidence of mild TBI in Ontario. Can J Neurol Sci. 2009;36(4):429–35.
60. Moppett IK. Traumatic brain injury: assessment, resuscitation and early management. Br J Anaesth. 2007;99:18–31.
61. Wajant H, Pfizenmaier K, Scheurich P. Tumor necrosis factor signaling. Cell Death Differ. 2003;10(1):45–65.
62. Grell M, Wajant H, Zimmermann G, Scheurich P. The type 1 receptor (CD120a) is the high-affinity receptor for soluble tumor necrosis factor. Proc Natl Acad Sci U S A. 1998;95(2):570–5.
63. Fontaine V, Mohand-Said S, Hanoteau N, Fuchs C, Pfizenmaier K, Eisel U. Neurodegenerative and neuroprotective effects of tumor necrosis factor (TNF) in retinal ischemia: opposite roles of TNF receptor 1 and TNF receptor 2. J Neurosci. 2002;22(7):RC216.
64. Yang L, Lindholm K, Konishi Y, Li R, Shen Y. Target depletion of distinct tumor necrosis factor receptor subtypes reveals hippocampal neuron death and survival through different signal transduction pathways. J Neurosci. 2002;22(8):3025–32.
65. Marchetti L, Klein M, Schlett K, Pfizenmaier K, Eisel UL. Tumor necrosis factor (TNF)-mediated neuroprotection against glutamate-induced excitotoxicity is enhanced by N-methyl-D-aspartate receptor activation. Essential role of a TNF receptor 2-mediated phosphatidylinositol 3-kinase-dependent NF-kappa B pathway. J Biol Chem. 2004;279(31):32869–81.
66. Grell M, Douni E, Wajant H, Löhden M, Clauss M, Maxeiner B, et al. The transmembrane form of tumor necrosis factor is the prime activating ligand of the 80 kDa tumor necrosis factor receptor. Cell. 1995;83(5):793–802.
67. Grell M. Tumor necrosis factor (TNF) receptors in cellular signaling of soluble and membrane-expressed TNF. J Inflamm. 1995–1996;47(1–2):8–17
68. Park KM, Bowers WJ. Tumor necrosis factor-alpha mediated signaling in neuronal homeostasis and dysfunction. Cell Signal. 2010;22(7):977–83.
69. Tweedie D, Sambamurti K, Greig NH. TNF-α inhibition as a treatment strategy for neurodegenerative disorders: new drug candidates and targets. Curr Alzheimer Res. 2007;4:378–85.
70. Ponsford J, Cameron P, Fitzgerald M, Grant M, Mikocka-Walus A. Long-term outcomes after uncomplicated mild traumatic brain injury: a comparison with trauma controls. J Neurotrauma. 2011;28:937–46.
71. Ghajar J, Ivry RB. Cognitive and Neurobiological Research Consortium. The predictive brain state: timing deficiency in traumatic brain injury? Neurorehabil Neural Repair. 2008;22(3):217–27.
72. Israelsson C, Bengtsson H, Kylberg A, Kullander K, Lewén A, Hillered L, et al. Distinct cellular patterns of upregulated chemokine expression supporting a prominent inflammatory role in traumatic brain injury. J Neurotrauma. 2008;25(8):959–74.
73. Israelsson C, Wang Y, Kylberg A, Pick CG, Hoffer BJ, Ebendal T. Closed head injury in a mouse model results in molecular changes indicating inflammatory responses. J Neurotrauma. 2009;26(8):1307–14.
74. Taupin V, Toulmond S, Serrano A, Benavides J, Zavala F. Increase in IL-6, IL-1 and TNF levels in rat brain following traumatic lesion: influence of pre- and post-traumatic treatment with Ro5 4864, a peripheral-type (p site) benzodiazepine ligand. J Neuroimmunol. 1993;42:177–85.
75. Shohami E, Novikov M, Bass R, Yamin A, Gallily R. Closed head injury triggers early production of TNF-α and IL-6 by brain tissue. J Cereb Blood Flow Metab. 1994;14:615–9.
76. Gourin CG, Shackford SR. Production of tumor necrosis factor-alpha and interleukin-1beta by human cerebral microvascular endothelium after percussive trauma. J Trauma. 1997;42(6):1101–7.
77. Knoblach SM, Fan L, Faden AI. Early neuronal expression of tumor necrosis factor-alpha after experimental brain injury contributes to neurological impairment. J Neuroimmunol. 1999;95(1–2):115–25.
78. Ross SA, Halliday MI, Campbell GC, Byrnes DP, Rowlands BJ. The presence of tumour necrosis factor in CSF and plasma after severe head injury. Br J Neurosurg. 1994;8(4):419–25.
79. Tweedie D, Ferguson RA, Fishman K, Frankola KA, Van Praag H, Holloway HW, et al. Tumor necrosis factor-α synthesis inhibitor 3,6′-dithiothalidomide attenuates markers of inflammation. Alzheimer pathology and behavioral deficits in animal models of neuroinflammation and Alzheimer's disease. J Neuroinflammation. 2012;9:106.
80. Gabbita SP, Srivastava MK, Eslami P, Johnson MF, Kobritz NK, Tweedie D, et al. Early intervention with a small molecule inhibitor for tumor necrosis factor-α prevents cognitive deficits in a triple transgenic mouse model of Alzheimer's disease. J Neuroinflammation. 2012;9:99.
81. Yoon JS, Lee JH, Tweedie D, Mughal MR, Chigurupati S, Greig NH, et al. 3,6′-Dithiothalidomide improves experimental stroke outcome by suppressing neuroinflammation. J Neurosci Res. 2013;91(5):671–80.
82. Tashlykov V, Katz Y, Volkov A, Gazit V, Schreiber S, Zohar O, et al. Minimal traumatic brain injury induce apoptotic cell death in mice. J Mol Neurosci. 2009;37(1):16–24.
83. Bussey TJ, Padain TL, Skillings EA, Winters BD, Morton AJ, Saksida LM. The touchscreen cognitive testing method for rodents: how to get the best out of your rat. Learn Mem. 2008;2008(15):516–23.
84. Tashlykov V, Katz Y, Gazit V, Zohar O, Schreiber S, Pick CG. Apoptotic changes in the cortex and hippocampus following minimal brain trauma in mice. Brain Res. 2007;1130(1):197–205.
85. Wakade C, Sukumari-Ramesh S, Laird MD, Dhandapani KM, Vender JR. Delayed reduction in hippocampal postsynaptic density protein-95 expression temporally correlates with cognitive dysfunction following controlled cortical impact in mice. J Neurosurg. 2010;113(6):1195–201.
86. Han X, Tong J, Zhang J, Farahvar A, Wang E, Yang J, et al. Imipramine treatment improves cognitive outcome associated with enhanced hippocampal neurogenesis after traumatic brain injury in mice. J Neurotrauma. 2011;28(6):995–1007.
87. Russo I, Caracciolo L, Tweedie D, Choi SH, Greig NH, Barlati S, et al. 3,6′-Dithiothalidomide, a new TNF-α synthesis inhibitor, attenuates the effect of Aβ1-42 intracerebroventricular injection on hippocampal neurogenesis and memory deficit. J Neurochem. 2012;122(6):1181–92.
88. Belarbi K, Jopson T, Tweedie D, Arellano C, Luo W, Greig NH, et al. TNF-α protein synthesis inhibitor restores neuronal function and reverses cognitive deficits induced by chronic neuroinflammation. J Neuroinflammation. 2012;9:23.
89. Starke RM, Chalouhi N, Jabbour PM, Tjoumakaris SI, Gonzalez LF, Rosenwasser RH, et al. Critical role of TNF-α in cerebral aneurysm formation and progression to rupture. J Neuroinflammation. 2014;11:77.
90. Ali MS, Starke RM, Jabbour PM, Tjoumakaris SI, Gonzalez LF, Rosenwasser RH, et al. TNF-α induces phenotypic modulation in cerebral vascular smooth muscle cells: implications for cerebral aneurysm pathology. J Cereb Blood Flow Metab. 2013;33(10):1564–73.
91. Chio CC, Lin JW, Chang MW, Wang CC, Kuo JR, Yang CZ, et al. Therapeutic evaluation of etanercept in a model of traumatic brain injury. J Neurochem. 2010;115(4):921–9.
92. Lee CJ, Kim KW, Lee HM, Nahm FS, Lim YJ, Park JH, et al. The effect of thalidomide on spinal cord ischemia/reperfusion injury in a rabbit model. Spinal Cord. 2007;45(2):149–57.
93. Koopmans GC, Deumens R, Buss A, Geoghegan L, Myint AM, Honig WH, et al. Acute rolipram/thalidomide treatment improves tissue sparing and

locomotion after experimental spinal cord injury. Exp Neurol. 2009;216(2):490–8.
94. Genovese T, Mazzon E, Esposito E, Di Paola R, Caminiti R, Meli R, et al. Effect of thalidomide on signal transduction pathways and secondary damage in experimental spinal cord trauma. Shock. 2008;30(3):231–40.
95. U.S. Department of Health and Human Services Food and Drug Administration Center for Drug Evaluation and Research (CDER). Guidance for industry: estimating the maximum safe starting dose in initial clinical trials for therapeutics in adult healthy volunteers. July 2005 <http://www.fda.gov/downloads/Drugs/Guidances/UCM078932.pdf> (viewed Nov. 19, 2014).
96. Mahony C, Erskine L, Niven J, Greig NH, Figg WD, Vargesson N. Pomalidomide is nonteratogenic in chicken and zebrafish embryos and nonneurotoxic in vitro. Proc Natl Acad Sci U S A. 2013;110(31):12703–8.
97. Vargesson N, Mahony C, Erskine L, Niven J, Greig NH, Figg WD. Reply to D'Amato et al. and Zeldis et al.: Screening of thalidomide derivatives in chicken and zebrafish embryos. Proc Natl Acad Sci U S A. 2013;110(50):E4820.
98. Shohami E, Bass R, Wallach D, Yamin A, Gallily R. Inhibition of tumor necrosis factor alpha (TNFalpha) activity in rat brain is associated with cerebroprotection after closed head injury. J Cereb Blood Flow Metab. 1996;16(3):378–84.
99. Sullivan PG, Bruce-Keller AJ, Rabchevsky AG, Christakos S, Clair DK, Mattson MP, et al. Exacerbation of damage and altered NF-kappaB activation in mice lacking tumor necrosis factor receptors after traumatic brain injury. J Neurosci. 1999;19:6248–56.
100. Becker RE, Greig NH, Giacobini E, Schneider LS, Ferrucci L. A new roadmap for drug development for Alzheimer's disease. Nat Rev Drug Discov. 2014;13(2):156.
101. Ignatowski TA, Spengler RN, Dhandapani KM, Folkersma H, Butterworth RF, Tobinick E. Perispinal etanercept for post-stroke neurological and cognitive dysfunction: scientific rationale and current evidence. CNS Drugs. 2014;28:679–97.
102. Morris GP, Clark IA, Zinn R, Vissel B. Microglia: a new frontier for synaptic plasticity, learning and memory, and neurodegenerative disease research. Neurobiol Learn Mem. 2013;105:40–53.

2

Omega-3 polyunsaturated fatty acid attenuates the inflammatory response by modulating microglia polarization through SIRT1-mediated deacetylation of the HMGB1/NF-κB pathway following experimental traumatic brain injury

Xiangrong Chen[1†], Chunnuan Chen[1†], Sining Fan[1], Shukai Wu[1], Fuxing Yang[1], Zhongning Fang[1], Huangde Fu[2*] and Yasong Li[1*]

Abstract

Background: Microglial polarization and the subsequent neuroinflammatory response are contributing factors for traumatic brain injury (TBI)-induced secondary injury. High mobile group box 1 (HMGB1) mediates the activation of the NF-κB pathway, and it is considered to be pivotal in the late neuroinflammatory response. Activation of the HMGB1/NF-κB pathway is closely related to HMGB1 acetylation, which is regulated by the sirtuin (SIRT) family of proteins. Omega-3 polyunsaturated fatty acids (ω-3 PUFA) are known to have antioxidative and anti-inflammatory effects. We previously demonstrated that ω-3 PUFA inhibited TBI-induced microglial activation and the subsequent neuroinflammatory response by regulating the HMGB1/NF-κB signaling pathway. However, no studies have elucidated if ω-3 PUFA affects the HMGB1/NF-κB pathway in a HMGB1 deacetylation of dependent SIRT1 manner, thus regulating microglial polarization and the subsequent neuroinflammatory response.

Methods: The Feeney DM TBI model was adopted to induce brain injury in rats. Modified neurological severity scores, rotarod test, brain water content, and Nissl staining were employed to determine the neuroprotective effects of ω-3 PUFA supplementation. Assessment of microglia polarization and pro-inflammatory markers, such as tumor necrosis factor (TNF)-α, interleukin (IL)-1β, IL-6, and HMGB1, were used to evaluate the neuroinflammatory responses and the anti-inflammatory effects of ω-3 PUFA supplementation. Immunofluorescent staining and western blot analysis were used to detect HMGB1 nuclear translocation, secretion, and HMGB1/NF-κB signaling pathway activation to evaluate the effects of ω-3 PUFA supplementation. The impact of SIRT1 deacetylase activity on HMGB1 acetylation and the interaction between HMGB1 and SIRT1 were assessed to evaluate anti-inflammation effects of ω-3 PUFAs, and also, whether these effects were dependent on a SIRT1-HMGB1/NF-κB axis to gain further insight into the mechanisms underlying the development of the neuroinflammatory response after TBI.

(Continued on next page)

* Correspondence: 303880058@qq.com
†Equal contributors
[2]Department of Neurosurgery, Affiliated Hospital of YouJiang Medical University for Nationalities, Baise 533000, Guangxi Province, China
[1]The Second clinical medical college, The Second Affiliated Hospital, Fujian Medical University, Quanzhou 362000, Fujian Province, China

(Continued from previous page)

Results: The results of our study showed that ω-3 PUFA supplementation promoted a shift from the M1 microglial phenotype to the M2 microglial phenotype and inhibited microglial activation, thus reducing TBI-induced inflammatory factors. In addition, ω-3 PUFA-mediated downregulation of HMGB1 acetylation and its extracellular secretion was found to be likely due to increased SIRT1 activity. We also found that treatment with ω-3 PUFA inhibited HMGB1 acetylation and induced direct interactions between SIRT1 and HMGB1 by elevating SIRT1 activity following TBI. These events lead to inhibition of HMGB1 nucleocytoplasmic translocation/extracellular secretion and alleviated HMGB1-mediated activation of the NF-κB pathway following TBI-induced microglial activation, thus inhibiting the subsequent inflammatory response.

Conclusions: The results of this study suggest that ω-3 PUFA supplementation attenuates the inflammatory response by modulating microglial polarization through SIRT1-mediated deacetylation of the HMGB1/NF-κB pathway, leading to neuroprotective effects following experimental traumatic brain injury.

Keywords: Traumatic brain injury, Omega-3 polyunsaturated fatty acid, Microglia polarization, Neuroinflammation, Sirtuin1, HMGB1/NF-κB pathway

Background

Neuronal inflammation induced by activation of microglia is a vital contributing factor of traumatic brain injury (TBI)-induced secondary injury [1–3]. After trauma, resident microglia and peripheral macrophages migrate to the site of injury and secrete a large number of inflammatory cytokines, such as tumor necrosis factor (TNF), interleukins (IL), and interferons (IFN) that cause acascade of inflammatory responses and neuronal apoptosis [4, 5]. Transition of microglia from the anti-inflammatory (M2) to the pro-inflammatory (M1) phenotype play a crucial role in microglial activation and the subsequent neuroinflammatory response. The M1 phenotype favors pro-inflammatory cytokine release that exacerbates neural damage while the M2 phenotype promotes neurotrophic factors that contribute to neural repair [6–8]. Wang et al. [6] found that microglia respond to TBI with a transient M2 phenotype, followed by a transition to M1, which is strongly correlated with the severity of TBI. Thus, inhibition of microglial dysfunction and its phenotypic switch to the M1 phenotype may offer new anti-inflammatory strategies to improve the recovery in TBI patients [2, 9].

High mobile group box 1 (HMGB1) is considered to be the central component of the late inflammatory response [10, 11]. Translocation and secretion of HMGB1 are important steps in HMGB1-induced inflammation [12]. After release, extracellular HMGB1 activates several cell surface receptors including advanced glycation end products, toll-like receptors, and chemokine (C-X-C motif) receptor 4, through both medullary differentiation factor (MyD88) and non-MyD88-dependent pathways. These pathways then trigger a signal cascade, either directly through the nuclear factor-κB (NF-κB) pathway or indirectly via the phosphatidylinositol 3-kinase or mitogen-activated protein kinase pathway [13–16]. Following nuclear translocation of NF-κB, cells release large numbers of inflammatory cytokines initiating a cascade amplification of inflammatory responses. Activation of the NF-κB pathway is associated with HMGB1 expression and the post-TBI inflammatory response [17, 18]. Our previous study [4] confirmed that inhibiting HMGB1 translocation and release, and also HMGB1-mediated activation of the NF-κB signaling pathway, led to a reduction in TBI-induced microglial activation and the subsequent inflammatory response, thus providing neuroprotection following TBI.

Activation of the HMGB1/NF-κB pathway is influenced by post-translational modifications, including acetylation levels, which are regulated by the balanced expression of histone deacetylases (HDACs) and histone acetyltransferases (HATs) [19, 20]. These in turn regulate HMGB1 intranuclear translocation and mobility by a lysine acetylation dependent mechanism. Thus, hyperacetylation of HMGB1 is also known to affect its DNA binding activity and intranuclear translocation [21]. The sirtuin (SIRT) family of proteins are a family of nicotinamide adenine dinucleotide (NAD+)-dependent class III HDACs, which include SIRT1through SIRT7 [22, 23]. Among the SIRT family, SIRT1 is one of the most studied deacetylases and has been shown to regulate the inflammatory response through deacetylation of lysine in HMGB1 which HMGB1 suppresses transcription [24–26]. Kim et al. [27] recently showed that SIRT1 promoted the deacetylation of HMGB1 and thus inhibited HMGB1 transcription and extracellular release in LPS-activated macrophages. These findings suggest that HMGB1 may be a novel deacetylation target of SIRT1, which in turn inhibits the HMGB1/NF-κB pathway through HMGB1 deacetylation, although, to date, the mechanism remains unclear.

Omega-3 polyunsaturated fatty acids (ω-3 PUFA) include eicosapentaenoic acid and docosahexaenoic acid, which are known to be biologically active compounds with antioxidative and anti-inflammatory effects, all of which influence the pathogenesis of many diseases, including Alzheimer's disease [28], acute pancreatitis [29], Parkinson's disease [30], and cerebral ischemia [31]. Accumulating evidence has demonstrated that ω-3 PUFA inhibits TBI-induced inflammatory responses and that this inhibitory mechanism may be related to microglial activation [32–34]. We previously reported that ω-3 PUFA supplementation inhibited TBI-induced microglial activation and the subsequent inflammatory response by regulating the HMGB1/NF-κB signaling pathway, which lead to neuroprotective effects [4]. In addition, we also found that SIRT1 levels were upregulated after ω-3 PUFA supplementation, indicating that ω-3 PUFA inhibited the expression, translocation, and release of HMGB1 in a SIRT1 deacetylation-mediated dependent manner [4]. To date, no studies have elucidated if ω-3 PUFA affects the HMGB1/NF-κB pathway through a HMGB1 deacetylation-dependent SIRT1 mechanism in a TBI-induced microglial activation model. Thus, in this present study, the neuroprotective effects of ω-3 PUFAs against TBI-induced inflammation were studied. In addition, the potential molecular mechanisms focusing on the phenotypic transition of microglia and the SIRT1-mediated HMGB1/NF-κB deacetylation were also investigated.

Methods

Animals

All animal experiments were approved by the Fujian Provincial Medical University Experimental Animal Ethics Committee (Fuzhou, China) and were performed under strict supervision. Adult male Sprague-Dawley rats, ranging between 230 and 260 g, were purchased from the Experimental Animal Facility in Fujian Medical University and housed in a temperature (23 ± 2 °C) and light (12-h light/dark cycle) controlled room with ad libitum access to food and water.

Experimental model and drug administration

All rats were randomly assigned into a sham group, sham + ω-3 PUFA supplementation group (sham + ω-3 group), TBI group, and TBI + ω-3 group. After injury, the groups were further divided into four subgroups: a 1 day group, a 3 day group, and a 7 day and 14 day group ($n = 12$ each). Six rats in each group were sacrificed for neurological evaluation and histological studies; the remaining six rats were used for molecular studies. TBI was induced in anesthetized (50 mg/kg sodium pentobarbital; intraperitoneally) rats as described previously [4]. Briefly, a midline incision was made over the skull, and a 5-mm craniotomy was drilled through the skull 2 mm caudal to the left coronal suture and 2 mm from the midline without disturbing the dura. TBI was induced using a weight-drop hitting device (ZH-ZYQ, Electronic Technology Development Co., Xuzhou, China) with a 4.5-mm-diameter cylinder bar weighing 40 g from a height of 20 cm. Bone wax was used to seal the hole, and the scalp was sutured. All procedures were the same for each group except in the sham group, in which no weight was dropped. Approximately 30 min after TBI, the TBI + ω-3 group was intraperitoneally injected with ω-3 PUFA (2 ml/kg; Sigma, St. Louis, MO, USA) once per day for 7 consecutive days [4]. To inhibit SIRT1 signaling, 30 ul/kg Sirtinol (2 mmol/l, diluted indimethyl sulfoxide) was administrated into the left lateral ventricle 24 h after intraperitoneal ω-3 PUFA injection, to clarify the role of SIRT1 in ω-3 PUFA-mediated neuroprotection [22]. The remaining groups were injected with same dose of vehicle as a control.

Measurement of neurological impairment score and rotarod test

Neurological deficit was calculated using neurological impairment score. Rats were subjected to exercise (muscular state and abnormal action), sensation (visual, tactile, and balance), and reflex examinations and assigned a modified neurological severity score (mNSS) [4] that was recorded when a task failed to be completed or when the corresponding reflex was lost. The mNSS test was graded on a scale of 0–18, where a total score of 18 points indicated severe neurological deficits and a score of 0 indicated normal performance, 13–18 points indicated severe injury, 7–12 indicated mean-moderate injury, and 1–6 indicated mild injury. Neurological function was measured at different time points by investigators who were blinded to group information.

The rotarod protocol was modified slightly from that in the previous report [35]. Briefly, rats underwent a 2-day testing phase with rotarod (IITC Life Science, Woodland Hills, CA, USA), which gradually accelerated from 5 to 45 rpm over 5 min. During the procedure, the latency to fall was recorded as the time before rats fell off the rod or gripped around for two successive revolutions from day 3 after TBI. The mean latency was measured at different time points by investigators who were blinded to group information.

Measurement of brain water content and blood-brain barrier (BBB) permeability

Brain water content was calculated using the wet weight-dry weight method [4]. Animals were sacrificed after the mNSS test, and their cortices were removed at the edge of the bone window (200 ± 20 mg). Filter paper was used to remove excess blood and cerebrospinal fluid. The wet weight was measured, and the brains were dried in an oven at 100 °C for 24 h until a constant weight was achieved, at which point the dry weight was measured. The % brain water content was calculated as: (wet weight – dry weight)/wet weight × 100%.

BBB permeability was investigated by measuring the extravasation of Evans blue (dye) (Sigma Aldrich) [36]. Evans blue (2% in saline; 4 mL/kg) was intravenously injected 2 h prior to sacrifice 3 days after TBI. Following sacrifice, mice were transcardially perfused with PBS followed by PBS containing 4% paraformaldehyde. Each tissue sample was immediately weighed and homogenized in a solution containing 1 mL 50% trichloroacetic acid. The samples were then centrifuged and the absorption of the supernatant was measured by a spectrophotometer (UV-1800 ENG 240V; Shimadzu Corporation, Japan) at a wave length of 620 nm. The quantity of Evans blue was calculated using a standard curve and expressed as micrograms of Evans blue/g of brain tissue using a standardized curve.

Nissl staining

Formaldehyde-fixed specimens were embedded in paraffin and cut into 4-μm-thick sections that were deparaffinized with xylene and rehydrated in a graded series of alcohol. Samples were treated with Nissl staining solution for 5 min. Damaged neurons were shrunken or contained vacuoles, whereas normal neurons had a relatively large, full soma and round, large nuclei. Average intensities or cell counts were calculated from the same sections in six rats per group with Image Pro Plus 7.0 by investigators who were blinded to the experimental groups.

Immunohistochemical analysis

Formaldehyde-fixed specimens were embedded in paraffin and cut into 4-μm-thick sections that were deparaffinized with xylene and rehydrated in a graded series of alcohol. Antigen retrieval was carried out by microwaving in citric acid buffer. Sections were incubated with an antibody against SIRT1 (1:100; Cell Signaling Technology, Danvers, MA, USA), washed, and then incubated with secondary antibody for 1 h at room temperature. The negative control was prepared without the addition of the anti-SIRT1 antibody. A total of five sections from each animal were used for quantification, and the signal intensity was evaluated as follows [4]: 0, no positive cells; 1, very few positive cells; 2, moderate number of positive cells; 3, large number of positive cells; and 4, the highest number of positive cells.

Immunofluorescence analysis

Formaldehyde-fixed specimens were embedded in paraffin and cut into 4-μm-thick sections that were deparaffinized with xylene and rehydrated in a graded series of alcohol, followed by antigen retrieval. Sections were incubated overnight at 4 °C with antibodies against CD16 (1:200, Abcam, Cambridge, UK), CD206 (1:200; Abcam), Neuronal nuclei (1:100; Boster Biotech, Wuhan, China), ionized calcium-binding adapter molecule (Iba)-1 (1:200; Santa Cruz Biotechnology, Santa Cruz, CA, USA), GFAP (1:200; Abcam), and HMGB1 (1:100; Cell Signaling Technology). After washing, the sections were incubated with secondary antibodies for 1 h at room temperature. Cell nuclei were stained with 4′,6-diamidino-2-phenylindole. Immunopositive cells in five selected fields were counted under a microscope (Leica, Wetzlar, Germany) at × 400 magnification by investigators who were blinded to the experimental groups.

Terminal deoxynucleotidyl transferase dUTP nick-end labeling (TUNEL) assay

Apoptotic cells were detected using a TUNEL kit (Roche Diagnostics, Indianapolis, IN, USA) according to the manufacturer's instructions. Indicators of apoptosis included a shrunken cell body, irregular shape, nuclear condensation, and brown diaminobenzidine staining, as observed by microscopy at × 400 magnification. The final average percentage of TUNEL-positive cells of the six sections was regarded as the data for each sample.

Enzyme-linked immunosorbent assay (ELISA)

Inflammatory factors in brain tissue were detected using ELISA kits for TNF-α, IL-1β, IL-6, HMGB1, and IL-10 (all from Boster Biotech, Wuhan, China). Measured OD values were converted into a concentration value.

Western blotting

Proteins were extracted with radioimmunoprecipitation assay lysis buffer (sc-24948; Santa Cruz Biotechnology). Proteins (30 μg) were separated by sodium dodecyl sulfate-polyacrylamide gel electrophoresis and transferred to a polyvinylidene difluoride membrane that was probed with primary antibodies against B cell lymphoma (Bcl)-2 (1:400), Bcl-2-associated X factor (Bax) (1:200), CD16 (1:200), CD206 (1:200); and GFAP (1:400) (all from Abcam); and cleaved caspase-3 (1:200), Iba-1 (1: 100), and NF-κB p65 (1:200) (all from Cell Signaling Technology), followed by incubation with appropriate secondary antibodies. Immunoreactivity was visualized with the ECL Western Blotting Detection System (Millipore, Billerica, MA, USA). Gray value analysis was conducted with the UN-Scan-It 6.1 software (Silk Scientific Inc., Orem, UT, USA). Expression levels were normalized against β-actin (1:5000, Boster Biotech) or laminin B1 (1:3000, Cell Signaling Technology).

Co-immunoprecipitation

Brain tissue from lesioned cortices were incubated with 1 μg of SIRT1 (Cell Signaling Technology) or HMGB1 anti-acetylated lysine antibody (Cell Signaling

Technology) for 2 h at 4 °C. A 10-μl volume of protein A/G agarose beads (Roche, Mannheim, Germany) was added to the samples and incubated overnight. After immunoprecipitation and centrifugation, agarose beads were washed three times with lysis buffer, and the degree of acetylation of SIRT1 or HMGB1 was analyzed by western blotting using an anti-acetylated lysine antibody (Cell Signaling Technology).

SIRT1 deacetylase activity and NF-κB DNA binding activity assay

Nucleoproteins were extracted, and their concentrations were determined using the bicinchoninic acid assay. The SIRT1/SIR2 Deacetylase Fluorometric Assay Kit (Cyclex, Nagano, Japan) was used to detect HDAC activity by measuring the absorbance at 460 nm on a microplate reader (2030 ARVO; PerkinElmer LifeSciences, Boston, MA, USA) according to the manufacturer's instructions. A transcription factor binding assay colorimetric ELISA kit (Cayman Chemical, Ann Arbor, MI) was used to detect NF-κB p65 DNA binding activity by measuring the absorbance at 450 nm on a microplate reader (2030 ARVO).

NAD+/NADH Quantification Colorimetric Kit

The NAD+/NADH ratio was measured using the NAD +/NADH Quantification Kit (Yusen Biotech, Shanghai, China) according to the manufacturer's instructions. The absorbance at 450 nm of the mixture was measured by a microplate reader (2030 ARVO).

Statistical analysis

All statistical analyses were performed using SPSS 18.0 statistical software (SPSS Inc., Chicago, IL, USA). The results were expressed as mean ± standard deviation. Statistical differences among the groups were assessed by one-way ANOVA, and post hoc multiple comparisons were performed using Student-Newman-Keuls tests. Values of $p < 0.05$ were considered statistically significant.

Results

Neuroprotective effects of ω-3 PUFA supplementation on TBI

The average blood pressure was lower during anesthesia with sodium pentobarbital than the baseline values throughout the sham group and sham + ω-3 group. However, there were no significant differences in the average blood pressure and arterial blood gas among the TBI groups (data not shown).

The neurological function scores of the sham and sham + ω-3 PUFA groups were unaltered at the corresponding time points (scored 1–3). However, neurological function was severely impaired 1 day after TBI (12.78 ± 0.69); from day 3 after TBI, rats in the TBI + ω-3 PUFA group showed significantly better neurological functions than rats in the TBI groups (10.69 ± 0.48 vs.12. 14 ± 0.52, $p < 0.05$) (Fig. 1a). Meanwhile, rats in the TBI + ω-3 PUFA group showed significantly improved rotarod performances than rats in the TBI groups from day 7 after TBI (Fig. 1b).

Brain water content is an important predictor of TBI prognosis [4]. Compared with sham group, the water content of brain tissue was higher (82.87%) in the TBI group 3 days after injury ($p < 0.05$). The water content of the TBI + ω-3 PUFA group was markedly lower than that of TBI group (81.54 ± 0.57% vs. 82.87 ± 0.73%, $p < 0.05$) (Fig. 1c).

BBB permeability was investigated by measuring the extravasation of Evans blue [37]. Results demonstrated that the TBI group had more Evans blue dye extravasation in the cortex 3 days after TBI compared to the sham and sham + ω-3 PUFA groups, respectively ($p < 0.05$ for each). Interestingly, compared to the TBI group, the TBI + ω-3 PUFA group had significantly decreased of Evans blue dye extravasation ($p < 0.05$) (Fig. 1e).

ω-3 PUFA supplementation protects neurons against TBI-induced neuronal apoptosis

Nissl staining was used to identify apoptotic neurons in lesioned cortices [4]. The sham group and the sham + ω-3 PUFA group showed a very low apoptotic fraction of neurons. The percentage of apoptotic cells was higher in the TBI group than in the sham group 3 days after TBI ($p < 0.05$), while the apoptotic fraction was significantly lower in the TBI + ω-3 PUFA than in the TBI group (42.49 ± 6.53% vs.66.23 ± 8.46%, $p < 0.05$) (Fig. 2a, b). Western blot analyses revealed that TBI resulted in the upregulation of apoptotic factors in the cortex 3 days after TBI; however, compared to the TBI group, cleaved caspase-3 and Bax levels were decreased, whereas the anti-apoptotic factor, Bcl-2, was increased in the TBI + ω-3 PUFA group ($p < 0.05$) (Fig. 2c). TUNEL staining further demonstrated that TUNEL-positive neurons were significantly decreased in the TBI + ω-3 group 3 days after TBI compared the TBI group (43.32 ± 6.03% vs.69.03 ± 7.31%, $p < 0.05$) (Fig. 2d). These results suggest that ω-3 PUFA supplementation has no obvious effect on the normal cortex, while it exerts a neuroprotective effect in the lesioned cortex.

ω-3 PUFA supplementation promotes M2 microglia polarization and alleviates the microglia-mediated inflammatory response

A microglial transition from the anti-inflammatory (M2) phenotype to the pro-inflammatory (M1) phenotype plays a crucial role both in the microglial activation and the subsequent neuroinflammatory response [1, 2]. To test for shifts in microglial polarization, we double-stained microglia with a pan microglial marker, Iba-1, and the M1-associated marker, CD16, or the M2-

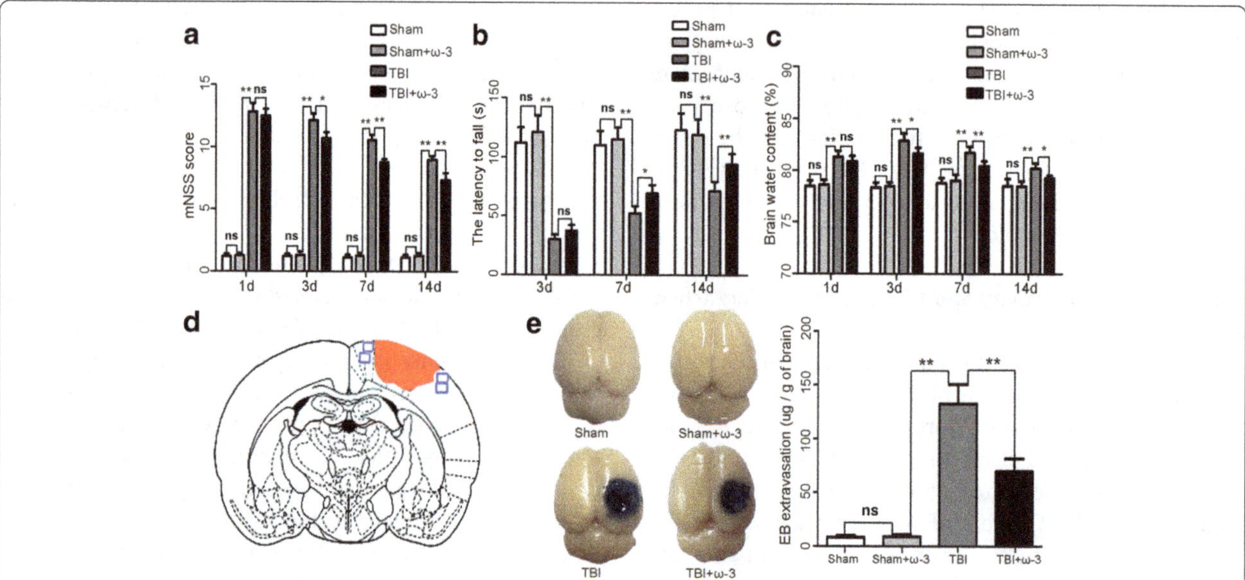

Fig. 1 ω-3 PUFA supplementation improves neurological function, brain edema, and BBB permeability after TBI. **a** ω-3 PUFA supplementation improved neurological functions 3 days after TBI (10.69 ± 0.48 vs. 12.14 ± 0.52, $p < 0.05$). **b** Rats in the TBI + ω-3 PUFA group showed significantly improved rotarod performances than rats in the TBI groups from day 7 after TBI. **c** ω-3 PUFA supplementation decreased brain water content 3 days after TBI (81.54 ± 0.57% vs. 82.87 ± 0.73%, $p < 0.05$). **d** A schematic of a brain section after TBI. Areas in red refer to lesioned sites and areas in blue refer to sample points. **e** The TBI group had more Evans blue dye extravasation in the cortex 3 days after TBI compared with the sham group ($p < 0.05$). Compared with the TBI group, the TBI + ω-3 PUFA group had significantly decreased Evans blue dye extravasation of ($p < 0.05$). Representative photos of Evans blue dye extravasation in the experimental groups. Values are expressed as mean ± standard deviation ($n = 6$ per group). N.S., $p > 0.05$, *$p < 0.05$, **$p < 0.01$

associated marker, CD206, 3 days after TBI. As expected, microglia labeled with the M1-associated marker (CD16+) were increased after TBI but significantly decreased by ω-3 PUFA supplementation, whereas the M2-associated marker (CD206+) increased after ω-3 PUFA supplementation. Therefore, ω-3 PUFA supplementation promoted a shift of microglia from the M1 phenotype to the M2 phenotype (Fig. 3a, b). Moreover, western blot analysis showed that CD16 was significantly inhibited, whereas CD206 was significantly increased after ω-3 PUFA supplementation (Fig. 3c). Expression levels of inflammatory factors (TNF-α, IL-1β, IL-6, and HMGB1) were measured after TBI using an ELISA kit, and results also showed that the TBI group had significantly higher expression levels of inflammatory factors compared with the sham group, while ω-3 PUFA supplementation decreased TBI-induced expression of these factors, and increased the expression of anti-inflammatory IL-10 ($p < 0.05$) (Fig. 3d). These findings suggest that ω-3 PUFA supplementation shifts microglia polarization toward the M2 phenotype and alleviates the microglial-mediated inflammatory response.

ω-3 PUFA supplementation inhibits HMGB1/NF-κB pathway in lesioned cortices

HMGB1 translocation and release play important roles in TBI-induced microglial activation and the subsequent inflammatory response [15, 37]. Using double immunofluorescent staining, HMGB1 expressions in neurons (NeuN+), microglia (Iba-1+), and astrocytes (GFAP+) were assessed in lesioned cortices 3 days after TBI. Compared with the sham group, the expression levels of HMGB1 were higher in the TBI group 3 days after injury. After ω-3 PUFA supplementation, HMGB1 expression was inhibited in both neurons and microglia, but not in astrocytes (Fig. 4a–c).

Western blot analyses demonstrated that expression levels of HMGB1 in the cytosol, nuclei, and in total protein of neurons and microglias from lesioned cortices increased after TBI, but ω-3 PUFA supplementation effectively decreased HMGB1 expression in the cytosol and in total protein of cells from lesioned cortices ($p < 0.05$), but not in nuclearprotein ($p > 0.05$) (Fig. 5a). Activation of the NF-κB pathway is associated with HMGB1 expression and the post-TBI inflammatory response [4]. A significant reduction in NF-κB p65 DNA binding activity was observed in the TBI + ω-3 group compared with the TBI group ($p < 0.05$) (Fig. 5b). Western blot and immunofluorescence staining further showed that compared with the TBI group, ω-3 PUFA supplementation significantly inhibited the translocation of NF-κB p65 from the cytosol to the nucleus, reduced NF-κB p65 expression, and attenuated NF-κB p65 DNA-binding activity (Fig. 5c, d). These results indicate that ω-3 PUFA supplementation can inhibit HMGB1 expression and extracellular secretion in both neurons and microglias,

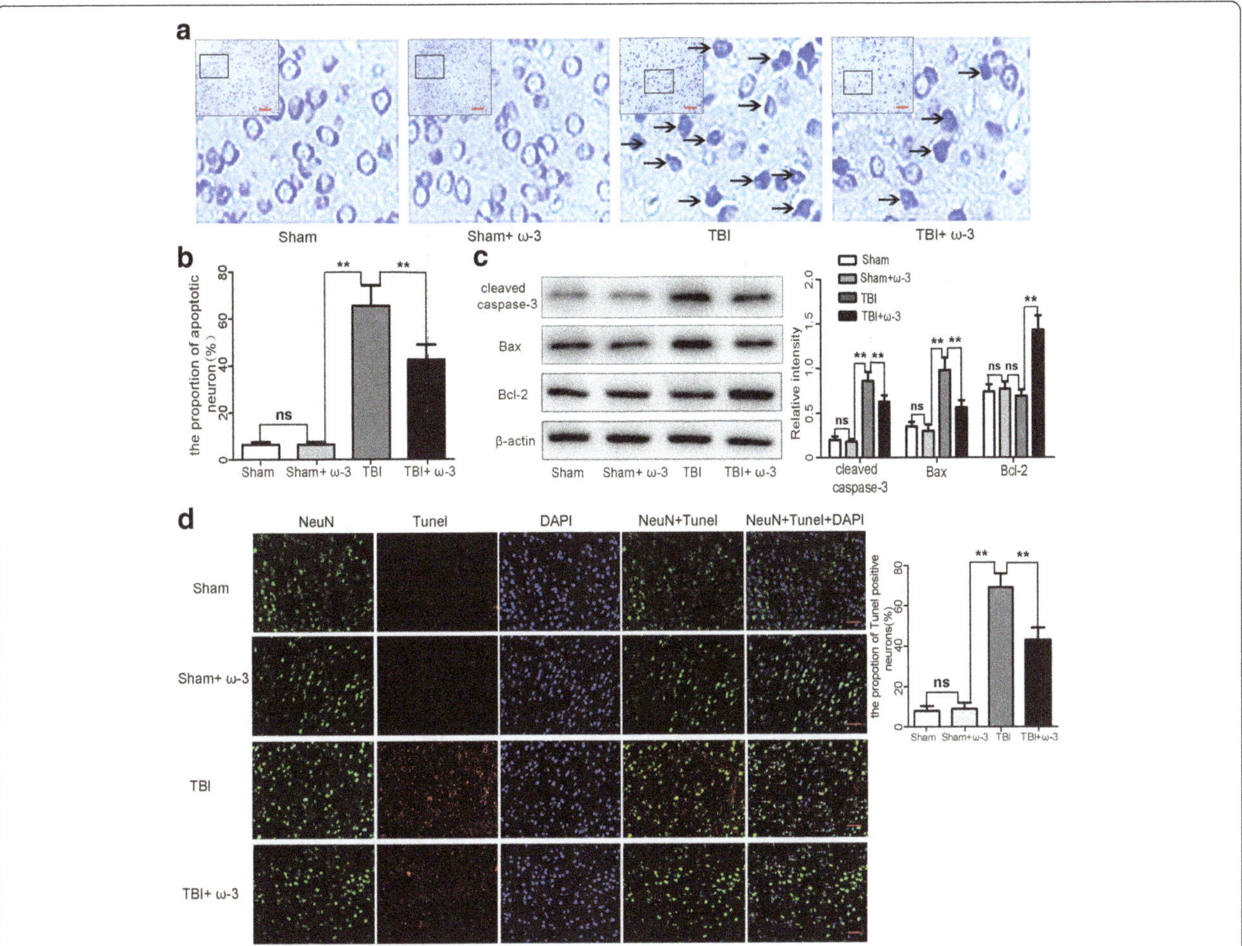

Fig. 2 ω-3 PUFA supplementation protects neurons against TBI-induced neuronal apoptosis in the lesioned cortex 3 day after TBI. **a**, **b** The sham group and the sham + ω-3 PUFA group had very low fractions of apoptotic neurons. The percentage of apoptotic cells was higher in the TBI group than in the sham group ($p < 0.05$); the apoptotic fraction was significantly lower in the TBI + ω-3 PUFA group than in the TBI group (42.49 ± 6.53% vs. 66.23 ± 8.46%, $p < 0.05$). Representative photomicrographs of Nissl-stained neurons are shown; arrows indicate apoptotic neurons. **c** Western blot analyses revealed that TBI resulted in the upregulation of apoptotic factors in the cortex; however, compared with the TBI group, cleaved caspase-3 and Bax levels were decreased, whereas the anti-apoptotic factor, Bcl-2, was increased in TBI + ω-3 PUFA group ($p < 0.05$). **d** TUNEL staining demonstrated that TUNEL-positive neurons were significantly decreased in the TBI + ω-3 group compared with the TBI group (43.32 ± 6.03% vs. 69.03 ± 7.31%, $p < 0.05$). Representative photomicrographs of TUNEL-positive neurons are shown; arrows indicate apoptotic neurons. Values are expressed as mean ± standard deviation ($n = 6$ per group). N.S., $p > 0.05$, *$p < 0.05$, **$p < 0.01$. Scale bars = 50 μm

thus inhibiting the NF-κB pathway and attenuating the inflammatory response after TBI.

ω-3 PUFA supplementation elevates SIRT1 expression and deacetylase activity

SIRTs are a family of deacetylases that require nicotinamide adenine dinucleotide (NAD+) as a cofactor for the deacetylation reaction [22, 23]. Consistent with our previous study, similar results were obtained by immunohistochemistry: SIRT1 immunoreactivity in both neurons and microglias from lesioned cortices was significantly increased after ω-3 PUFA supplementation (2.92 ± 0.52 vs. 1.86 ± 0.29, $p < 0.05$) (Fig. 6a). SIRT1 protein levels were also upregulated after ω-3 PUFA supplementation ($p < 0.05$) (Fig. 6b). As SIRT1 is a NAD +-dependent histone deacetylase that affects NAD+ metabolism [24, 38], we also measured the NAD+/NADH ratio to detect SIRT1 activity. Treatment with ω-3 PUFA significantly increased the NAD+/NADH ratio ($p < 0.05$) (Fig. 6c).

ω-3 PUFA supplementation suppresses the HMGB1 pathway by elevating SIRT1 activity

Posttranslational modifications such as acetylation are critical for HMGB1 transcription and extracellular secretion [21]. SIRT1 inhibits HMGB1 transcription and extracellular secretion by keeping HMGB1 in a deacetylated (inactive) state which sequesters the inflammatory response [21, 26]. Co-immunoprecipitation (Co-IP) analysis showed that both HMGB1 and NF-κB acetylation

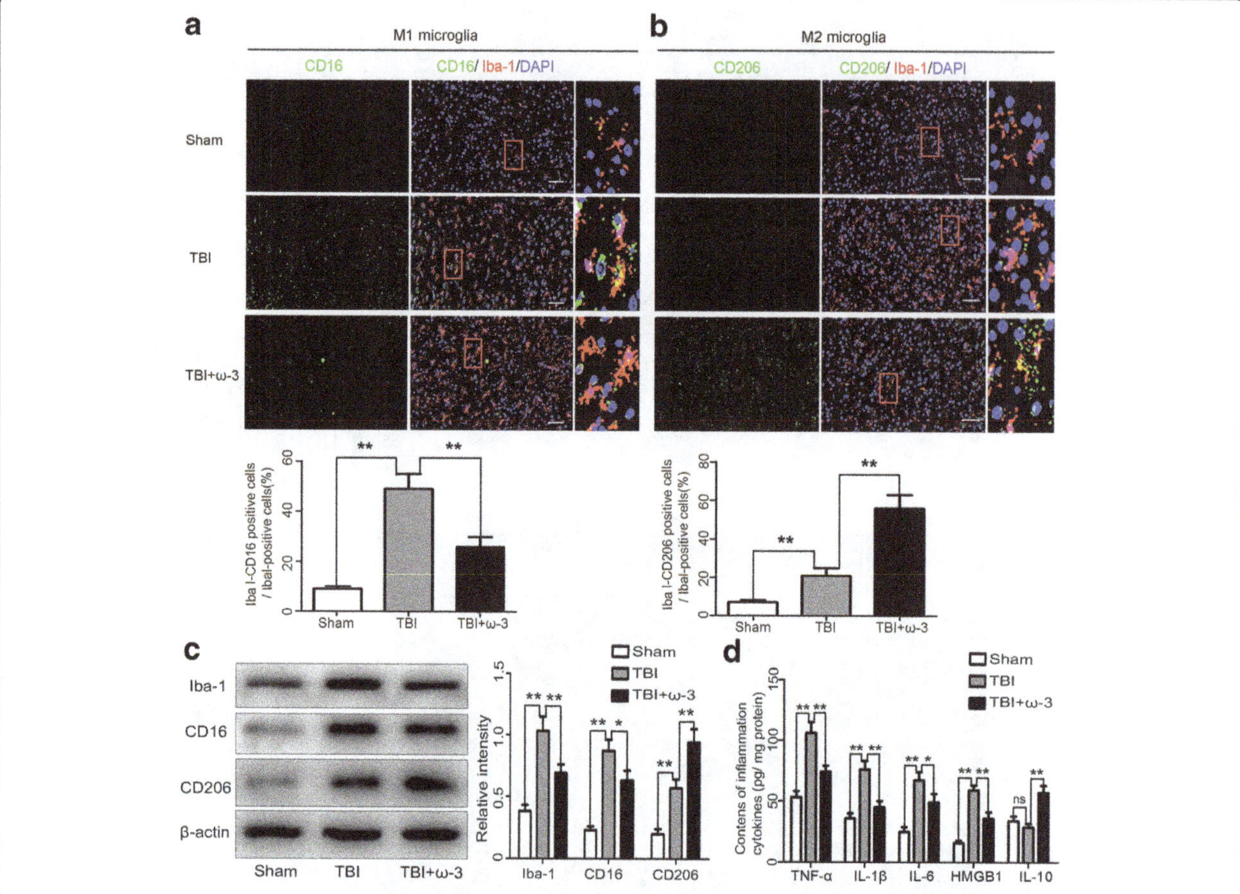

Fig. 3 ω-3 PUFA supplementation promotes microglia polarization toward M2 and alleviatesmicroglial-mediated inflammatory responses. **a**, **b** Double staining was used to assess microglia (Iba1+) and a M1-associated marker (CD16+) or a M2-associated marker (CD206+) in the lesioned cortex 3 days after TBI. CD16+-positive microglia increased after TBI but significantly decreased following ω-3 PUFA supplementation, whereas CD206+-positive microglia increased following ω-3 PUFA supplementation. Representative photomicrographs of CD16- or CD206-positive microglias are shown. **c** Western blot analysis showed that CD16 was significantly inhibited, but CD206 was significantly increased after ω-3 PUFA supplementation. **d** ω-3 PUFA supplementation significantly decreased TBI-induced enhancement of TNF-α, IL-1β, IL-6, and HMGB1, while increased the expression of anti-inflammatory IL-10 ($p < 0.05$). Values are expressed as mean ± standard deviation ($n = 6$ per group). N.S., $p > 0.05$, *$p < 0.05$, **$p < 0.01$. Scale bars = 50 μm

were decreased in acetyl-lysine immunoprecipitate fractions after ω-3 PUFA supplementation compared with the TBI group ($p < 0.05$) (Fig. 7a, b). To verify whether HMGB1 acetylation formed a direct complex with SIRT1, we assessed the impact of SIRT1 deacetylase activity on the interaction between HMGB1 and SIRT1. Co-IP analysis further showed that the acetylation of HMGB1 caused it to dissociate from SIRT1, thereby promoting HMGB1 extracellular secretion after TBI; ω-3 PUFA supplementation induced direct interactions between SIRT1 and HMGB1 ($p < 0.05$) (Fig. 7c). The inhibitory effects of ω-3 PUFA supplementation on the inflammatory response and on SIRT1-HMGB1/NF-κB axis activation were reversed by pharmacological inhibition of SIRT1, suggesting that the anti-inflammatory effect of ω-3 PUFA was dependent on SIRT1 activity (Fig. 7d, e).

Discussion

Accumulating evidence has demonstrated the benefits of ω-3 PUFA or its constituents against TBI-induced neural damage and secondary pathological processes [32–34]. We previously reported that ω-3 PUFA supplementation inhibited TBI-induced microglial activation and the subsequent inflammatory response, leading to neuroprotective effects [4]. Taken together with our previously reported findings, the present study supports the view that ω-3 PUFA is a suitable therapeutic candidate against trauma-induced mechanical injury and secondary neuronal apoptosis. Furthermore, ω-3 PUFA supplementation reduced brain edema and BBB permeability, and improved neurological function in lesioned cortices by inhibiting the expression of the pro-apoptotic factors, cleaved caspase-3 and Bax, and increasing expression of the anti-apoptotic factor, Bcl-2 (Fig. 8).

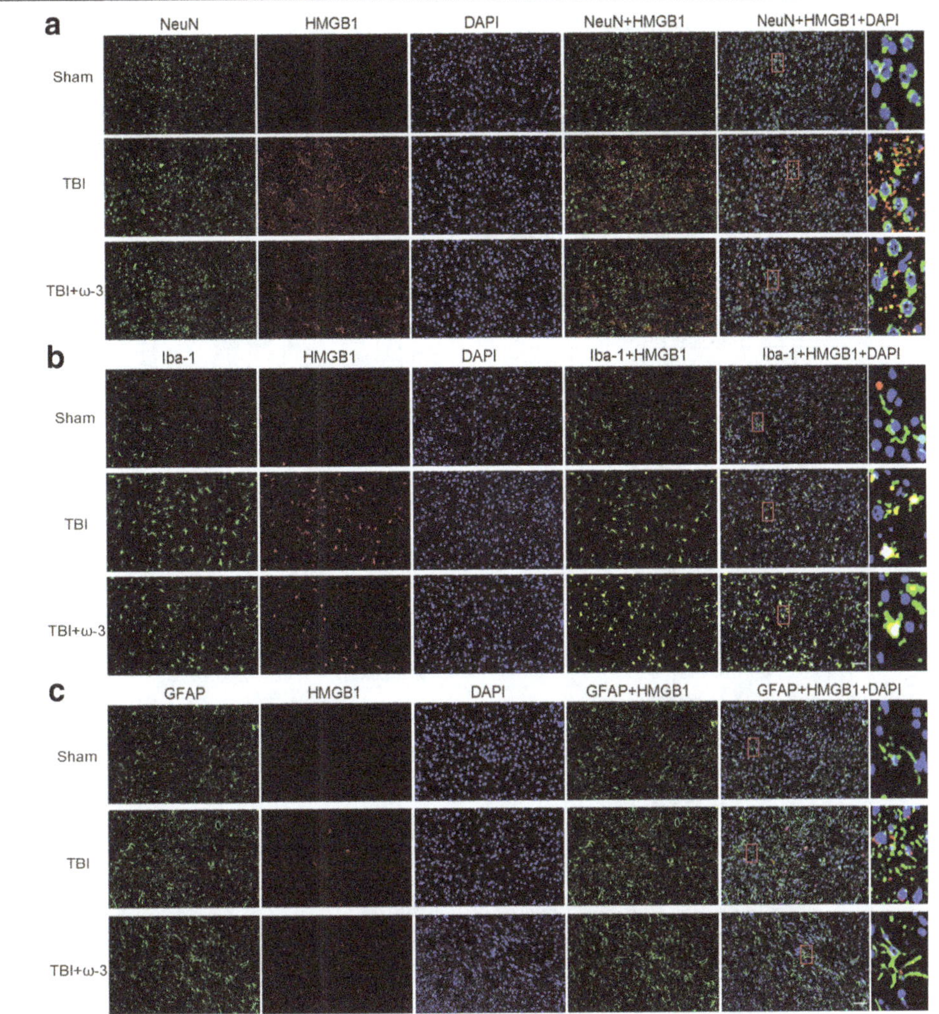

Fig. 4 ω-3 PUFA supplementation inhibits HMGB1 expression in lesioned cortices 3 days after TBI. Double staining was used to assessneurons (NeuN +), microglia (Iba-1+), and astrocytes (GFAP+) in the lesioned cortex. **a** TBI enhanced the expression of HMGB1 in neurons, which was significantly decreased by ω-3 PUFA supplementation. Representative photomicrographs of HMGB1-positive neurons are shown. **b** TBI enhanced the expression of HMGB1 in microglia, which was significantly decreased by ω-3 PUFA supplementation. Representative photomicrographs of HMGB1-positive microglias are shown. **c** ω-3 PUFA supplementation had no obvious effect on the expression of HMGB1 in astrocytes. Representative photomicrographs of HMGB1-positive astrocytes are shown. Scale bars = 50 μm

Microglial activation and the subsequent neuroinflammatory response were reported to be associated with decreased mitochondrial membrane potential and increased release of cytochrome C. Caspase activity contributes to neuronal apoptosis [39, 40]. Apoptotic event can cause further damage within the brain through the process of microglial activation, which is a vital contributing factor of TBI-induced secondary injury [1–3]. A transition from an anti-inflammatory M2 phenotype to a pro-inflammatory M1 phenotype plays a crucial role in microglial activation and the resulting neuroinflammatory response [1, 2, 7]. Our study showed that activation of microglia and expression of inflammatory factors (TNF-α, IL-1β, IL-6, and HMGB1) were significantly enhanced in brain tissue after TBI, which were associated with brain edema and neurological deficits. In addition, ω-3 PUFA supplementation promoted a shift from the M1 to the M2 phenotype and inhibited microglial activation, thus reducing TBI-induced inflammatory factors. These findings were consistent with the observation that ω-3 PUFA supplementation reduced neuronal apoptosis following TBI. Our results suggest that ω-3 PUFA supplementation may modulate microglial polarization, decrease microglial activation and the subsequent inflammatory response, reduce brain edema, inhibit apoptosis, and improve neurological functions.

HMGB1 translocation, release, and activation of the NF-κB signaling pathway are considered to be pivotal in the TBI-induced inflammatory response due to the secretion of pro-inflammatory factors [41, 42]. An

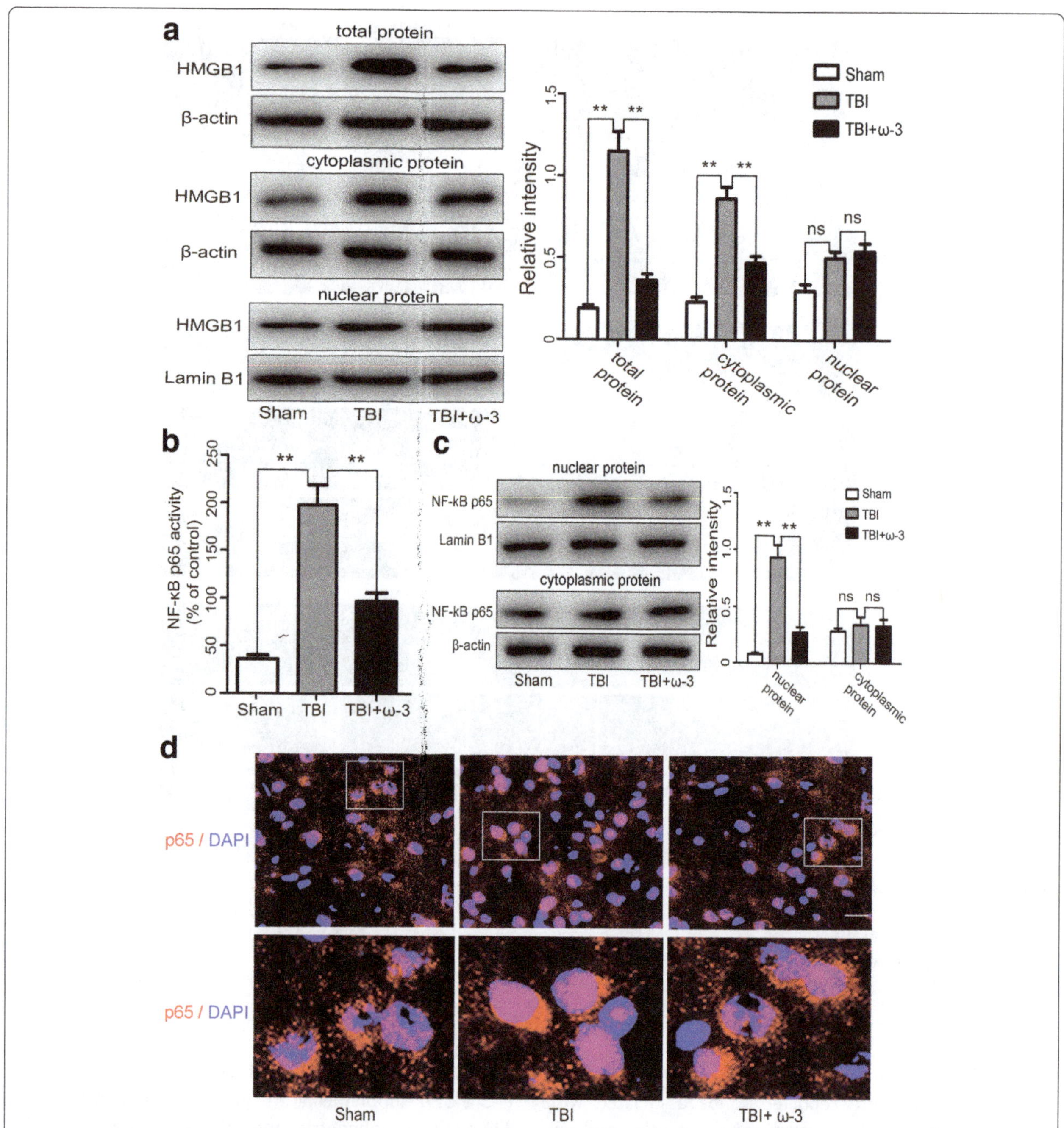

Fig. 5 ω-3 PUFA supplementation inhibits the HMGB1/ NF-κB pathway in lesioned cortices 3 days after TBI. **a** Western blot analysis demonstrated that expression levels of HMGB1 in the cytosol, nuclei and in total protein of neurons and microglias from lesioned cortices increased after TBI. ω-3 PUFA supplementation significantly decreased HMGB1 expression in cytosolic and total cellular protein levels ($p < 0.05$), but not nuclearprotein ($p > 0.05$). **b** A significant reduction in NF-κB p65 DNA binding activity was observed in the TBI + ω-3 group compared with the TBI group ($p < 0.05$). **c** ω-3 PUFA supplementation significantly inhibited the translocation of NF-κB p65 from the cytosol to the nucleus and reduced NF-κB p65 expression ($p < 0.05$). ω-3 PUFA supplementation inhibited NF-κB p65 translocation to the nucleus ($p < 0.05$). **d** Representative photomicrographs of NF-κB p65 staining in the experimental groups. Values are expressed as mean ± standard deviation ($n = 6$ per group). N.S., $p > 0.05$, $*p < 0.05$, $**p < 0.01$. Scale bars = 50 μm

increase in HMGB1 nucleocytoplasmic translocation and extracellular secretion, and the activation of HMGB1/NF-κB, coupled with increased expression of pro-inflammatory factors, were detected after TBI [4]. Furthermore, clinical evidence suggests that elevation of HMGB1 in cerebrospinal fluid was correlated with neurologic outcome in TBI patients [43]. Measuring HMGB1 might represent a potentially predictive biomarker in the early detection of post-trauma complications, suggesting inhibition of HMGB1 and extracellular

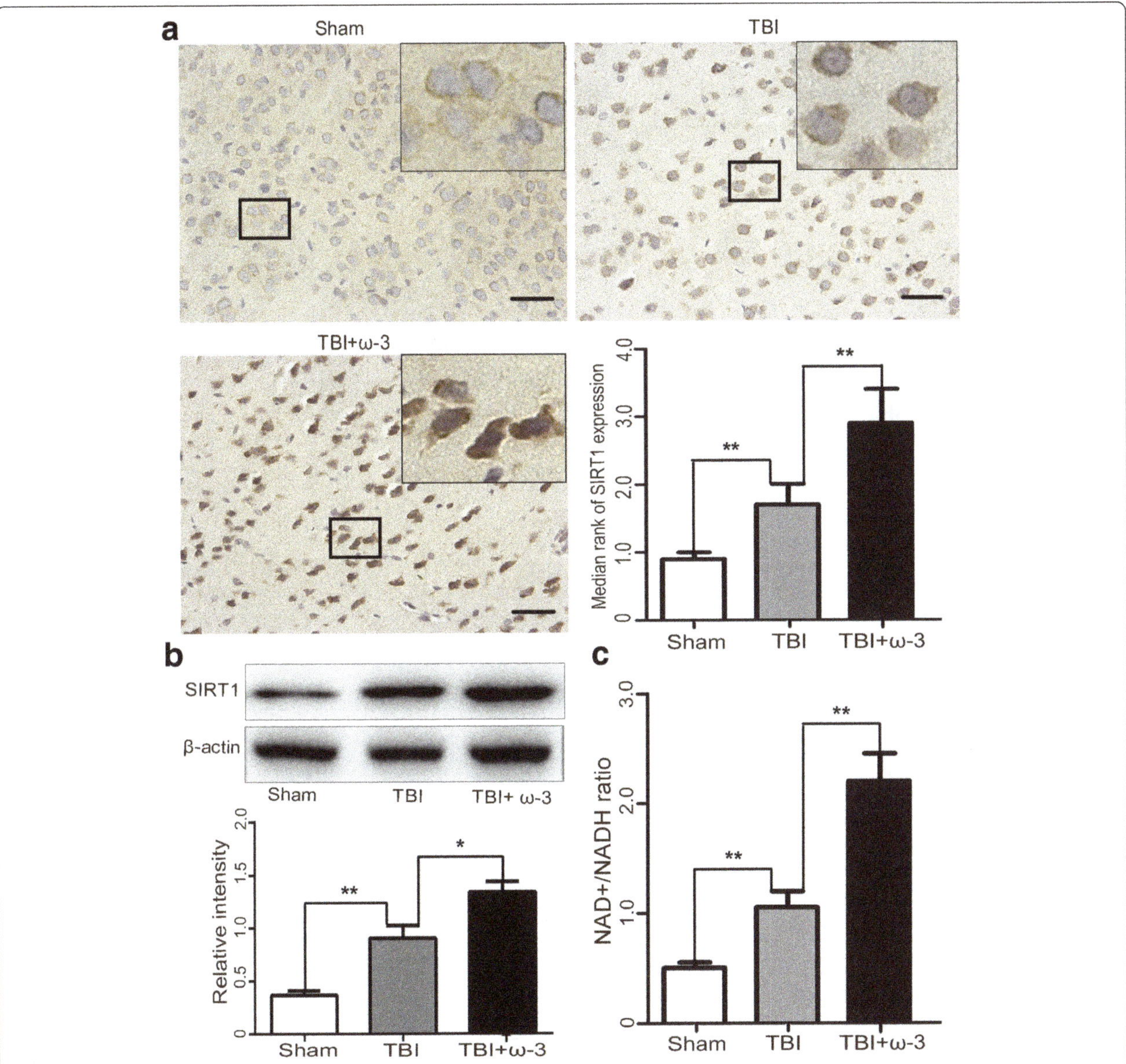

Fig. 6 ω-3 PUFA supplementation elevates SIRT1 expression and deacetylase activity in lesioned cortices 3 days after TBI. **a** SIRT1 immunoreactivity in both neurons and microglias from lesioned cortices was significantly increased by ω-3 PUFA supplementation (2.92 ± 0.52 vs. 1.86 ± 0.29, $p < 0.05$). **b** SIRT1 levels were also upregulated after ω-3 PUFA supplementation ($p < 0.05$). **c** The NAD+/NADH ratio was measured to detect SIRT1 activity. Treatment with ω-3 PUFA significantly increased the NAD+/NADH ratio ($p < 0.05$). Values are expressed as mean ± standard deviation ($n = 6$ per group). N.S., $p > 0.05$, *$p < 0.05$, **$p < 0.01$. Scale bars = 50 μm

secretion might offer a novel anti-inflammatory strategy to protect against TBI [43]. Our previous study [4] confirmed that inhibition of HMGB1 translocation release and activation of the NF-κB signaling pathway led to a reduction in TBI-induced microglial activation and the subsequent inflammatory response, thus providing neuroprotection following TBI. Consistent with our previous findings [4], we showed that expression levels of HMGB1 in both neurons and microglia were higher in the TBI group 3 days after injury. We also found that after ω-3 PUFA supplementation, HMGB1 expression was inhibited in both neurons and microglia in lesioned cortices. Moreover, ω-3 PUFA supplementation inhibited HMGB1 translocation, release, and NF-κB pathway activation after TBI. These results suggest that HMGB1 has important roles in microglial polarization and the neuroinflammatory response after TBI.

Activation of the HMGB1/NF-κB pathway is closely related to HMGB1 acetylation, which is regulated by the balance of HDACs and HATs [19, 20]; furthermore, HMGB1 mediates late inflammatory responses, which are related to protein acetylation levels [12, 44]. HMGB1

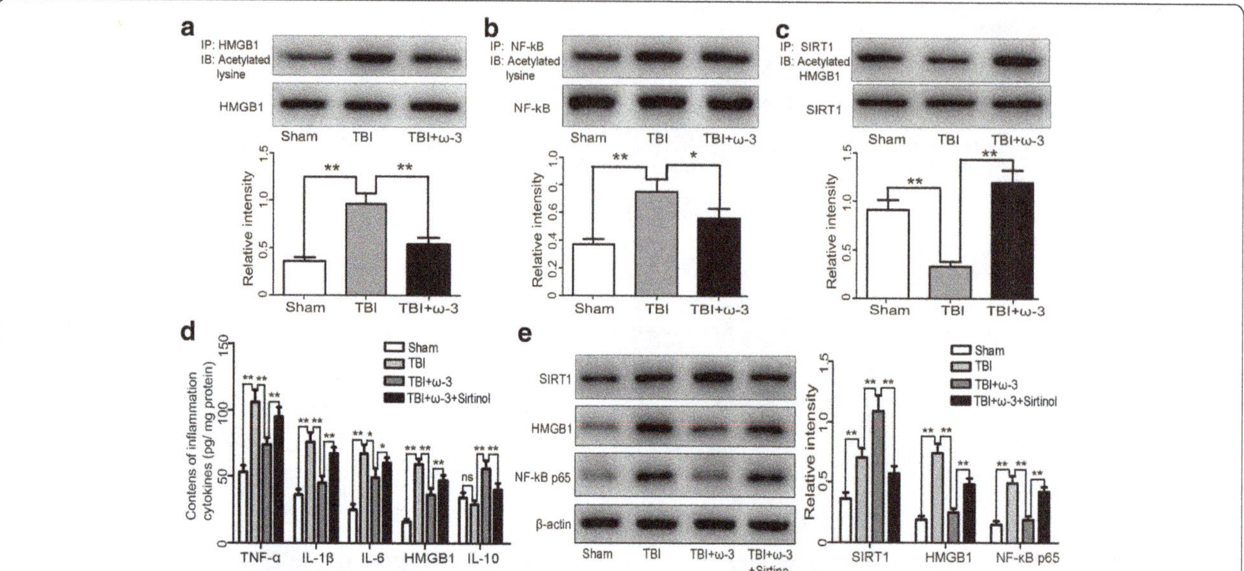

Fig. 7 ω-3 PUFA supplementation suppressed HMGB1 pathway via elevating SIRT1 activity in lesioned cortices 3 days after TBI. **a** Co-IP analysis showed that a reduction in HMGB1 acetylation following ω-3 PUFA supplementation compared with the TBI group ($p < 0.05$). **b** Co-IP analysis showed a reduction in NF-κB acetylation following ω-3 PUFA supplementation compared with the TBI group ($p < 0.05$). **c** HMGB1 acetylation caused it to dissociate from SIRT1, thereby promoting HMGB1 extracellular secretion after TBI; ω-3 PUFA supplementation also induced direct interactions between SIRT1 and HMGB1 ($p < 0.05$). **d** The inhibitory effect of ω-3 PUFA supplementation on the neuroinflammatory response was reversed by pharmacological inhibition of SIRT1. **e** The inhibitory effect of ω-3 PUFA supplementation on HMGB1/NF-κB pathway activation was reversed by pharmacological inhibition of SIRT1. Values are expressed as mean ± standard deviation ($n = 6$ per group). N.S., $p > 0.05$, *$p < 0.05$, **$p < 0.01$. Scale bars = 50 μm

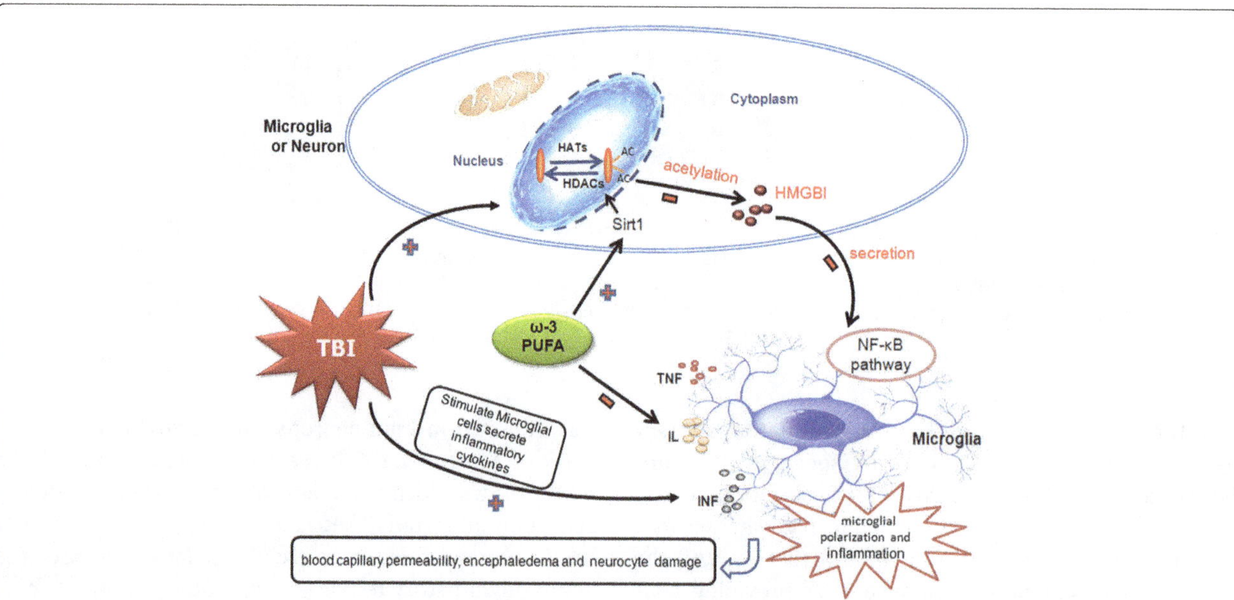

Fig. 8 Schematic illustration of the possible neuroprotective mechanisms of ω-3 PUFA supplementation after TBI. As illustrated, TBI-induced microglial activation initiates a neuronal-glial neuroinflammatory response by producing a wide array of pro-inflammatory factors or mediators such as TNF, ILs, and IFN. Under inflammatory conditions, activation of the HMGB1/NF-κB pathway is closely related to its acetylation levels, which is regulated by SIRT1. Supplementation with ω-3PUFA attenuates the inflammatory response by modulating microglial polarization through SIRT1-mediated deacetylation of HMGB1/NF-κB pathway, leading to neuroprotective effects following experimental traumatic brain injury

acetylation was previously found to promote the cytoplasmic accumulation and secretion of lysosomes [19, 20, 45]. SIRTs are a family of deacetylases that require NAD+ as a cofactor for the deacetylation reaction [22]. Our previous study [4] confirmed that the expression of acetylated HMGB1 and SIRT1 activity were involved in inflammatory mechanisms after TBI. In addition, we also found that SIRT1 levels were upregulated after ω-3 PUFA supplementation, indicating that ω-3 PUFA inhibited the expression and release of HMGB1 in a SIRT1 deacetylation-mediated dependent manner. Despite an increasing number of studies [24–26] showing that SIRT1 promotes the deacetylation of HMGB1, thus inhibiting HMGB1 transcription and extracellular release, the anti-inflammatory effect of the SIRT1-HMGB1 axis underlying TBI remains relatively under explored.

As SIRT1 is an NAD+-dependent histone deacetylase that affects the NAD+ metabolism, the NAD+/NADH ratio was measured to detect SIRT1 activity [24, 38]. We showed that treatment with ω-3 PUFA significantly increased the NAD+/NADH ratio and SIRT1 activity following TBI. Posttranslational modifications such as acetylation are critical for HMGB1 transcription and its extracellular secretion [21]. SIRT1 was also shown to inhibit HMGB1 transcription and extracellular secretion by maintaining HMGB1 in a deacetylated state, hence repressing the inflammatory response [21, 26]. Here, we found a novel counter-regulatory relationship between the attenuation of TBI-mediated HMGB1/NF-kB p65 pathway activity and regulation of SIRT1 overexpression. Our co-IP analysis also showed the presence of HMGB1 in acetyl-lysine immunoprecipitate fractions, confirming a decrease in HMGB1 acetylation after ω-3 PUFA supplementation. To verify whether acetylated HMGB1 formed a direct complex with SIRT1, we assessed the impact of SIRT1 deacetylase activity on the interaction between HMGB1 and SIRT1. Results showed that HMGB1 acetylation caused it to dissociate from SIRT1, thereby promoting HMGB1 extracellular secretion after TBI. Furthermore, ω-3 PUFA supplementation not only increased SIRT1 expression and HMGB1 deacetylation but also induced direct interactions between the two. The downregulation of acetylated HMGB1 promoted the formation of a complex with nuclear SIRT1, thereby inhibiting HMGB1 release and attenuating the central inflammatory response following TBI. These results indicate that ω-3 PUFA-mediated downregulation of HMGB1 acetylation and its complex with SIRT1 were likely due to an upregulation of SIRT1 (Fig. 8).

Activation of the NF-κB pathway is associated with HMGB1 expression and the post-TBI inflammatory response [17, 18]. Treatment with ω-3 PUFA significantly inhibited the translocation of NF-κB p65 from the cytosol to the nucleus, reduced NF-κB p65 acetylation, and attenuated NF-κB p65 DNA-binding activity, thus modulating downstream inflammatory responses. Sirtinol has many off-target effects, as there are iron chelation and biological effects below the SIRT protein inhibition levels. However, as a pharmacological inhibition of SIRT1, Sirtinol effectively inhibited the expressions of SIRT1 and SIRT2 and was used to inhibit SIRT1 signaling in several studies [22, 46, 47]. In our study, we also showed intervention with SIRT1 significantly decreased the SIRT1 expression following TBI. Moreover, the inhibitory effects of ω-3 PUFA supplementation on the inflammatory response and on SIRT1-HMGB1/NF-κB axis activation were reversed by Sirtinol, suggesting the anti-inflammation effects of ω-3 PUFAs were SIRT1 dependent. Future studies involving HMGB1 knockout mice are warranted to further investigate the mechanisms involved in ω-3 PUFA-mediated inhibition of HMGB1 and subsequent activation of the NF-κB pathway. Meanwhile, additional in vitro experiments are also needed to confirm the direct effects of ω-3 PUFA supplementation on neuronal and microglial activation.

Conclusions

In summary, ω-3 PUFA supplementation promoted a shift of microglia from the M1 to the M2phenotype, inhibited microglial activation, and thus reduced TBI-induced inflammatory factors. In addition, ω-3 PUFA-mediated downregulation of HMGB1 acetylation and its extracellular secretion were likely due to increased SIRT1 activity. This indicates that treatment with ω-3 PUFA inhibited HMGB1 acetylation and induced direct interactions between SIRT1 and HMGB1 by increasing SIRT1 activity following TBI. These interactions then led to inhibition of HMGB1 nucleocytoplasmic translocation/extracellular secretion, which sequestered HMGB1-mediated activation of the NF-κB signaling pathway following TBI-induced microglial activation and thus inhibited the subsequent inflammatory response (Fig. 8).

Abbreviations

BBB: Blood-brain barrier; co-IP: Co-immunoprecipitation; DHA: Docosahexaenoic acid; ELISA: Enzyme-linked immunosorbent assay; EPA: Eicosapentaenoic acid; HATs: Histone acetyltransferases; HDACs: Histone deacetylases; HMGB1: High mobile group box 1; IFN: Interferon; IL: Interleukin; MAPK: Mitogen-activated protein kinase; mNSS: Modified neurological severity scores; NAD: Nicotinamide adenine dinucleotide; NF-κB: Nuclear factor-κB; PI3K: Phosphatidylinositol 3-kinase; RAGE: Glycation end products; SIRT: Sirtuin; TBI: Traumatic brain injury; TLRs: Toll-like receptors; TNF: Tumor necrosis factor; TUNEL: Terminal deoxynucleotidyl transferase dUTP nick-end labelling; ω-3 PUFA: Omega-3 polyunsaturated fatty acid

Acknowledgements

We would like to thank Dr. Hongzhi Gao (Department of Central Laboratory, the Second Affiliated Hospital, Fujian Medical University) for advice and expert technical support. Sincere appreciation is also given to the teachers and our colleagues from the Second Affiliated Hospital of Fujian Medical University, who participated in this study with great cooperation.

Funding
This work was supported by grants from the funds for Fujian Province Scientific Foundation (no. 2015J01443) and Fujian Province Hygiene Innovation Foundation (no. 2015-CXB-20) from Dr. Xiangrong Chen.

Authors' contributions
XC contributed to the conception and design and writing of the manuscript. CC, SW, YF, and ZF supported several experiments and helped in the acquisition of data and analysis and interpretation of data. SF and YL helped in the statistical analysis and revision of the manuscript. XC and HF helped in the technical support, obtaining of funding, conception and design, and revision of the manuscript. All authors read and approved the final manuscript.

Competing interests
The authors declare that they have no competing interests.

References

1. Xu H, Wang Z, Li J, Wu H, Peng Y, Fan L, Chen J, Gu C, Yan F, Wang L, et al. The polarization states of microglia in TBI: a new paradigm for pharmacological intervention. Neural Plast. 2017;2017:5405104.
2. Kumar A, Alvarez-Croda DM, Stoica BA, Faden AI, Loane DJ. Microglial/macrophage polarization dynamics following traumatic brain injury. J Neurotrauma. 2016;33:1732–50.
3. Fu R, Shen Q, Xu P, Luo JJ, Tang Y. Phagocytosis of microglia in the central nervous system diseases. Mol Neurobiol. 2014;49:1422–34.
4. Chen X, Wu S, Chen C, Xie B, Fang Z, Hu W, Chen J, Fu H, He H. Omega-3 polyunsaturated fatty acid supplementation attenuates microglial-induced inflammation by inhibiting the HMGB1/TLR4/NF-κB pathway following experimental traumatic brain injury. J Neuroinflammation. 2017;14:143–55.
5. Ma Y, Matsuwaki T, Yamanouchi K, Nishihara M. Progranulin protects hippocampal neurogenesis via suppression of neuroinflammatory responses under acute immune stress. Mol Neurobiol. 2017;54:3717–28.
6. Wang G, Shi Y, Jiang X, Leak RK, Hu X, Wu Y, Pu H, Li W, Tang B, Wang Y, et al. HDAC inhibition prevents white matter injury by modulating microglia/macrophage polarization through the GSK3β/PTEN/Akt axis. Proc Natl Acad Sci. 2015;112:2853–8.
7. Yao X, Liu S, Ding W, Yue P, Jiang Q, Zhao M, Hu F, Zhang H. TLR4 signal ablation attenuated neurological deficits by regulating microglial M1/M2 phenotype after traumatic brain injury in mice. J Neuroimmunol. 2017;310:38–45.
8. Aryanpour R, Pasbakhsh P, Zibara K, Namjoo Z, Beigi BF, Shahbeigi S, Kashani IR, Beyer C, Zendehdel A. Progesterone therapy induces an M1 to M2 switch in microglia phenotype and suppresses NLRP3 inflammasome in a cuprizone-induced demyelination mouse model. Int Immunopharmacol. 2017;51:131–9.
9. Kumar A, Stoica BA, Loane DJ, Yang M, Abulwerdi G, Khan N, Kumar A, Thom SR, Faden AI. Microglial-derived microparticles mediate neuroinflammation after traumatic brain injury. J Neuroinflammation. 2017;14:47.
10. Braun M, Vaibhav K, Saad NM, Fatima S, Vender JR, Baban B, Hoda MN, Dhandapani KM. White matter damage after traumatic brain injury: a role for damage associated molecular patterns. Biochim Biophys Acta. 1863;2017:2614–26.
11. Fang P, Schachner M, Shen YQ. HMGB1 in development and diseases of the central nervous system. Mol Neurobiol. 2012;45:499–506.
12. Wang D, Liu K, Wake H, Teshigawara K, Mori S, Nishibori M. Anti-high mobility group box-1 (HMGB1) antibody inhibits hemorrhage-induced brain injury and improved neurological deficits in rats. Sci Rep. 2017;7:46243.
13. Ding J, Cui X, Liu Q. Emerging role of HMGB1 in lung diseases: friend or foe. J Cell Mol Med. 2017;21:1046–57.
14. Qiu Y, Chen Y, Zeng T, Guo W, Zhou W, Yang X. High-mobility group box-B1 (HMGB1) mediates the hypoxia-induced mesenchymal transition of osteoblast cells via activating ERK/JNK signaling. Cell Biol Int. 2016;40:1152–61.
15. Laird MD, Shields JS, Sukumari-Ramesh S, Kimbler DE, Fessler RD, Shakir B, Youssef P, Yanasak N, Vender JR, Dhandapani KM. High mobility group box protein-1 promotes cerebral edema after traumatic brain injury via activation of toll-like receptor 4. Glia. 2014;62:26–38.
16. Wang TH, Xiong LL, Yang SF, You C, Xia QJ, Xu Y, Zhang P, Wang SF, Liu J. LPS pretreatment provides neuroprotective roles in rats with subarachnoid hemorrhage by downregulating MMP9 and Caspase3 associated with TLR4 signaling activation. Mol Neurobiol. 2017;54:7746–60.
17. Leus NG, Zwinderman MR, Dekker FJ. Histone deacetylase 3 (HDAC 3) as emerging drug target in NF-kappaB-mediated inflammation. Curr Opin Chem Biol. 2016;33:160–8.
18. Schuliga M. NF-kappaB signaling in chronic inflammatory airway disease. Biomol Ther. 2015;5:1266–83.
19. Chi J, Seo GS, Cheon JH, Lee SH. Isoliquiritigenin inhibits TNF-α-induced release of high-mobility group box 1 through activation of HDAC in human intestinal epithelial HT-29 cells. Eur J Pharmacol. 2017;796:101–9.
20. Zou JY, Crews FT. Release of neuronal HMGB1 by ethanol through decreased HDAC activity activates brain neuroimmune signaling. PLoS One. 2014;9:e87915.
21. Lan K, Chao S, Wu H, Chiang C, Wang C, Liu S, Weng T. Salidroside ameliorates sepsis-induced acute lung injury and mortality via downregulating NF-κB and HMGB1 pathways through the upregulation of SIRT1. Sci Rep-Uk. 2017;7:12026.
22. Zhang X, Wu Q, Wu L, Ye Z, Jiang T, Li W, Zhuang Z, Zhou M, Zhang X, Hang C. Sirtuin 1 activation protects against early brain injury after experimental subarachnoid hemorrhage in rats. Cell Death and Disease. 2016;7:e2416.
23. Xie XQ, Zhang P, Tian B, Chen XQ. Downregulation of NAD-dependent deacetylase SIRT2 protects mouse brain against ischemic stroke. Mol Neurobiol. 2016;54:7251–61.
24. Wang T, Yang B, Ji R, Xu W, Mai K, Ai Q. Omega-3 polyunsaturated fatty acids alleviate hepatic steatosis-induced inflammation through Sirt1-mediated nuclear translocation of NF-kappaB p65 subunit in hepatocytes of large yellow croaker (Larmichthys crocea). Fish Shellfish Immunol. 2017;71:76–82.
25. Cai Y, Xu L, Xu H, Fan X. SIRT1 and neural cell fate determination. Mol Neurobiol. 2016;53:2815–25.
26. Godoy JA, Zolezzi JM, Braidy N, Inestrosa NC. Role of Sirt1 during the ageing process: relevance to protection of synapses in the brain. Mol Neurobiol. 2014;50:744–56.
27. Kim YM, Park EJ, Kim JH, Park SW, Kim HJ, Chang KC. Ethyl pyruvate inhibits the acetylation and release of HMGB1 via effects on SIRT1/STAT signaling in LPS-activated RAW264.7 cells and peritoneal macrophages. Int Immunopharmacol. 2016;41:98–105.
28. Serini S, Calviello G. Reduction of oxidative/Nitrosative stress in brain and its involvement in the neuroprotective effect of n-3 PUFA in Alzheimer's disease. Curr Alzheimer Res. 2016;13:123–34.
29. Wang B, Wu X, Guo M, Li M, Xu X, Jin X, Zhang X. Effects of ω-3 fatty acids on toll-like receptor 4 and nuclear factor-κB p56 in lungs of rats with severe acute pancreatitis. World J Gastroentero. 2016;22:9784–93.
30. Delattre AM, Carabelli B, Mori MA, Kempe PG, Rizzo DSL, Zanata SM, Machado RB, Suchecki D, Andrade DCB, Lima M, et al. Maternal omega-3 supplement improves dopaminergic system in pre- and postnatal inflammation-induced neurotoxicity in Parkinson's disease model. Mol Neurobiol. 2017;54:2090–106.
31. Chang CY, Kuan YH, Li JR, Chen WY, Ou YC, Pan HC, Liao SL, Raung SL, Chang CJ, Chen CJ. Docosahexaenoic acid reduces cellular inflammatory response following permanent focal cerebral ischemia in rats. J Nutr Biochem. 2013;24:2127–37.
32. Harvey LD, Yin Y, Attarwala IY, Begum G, Deng J, Yan HQ, Dixon CE, Sun D. Administration of DHA reduces endoplasmic reticulum stress-associated inflammation and alters microglial or macrophage activation in traumatic brain injury. Asn Neuro. 2015;7:1759091415618969.
33. Kurtys E, Eisel UL, Verkuyl JM, Broersen LM, Dierckx RA, de Vries EF. The combination of vitamins and omega-3 fatty acids has an enhanced anti-inflammatory effect on microglia. Neurochem Int. 2016;99:206–14.
34. Pu H, Guo Y, Zhang W, Huang L, Wang G, Liou AK, Zhang J, Zhang P, Leak RK, Wang Y, et al. Omega-3 polyunsaturated fatty acid supplementation improves neurologic recovery and attenuates white matter injury after experimental traumatic brain injury. J Cereb Blood Flow Metab. 2013;33:1474–84.
35. Yang X, Wu Q, Zhang L, Feng L. Inhibition of histone deacetylase 3 (HDAC3) mediates ischemic preconditioning and protects cortical neurons against ischemia in rats. Front Mol Neurosci. 2016;9:131.
36. Hopp S, Nolte MW, Stetter C, Kleinschnitz C, Sirén A, Albert-Weissenberger C. Alleviation of secondary brain injury, posttraumatic inflammation, and brain edema formation by inhibition of factor XIIa. J Neuroinflamm. 2017;14:39.
37. Parker TM, Nguyen AH, Rabang JR, Patil AA, Agrawal DK. The danger zone: systematic review of the role of HMGB1 danger signalling in traumatic brain injury. Brain Inj. 2017;31:2–8.
38. Ma Y, Nie H, Chen H, Li J, Hong Y, Wang B, Wang C, Zhang J, Cao W, Zhang M, et al. NAD(+)/NADH metabolism and NAD(+)-dependent enzymes in cell death and ischemic brain injury: current advances and therapeutic implications. Curr Med Chem. 2015;22:1239–47.

39. Logsdon AF, Lucke-Wold BP, Turner RC, Huber JD, Rosen CL, Simpkins JW. Role of microvascular disruption in brain damage from traumatic brain injury. Compr Physiol. 2015;5:1147–60.
40. Hamblin MR. Photobiomodulation for traumatic brain injury and stroke. J Neurosci Res. 2018;96:731–43.
41. Foglio E, Puddighinu G, Germani A, Russo MA, Limana F. HMGB1 inhibits apoptosis following MI and induces autophagy via mTORC1 inhibition. J Cell Physiol. 2017;232:1135–43.
42. Takizawa T, Shibata M, Kayama Y, Shimizu T, Toriumi H, Ebine T, Unekawa M, Koh A, Yoshimura A, Suzuki N. High-mobility group box 1 is an important mediator of microglial activation induced by cortical spreading depression. J Cereb Blood Flow Metab. 2017;37:890–901.
43. Polito F, Cicciu M, Aguennouz M, Cucinotta M, Cristani M, Lauritano F, Sindoni A, Gioffre-Florio M, Fama F. Prognostic value of HMGB1 and oxidative stress markers in multiple trauma patients: a single-centre prospective study. Int J Immunopath Ph. 2016;29:504–9.
44. Kang KA, Piao MJ, Ryu YS, Kang HK, Chang WY, Keum YS, Hyun JW. Interaction of DNA demethylase and histone methyltransferase upregulates Nrf2 in 5-fluorouracil-resistant colon cancer cells. Oncotarget. 2016;7:40594–620.
45. Bai Y, Du S, Li F, Huang F, Deng R, Zhou J, Chen D. Histone deacetylase-high mobility group box-1 pathway targeted by hypaconitine suppresses the apoptosis of endothelial cells. Exp Biol Med (Maywood). 2017;242:527–35.
46. Garmpis N, Damaskos C, Garmpi A, Dimitroulis D, Spartalis E, Margonis GA, Schizas D, Deskou I, Doula C, Magkouti E. Targeting histone deacetylases in malignant melanoma: a future therapeutic agent or just great expectations? Anticancer Res. 2017;37:5355–62.
47. Villalba JM, Alcain FJ. Sirtuin activators and inhibitors. Biofactors. 2012; 38:349–59.

3

Multivariate projection method to investigate inflammation associated with secondary insults and outcome after human traumatic brain injury

Anna Teresa Mazzeo[1], Claudia Filippini[2], Rosalba Rosato[3], Vito Fanelli[1], Barbara Assenzio[1], Ian Piper[4], Timothy Howells[5], Ilaria Mastromauro[1], Maurizio Berardino[6], Alessandro Ducati[7] and Luciana Mascia[8*]

Abstract

Background: Neuroinflammation has been proposed as a possible mechanism of brain damage after traumatic brain injury (TBI), but no consensus has been reached on the most relevant molecules. Furthermore, secondary insults occurring after TBI contribute to worsen neurological outcome in addition to the primary injury. We hypothesized that after TBI, a specific pattern of cytokines is related to secondary insults and outcome.

Methods: A prospective observational clinical study was performed. Secondary insults by computerized multimodality monitoring system and systemic value of different cytokines were collected and analysed in the first week after intensive care unit admission. Neurological outcome was assessed at 6 months (GOSe). Multivariate projection technique was applied to analyse major sources of variation and collinearity within the cytokines dataset without a priori selecting potential relevant molecules.

Results: Twenty-nine severe traumatic brain injury patients undergoing intracranial pressure monitoring were studied. In this pilot study, we demonstrated that after TBI, patients who suffered of prolonged and severe secondary brain damage are characterised by a specific pattern of cytokines. Patients evolving to brain death exhibited higher levels of inflammatory mediators compared to both patients with favorable and unfavorable neurological outcome at 6 months. Raised ICP and low cerebral perfusion pressure occurred in 21 % of good monitoring time. Furthermore, the principal components selected by multivariate projection technique were powerful predictors of neurological outcome.

Conclusions: The multivariate projection method represents a valuable methodology to study neuroinflammation pattern occurring after secondary brain damage in severe TBI patients, overcoming multiple putative interactions between mediators and avoiding any subjective selection of relevant molecules.

Keywords: Traumatic brain injury, Intracranial hypertension, Secondary insults, Neuroinflammation, Cytokines, Principal component analysis

* Correspondence: luciana.mascia@uniroma1.it
[8]Dipartimento di Scienze e Biotecnologie Medico Chirurgiche, Sapienza University of Rome, Rome, Italy
Full list of author information is available at the end of the article

Background

Neuroinflammation is recognized as a key feature occurring after traumatic brain injury (TBI), and both localized and systemic inflammatory reactions have been proposed as potential mechanisms of damage or as putative beneficial responses to injury, depending on timing and severity [1–7]. Several cytokines, chemokines, and cell adhesion molecules have been identified in blood, cerebrospinal fluid (CSF), or brain microdialysate of patients with TBI with a highly variable profile in terms of peak and duration [5, 7–10].

After TBI, the injured brain is vulnerable to secondary damage which may be exacerbated by damaging events known as secondary insults contributing to worsen neurological outcome [11–15]. These harmful complications, occurring both in the prehospital phase and after intensive care unit (ICU) admission, include hypotension, hypoxia, high intracranial pressure, and nosocomial infection whose occurrence can be determined only if rigorously pursued after TBI [15–19]. The use of a minute by minute recording of physiological variables with a computerised multimodality monitoring system [18] can be applied to investigate basic mechanisms underlying secondary brain damage. These complications are indicative of secondary central nervous system (CNS) injury eventually occurring as a result of prolonged inflammation. Although several studies [1, 2, 4, 5, 7, 9, 20–23] have investigated the role of some given cytokines in the pathophysiology of TBI, there is no consensus on those who may serve as biomarkers of brain injury. Previous studies separately evaluated the relationship between selected cytokines and intracranial hypertension [22], hypoxemia [24], or the prognostic value of these mediators [25]. Among the main limitations of these studies on neuroinflammation, there are the multiple putative interactions between mediators which may vary together after TBI, and the limit of "a priori" selection of the potential relevant molecules [5, 8, 10]. Multivariate regression techniques are indeed limited to comparison of multivariate data in a large number of patients to prevent overfitting.

Multivariate projection methods, such as principal component analysis (PCA), and partial least squares (PLS), are data reduction techniques that allow the major sources of variation in a multi-dimensional dataset to be analysed avoiding the "a priori" selection of the potential relevant variables in a relatively small number of observations. PCA has been first proposed by Helmy et al. [9] in TBI patients to explore the pattern of production, time profile, and differing patterns of response of cytokines in brain and peripheral blood and then by Kumar et al. [5], who studied the prognostic value of a combination of CSF inflammatory molecules taking into account the variability across patients.

In the present study, we hypothesised that in patients with TBI, a specific pattern of cytokines and chemokines is related to secondary insults and may identify patients who die early because of brain herniation. To address the issue of mediators covariance we applied the multivariate projection techniques, including PCA and PLS analyses.

Methods

Patient population

The Institutional Review Board (Comitato Etico Interaziendale AOU Citta' della Salute e della Scienza di Torino, Italy) approved the study protocol. At enrollment, patients were unconscious and unable to give consent, therefore the family was informed of the study, and consent was delayed until the patient was able to provide valid informed consent. Written permission for using collected data was then obtained from the patient or from the family (in case of death or if the patient remained incompetent to give consent). All patients with severe TBI consecutively admitted to the NeuroICU at the Azienda Ospedaliera Universitaria Citta' della Salute e delle Scienza di Torino were prospectively recruited over a period of 3 years, according to the following inclusion criteria: age older than 18 years, severe head injury (Glasgow Coma Score (GCS) < 9) at ICU admission, placement of intracranial pressure (ICP) monitoring, and admission within 24 h after injury. Exclusion criteria were: both pupils fixed and dilated, history of immunosuppression, pregnancy, and lack of consent.

Clinical management

All the patients were sedated, intubated, mechanically ventilated, and managed according to the Brain Trauma Foundation Guidelines [26]. The GCS at the time of admission was recorded, and the Injury Severity Score (ISS) was used for the assessment of multiple injuries. Apache II score (Acute Physiology And Chronic Health Evaluation) was used for a quantification of the severity of illness and Marshall scale was used to classify head CT scan on admission. As part of the clinical management mean arterial pressure (MAP), intracranial pressure (ICP), cerebral perfusion pressure (CPP), oxygen saturation measured by pulse oximetry (SpO_2), and temperature were continuously recorded.

Multimodality monitoring system for secondary insults detection

A computerized multimodality monitoring system was used for the collection of physiological parameters. A bedside laptop computer with specialized software displayed and saved one value per minute for each monitored physiological parameter. For the purpose of the study, data monitoring was started at the time of ICP placement and collected until ICP monitoring was discontinued for clinical reasons. Data were collected as part of a European network for collection and analysis of higher resolution data after TBI, the Brain Monitoring with Information Technology (BrainIT group) [27]. The Odin browser software was used for data analysis. Thresholds for secondary insults were derived from EUSIG [13]. The secondary insults analysed were raised ICP, low CPP, hypotension, hypoxia and pyrexia. Secondary insult thresholds, for grades 1, 2, and 3 were, respectively: ICP $\geq$ 20, $\geq$ 30, $\geq$ 40 mmHg for raised ICP insult; CPP $\leq$ 60, $\leq$50, $\leq$40 mmHg for low CPP insult; MAP $\leq$ 70, $\leq$ 55, $\leq$ 40 mmHg for hypotension insult; SaO2 $\leq$ 90, $\leq$85, $\leq$ 80 % for hypoxia insult; Temperature $\geq$ 38, $\geq$39, $\geq$ 40 °C for pyrexia insult. Each derangement had to be sustained for at least 5 min to be deemed a secondary insult, for 60 min in the case of pyrexia. The amount of secondary insult was calculated as the time spent within the insult threshold level divided by the good monitoring time (GMT) for that patient and presented as proportion of GMT [13, 18, 28, 29]. GMT is described as total monitoring time minus invalid monitoring or gaps in data collection for procedures, computerized tomography (CT) scan or system failures. All monitoring data were screened manually to disclose artifacts.

Neurological outcome

For evaluation of neurological outcome at 6 months the Glasgow Outcome Scale-extended (GOSe) was used, with a score ranging from 1 (death) to 8 (upper good recovery) [30, 31]. Dichotomization of outcome in favorable (GOSe 5–8) and unfavorable (GOSe1-4) was used; patients evolving to brain death in the early phase of ICU stay were identified as a separate group.

Inflammatory mediators analysis

Blood samples for cytokine analysis were collected at the time of ICP placement (T0), 24 (T1), 48 (T2), and 72 h (T3) later. Samples were centrifuged for 10 min at 3000 RPM at 4 °C and plasma was then frozen at −80 ° C until analysed. The cytokine analysis was performed with the Bioplex technology (BioRad Laboratories), which combines the principle of a sandwich immunoassay with fluorescent bead-based technology [32]. The Bioplex assay analyses 27 cytokines: Interleukin-1 beta (IL-1β), IL-1 receptor antagonist (IL-1ra), IL-2, IL-4, IL-5, IL-6, IL-7, IL-8, IL-9, IL-10, IL-12 subunit p70 (IL-12p70), IL-13, IL-15, IL-17, basic Fibroblast growth factor (basic FGF), eotaxin, granulocyte colony-stimulating factor (G-CSF), granulocyte-macrophage colony-stimulating factor (GM-CSF), interferon gamma (IFN-γ), interferon gamma-induced protein 10 (IP-10), monocyte chemoattractant protein 1 (MCP-1), macrophage inflammatory protein 1 alpha (MIP-1α), MIP-1β, Platelet-derived growth factor BB (PDGF-BB), Regulated upon Activation Normal T-cell Expressed (RANTES), Tumor necrosis factor alpha (TNF-α), Vascular endothelial growth factor (VEGF) and was carried out in 96-well microplates using the Bio-Plex Pro Human Cytokine 27-plex Assay kit following manufacture instruction (Code M50-0KCAF0Y, Bio-Rad Laboratories) at the Bioclarma-Research and Molecular Diagnostics, Torino, Italy. The intra-plate % coefficient of variance (CV) ranged from 1.11 to 9.96 %, while the inter-plate % CV ranged from 3 to 11 % for these assays.

All cytokine determinations on plasma samples were carried out in duplicate using Bio-Plex Manager software (vers 6.1). Soluble TNF-α receptors (TNF-RI and TNF-RII) was carried out using a solid-phase enzyme-linked immunosorbent assay method (ELISA) based on the quantitative immunometric sandwich enzyme immunoassay technique following the manifacture instruction (R&D Systems, Abingdon, UK). The intra-plate CV% was less than 4.8, while the inter-plate CV% was less than 5.1 for these assays. Plasma samples from 10 healthy volunteers were used as controls.

Statistical analysis

In view of the inherent variation in absolute cytokine concentrations between patients, the median value for each cytokine was chosen for univariate analyses. Continuous data are presented as mean and standard deviation (SD) or median and interquartile range (IQR) depending on data distribution, while categorical data are presented as rate and proportion. Correlation between each cytokine and different secondary insults expressed as proportion of GMT was performed by linear regression analysis; differences among demographic data and cytokines level in the three outcome categories were tested using analysis of variance (ANOVA) or chi-squared test as appropriate and considered significant for $p < 0.05$. If ANOVA was significant, post-hoc analysis by Bonferroni was applied.

Multivariate projection is a data reduction technique that allows the major sources of variation in a multi-dimensional dataset to be analysed without introducing inherent bias. Principal component analysis (PCA) is used to identify principal components which account for the majority of the variation within the dataset. Number of principal components have been identified using Kaiser criteria (Eigenvalue >1).

Partial least squares (PLS) is a linear predictive model to maximize both the variation within the dataset and to the response variable. For multivariate projection techniques all cytokines values (T0, T1, T2 and T3) have been used after log-tranformation. The most significant cytokines in the PLS model were identified by the Variable Importance Projection (VIP). VIP is a measure of a variable's importance in modeling both variation of cytokines, explained by each partial least squares factor, and variation of raised ICP insult. If a variable has a small coefficient and a small

VIP (<0.8 -Wold's criterion), then it is a candidate for deletion from the model.

In our study, PCA was applied to explore any intrinsic variation in the cytokine dataset while PLS was used to test the correlation between raised ICP (response variable) and cytokines. Finally, a multinomial generalized equation estimated (GEE) logistic regression model was applied to verify the predictive value of the principal components adjusted for clinical variables on neurological outcome. In order to correct for repeated measurements a robust sandwich standard error estimate was used. (SAS vers 9.3).

Results

Clinical data and occurrence of secondary insults

Twenty nine adult severe TBI patients (25 males and 4 females) were enrolled in the study. Demographic data of patients classified according to neurological outcome are presented in Table 1. Three patients presenting at admission with a GCS > 8 where included in the study as they suddenly deteriorated and met inclusion criteria. Difference in admission characteristics among favorable, unfavorable outcome at 6 months and brain-dead patients were not significant. Seventeen of the 29 enrolled patients suffered a polytrauma. The severity of trauma, assessed by ISS revealed a serious injury (ISS 9–15) in thre patients, a severe injury (ISS 16–24) in four patients, and a critical injury (ISS 25–75) in 22 patients. Five patients evolved to brain death within the first 3 days. GOSe at 6 months revealed: seven deaths including brain death (24 %), one persistent vegetative state (3 %), six upper or lower severe disability (21 %), eigth upper or lower moderate disability (28 %), seven lower or upper good recovery (24 %).

Median duration of GMT in the studied population was 7350 min (range 1191–13040). Occurrence of secondary insults during early phase of ICU stay, expressed as proportion of GMT for each grade, in each insult category is presented in Fig. 1. Raised ICP insult occurred in 21.9 % of GMT (CI 10.96; 32.75), low CPP insult in

Table 1 Demographic data of the patient population in the three outcome groups ($n = 29$ Patients)

Variables	Favorable outcome 6M[a]	Unfavorable outcome 6M[a]	Brain death
	$n = 15$	$n = 9$	$n = 5$
Age (years), mean (SD)	35.9 (16.6)	40.8 (23.3)	42.2 (19.8)
Apache II, mean (SD)	14.1 (3.6)	15.6 (2.6)	16.6 (2.3)
GCS, median (IQR)	6 (3; 8)	4 (3; 5)	3 (3; 4)
GCSm, median (IQR)	4 (1; 4)	2 (1; 3)	1 (1; 1)
Marshall, median (IQR)	3 (2; 5)	3 (3; 5)	5 (4; 5)
Isolated TBI, *n* (%)	6 (40)	3 (33)	3 (60)
TBI in politrauma, *n* (%)	9 (60)	6 (67)	2 (40)
ISS, mean (SD)	27.5 (12.3)	28.3 (10.6)	26.2 (1.8)
AIS head, median (IQR)	4 (3; 4)	4 (3; 5)	5 (4; 5)
Focal injury, *n* (%)	4 (27)	3 (33)	3 (60)
Diffuse injury, *n* (%)	11 (73)	6 (67)	2 (40)
Main intracranial lesion, *n* (%)			
Epidural hematoma	2 (13)	0 (0)	1 (20)
Subdural hematoma	1 (7)	2 (22)	3 (60)
Traumatic subarachnoid hemorrhage	3 (20)	1 (11)	0 (0)
Contusions	7 (47)	2 (22)	1 (20)
Intracerebral mass lesion	1 (7)	2 (22)	0 (0)
Brain swelling	1 (7)	1 (11)	0 (0)
Diffuse axonal injury	0 (0)	1 (11)	0 (0)
Mechanism of injury, *n* (%)			
Fall	7 (47)	3 (33)	4 (80)
Motor vehicle collision	3 (20)	2 (22)	0 (0)
Motorcycle	1 (7)	3 (33)	1 (20)
Bicycle crash	2 (13)	0 (0)	0 (0)
Pedestrian	2 (13)	1 (11)	0 (0)

[a]At 6 months. *GCS* Glasgow coma scale, *GCSm* Glasgow coma scale, motor score, *TBI* traumatic brain injury, *ISS* injury severity score, *AIS* abbreviated injury scale

21.1 % (CI 11.69; 30.59), pyrexia insult in 14.2 % (CI 9.23; 19.19), hypotension insult in 9.5 % (CI 4.61; 14.41) and hypoxia insult in 1.5 % (CI 0; 3.61). The majority of insults were of grade 1 and occurred in 11.9, 11.1, 13.8, and 7.9 % of GMT for raised ICP, low CPP, pyrexia and hypotension insult, respectively. Hypoxia insult in the early phase of ICU was rare but severe (grade 3). Median and range of secondary insults duration in the studied population were: raised ICP insult equal to 833 min (range 0–3513), low CPP insult equal to 904 (0–4095), pyrexia insult equal to 660 (0–3329), hypotension insult equal to 258 (0–2242), hypoxia insult equal to 0 (0–1637).

Relationship between plasma cytokines level and secondary insults

A several-fold variation in the cytokine concentrations recovered was observed among patients. All cytokines were detectable in the analysed samples and increased from control levels while IL-2, MIP1α, IL-15, IL-17, and basic FGF were under detection limit in several patients. To deal with the repeated measures obtained from T0 to T3, we presented cytokines as median values over time. One patient died at T1 and had only two determinations.

Il-6, IL-2, Il-10, IL-12, IL-15, VEGF, and MIP1β were the cytokines with the strongest correlation with secondary insults ($R^2 > 0.5$ and $p < 0.01$). IL-6, IL-15 and VEGF were associated with ICP and low CPP insult, MIP1β with CPP insult, and IL-2, IL-10, and IL-12 with hypoxia insult (Fig. 2). IL-6 was the most important cytokine associated with raised ICP ($R^2 = 0.574$, $p < 0.0001$) and low CPP insult ($R^2 = 0.587$, $p = 0.0001$) (Fig. 3). All the correlations were confirmed when absolute numbers of minutes of insults were considered for analysis.

Correlations were found between plasma cytokine levels and demographic or severity scores at admission: age correlated with TNF-RI ($R^2 = 0.224$, $p = 0.009$), TNF-RII ($R^2 = 0.270$, $p = 0.004$) and VEGF ($R^2 = 0.129$, $p = 0.05$); GCS motor score (GCSm) correlated with basicFGF ($R^2 = 0.146$, $p = 0.041$), GCSF ($R^2 = 0.132$, $p = 0.05$) and IP-10 ($R^2 = 0.167$, $p = 0.028$); APACHE II score correlated with IP-10 ($R^2 = 0.154$, $p = 0.035$), MIP1β ($R^2 = 0.134$, $p = 0.05$), TNF-RII ($R^2 = 0.257$, $p = 0.005$), and VEGF ($R^2 = 0.161$, $p = 0.031$); Marshall scale correlated with IL-7 ($R^2 = 0.131$, $p = 0.05$), IL-13 ($R^2 = 0.130$, $p = 0.05$), IP-10 ($R^2 = 0.157$, $p = 0.033$), and VEGF ($R^2 = 0.153$, $p = 0.036$).

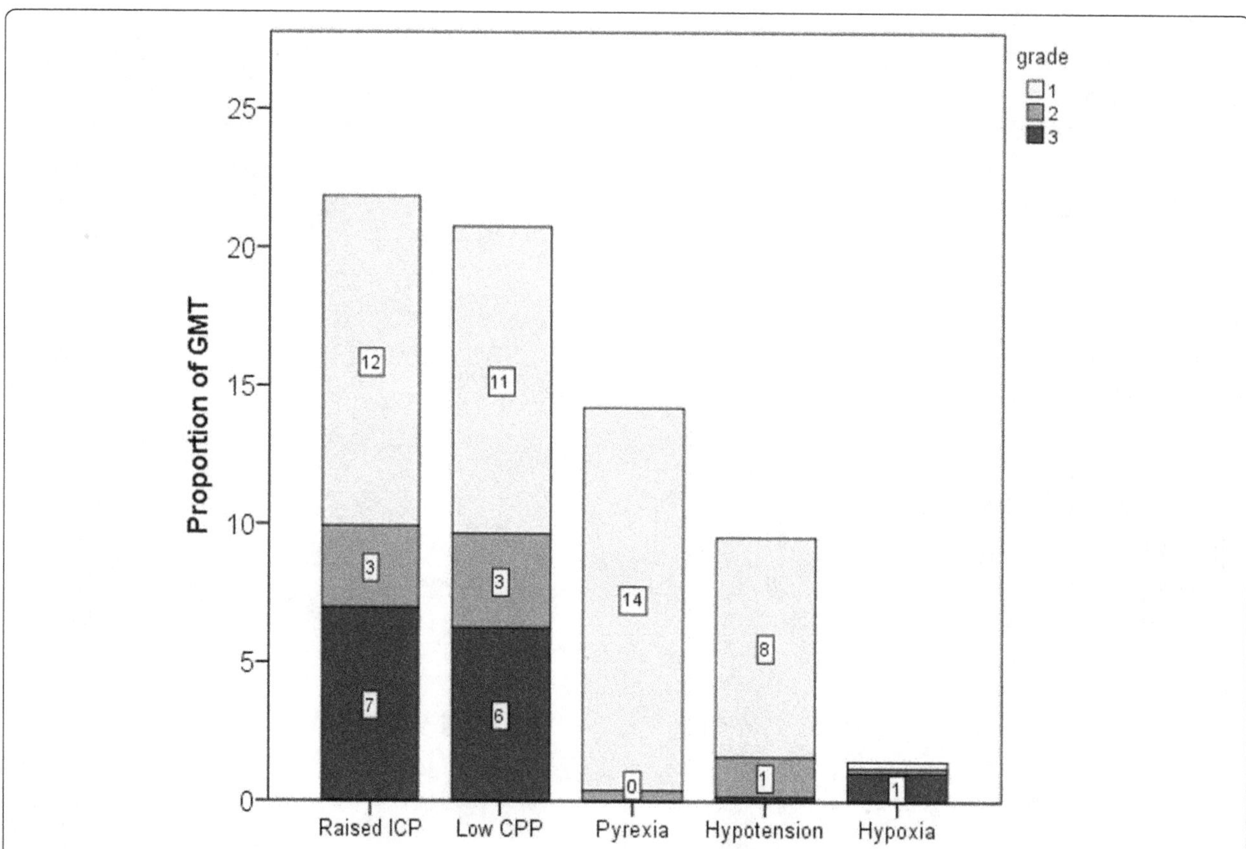

Fig. 1 Occurrence of secondary insults, expressed as proportion of good monitoring time (GMT), for each insult category and each grade of severity. *ICP* intracranial pressure, *CPP* cerebral perfusion pressure. *Tags* inside *bars* indicate proportion of GMT for each insult grade

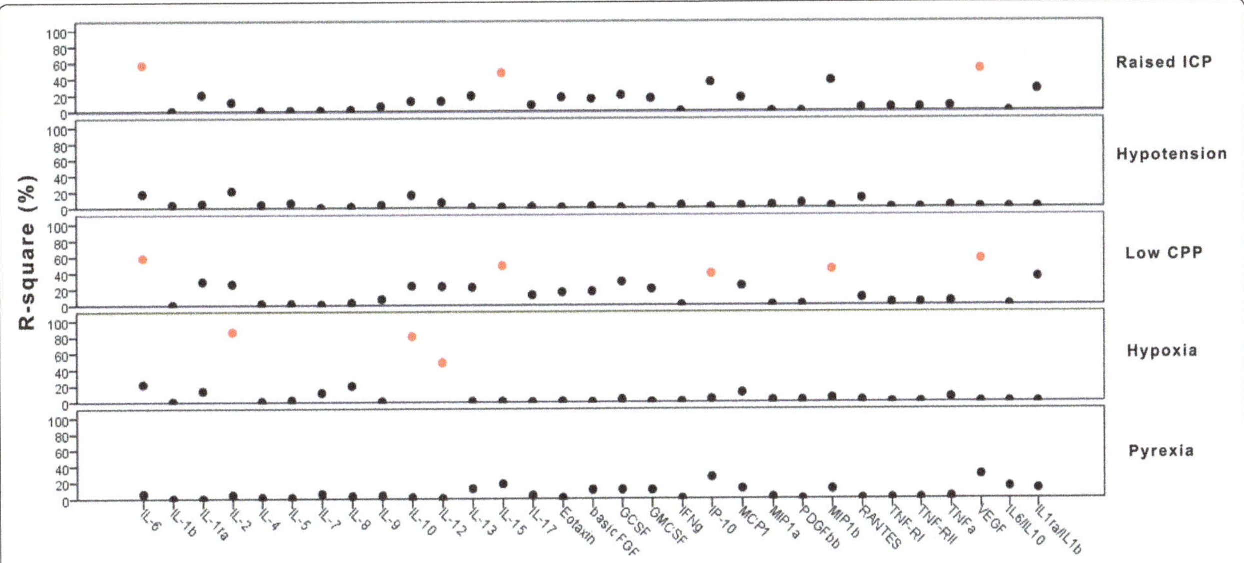

Fig. 2 Linear regression analysis between median plasma levels of cytokines and secondary insults. The results are presented as percentage of R square between cytokines and secondary insults. $R^2 > 0.5$ and $p < 0.01$ are red colored. *ICP* intracranial pressure, *CPP* cerebral perfusion pressure

Relationship between plasma cytokine levels and neurological outcome

Median plasma cytokine levels were significantly higher in patients evolving to brain death when compared to the other two groups (Table 2). Raised ICP, hypotension, low CPP, hypoxia insults (Fig. 4a) and IL-6 level (Fig. 4b) were significantly ($p < 0.05$) higher in patients early evolving to brain death compared to both patients with unfavorable and favorable outcome at 6 months.

Multivariate projection method

PCA was performed to examine the presence of covariance in the cytokine dataset. According to Kaiser criteria, the first five PCs generated by the model explained 72 % of the cumulative variation within the dataset. Figure 5a shows the scores plot for each observation of PC1 and PC2 which explained 53 % of the cumulative variation within data set. The ellipse on the plot (Hotelling ellipse) represents the 95 % CI for the model and no outlier was detected. The loading plot (Fig. 5b) illustrates the relative contribution of each cytokine to the two PCs. The first component was strongly correlated with the following cytokines: GCSF, IL-4, IL-12, IL-10, basic FGF, IL-17, IFNγ, IL-8, MIP1α, VEGF, IL-1ra, IL-9, IL-7, PDGFbb, IP10, RANTES, IL-13, and IL-5. The second component was strongly correlated with IL-6, MIP1β, TNF-RII, Eotaxin, TNF-RI, MCP1, and IL-15. IL1β and TNFα were the cytokines which showed the highest coefficient of correlation within the third principal component; that explained the 8 % of variation within the dataset.

Overall PLS analysis including the first five factors explained 63 % of cytokines variation and 53 % of raised ICP. According to the Wold's criterion, in the PLS analysis IL-6, basic FGF, MIP1α, RANTES, IP10, MIP1β, explained most of the variation in the dataset and were the most powerful predictors for raised ICP (Fig. 6a and b).

To verify the predictive power of cytokine data on neurological outcome, the first two PCs, which explained most of the variability in the dataset, were entered in the multinomial logistic regression model together with demographic clinical variables (age, GCSm and Marshall score). GCSm was a powerful predictor discriminating patients with favorable outcome versus those who early died because of brain death. The first two PCs were significant predictors discriminating patients with favorable outcome versus both brain dead (OR = 1.91 [1.24; 2.94] and 4.64 [1.79; 12.05]) and unfavorable outcome (OR = 1.80 [1.34; 2.42] and 1.62 [1.02; 2.59], for PC1 and PC2 respectively, Table 3). The odds to evolve in brain death rather than favorable outcome increased 91 % for each unit increase in PC1.

Discussion

In this pilot study, we used a multivariate projection technique to identify distinct pattern of inflammatory response in TBI patients suffering of secondary insults. With this methodology, we demonstrated that patients who suffered from prolonged and severe secondary brain damage were characterized by a specific pattern of cytokines. Interestingly, in patients early evolving to brain death higher levels of inflammatory mediators were detected compared to both patients with long term favorable and unfavorable outcome. Keeping in mind the relatively small number of patients, the large number of cytokines and their putative statistical interactions, we applied the PCA to objectively identify the most relevant

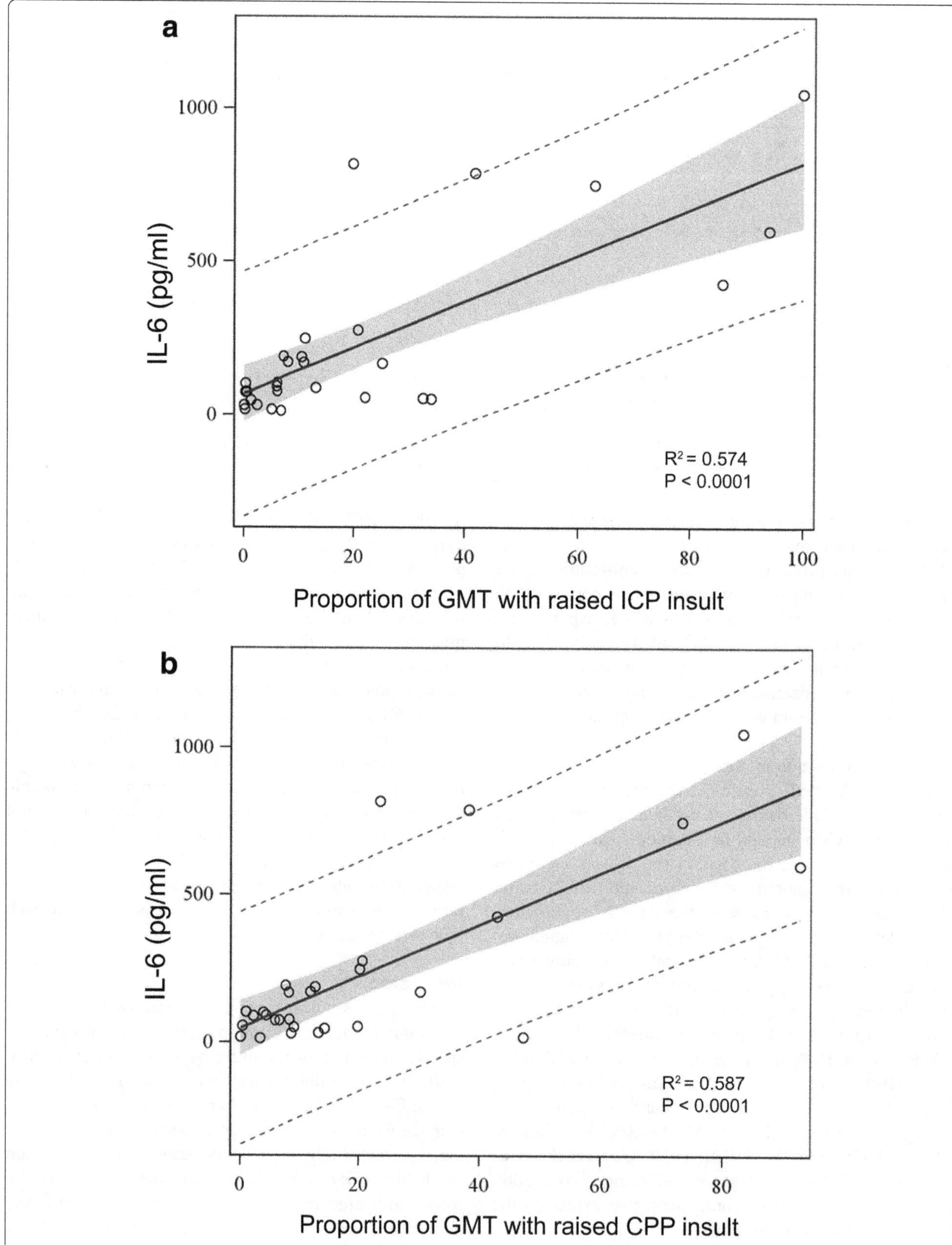

Fig. 3 Linear regression analysis between median plasma levels of IL-6 and proportion of raised ICP **a** and low CPP **b** insults. Insults are expressed as proportion of good monitoring time (GMT). *Grey shadow* represents 95 % confidence limits. *Dotted lines* represent 95 % prediction limits. *ICP* intracranial pressure, *CPP* cerebral perfusion pressure

Table 2 Median plasma level of inflammatory mediators in the 3 outcome groups

	Favorable outcome 6M[a]	Unfavorable outcome 6M[a]	Brain death	*p* value
IL-6	75.08 (31.81; 104.76)	169.95 (79.17; 188.3)	750 (602; 817)	*<0.0001*
IL-1β	0.66 (0.1; 1.05)	1.04 (0.6; 5.78)	1.32 (1.1; 1.97)	0.179
IL-1ra	66.92 (34.68; 226.97)	82.02 (70; 384.13)	532.66 (399; 2078.5)	0.078
IL-2	0.8 (0.8; 0.8)	0.8 (0.8; 0.8)	0.8 (0.8; 29.5)	*0.041*
IL-4	0.21 (0.01; 1.32)	0.6 (0.42; 5.31)	0.93 (0.8; 1.34)	0.304
IL-5	0.85 (0.13; 5.24)	1.14 (0.28; 15.36)	0.5 (0.29; 0.62)	0.415
IL-7	9.27 (1.38; 31.41)	45.4 (7.23; 141.17)	58.98 (16.25; 92.5)	0.215
IL-8	19.39 (3.99; 39.64)	60.29 (39; 104.58)	125.55 (37.02; 129)	*0.013*
IL-9	12.13 (2.35; 20.13)	32.91 (28; 46.86)	23.68 (20.5; 48.26)	*0.022*
IL-10	11.52 (1.57; 20.14)	20 (7.83; 57.02)	39.47 (12.37; 108.5)	*0.029*
IL-12	5.64 (0.81; 22.2)	11.82 (5.33; 42.48)	20.15 (17; 109.5)	*0.043*
IL-13	2.97 (0.62; 5.27)	7.4 (1.92; 11.27)	12.06 (5.78; 30)	*0.047*
IL-15	1.05 (0.06; 4.6)	0.06 (0.06; 6.16)	22.75 (3.7; 44.9)	*0.001*
IL-17	0.9 (0.9; 9.58)	49.06 (0.9; 75.33)	67.84 (28; 77.42)	0.162
Eotaxin	0.35 (0.35; 18.45)	19 (0.35; 29.31)	24.49 (10.5; 34.42)	0.094
basic FGF	3 (3; 24.45)	48.73 (3; 66.79)	49.61 (49.49; 131)	*0.053*
GCSF	50.95 (8.99; 138.65)	156.61 (107.5; 368.77)	483.17 (165; 491.86)	0.012
GMCSF	48 (2.29; 78.14)	39.18 (0.21; 91.61)	99.55 (83.84; 113)	0.084
IFNγ	4.15 (1.08; 25.73)	14.97 (11.99; 110.33)	25 (24.74; 29.08)	0.230
IP-10	111.06 (29; 256.19)	248.22 (215.09; 459.34)	2081.5 (528.43; 2232.08)	*<0.0001*
MCP1	162.16 (44.12; 307.83)	196.04 (77.78; 657.25)	690.82 (600; 2210)	*0.001*
MIP1α	1.5 (0.05; 2.33)	3.07 (1.2; 6.49)	3.71 (0.05; 11)	0.209
PDGFbb	141.57 (58.58; 229.67)	271.36 (195.11; 372.25)	104.64 (93.1; 210.46)	0.324
MIP1β	87.27 (55.98; 134.88)	123.05 (98; 133.01)	416 (275.42; 594)	*0.001*
RANTES	5193.61 (1952.35; 8553.06)	8903.57 (4098.28; 11442.69)	3570.05 (2309.71; 3831.31)	0.564
TNF-RI	1252.27 (522.38; 1568.18)	1320.45 (970.33; 1513.64)	1957 (1543.13; 2679)	0.394
TNF-RII	2190 (730; 4723.08)	4161.9 (3707.69; 5368.54)	5678 (4919; 6564.78)	*0.021*
TNFα	8 (5.58; 50.59)	5.5 (3.9; 93.05)	9.78 (8.12; 18.45)	0.262
VEGF	6.04 (0.08; 27.12)	29.79 (8.12; 42.22)	60.22 (34.28; 322)	*0.002*
IL6/IL10	57 (30.39; 324.61)	59.24 (39.89; 104.28)	277.07 (126.7; 1598.89)	0.765
IL1ra/IL1β	7.92 (3.66; 19.53)	8.9 (3.77; 22.4)	27.11 (5; 32.29)	0.064

[a]At 6 months. Values are median (IQR). *IQR* interquartile range. Significant correlations are reported in italics

molecules in the early phase after TBI. The first 2 principal components explained 72 % of the variation within the dataset and were independently associated with poor neurological outcome. In the two components, the most relevant proinflammatory cytokines (GCSF, IL-6, IL-15), anti-inflammatory cytokines (IL-10, IL-1ra), chemokines, and growth factors (basicFGF, MIP1α, MIP1β, VEGF) were recognised by high coefficients. The PLS analysis identified IL-6, basic FGF, MIP1α, MIP1β, RANTES and IP10, as the main cytokines able to explain most of the variation in the dataset and to predict raised ICP.

Detrimental effects of secondary insults on TBI prognosis has been extensively investigated, but the exact mechanism leading to the exacerbation of brain damage remains unclear. Post-traumatic neuroinflammation, proposed as a potential mechanism of damage and repair, is characterised by glial activation, leukocyte recruitment and upregulation and secretion of mediators such as cytokines and chemotactic cytokines (chemokines) [3, 21, 22, 33, 34]. Inflammatory mediators have been measured in plasma, CSF and in brain microdialysate, suggesting a cerebral production of pro and anti-inflammatory cytokines [9]. In cases of brain injury complicated by multiple traumas, plasmatic levels of inflammatory mediators may reflect the effect of peripheral immune response [7]. Indeed recently Santarsieri et al. [6], demonstrated an association between CSF levels of inflammatory mediators in the first 6 days after injury and outcome modulated by

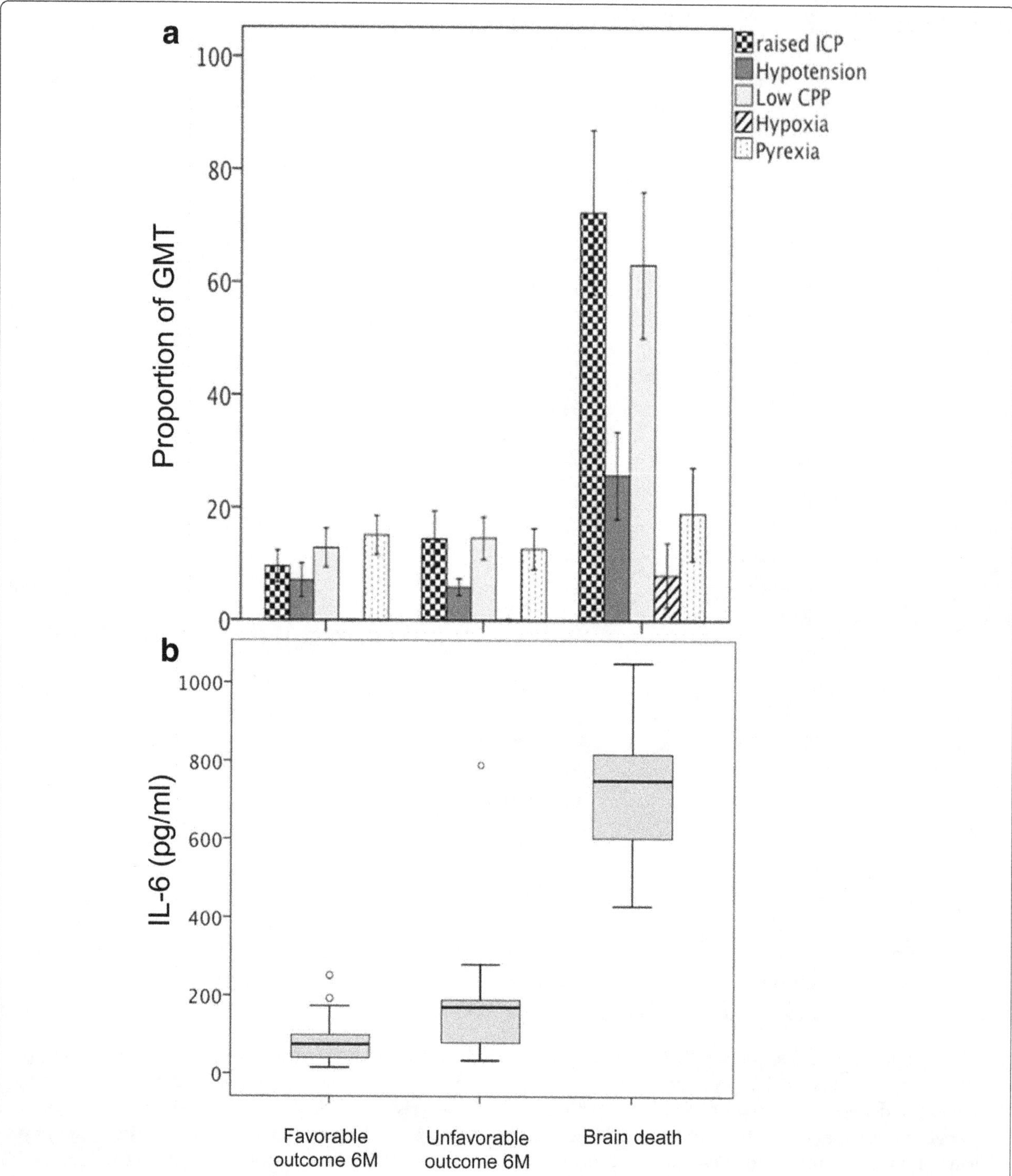

Fig. 4 The incidence of secondary insults, expressed as proportion of good monitoring time (GMT) is described in each outcome group (**a**). Difference among groups was significant for raised ICP, hypotension, low CPP, and hypoxia insults (ANOVA, $p < 0.01$). Post-hoc analysis revealed that differences were significant between brain death and both favorable and unfavorable outcome (*$p < 0.05$). Data are expressed as mean and standard error. *ICP* intracranial pressure, *CPP* cerebral perfusion pressure. **b** Boxplots of IL-6 level in each outcome group. Difference among groups was significant (ANOVA, $p < 0.001$). Post-hoc analysis revealed that differences were significant between brain death and both favorable and unfavorable outcome (*$p < 0.05$). *Circles* represent outliers

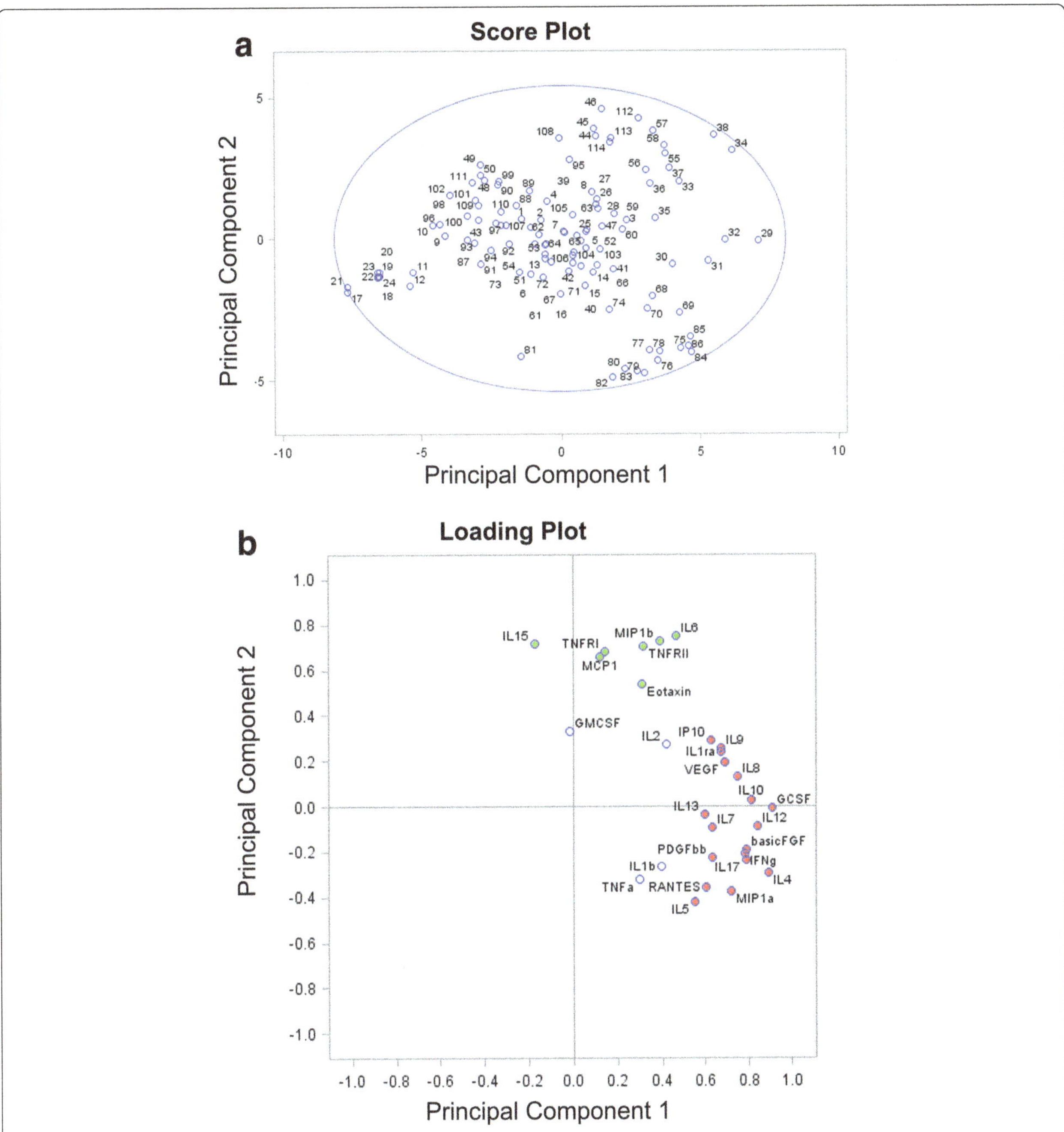

Fig. 5 Panel **a**: Scores plot shows the scores on each principal component for each observation. The ellipse on the plot (Hotelling ellipse) is the 95 % CI for the model. **b** Loading plot shows the cytokines which load on the respective principal components. Cytokines which better explain Principal Components 1 and 2 are marked in *red* and *green*, respectively

cortisol levels. Recent experimental and clinical investigations data have also documented the role of microglia as source and target of inflammatory response [10, 35].

Cytokines produced by different CNS cells may have both beneficial and detrimental roles. Clear benefit can be achieved if the inflammation is controlled in a regulated manner and for a defined period of time; when sustained or excessive, however, inflammation is detrimental [36]. Unfortunately conflicting results have been reported on the role of different cytokines as repair mechanisms or exacerbation of the pathophysiology of brain trauma.

IL-6 is a multifunctional factor widely investigated in both experimental and clinical studies. Hergenroeder et al. [21] found that serum IL-6 levels within the first 24 h were significantly higher in patients who developed high ICP compared with patients with normal ICP. Minambres et al. [25] demonstrated that transcranial IL-6 gradient at admission correlated with poor prognosis at 6 months,

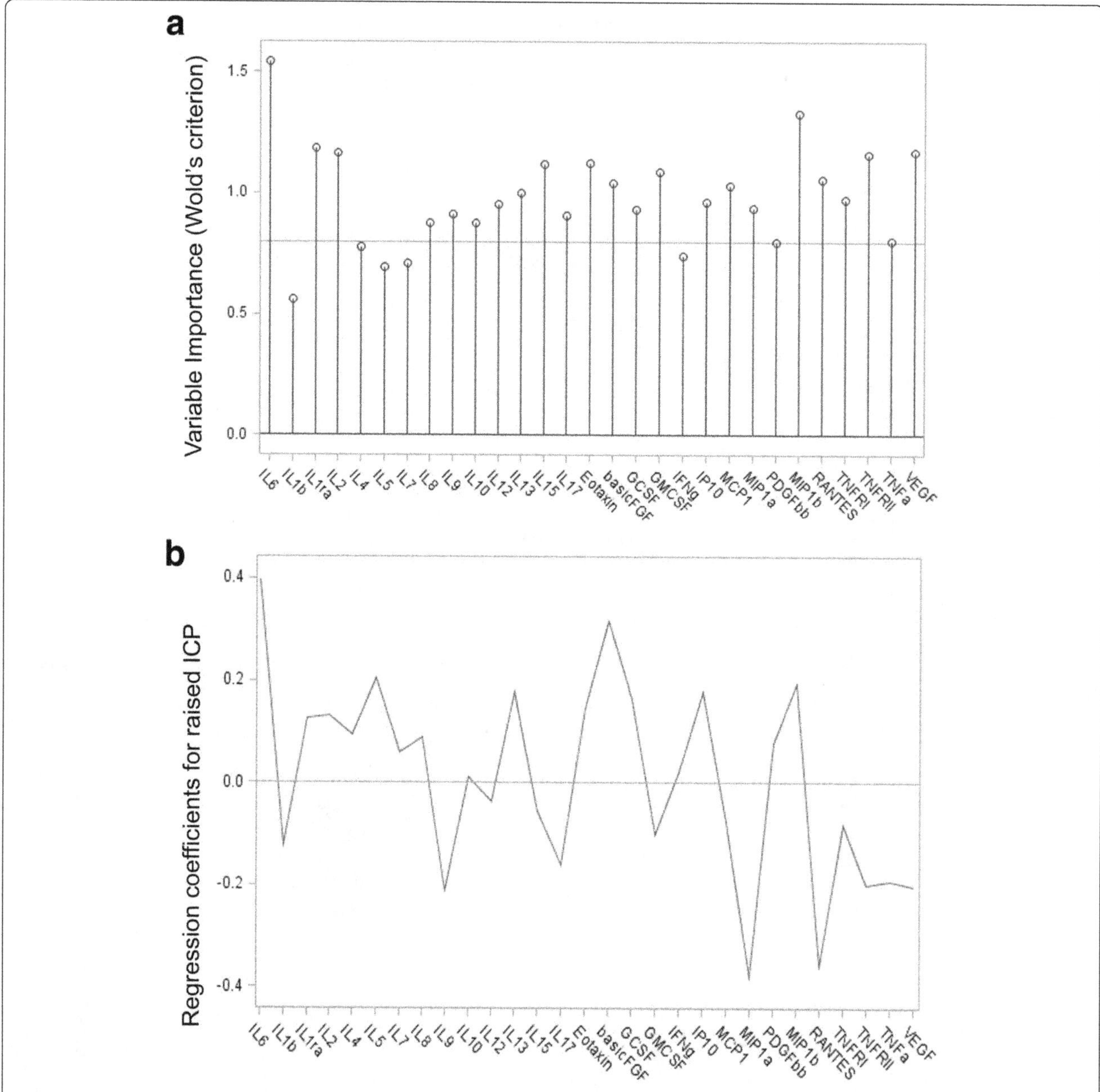

Fig. 6 Panel **a** shows the variable importance projection (VIP) scores. A VIP score is a measure of a variable's importance in modeling both variation of cytokines and variation of raised ICP insult. A value of 0.8 is generally considered to be a small VIP and a line is drawn on the plot at 0.8. Panel **b** is a regression coefficient profile indicating which cytokines better predict raised ICP insult. The regression coefficients represents the importance that each cytokine has in the prediction of raised ICP insult

and was significantly higher in patients evolving to brain death. Conversely Perez-Barcena et al. [37] did not identify a clear relationship between the temporal profile of IL-6 and ICP elevation, brain tissue oxygenation and the presence of brain swelling on CT scan. More recently, Kumar et al. using the group-based trajectory analysis demonstrated that patients with a high CSF IL-6 trajectory profile had worst outcome [5].

IL-1 cytokine family has been described as an important determinant of inflammation: IL-1α and IL-1β appear pro-inflammatory, while the endogenous IL-1ra appears anti-inflammatory. Thus elevation of IL-1ra/IL-1β ratio is seen as an anti-inflammatory indicator and in an elegant microdialysis study has been shown to be associated with better outcome [34, 38].

Chemokines contribution to secondary injury is mediated by accumulation of active leukocytes that perpetuates inflammation and neurotoxic cascades. In an observational clinical study the occurrence of hypoxemia after TBI was not associated with increased levels of IL-2, IL-6,

Table 3 Multinomial logistic regression model of neurological outcome

Variables	OR [CI 95 %] vs favorable outcome	*p* value
Age		
Brain dead	0.96 [0.91; 1.02]	0.226
Unfavorable	0.98 [0.93; 1.04]	0.523
Marshall		
Brain dead	1.27 [0.28; 5.81]	0.762
Unfavorable	1.18 [0.46; 3.04]	0.730
GCSm		
Brain dead	0.37 [0.16; 0.85]	0.018
Unfavorable	0.98 [0.48; 2.01]	0.958
Principal component 1		
Brain dead	1.91 [1.24; 2.94]	0.003
Unfavorable	1.80 [1.34; 2.42]	<0.0001
Principal component 2		
Brain dead	4.64 [1.79; 12.05]	0.002
Unfavorable	1.62 [1.02; 2.59]	0.041

GCSm Glasgow Coma Scale, motor score. Unfavorable = unfavorable outcome at 6 months
Brain dead = brain dead patients

and IL-10 but only with GM-CSF, S100 and myelin basic protein levels measured in CSF [24] while Stein et al. demonstrated that TNF-α and IL-8 were good predictors of both high ICP and low CPP recorded hourly by the chart [22, 33]. Recently Di Battista et al. [7] demonstrated the association between elevated IL-8, IL-10, TNF-α, MIP 1β, and MCP-1, hyperadrenergic state and poor outcome. The differences in study design, time window, and parameters analysed may account for much of the variability in these results.

Recently, the Wagner group [5] suggested that individual inflammatory markers may not be as informative of TBI pathology or predictive of outcome as an aggregated inflammatory score. In this perspective, they proposed a novel cytokine load score (CLS) and found a persistent inflammatory state with elevated serum IL-1β, IL-6, IL-8, IL-10, and TNFα levels over the first year post-injury, possibly as a result of a spillover effect from acute elevation after TBI; the proposed CLS was predictive of outcome at 6 and 12 months [5].

The main limitation in studies on neuroinflammation is indeed that authors mainly investigated the relationship between "a priori" selected cytokines and clinical variables, such as intracranial hypertension, hypoxemia or the prognostic value of these mediators. In these studies univariate correlations between a given mediator and a clinical outcome was applied to draw inferences regarding the biological action of the selected cytokine. From the pathophysiological point of view, this approach may be flawed because the primary injury is the common trigger for cytokines production and therefore is likely that these mediators will correlate with each other, particularly those cytokines that are directly antagonistic to one another at the same receptor.

The possible multiple collinearity among variables can be managed by data reduction methods but to prevent overfitting, large numbers of subjects in relation to the number of variables are required. Disentangling the profile and the inter-relationship between these mediators and avoiding the "a priori" selection of the potential relevant molecules is crucial to investigate their mechanistic role in the pathophysiology of TBI.

To overcome the problem of multiple variables with putative statistical interactions, multivariate projection techniques have been recently proposed. Helmy et al. used the PCA [8] to simplify multivariate data into few PCs that contains the main sources of variation within the dataset as a whole. These PCs are made up of a linear combination of the original variables, each of which contributes to a varying degree, termed the "loading". The first PC is a linear combination of each of the original variables which incorporate the greatest source of variation within the dataset and will have a larger magnitude of coefficient than those contributing to a lesser degree. The second and subsequent PCs are further variables that explain the greatest sources of variation left over beyond the first PC. This analysis was used by Helmy et al. to demonstrate the different pattern of response in brain and peripheral blood of cytokines production and to demonstrate difference in cytokines profile after recombinant human IL-1ra administration in a phase II randomized control trial [10, 38].

In coherence with previous literature, in our study Il-6, IL-1ra, Il-8, IL-10, IL-15, MCP-1, MIP-1β, and IP10 were selected in the first two components of PCA as strong predictors of outcome confirming their role in the pathophysiology of brain injury. Among them IL-6, IP10, and MIP-1β remained in the predictive model for raised ICP. PCA analysis has also been recently used by Kumar et al. to explore the pattern of markers that contribute independently to variability in CSF inflammatory response. They found that Il-1β and TNFα provided limited contribution to variance suggesting that even if elevated, these markers had low discriminative capacity in inter-individual variability after TBI [5].

In our study, we collected data from ICU admission for the first 5 days and included also multiple trauma patients. It is therefore possible that an inflammatory response occurring within few hours from injury or after the first 5 days was missed in our database. Finally, the coexisting multiple trauma may have affected the extent of systemic inflammatory response in our patients and their impact on outcome.

A novel aspect of our study is related to the rigorous methodology that we used to record and collect secondary insults occurring early after ICU admission. In TBI patients following the initial event, secondary insults such as high ICP, low CPP, hypoxemia and pyrexia amplify the secondary damage and have been widely demonstrated to affect outcome. We resorted to the EUSIG scale proposed by Miller et al. [18] which is based on physiological thresholds to quantify occurrence and severity of secondary insults [13]. As part of the BrainIT group [27] in the present study, we collected high quality minute-by-minute physiological monitoring data using a standardized data collection equipment. Raised ICP and low CPP were the most frequent secondary insults occurring in almost 21 % of GMT. These results are consistent with literature, with intracranial hypertension occurring in 5–39 % of monitoring time depending on systems used to capture the insults and applied thresholds [28, 39, 40]. The strong predictive power of raised ICP on neurological outcome has been further confirmed by Güiza et al. [41]. Pyrexia occurred in 14 % of GMT, similarly to data reported with the same methodology [13, 42]. The occurrence of hypoxemia was rare (1.5 % of GMT) in our study, since patients were included after initial ICU stabilization. In the present study we separately analysed those patients who died because of brain herniation from those who had a poor outcome at 6 months. Those who evolved to brain death clearly represented the group with the worst secondary insults. Indeed intracranial hypertension was present for almost 70 % of the GMT. On the other hand, in the same time window, occurrence of secondary insults was not significantly different between patients with favorable and unfavorable outcome at 6 months. This result suggests that different factors such as late secondary insults [43] and non neurological complications may play a major role in determining long-term neurological outcome [44].

Due to the observational design of the study, we were not able to conclude if the inflammatory reaction should be considered as marker of severity or mediator of the secondary insults. However the multivariate projection method identified a specific pattern of inflammation overcoming putative interactions and avoiding any subjective selection of relevant molecules.

Conclusions

With the use of multivariate projection method, we showed that patients with severe TBI were characterized by a specific pattern of inflammatory reaction associated with the occurrence of raised ICP. This pattern of cytokines was selected by the PCA as powerful predictor of both the conditions of unfavorable outcome and early brain death. Even if this preliminary analysis requires confirmation in larger studies, our results shed more light on the correlation between secondary insults, systemic inflammation and neurological outcome after TBI, and may help in the future to identify specific therapeutic targets that modulate inflammation.

Abbreviations

Apache, Acute Physiology And Chronic Health Evaluation; Basic FGF, basic Fibroblast growth factor; BrainIT, Brain Monitoring with Information Technology; CLS, cytokine load score; CPP, cerebral perfusion pressure; CSF, cerebrospinal fluid; CT, computerized tomography; EUSIG, Edinburgh University secondary insult grading; GCS, Glasgow Coma Score; G-CSF, granulocyte colony-stimulating factor; GCSm, GCS motor score; GM-CSF, granulocyte-macrophage colony-stimulating factor; GMT, good monitoring time; GOSe, Glasgow Outcome Scale-extended; ICP, intracranial pressure; ICU, intensive care unit; IFN-γ, interferon gamma; IL-12p70, IL-12 subunit p70; IL-1ra,IL-1 receptor antagonist; IL-1β, Interleukin-1 beta; IP-10, interferon gamma-induced protein 10; IQR, interquartile range; ISS, Injury Severity Score; MAP, mean arterial pressure; MCP-1, monocyte chemoattractant protein 1; MIP-1α, macrophage inflammatory protein 1 alpha; PC, principal component; PCA, Principal component analysis; PDGF-BB, Platelet-derived growth factor BB; PLS, Partial Least Squares; RANTES, Regulated upon Activation Normal T-cell Expressed; SD, standard deviation; SpO_2, oxygen saturation measured by pulse oximetry; TBI, traumatic brain injury; TCDB, Traumatic Coma Data Bank; TNF-RI, TNF-α receptors; TNF-α, Tumor necrosis factor alpha; VEGF, Vascular endothelial growth factor.

Acknowledgements

The authors acknowledge students and residents at Department of Anesthesia and Intensive care of the University of Torino for their role in data collection. The authors thank Dr Federica Civiletti for her technical laboratory support.

Funding

This work was supported by the University of Torino (grant no.:MASL1RIL12) for data collection, mining and analysis.

Authors' contributions

ATM participated in the design of the study and data analysis and wrote the manuscript. CF participated in the design of the study and performed the statistical analysis. RS participated in the design of the study and performed the statistical analysis. VF participated in the design of the study and interpretation of data. BA was involved in inflammatory mediators analysis. IP carried out secondary insults analysis. TH carried out secondary insults analysis. IM was involved in data analysis and interpretation. MB involved in data acquisition and interpretation. AD, involved in data acquisition and interpretation. LM designed the study, participated in data analysis and interpretation and wrote the manuscript. All authors read and approved the final manuscript.

Competing interests

The authors declare that they have no competing interests.

Consent for publication

Not applicable.

Author details

[1]Anesthesia and Intensive Care Unit, Department of Surgical Sciences, University of Torino, Torino, Italy. [2]Department of Surgical Sciences, University of Torino, Torino, Italy. [3]Department of Psychology, University of Torino, Torino, Italy. [4]Department of Clinical Physics, Southern General Hospital, Glasgow, UK. [5]Section of Neurosurgery, Department of Neuroscience, Uppsala University, Uppsala, Sweden. [6]Anesthesia and Intensive Care Unit,

AOU Citta' della Salute e della Scienza di Torino, Presidio CTO, Torino, Italy. [7]Neurosurgery Unit, Department of Neuroscience, University of Torino, Torino, Italy. [8]Dipartimento di Scienze e Biotecnologie Medico Chirurgiche, Sapienza University of Rome, Rome, Italy.

References

1. Kossmann T, Hans V, Imhof HG, Trentz O, Morganti-Kossmann MC. Interleukin-6 released in human cerebrospinal fluid following traumatic brain injury may trigger nerve growth factor production in astrocytes. Brain Res. 1996;713(1–2):143–52.
2. Kossmann T, Stahel PF, Lenzlinger PM, Redl H, Dubs RW, Trentz O, et al. Interleukin-8 released into the cerebrospinal fluid after brain injury is associated with blood–brain barrier dysfunction and nerve growth factor production. J Cereb Blood Flow Metab. 1997;17(3):280–9. doi:10.1097/00004647-199703000-00005.
3. Morganti-Kossmann MC, Rancan M, Stahel PF, Kossmann T. Inflammatory response in acute traumatic brain injury: a double-edged sword. Curr Opin Crit Care. 2002;8(2):101–5.
4. Woodcock T, Morganti-Kossmann MC. The role of markers of inflammation in traumatic brain injury. Front Neurol. 2013;4:18. doi:10.3389/fneur.2013.00018.
5. Kumar RG, Boles JA, Wagner AK. Chronic Inflammation After Severe Traumatic Brain Injury: Characterization and Associations With Outcome at 6 and 12 Months Postinjury. J Head Trauma Rehabil. 2015;30(6):369–81. doi:10.1097/HTR.0000000000000067.
6. Santarsieri M, Kumar RG, Kochanek PM, Berga S, Wagner AK. Variable neuroendocrine-immune dysfunction in individuals with unfavorable outcome after severe traumatic brain injury. Brain Behav Immun. 2015;45.
7. Di Battista AP, Rhind SG, Hutchison MG, Hassan S, Shiu MY, Inaba K, et al. Inflammatory cytokine and chemokine profiles are associated with patient outcome and the hyperadrenergic state following acute brain injury. J Neuroinflammation. 2016;13(1):40. doi:10.1186/s12974-016-0500-3.
8. Helmy A, Antoniades CA, Guilfoyle MR, Carpenter KL, Hutchinson PJ. Principal component analysis of the cytokine and chemokine response to human traumatic brain injury. PLoS One. 2012;7(6):e39677. doi:10.1371/journal.pone.0039677PONE-D-12-05243.
9. Helmy A, Carpenter KL, Menon DK, Pickard JD, Hutchinson PJ. The cytokine response to human traumatic brain injury: temporal profiles and evidence for cerebral parenchymal production. J Cereb Blood Flow Metab. 2011;31(2):658–70.
10. Helmy A, Guilfoyle MR, Carpenter KL, Pickard JD, Menon DK, Hutchinson PJ. Recombinant human interleukin-1 receptor antagonist promotes M1 microglia biased cytokines and chemokines following human traumatic brain injury. Journal of cerebral blood flow and metabolism : official journal of the International Society of Cerebral Blood Flow and Metabolism. 2015; doi:0271678X15620204 .
11. Miller JD, Sweet RC, Narayan R, Becker DP. Early insults to the injured brain. JAMA. 1978;240(5):439–42.
12. Andrews PJ, Piper IR, Dearden NM, Miller JD. Secondary insults during intrahospital transport of head-injured patients. Lancet. 1990;335(8685):327–30.
13. Jones PA, Andrews PJ, Midgley S, Anderson SI, Piper IR, Tocher JL, et al. Measuring the burden of secondary insults in head-injured patients during intensive care. J Neurosurg Anesthesiol. 1994;6(1):4–14.
14. Stocchetti N, Colombo A, Ortolano F, Videtta W, Marchesi R, Longhi L, et al. Time course of intracranial hypertension after traumatic brain injury. J Neurotrauma. 2007;24(8):1339–46. doi:10.1089/neu.2007.0300.
15. McHugh GS, Engel DC, Butcher I, Steyerberg EW, Lu J, Mushkudiani N, et al. Prognostic value of secondary insults in traumatic brain injury: results from the IMPACT study. J Neurotrauma. 2007;24(2):287–93. doi:10.1089/neu.2006.0031.
16. Bullock R, Zauner A, Woodward JJ, Myseros J, Choi SC, Ward JD, et al. Factors affecting excitatory amino acid release following severe human head injury. J Neurosurg. 1998;89(4):507–18. doi:10.3171/jns.1998.89.4.0507.
17. Chesnut RM, Marshall LF, Klauber MR, Blunt BA, Baldwin N, Eisenberg HM, et al. The role of secondary brain injury in determining outcome from severe head injury. J Trauma. 1993;34(2):216–22.
18. Signorini DF, Andrews PJ, Jones PA, Wardlaw JM, Miller JD. Adding insult to injury: the prognostic value of early secondary insults for survival after traumatic brain injury. J Neurol Neurosurg Psychiatry. 1999;66(1):26–31.
19. Mazzeo AT, Kunene NK, Choi S, Gilman C, Bullock RM. Quantitation of ischemic events after severe traumatic brain injury in humans: a simple scoring system. J Neurosurg Anesthesiol. 2006;18(3):170–8. doi:10.1097/01.ana.0000210999.18033.f600008506-200607000-00002.
20. McKeating EG, Andrews PJ, Signorini DF, Mascia L. Transcranial cytokine gradients in patients requiring intensive care after acute brain injury. Br J Anaesth. 1997;78(5):520–3.
21. Hergenroeder GW, Moore AN, McCoy Jr JP, Samsel L, Ward III NH, Clifton GL, et al. Serum IL-6: a candidate biomarker for intracranial pressure elevation following isolated traumatic brain injury. J Neuroinflammation. 2010;7:19.
22. Stein DM, Lindell A, Murdock KR, Kufera JA, Menaker J, Keledjian K, et al. Relationship of serum and cerebrospinal fluid biomarkers with intracranial hypertension and cerebral hypoperfusion after severe traumatic brain injury. J Trauma. 2011;70(5):1096–103. doi:10.1097/TA.0b013e318216930d00005373-201105000-00012.
23. Mussack T, Biberthaler P, Kanz KG, Wiedemann E, Gippner-Steppert C, Mutschler W, et al. Serum S-100B and interleukin-8 as predictive markers for comparative neurologic outcome analysis of patients after cardiac arrest and severe traumatic brain injury. Crit Care Med. 2002;30(12):2669–74. doi:10.1097/01.CCM.0000037963.51270.44.
24. Yan EB, Satgunaseelan L, Paul E, Bye N, Nguyen P, Agyapomaa D, et al. Post-traumatic hypoxia is associated with prolonged cerebral cytokine production, higher serum biomarker levels, and poor outcome in patients with severe traumatic brain injury. J Neurotrauma. 2014;31(7):618–29. doi:10.1089/neu.2013.3087.
25. Minambres E, Cemborain A, Sanchez-Velasco P, Gandarillas M, Diaz-Reganon G, Sanchez-Gonzalez U, et al. Correlation between transcranial interleukin-6 gradient and outcome in patients with acute brain injury. Crit Care Med. 2003;31(3):933–8. doi:10.1097/01.CCM.0000055370.66389.59.
26. Brain Trauma Foundation A, CNS, AANS/CNS. Guidelines for the Management of Severe Traumatic Brain Injury. J Neurotrauma. 2007;24:S1–S106.
27. Piper I, Citerio G, Chambers I, Contant C, Enblad P, Fiddes H, et al. The BrainIT group: concept and core dataset definition. Acta Neurochir (Wien). 2003;145(8):615–28. doi:10.1007/s00701-003-0066-6. discussion 28–9.
28. Nyholm L, Howells T, Enblad P, Lewen A. Introduction of the Uppsala Traumatic Brain Injury register for regular surveillance of patient characteristics and neurointensive care management including secondary insult quantification and clinical outcome. Ups J Med Sci. 2013;118(3):169–80. doi:10.3109/03009734.2013.806616.
29. Elf K, Nilsson P, Ronne-Engstrom E, Howells T, Enblad P. Cerebral perfusion pressure between 50 and 60 mm Hg may be beneficial in head-injured patients: a computerized secondary insult monitoring study. Neurosurgery. 2005;56(5):962–71. discussion –71.
30. Wilson JT, Pettigrew LE, Teasdale GM. Emotional and cognitive consequences of head injury in relation to the glasgow outcome scale. J Neurol Neurosurg Psychiatry. 2000;69(2):204–9.
31. Wilson JT, Pettigrew LE, Teasdale GM. Structured interviews for the Glasgow Outcome Scale and the extended Glasgow Outcome Scale: guidelines for their use. J Neurotrauma. 1998;15(8):573–85.
32. Vignali DA. Multiplexed particle-based flow cytometric assays. J Immunol Methods. 2000;243(1–2):243–55.
33. Stein DM, Lindel AL, Murdock KR, Kufera JA, Menaker J, Scalea TM. Use of serum biomarkers to predict secondary insults following severe traumatic brain injury. Shock. 2012;37(6):563–8. doi:10.1097/SHK.0b013e3182534f93.
34. Hutchinson PJ, O'Connell MT, Rothwell NJ, Hopkins SJ, Nortje J, Carpenter KL, et al. Inflammation in human brain injury: intracerebral concentrations of IL-1alpha, IL-1beta, and their endogenous inhibitor IL-1ra. J Neurotrauma. 2007;24(10):1545–57. doi:10.1089/neu.2007.0295.
35. Das M, Mohapatra S, Mohapatra SS. New perspectives on central and peripheral immune responses to acute traumatic brain injury. J Neuroinflammation. 2012;9:236.
36. Ziebell JM, Morganti-Kossmann MC. Involvement of pro- and anti-inflammatory cytokines and chemokines in the pathophysiology of traumatic brain injury. Neurotherapeutics. 2010;7(1):22–30.
37. Perez-Barcena J, Ibanez J, Brell M, Crespi C, Frontera G, Llompart-Pou JA, et al. Lack of correlation among intracerebral cytokines, intracranial pressure, and brain tissue oxygenation in patients with traumatic brain injury and diffuse lesions. Crit Care Med. 2011;39(3):533–40. doi:10.1097/CCM.0b013e318205c7a4.
38. Helmy A, Guilfoyle MR, Carpenter KL, Pickard JD, Menon DK, Hutchinson PJ. Recombinant human interleukin-1 receptor antagonist in severe traumatic brain injury: a phase II randomized control trial. J Cereb Blood Flow Metab. 2014;34(5):845–51.
39. Stocchetti N, Zanaboni C, Colombo A, Citerio G, Beretta L, Ghisoni L, et al.

Refractory intracranial hypertension and "second-tier" therapies in traumatic brain injury. Intensive Care Med. 2008;34(3):461–7. doi:10.1007/s00134-007-0948-9.

40. Zanier ER, Ortolano F, Ghisoni L, Colombo A, Losappio S, Stocchetti N. Intracranial pressure monitoring in intensive care: clinical advantages of a computerized system over manual recording. Crit Care. 2007;11(1):R7.
41. Guiza F, Depreitere B, Piper I, Citerio G, Chambers I, Jones PA, et al. Visualizing the pressure and time burden of intracranial hypertension in adult and paediatric traumatic brain injury. Intensive Care Med. 2015;41: 1067–76. doi:10.1007/s00134-015-3806-1.
42. Stocchetti N, Rossi S, Zanier ER, Colombo A, Beretta L, Citerio G. Pyrexia in head-injured patients admitted to intensive care. Intensive Care Med. 2002; 28(11):1555–62. doi:10.1007/s00134-002-1513-1.
43. Unterberg A, Kiening K, Schmiedek P, Lanksch W. Long-term observations of intracranial pressure after severe head injury. The phenomenon of secondary rise of intracranial pressure. Neurosurgery. 1993;32(1):17–23. discussion –4.
44. Mascia L, Sakr Y, Pasero D, Payen D, Reinhart K, Vincent JL. Extracranial complications in patients with acute brain injury: a post-hoc analysis of the SOAP study. Intensive Care Med. 2008;34(4):720–7. doi:10.1007/s00134-007-0974-7.

4

Cell cycle inhibition reduces inflammatory responses, neuronal loss, and cognitive deficits induced by hypobaria exposure following traumatic brain injury

Jacob W. Skovira[1,2†], Junfang Wu[1*†], Jessica J. Matyas[1], Alok Kumar[1], Marie Hanscom[1], Shruti V. Kabadi[1], Raymond Fang[3] and Alan I. Faden[1*]

Abstract

Background: Traumatic brain injury (TBI) patients in military settings can be exposed to prolonged periods of hypobaria (HB) during aeromedical evacuation. Hypobaric exposure, even with supplemental oxygen to prevent hypoxia, worsens outcome after experimental TBI, in part by increasing neuroinflammation. Cell cycle activation (CCA) after TBI has been implicated as a mechanism contributing to both post-traumatic cell death and neuroinflammation. Here, we examined whether hypobaric exposure in rats subjected to TBI increases CCA and microglial activation in the brain, as compared to TBI alone, and to evaluate the ability of a cyclin-dependent kinase (CDK) inhibitor (CR8) to reduce such changes and improve behavioral outcomes.

Methods: Adult male Sprague Dawley rats were subjected to fluid percussion-induced injury, and HB exposure was performed at 6 h after TBI. Western blot and immunohistochemistry (IHC) were used to assess cell cycle-related protein expression and inflammation at 1 and 30 days after injury. CR8 was administered intraperitoneally at 3 h post-injury; chronic functional recovery and histological changes were assessed.

Results: Post-traumatic hypobaric exposure increased upregulation of cell cycle-related proteins (cyclin D1, proliferating cell nuclear antigen, and CDK4) and microglial/macrophage activation in the ipsilateral cortex at day 1 post-injury as compared to TBI alone. Increased immunoreactivity of cell cycle proteins, as well as numbers of Iba-1$^+$ and GFAP$^+$ cells in both the ipsilateral cortex and hippocampus were found at day 30 post-injury. TBI/HB significantly increased the numbers of NADPH oxidase 2 (gp91^{phox}) enzyme-expressing cells that were co-localized with Iba-1$^+$. Each of these changes was significantly reduced by the administration of CR8. Unbiased stereological assessment showed significantly decreased numbers of microglia displaying the highly activated phenotype in the ipsilateral cortex of TBI/HB/CR8 rats compared with TBI/HB/Veh rats. Moreover, treatment with this CDK inhibitor also significantly improved spatial and retention memory and reduced lesion volume and hippocampal neuronal cell loss.

Conclusions: HB exposure following TBI increases CCA, neuroinflammation, and associated neuronal cell loss. These changes and post-traumatic cognitive deficits are reduced by CDK inhibition; such drugs may therefore serve to protect TBI patients requiring aeromedical evacuation.

Keywords: Traumatic brain injury, Inflammation, Neuronal cell death, Aeromedical evacuation, Hypobaria

* Correspondence: jwu@anes.umm.edu; afaden@anes.umm.edu
†Equal contributors
[1]Department of Anesthesiology and Center for Shock, Trauma and Anesthesiology Research (STAR), University of Maryland School of Medicine, Baltimore, MD 21201, USA
Full list of author information is available at the end of the article

Background

Traumatic brain injury (TBI) is a major cause of morbidity and mortality in civilian populations [1] and has been a serious concern for US military forces, where the number of cases has nearly tripled over the last decade [2]. TBI casualties are moved from the battlefield to the appropriate level of care through the military aeromedical evacuation (AE) system [3]. During transport, patients can be exposed to long periods of hypobaria (HB), as military flights are often pressurized only to 8000 ft, substantially different from commercial air travel [3, 4]. It has been recently shown in a rat TBI model that hypobaria during simulated AE worsens cognitive and pathological outcomes [5]; this report and an earlier one using a mouse TBI model also suggest that hypobaria can increase post-traumatic inflammatory responses [6].

TBI-related neuropathology reflects both direct mechanical damage (primary injury) and delayed induced molecular and cellular cascades (secondary injury)—leading to neuronal cell death, axonal disruption, demyelination, astrogliosis, and inflammation [7]. Cell cycle activation (CCA) occurs after TBI in both neurons and glial cells and contributes to secondary injury [8–10]. In post-mitotic cells such as neurons, CCA contributes to programmed cell death. In glia, CCA induces astrocyte and microglial proliferation/reactivation, leading to astroglial scar formation, release of pro-inflammatory cytokines and reactive oxygen species (ROS), and ultimately neuronal degeneration [8–10]. Administration of cell cycle inhibitors after TBI increases neuronal survival and reduces both microglial and astroglial activation; the latter includes multiple studies utilizing the rat LFP injury model [11–15].

TBI-induced neuroinflammation appears to play a pivotal role in secondary injury severity and progression. Although the neuroinflammatory response to injury may have either beneficial or detrimental actions [16], both pre-clinical and clinical studies show that chronic microglial activation after TBI contributes to both progressive neurodegeneration and related neurological deficits [17–19]. As sustained post-traumatic CCA appears to contribute to chronic neuroinflammation, this study was designed to evaluate whether HB following TBI increases both CCA and related neuroinflammation and whether CCA inhibition can limit these harmful consequences of hypobaric exposure and reduce cognitive dysfunction.

Methods

Animals

Male Sprague Dawley rats (Harlan Labs, Frederick, MD) weighing 325 g (±25 g) were utilized for this study. Animals were fed a standard laboratory diet with food and water ad libitum. All procedures and experiments were carried out in accordance with protocols approved by the Animal Care and Use Committee at the University of Maryland and the United States Air Force.

Micro-fluid percussion and hypobaric animal experiments

Rats were anesthetized with isoflurane (4% induction, 2% maintenance), and a 5-mm craniotomy was made over the left parietal cortex midway between the lambda and bregma as previously described [5, 20]. Using our custom micro-fluid percussion (FP) device, a 1.5–1.9-atmosphere (atm) pressure was used to produce a mild injury with regard to neurologic and histologic deficits [20]. Sham animals underwent the same procedures without injury. Hypobaria was induced using a steel cylindrical chamber with interior dimensions of 46 cm wide and 112 cm long equipped with internal temperature, oxygen, carbon dioxide, and pressure gauges and connected to a vacuum pump. Animals were placed into the chamber in their home cages with access to water and food to reduce stress from acclimation to the HB chamber. Multiple animals in various groups were randomly exposed simultaneously. The chamber was de-pressurized over 30 min to reach 568 mmHg (=8000 ft. altitude)—approximating the cabin pressure during military AE with cruising altitudes of 30,000–40,000 ft. To account for the mean oxygen saturation decrease of 5.5% experienced at this pressure, 28% O_2 was continuously delivered to the chamber to maintain pO_2 at sea level despite the drop in atmospheric pressure. Chamber gases were continuously monitored to validate concentration of O_2 delivered, as well as to verify that CO_2 was not accumulating in the chamber. At 5.5 h of "flight," the chamber was re-pressurized over 30 min to 1 atm (765 mmHg), and the animals were then removed. Interior chamber temperature was monitored continuously and maintained at 22 ± 2 °C.

Experimental procedure

An inhibitor of cell cycle activation—(2-(R)-(1-ethyl-2-hydroxyethylamino)-6-(4-(2-pyridyl)benzyl)-9-isopropyl-purine trihydrochloride (CR8, Tocris Bioscience, Minneapolis, MN), was evaluated for its effects on cellular inflammatory reactions (microglial and astrocyte activation) as well as on histologic and neurologic outcome after TBI. For tissue collection experiments, male rats were randomized to one of four groups: sham injury, TBI alone, TBI + HB + vehicle (Veh), and TBI + HB + CR8 (Fig. 1). For behavioral analysis and stereology experiments, male rats were randomized to one of three groups: sham injury, TBI + HB + Veh, and TBI + HB + CR8 (Fig. 1). We have previously reported a TBI-alone group for behavioral analysis [5]. Animals in the treatment groups received a dose of CR8 (5 mg/kg in saline, IP) or an equal volume of vehicle (saline) 3 h following the induction of a TBI. Six hours after the induction of TBI (1.5–1.9 atm), the animals were exposed to HB for 6 h at 0.75 atm. This

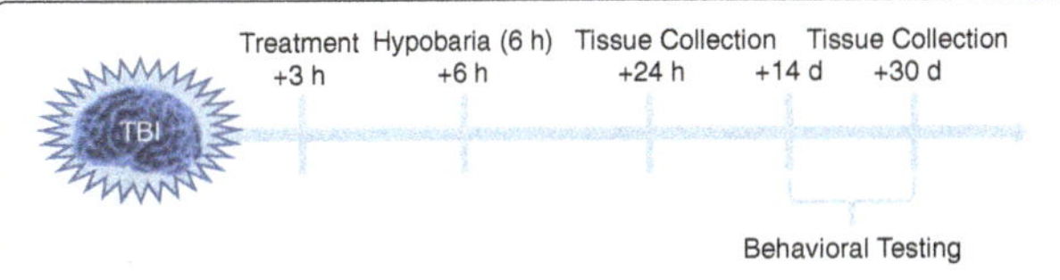

Fig. 1 Experimental timeline for evaluating CR8 treatment on simulated AE-induced cell cycle activation and inflammatory responses following TBI

dose and timing of administration was based on previous studies using this compound in experimental animal models of TBI—which have shown neuroprotection by limiting microglial activation, astrocytosis, and neuronal loss [5, 15]. Behavioral tests were conducted over 30 days post-HB. This experimental timeline was chosen to be consistent and comparable to established procedures for accurate assessment of behavioral and histological outcomes following TBI [5, 15]. All behavioral tests were conducted by an experimenter blinded to the experimental groups. Behavioral testing included Morris water maze tests for learning and memory (post-HB days 14–18), novel object recognition test for retention memory (post-HB day 21), and the forced swim test (post-HB day 26) for depressive-like behaviors. Brains were collected at 24 h post-injury or on post-HB day 30 for pathologic or immunohistochemical analysis. The number of rats in each group or subgroup is indicated in Table 1.

Tissue collection and western blot

At 24 h post-injury, rats were anesthetized with sodium pentobarbital (100 mg/kg, IP). A blunt 21-gauge needle connected to a peristaltic pump (Harvard Apparatus, Holliston, MA) primed with 0.9% sodium chloride (saline) was pierced through the left lateral ventricle and inserted diagonally into the ascending aorta. An incision was then made in the right atrium to allow the fluid to flow through. The brain was perfused with saline at a rate of 50 ml/min for 10 min before being removed. A 5-mm area surrounding the lesion epicenter on the ipsilateral cortex was rapidly dissected placed in a 1-ml microcentrifuge tube and flash frozen with liquid nitrogen. Frozen tissue samples were stored at −80 °C prior to analysis.

Table 1 Definition of the groups

Groups/rats #	Functional assessment	Outcome measures in subgroups (subgroups, randomly selected)
24 h TBI		
Sham	7	WB
TBI	9	WB
TBI/Veh/HB	10	WB
TBI/CR8/HB	7	WB
30 days TBI		
Sham	16	Behavioral tests, IHC
TBI	6	IHC
TBI/Veh/HB	14	Behavioral tests, IHC, lesion volume, stereology
TBI/CR8/HB	15	Behavioral tests, IHC, lesion volume, stereology

TBI traumatic brain injury, *WB* western blot, *HB* hypobaria, *Veh* vehicle, *IHC* immunohistochemistry

For all immunoblot samples, the cortical tissue was homogenized in radioimmunoprecipitation assay (RIPA) buffer and centrifuged at 15,000 rpm for 15 min at 4 °C to isolate proteins, and the protein concentration was determined using the Pierce BCA Protein Assay kit (Thermo Scientific, Rockford, IL). Twenty-five microgram of protein was run on sodium dodecyl sulfate (SDS) polyacrylamide gel electrophoresis and transferred onto nitrocellulose membrane ($n = 6–10$/group). The blots were probed with antibodies against cyclin-dependent kinase (CDK)4 (1:1000, Santa Cruz Biotechnology, Inc., Santa Cruz, CA); cyclin D1 (1:500, Santa Cruz Biotechnology, Inc., Santa Cruz, CA); proliferating cell nuclear antigen (PCNA; 1:500, Santa Cruz Biotechnology); and ionized calcium-binding adapter molecule 1 (Iba-1; 1:1000, Wako Chemicals, Richmond, VA), and GAPDH (1:2000; Sigma-Aldrich, St. Louis, MO) was used as an endogenous control. Immune complexes were detected with the appropriate horseradish peroxidase (HRP)-conjugated secondary antibodies (KPL, Inc., Gaithersburg, MD) and visualized using SuperSignal West Dura Extended Duration Substrate (Thermo Scientific, Rockford, IL). Chemiluminescence was captured on a Kodak Image Station 4000R station (Carestream Health, Rochester, NY), and protein bands were quantified by densitometric analysis using Carestream Molecular Imaging Software. The data presented reflect the intensity of the target protein band compared to the control and were normalized based on the intensity of the endogenous control for each sample.

Functional assessment

Morris water maze

Spatial learning and memory were assessed using the acquisition paradigm of the Morris water maze (MWM) test as previously described [15]. A circular pool (1.5 m in diameter) was divided into four quadrants using computer-based AnyMaze video tracking system (Stoelting Co., Wood Dale, IL). Each rat was subjected to four trials to locate the hidden platform every day from post-HB days 14 to 17 (acquisition phase). Latency (seconds) to locate the hidden platform was measured, with a 90-s limit per trial, and swimming velocities assessed. Water maze search strategy analysis was also performed as previously described [15]. Reference memory was assessed by a probe trial carried out on post-HB day 18. A visual cue test was also performed on post-HB day 18.

Novel object recognition

Nonspatial retention and recognition memory was assessed by the novel object recognition test as previously described [5, 15]. On post-HB day 20, animals were placed into the open field and allowed to explore for 10 min each without any of the objects present for habituation and familiarization. On the testing day (post-HB day 21), two trials of 5 min each were performed. The first trial (training phase) involved placing identical square-shaped "old objects" in both zones of the open field. The second trial (testing phase) involved placing one square-shaped "old object" and one triangular-shaped "novel object" in the respective zones of the open field. The time that was spent exploring each object during both trials was recorded. In addition, time spent in the novel object and old object zones was analyzed and compared between groups separately. The cognitive outcomes were calculated as the "discrimination index" (D.I.) for the second trial using the following formula: % D.I. = (time spent exploring novel object / (total time spent exploring both objects)) × 100.

Forced swim test

The forced swim test was used to examine depressive-like behaviors [5, 15]. On post-HB day 26, rats were individually forced to swim inside a vertical plastic container (height 60 cm; diameter 25 cm) containing 30 cm of water for a time period of 6 min. The total duration of immobility (passive floating, slightly hunched, upright position, the head just above the surface) vs. struggle (diving, jumping, strongly moving all four limbs, scratching the walls) was recorded.

Tissue processing, immunohistochemistry, image acquisition, and quantification

At 30 days after injury, rats were anesthetized and intracardially perfused with 200 ml of saline followed by 300 ml of 4% paraformaldehyde. The dissected brains were post-fixed for overnight and cryoprotected through a sucrose gradient. The coronal sections were cut, serially collected (3 × 60 μm followed by 3 × 20 μm sections) throughout the brain and mounted onto glass slides for histology and immunohistochemistry.

Standard fluorescent immunohistochemistry on serial, 20-μm-thick sections was performed as described previously [21]. The following primary antibodies were used: rabbit anti-CDK4 (1:500, Santa Cruz Biotechnology); mouse anti-cyclin D1 (1:500, Neomarker); rabbit anti-PCNA (1:500, Santa Cruz Biotechnology); rabbit or mouse anti-GFAP (1:1000, Chemicon); rabbit anti-Iba-1 (1:1000, Wako Chemicals); mouse anti-gp91^{phox} (1:500; BD Transduction Laboratories, Franklin Lakes, NJ); and galectin 3 (1:500, Santa Cruz Biotechnology). Fluorescent-conjugated secondary antibodies (1:1000, Alexa 488-conjugated goat anti-mouse or rabbit, Alexa Fluor 546 goat anti-mouse, Alexa Fluor 633 goat anti-mouse, Molecular Probes) were incubated with tissue sections for 1 h at room temperature. Counterstaining was performed with 4′,6-diamidino-2-phenylindole (DAPI) (1 μg/ml; Sigma-Aldrich). All immunohistological staining experiments were carried out with appropriate positive control tissue as well as primary/secondary-only negative controls.

For quantitative image analysis, images were acquired using a fluorescent Nikon Ti-E inverted microscope, at ×20 (CFI Plan APO VC 20× NA 0.75 WD 1 mm) magnification. Exposure times were kept constant for all sections in each experiment. Background for all images was subtracted using Elements. All images were quantified using Elements: nuclei were identified using Spot Detection algorithm based on DAPI staining; cells positive for any of the immunofluorescence markers were identified using Detect Regional Maxima or Detect Peaks algorithms, followed by global thresholding. The intensity of cyclin D1, PCNA, and CDK4 was normalized to the total area imaged. The number of positive cells was normalized to the total number of cells based on DAPI staining. All quantifications were performed in the ipsilateral cortex and hippocampus. For each experiment, data from all images from one region in each animal were summated and used for statistical analysis [22, 23]. At least 1000–2000 cells were quantified for each rat per area per experiment.

Stereological quantification of microglial phenotypes in the ipsilateral cortex

Every fourth 60-μm brain section was immunostained for Iba-1 and DAB and analyzed using a Leica DM4000B microscope (Leica Micro-systems Inc., Buffalo Grove, IL, USA). The number of cortical microglia in either activated (hypertrophic and bushy) or resting (ramified) morphologic phenotypes were counted using the optical fractionator method with the Stereo Investigator software (MBF Biosciences) as described previously [5, 15]. Microglial phenotypic classification was based on the length and thickness of the projections, the number of branches, and the size of the cell body, as previously described [5]. The sampling region was between −2.04 and −4.56 mm from the bregma in the ipsilateral cortex with a dorsal depth of 2.0 mm from the surface. The volume of the region of interest was measured using the Cavalieri estimator method. The estimated number of microglia in each phenotypic class was divided by the volume of the region of interest to obtain cellular density expressed in counts per cubic millimeters (mm^3).

Lesion volume and neuronal survival in the hippocampal subregions

Sections were stained with cresyl violet (FD Neuro-Technologies, Baltimore, MD), dehydrated, and mounted for analysis. Lesion volume was quantified based on the Cavalieri method of unbiased stereology using Stereologer 2000 program software (Systems Planning and Analysis, Alexandria, VA). The lesion volume was quantified by outlining the missing tissue on the injured hemisphere using the Cavalieri estimator with a grid spacing of 0.1 mm. Every fourth 60-μm section between −2.04 and −4.56 mm from the bregma was analyzed beginning from a random start point.

The total number of surviving neurons in the cornus ammonis (CA)1, CA2, CA3, and dentate gyrus (DG) subregions of the hippocampus was assessed using the optical fractionator method [5, 15]. Every fourth 60-μm section between −2.04 and −4.56 mm from the bregma was analyzed, beginning from a random start point. The volume of each hippocampal subfield was measured using the Cavalieri estimator method. The estimated number of surviving neurons in each field was divided by the volume of the region of interest to obtain the neuronal cellular density, expressed as counts/mm^3.

Statistical analysis

Quantitative data were expressed as mean ± standard error of the mean (SEM). Analysis of histological data was conducted using a one-way ANOVA followed by the Student-Newman-Keuls post hoc test. Functional data (latency to find the platform in seconds) for the acquisition phase of the MWM were analyzed by repeated measure (trial over time) two-way ANOVA (TBI + Veh + HB vs. TBI + CR8 + HB) to determine the interactions of post-injury days and groups, followed by post hoc adjustments using the Student-Newman-Keuls test. As we are only interested in whether CR8 treatment improves outcomes over TBI + HB with vehicle treatment, further analysis of behavioral outcomes was conducted using a one-tailed unpaired Student's t test to determine the differences between groups within each trial day. The comparison of search strategies during the final day of the trials of the MWM acquisition phase was analyzed using a chi-square test. As we are only interested in whether CR8 treatment improves outcomes over TBI + HB with vehicle treatment, all other analyses (MWM probe, novel object, forced swim, stereological assessments, lesion volume) were conducted using a one-tailed unpaired Student's t test (TBI + Veh + HB vs. TBI + CR8 + HB). All tests were performed using either SigmaPlot 12 (Systat Software, San Jose, CA) or GraphPad Prism program; version 4.0 (GraphPad Software; San Diego, CA). A p value of less than 0.05 was considered statistically significant.

Results

Post-traumatic hypobaria exposure increases CCA as compared to TBI alone

To evaluate the effect of HB on cell cycle activation, we first examined cell cycle pathway changes in the ipsilateral cortex at day 1 after TBI. Western blotting was performed for the markers of cell cycle-related proteins cyclin D1, PCNA, and CDK4 (Fig. 2). At 24 h post-injury, a significant increase in the protein expression of these markers was observed in the injured/no-HB exposure group ($n = 9$) in comparison to the sham injury group ($n = 7$, $p < 0.001$, TBI/no-HB vs. sham injury). HB exposure following TBI ($n = 10$) significantly further increased the protein expression of cyclin D1, PCNA, and CDK4 in comparison to the TBI/no-HB exposure group ($p < 0.001$ for CDK4, $p < 0.05$ for cyclin D1, TBI + HB vs. TBI/no-HB). In contrast, cell cycle inhibition by administration of CR8 ($n = 7$) limited the TBI + HB-induced increase in the expression of these cell cycle proteins at 1 day post-injury ($p < 0.05$ for cyclin D1 and PCNA, $p < 0.001$ for CDK4, TBI + Veh + HB vs. TBI + CR8 + HB).

We also examined immunoreactivity of cyclin D1, PCNA, and CDK4 in the ipsilateral cortex and hippocampus from sham ($n = 4$), TBI alone ($n = 6$), TBI + Veh + HB ($n = 6$), and TBI + CR8 + HB ($n = 6$) rats at 30 days post-injury. Quantification of pixel intensity for these markers showed significant increases in the TBI + Veh + HB group in contrast to the TBI-alone tissue (Figs. 3, 4, and 5). Cyclin D1 was predominantly expressed by GFAP$^+$ astrocytes (Fig. 3d). Most of the PCNA$^+$ cells in the injured cortex were co-labeled with galectin 3-expressing microglia/macrophages (Fig. 4d). Some of the CDK4$^+$ cells displayed neuronal morphology and co-labeled with NeuN (Fig. 5a, d). In addition, CDK4 was also expressed by astrocytes (data not shown). The post-traumatic upregulation of these proteins was attenuated by CR8 treatment.

Cell cycle inhibition reduces microglial activation and astrogliosis induced by hypobaria exposure following TBI

To examine whether HB-induced activation of microglia and astrocytes were attenuated by inhibiting CCA, rats were treated with CR8 or saline by ip injection at 3 h post injury and the ipsilateral cerebral cortical tissue was collected at 24 h after TBI. Quantitative analysis of western blots showed that Iba-1 expression in TBI ($n = 9$) or TBI + Veh + HB ($n = 10$) groups increased by approximately 1.5- or 2.1-fold, respectively, as compared to sham-injured animals ($n = 7$, Fig. 6a, b). Notably, CR8 treatment ($n = 7$) significantly attenuated (TBI + Veh + HB)-induced increase of Iba-1 expression. Moreover, immunohistochemical analysis demonstrated that TBI + Veh + HB ($n = 6$), in contrast to TBI-alone tissue ($n = 6$), caused a 1.4-fold of the total number of Iba-1$^+$ microglia/macrophages at 30 days post-injury in both the ipsilateral cortex and

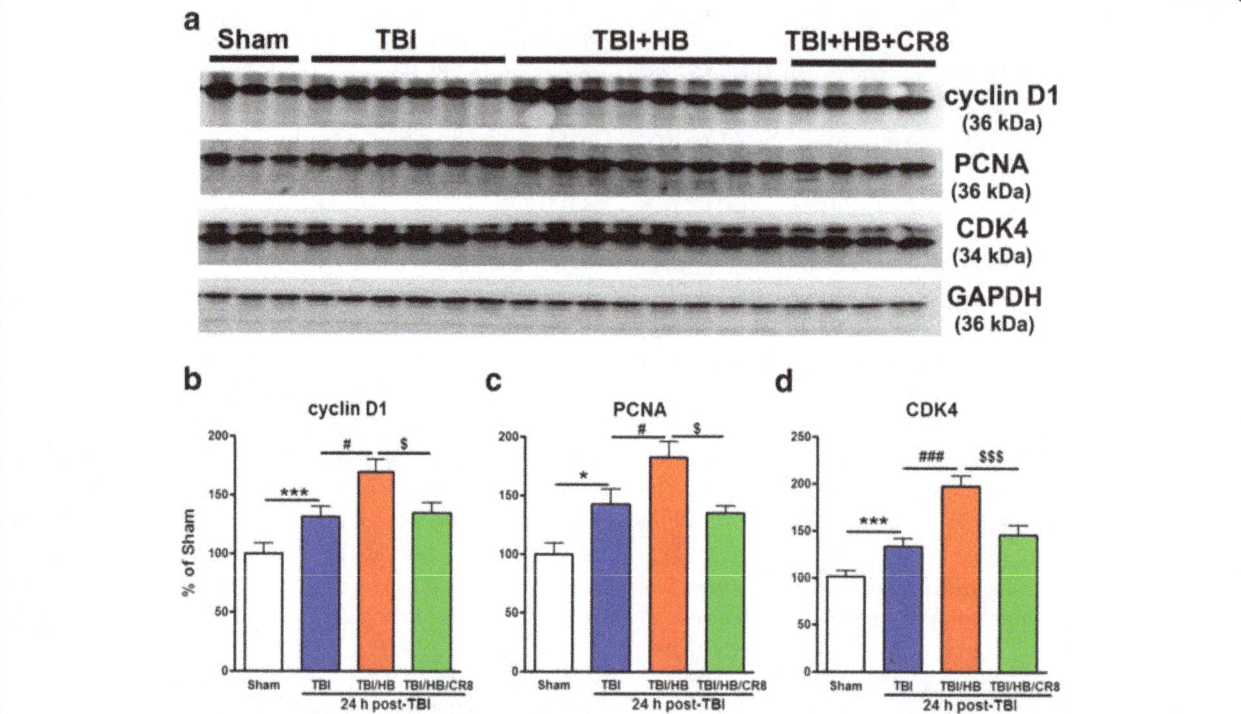

Fig. 2 Hypobaria exposure increases markers of cell cycle activation at 24 h after TBI. **a** Representative immunoblots for cell cycle-related proteins (cyclin D1, PCNA, and CDK4) and the loading control (GAPDH). **b–d** Expression levels of cell cycle proteins were normalized by GAPDH, as estimated by optical density measurements, and expressed as a percentage of sham tissue. At 24 h post-injury, a significant increase in the protein expression of cyclin D1, PCNA, and CDK4 was observed in the TBI/no-HB exposure group in comparison to the sham injury group. HB exposure following TBI significantly increased the protein expression of all three markers in comparison to the TBI-alone group. A significant decrease in the protein expression of all three markers was observed in the CR8 treatment group in comparison to the TBI/Veh/HB group. $N = 7$ (sham), 9 (TBI), 10 (TBI/Veh/HB), 7 (TBI/CR8/HB). $^{*}p < 0.05$, $^{***}p < 0.001$, TBI vs. sham injury; $^{\#}p < 0.05$, $^{\#\#\#}p < 0.001$, TBI/Veh/HB vs. TBI/no-HB; $^{\$}p < 0.05$, $^{\$\$\$}p < 0.001$, TBI/CR8/HB vs. TBI/Veh/HB

hippocampus (Fig. 6c–e). CR8-treated rats ($n = 6$) showed significantly reduced total numbers of Iba-1$^+$ cells.

It is well known the TBI significantly increases microglial activation [7–15]. In our previous study, we have shown that TBI + HB further increases activated microglia at 30 days in comparison to TBI alone [5]. In order to examine if CR8 treatment reduced the neuroinflammatory response associated with TBI + HB, stereological quantifications of resting and activated microglia cell numbers in the injured cortex were evaluated at 30 days post-HB. CR8 treatment ($n = 6$, Fig. 7) significantly reduced the total number of microglia and number of activated microglia in comparison to the TBI + HB group ($p < 0.01$, TBI + CR8 + HB vs. TBI + Veh + HB).

In addition, we evaluated the effect of HB on the expression of NADPH oxidase membrane component gp91^{phox} after TBI. Immunohistochemistry at 30 days post-injury demonstrated that TBI + Veh + HB ($n = 6$) significantly increased the total numbers of gp91^{phox}-positive cells in contrast to TBI-alone tissue ($n = 6$, Fig. 8a–c). Moreover, double-labeling immunohistochemistry revealed that large numbers of gp91^{phox}-positive cells in the injured coronal sections were colabeled with Iba-1 (Fig. 8d). Notably, there were fewer gp91^{phox}-positive cells in the CR8-treated TBI + HB samples ($n = 6$), and Iba-1 expression was also reduced in these cells.

Quantitative immunofluorescence image analysis also showed significant increases in the total numbers of GFAP$^+$ astrocytes in the TBI + Veh + HB group ($n = 6$) in contrast to the TBI-alone tissue ($n = 6$, $P < 0.01$; Fig. 9). Notably, there were significant reductions in the positively stained cells in both the ipsilateral cortex and hippocampus in CR8-treated animals ($n = 6$, $P < 0.01$).

Cell cycle inhibition by CR8 improves functional outcomes following TBI + HB

The MWM was used to evaluate if CR8 treatment attenuates deficits in spatial learning caused by HB exposure following TBI (Fig. 10a). The factors of "post-injury days" ($F(3126) = 102.803$; $p < 0.001$) and "groups" ($F(2126) = 12.576$; $p < 0.001$) were found to be significant. The interaction of "post-injury days × groups" ($F(6126) = 7.730$; $p < 0.01$; repeated measures two-way ANOVA) was significant. Further analysis of differences between groups for each trial day was conducted using a one-tailed unpaired Student's t test. The TBI + CR8 + HB group showed significant improvement in the spatial learning deficits in comparison to the TBI + Veh + HB

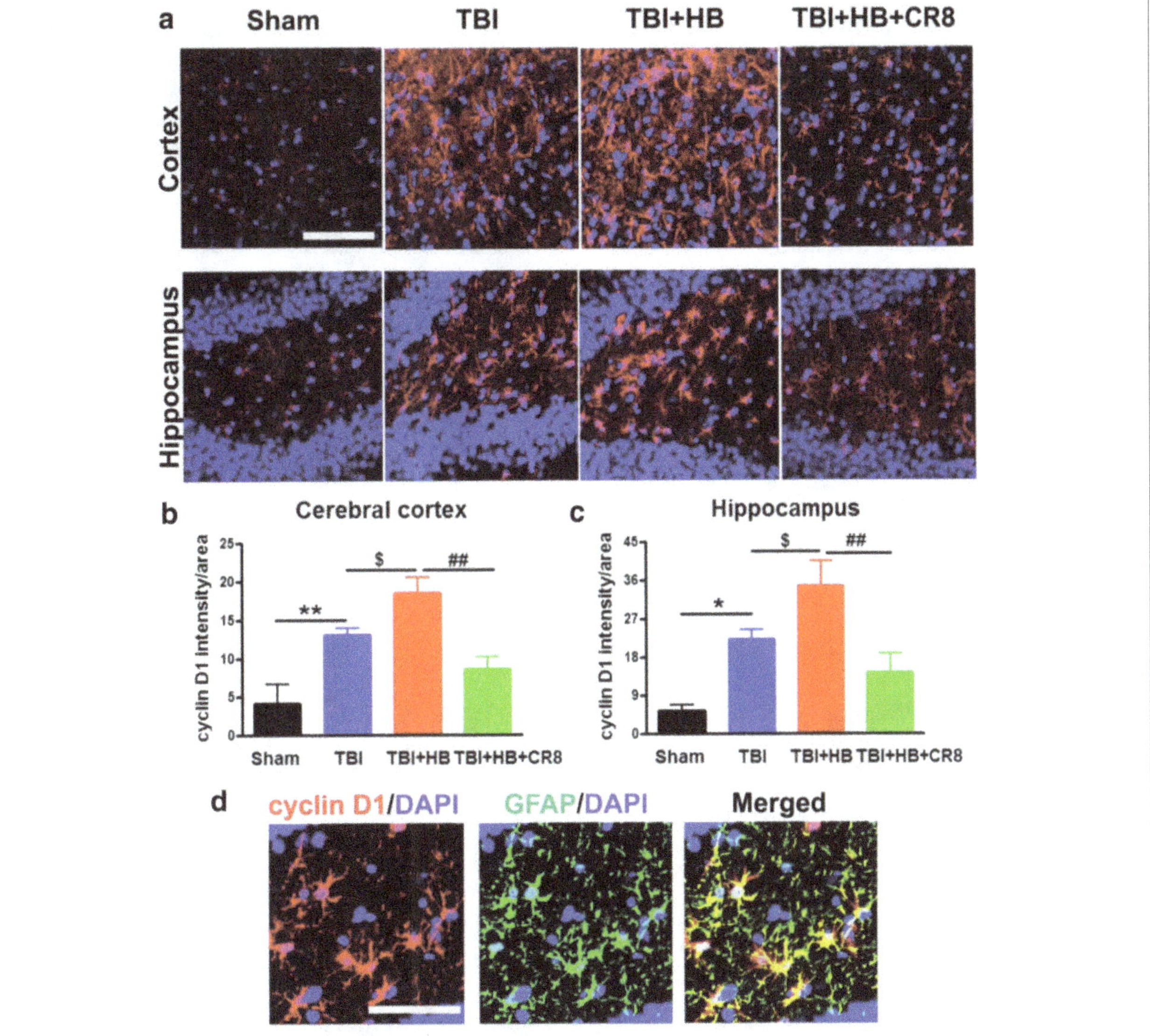

Fig. 3 Hypobaria exposure upregulates the expression of cyclin D1 in the ipsilateral cortex and hippocampus at 30 days after TBI. **a** Representative immunofluorescent staining for cyclin D1 (*red*) and DAPI (*blue*). **b**, **c** Quantification of pixel intensity for cyclin D1 revealed significant increases in the TBI + HB group in contrast to the TBI-alone tissue. A significant decrease of cyclin D1 expression was observed in the CR8 treatment group in comparison to the TBI/Veh/HB group. *N* = 4 (sham), 6 (TBI), 6 (TBI/Veh/HB), 6 (TBI/CR8/HB). **p* < 0.05, ***p* < 0.01, TBI vs. sham injury; $^{\$}p < 0.05$, TBI/Veh/HB vs. TBI; $^{\#\#}p < 0.01$, TBI/CR8/HB vs. TBI/Veh/HB. **d** Cyclin D1 (*red*) predominantly expressed by GFAP$^+$ astrocytes (*green*; DAPI, *blue*). *Scale bar* = 50 μm in **a** and **d**

group on trial day 4 (Fig. 10a: $p < 0.05$). The mean escape latency on the last day of training was 30.2 ± 3.9 s for the sham-injured group, 68.6 ± 6.7 for the Veh + HB group, and 51.0 ± 6.7 for the CR8-treated group.

The swimming patterns during all trials on the fourth day of the acquisition phase were analyzed to assess the search strategies utilized by the animals to locate the hidden platform (Fig. 10b). A chi-square analysis was used to compare strategies between groups ($p < 0.001$; $\chi^2 = 57.79$, $df = 4$). HB-exposed animals were less efficient in their search strategy while attempting to locate the hidden platform with only 32% of the day 4 trials reflecting a spatial strategy. CR8-treated animals utilized a spatial search strategy on day 4 in a higher percentage of trials 61% than untreated injured animals. Spatial memory was assessed using the MWM probe trial on day 18 after HB by examining the number of entries into the target quadrant (Fig. 10c). CR8 treatment increased the number of target quadrant entries in comparison to the TBI + Veh + HB group indicating a reduction in spatial memory deficits in the probe trial ($p < 0.05$ vs. Veh + HB). Swim speeds did not differ across groups (Fig. 10d; $p = 0.4382$).

Nonspatial memory was assessed using the novel object recognition test on post-HB day 21 to evaluate if CR8 treatment improves non-hippocampal-dependent

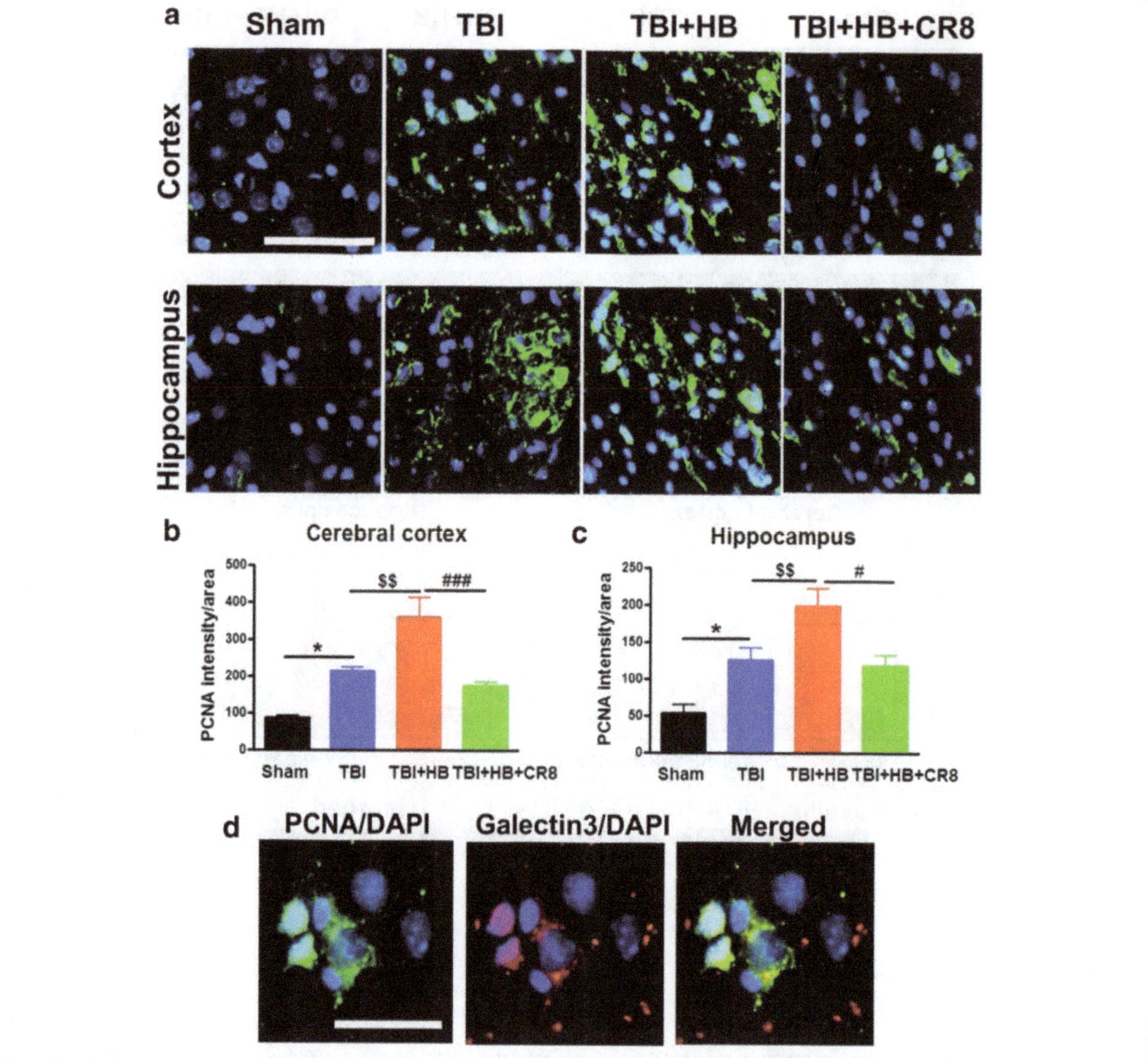

Fig. 4 Hypobaria exposure upregulates the expression of PCNA in the ipsilateral cortex and hippocampus at 30 days after TBI. **a** Representative immunofluorescent staining for PCNA (*green*) and DAPI (*blue*). **b**, **c** Quantification of pixel intensity for PCNA revealed significant increases in the TBI + Veh + HB group in contrast to the TBI-alone tissue. A significant decrease of cyclin D1 expression was observed in the CR8 treatment group in comparison to the TBI/Veh/HB group. $N = 4$ (sham), 6 (TBI), 6 (TBI/Veh/HB), 6 (TBI/CR8/HB). $^{*}p < 0.05$, TBI vs. sham injury; $^{\$\$}p < 0.01$, TBI/Veh/HB vs. TBI; $^{\#}p < 0.05$, $^{\#\#\#}p < 0.001$, TBI/CR8/HB vs. TBI/Veh/HB. **d** Most of the PCNA^{+} cells (*green*) in the injured cortex were co-labeled with galectin 3-expressing microglia/macrophages (*red*; DAPI, *blue*). *Scale bar* = 50 μm in **a** and 25 μm in **d**

memory (Fig. 10e). Animals showed an equal preference for the two identical objects during the training phase. CR8 treatment significantly increased the discrimination index in comparison to the TBI + vehicle + HB group indicating an improvement in nonspatial memory ($p < 0.01$ vs. TBI + Veh + HB).

The forced swim test was performed on post-HB day 26 to determine if CR8 treatment reduces depressive-like behaviors induced by TBI + HB (Fig. 10f). CR8 treatment did not significantly reduce the depressive-like behavior caused by TBI + HB ($p > 0.05$ TBI + Veh + HB vs. TBI + CR8 + HB).

CR8 treatment reduced lesion volume induced by hypobaria exposure following TBI

TBI-induced lesion volume was measured by unbiased stereological techniques (Fig. 11). Histological assessment showed that CR8 treatment (0.71 ± 0.17 mm^3, $n = 5$) resulted in a significant reduction in lesion size after injury as compared with TBI + Veh + HB (2.8 ± 0.74 mm^3; $n = 5$; $P < 0.05$).

Loss of hippocampal neurons and cell cycle inhibition following TBI/HB

It is well known the TBI causes hippocampal neuronal loss [7–15]. In our previous study, we have shown that

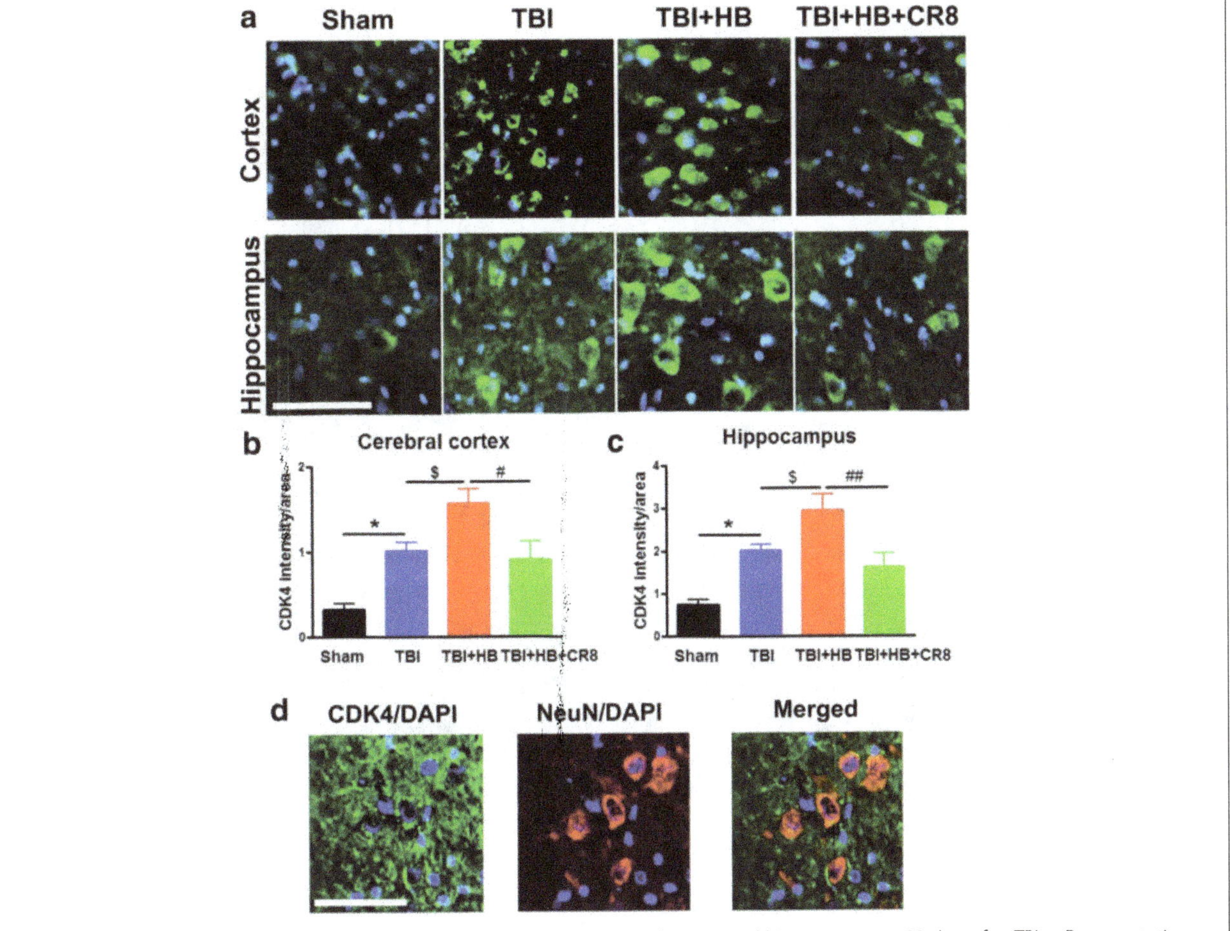

Fig. 5 Hypobaria exposure upregulates the expression of CDK4 in the ipsilateral cortex and hippocampus at 30 days after TBI. **a** Representative immunofluorescent staining for CDK4 (*green*) and DAPI (*blue*). **b**, **c** Quantification of pixel intensity for CDK4 revealed significant increases in the TBI + Veh + HB group in contrast to the TBI-alone tissue. A significant decrease of CDK4 expression was observed in the CR8 treatment group in comparison to the TBI/Veh/HB group. $N = 4$ (sham), 6 (TBI), 6 (TBI/Veh/HB), 6 (TBI/CR8/HB). $^{*}p < 0.05$, TBI vs. sham injury; $^{\$}p < 0.05$, TBI/CR8/HB vs. TBI; $^{\#}p < 0.05$, $^{\#\#\#}p < 0.001$, TBI/HB/CR8 vs. TBI/Veh/HB. **d** Some of the $CDK4^{+}$ cells (*green*) in the injured cortex were co-labeled with NeuN-expressing neurons (*red*; DAPI, *blue*). *Scale bar* = 50 μm in **a** and 25 μm in **d**

TBI + HB further increases hippocampal neuronal loss at 30 days in comparison to TBI alone [5]. Here, we evaluated whether improvements in cognitive memory function following CR8 treatment were associated with increased hippocampal neuronal survival and total neuronal cell numbers in the ipsilateral hippocampus at post-HB day 30 (Fig. 12). The CR8-treated TBI/HB group showed a significant increase in the total number of surviving hippocampal neurons and number of surviving neurons in the hippocampal DG region compared to the TBI + vehicle + HB group ($p < 0.05$).

Discussion

Only two prior experimental studies have evaluated the effects of hypobaria following rodent TBI. We recently reported that hypobaria during simulated AE in a rat TBI model, even with oxygen levels maintained in the normal physiological range, worsens cognitive outcome and increases progressive delayed neurodegeneration and associated chronic inflammatory responses [5]. The other study showed that hypobaric exposure increased cytokine levels acutely after mouse TBI, but that group did not control for the hypoxic effects of hypobaria [6]. The present study is the first to evaluate treatment to limit the negative consequences of post-traumatic hypobaria in an animal model that simulates AE following TBI. Treatment with the CDK inhibitor CR8 reduced hypobaric-induced increases in CCA, post-traumatic microglial activation, and neurodegeneration.

CCA in the brain has been well demonstrated experimentally in models of TBI [11–15], spinal cord injury [21, 24–29], stroke [30, 31], and Alzheimer's disease (AD) [32–35]; it has also been reported in clinical AD [36, 37]. Both neurons and glial cells show increased expression after CNS injury, and such changes may persist for weeks to months [8–10]. Chronic proliferation/

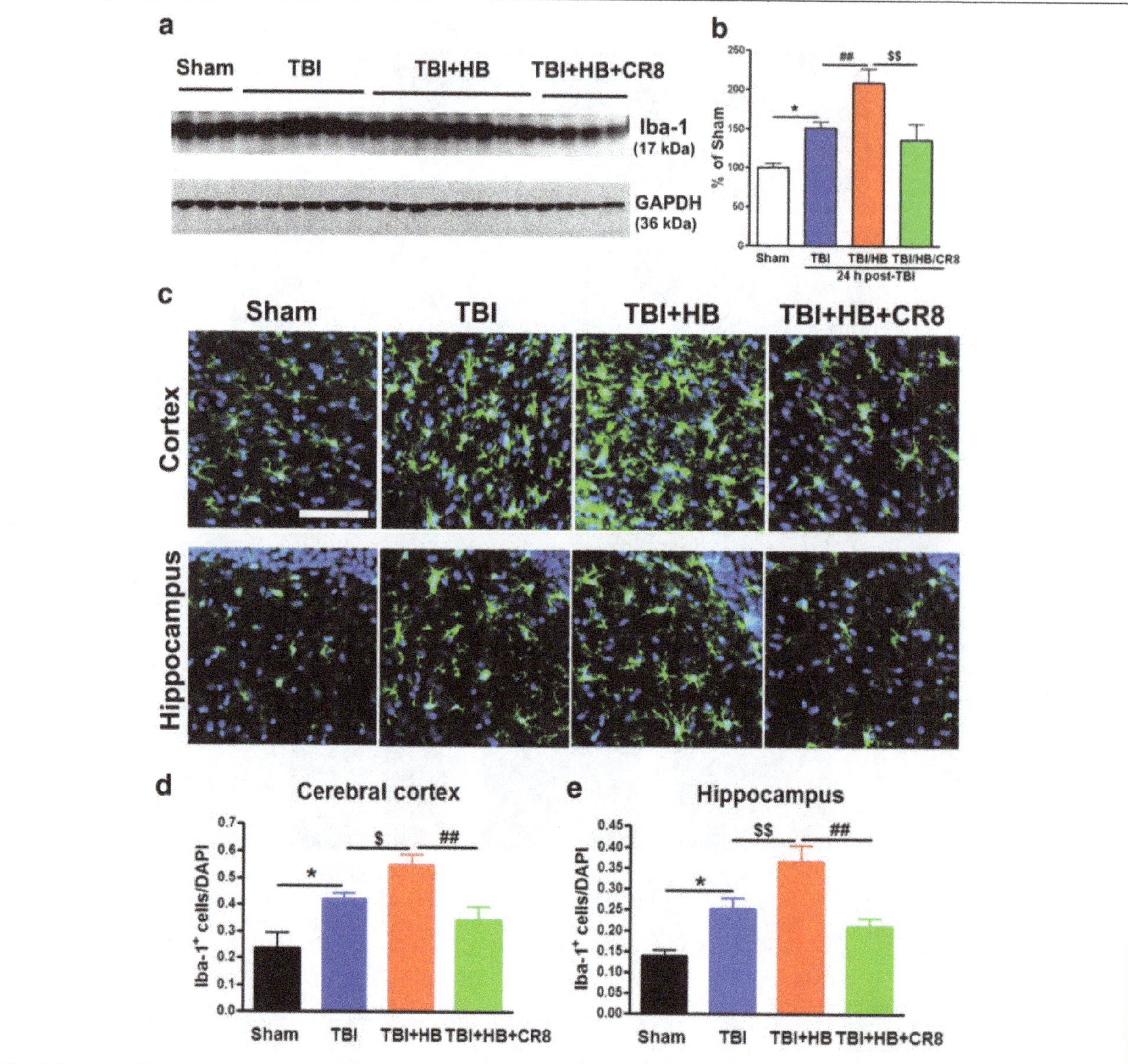

Fig. 6 Cell cycle inhibition reduces protein expression of microglial/macrophages marker Iba-1 induced by hypobaria exposure after TBI. **a** Representative immunoblots for Iba-1 and the loading control (GAPDH). **b** Quantification of the expression levels of Iba-1 protein revealed significant increases in the TBI + Veh + HB group in contrast to the TBI-alone group in the ipsilateral cortex at day 1 after TBI. A significant decrease of Iba-1 expression was observed in the CR8 treatment group in comparison to the TBI/Veh/HB group. $N = 7$ (sham), 9 (TBI), 10 (TBI//Veh/HB), 7 (TBI/CR8/HB). $^{*}p < 0.05$, TBI vs. sham injury; $^{\#\#}p < 0.01$, TBI/Veh/HB vs. TBI no HB; $^{\$\$}p < 0.01$, TBI/CR8/HB vs. TBI/Veh/HB. **c** Representative immunofluorescent staining for Iba-1 (*green*) at 30 days post-injury and DAPI (*blue*). **d**, **e** Quantification of Iba-1$^+$ cells revealed significant increases in the TBI + Veh + HB group in contrast to the TBI-alone group. A significant decrease of Iba-1$^+$ cells was observed in the CR8 treatment group in comparison to the TBI/Veh/HB group. $N = 4$ (sham), 6 (TBI), 6 (TBI/Veh/HB), 6 (TBI/CR8/HB). $^{*}p < 0.05$, TBI vs. sham injury; $^{\$}p < 0.05$, $^{\$\$}p < 0.01$, TBI/Veh/HB vs. TBI; $^{\#\#\#}p < 0.001$, TBI/CR8/HB vs. TBI/Veh/HB. *Scale bar* = 50 μm

activation of astrocytes and microglia resulting from CCA may contribute to secondary injury and limit neurorestoration [15, 18]. Reactive astrocytes are involved in the formation of the glial scar, which can inhibit axonal regeneration [38]. Activated microglia can produce pro-inflammatory cytokines and ROS, leading to neuronal degeneration [18]. Adult differentiated post-mitotic neurons can re-enter the cell cycle; however, such re-entry is associated with caspase-mediated neuronal apoptosis [11, 39–41].

CCA is an intricate and highly regulated process [8–10]. Through each phase in the cycle, there is a systematic progression of synthesis and degradation of phase-specific cyclin proteins. Cyclins bind and activate Ser/Thr kinases known as cyclin-dependent kinases (CDKs), which in turn phosphorylate additional

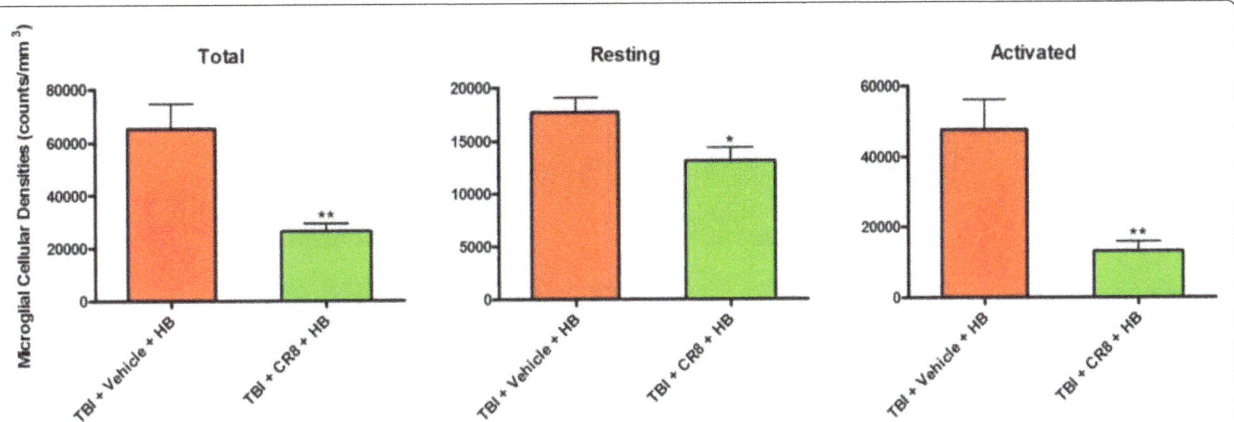

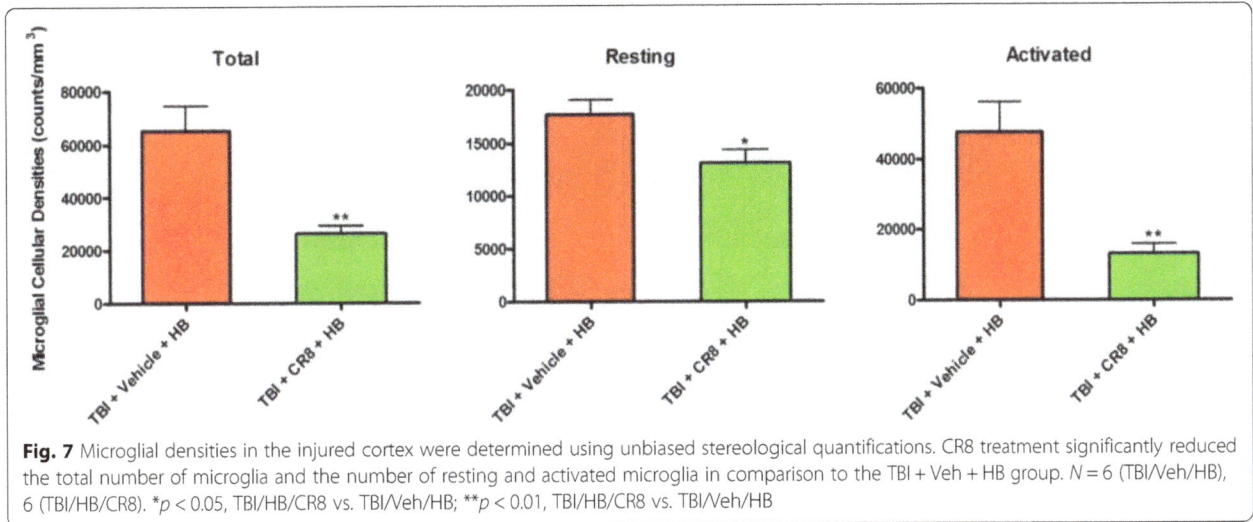

Fig. 7 Microglial densities in the injured cortex were determined using unbiased stereological quantifications. CR8 treatment significantly reduced the total number of microglia and the number of resting and activated microglia in comparison to the TBI + Veh + HB group. $N = 6$ (TBI/Veh/HB), 6 (TBI/HB/CR8). $^{*}p < 0.05$, TBI/HB/CR8 vs. TBI/Veh/HB; $^{**}p < 0.01$, TBI/HB/CR8 vs. TBI/Veh/HB

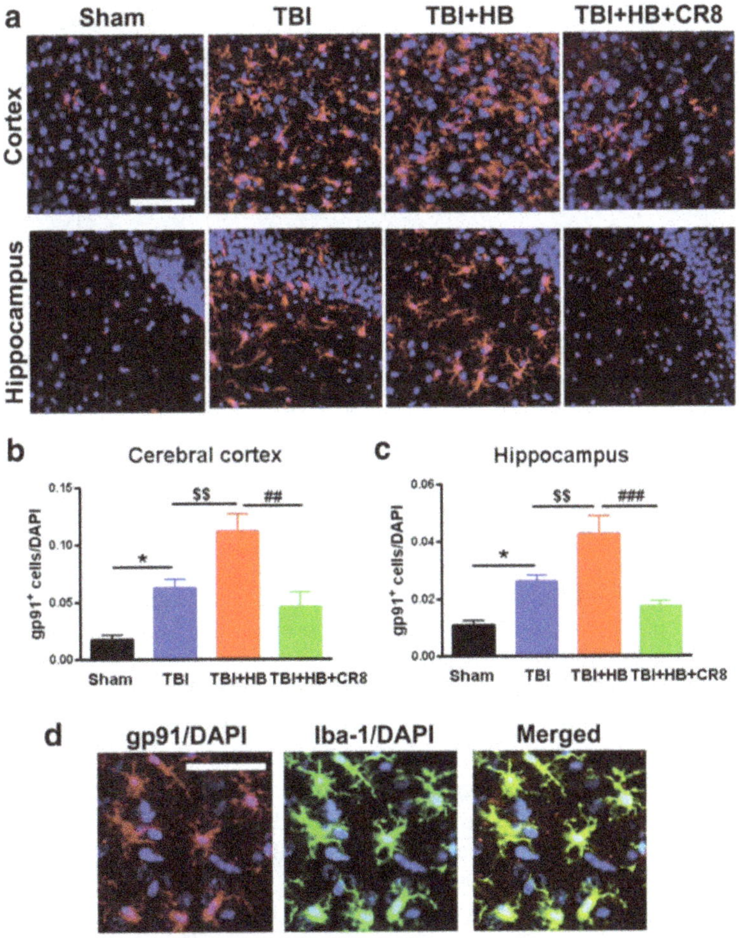

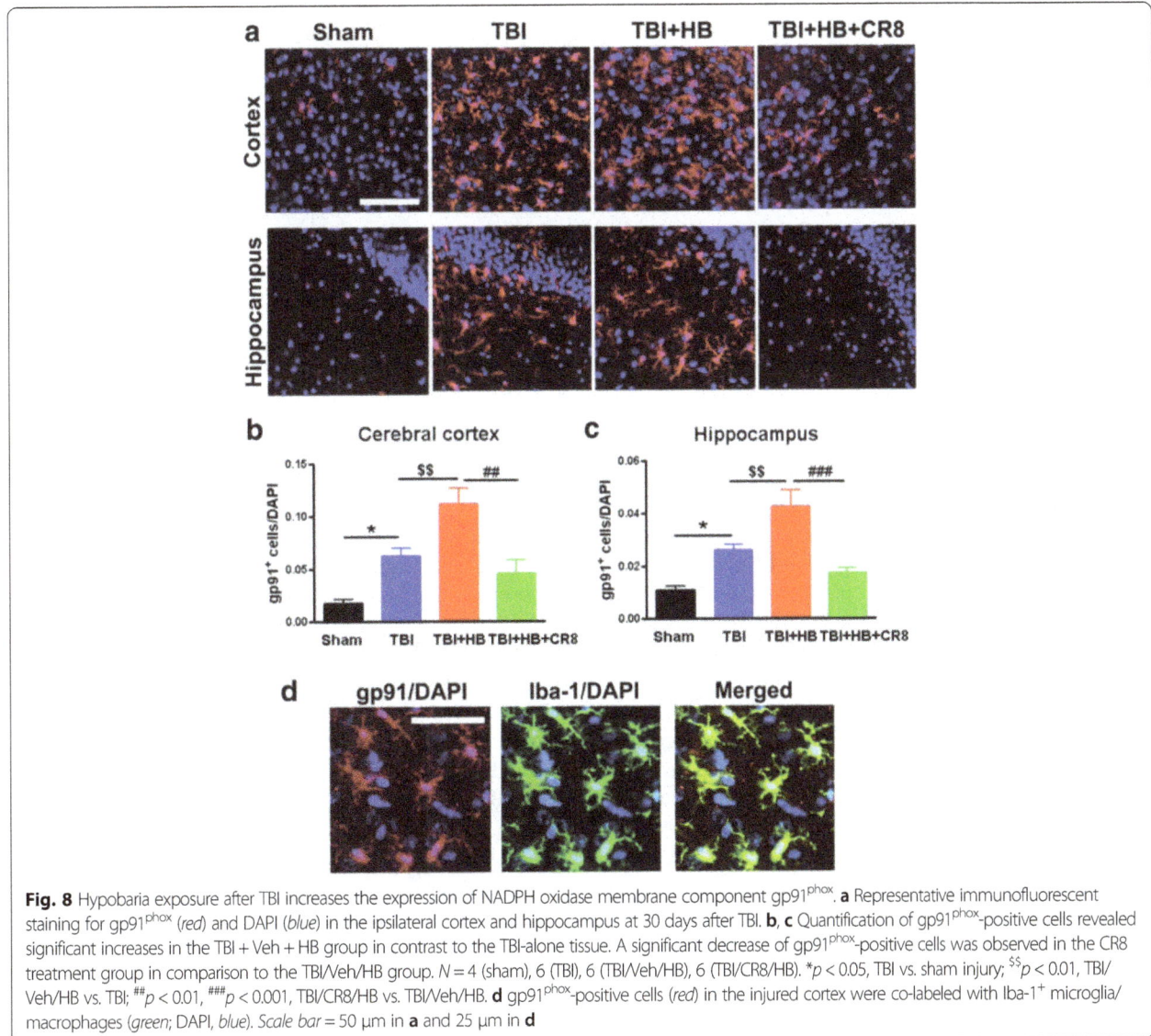

Fig. 8 Hypobaria exposure after TBI increases the expression of NADPH oxidase membrane component gp91^{phox}. **a** Representative immunofluorescent staining for gp91^{phox} (*red*) and DAPI (*blue*) in the ipsilateral cortex and hippocampus at 30 days after TBI. **b**, **c** Quantification of gp91^{phox}-positive cells revealed significant increases in the TBI + Veh + HB group in contrast to the TBI-alone tissue. A significant decrease of gp91^{phox}-positive cells was observed in the CR8 treatment group in comparison to the TBI/Veh/HB group. $N = 4$ (sham), 6 (TBI), 6 (TBI/Veh/HB), 6 (TBI/CR8/HB). $^{*}p < 0.05$, TBI vs. sham injury; $^{\$\$}p < 0.01$, TBI/Veh/HB vs. TBI; $^{\#\#}p < 0.01$, $^{\#\#\#}p < 0.001$, TBI/CR8/HB vs. TBI/Veh/HB. **d** gp91^{phox}-positive cells (*red*) in the injured cortex were co-labeled with Iba-1^{+} microglia/macrophages (*green*; DAPI, *blue*). *Scale bar* = 50 μm in **a** and 25 μm in **d**

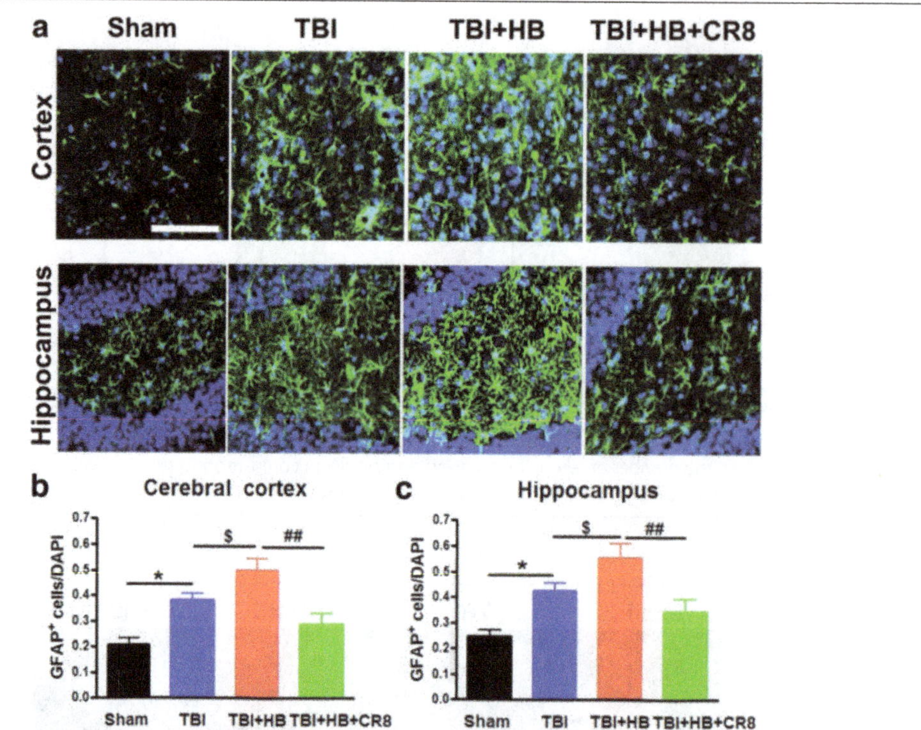

Fig. 9 Cell cycle inhibition reduces protein expression of astrocytes marker GFAP induced by hypobaria exposure following TBI. **a** Representative immunofluorescent staining for GFAP (*green*) and DAPI (*blue*). **b**, **c** Quantification of $GFAP^+$ cells revealed significant increases in the TBI + Veh + HB group in contrast to the TBI-alone tissue. A significant decrease of $GFAP^+$ cells was observed in the CR8 treatment group in comparison to the TBI/HB group. $N = 4$ (sham), 6 (TBI), 6 (TBI/Veh/HB), 6 (TBI/CR8/HB). $^*p < 0.05$, TBI vs. sham injury; $^{\$}p < 0.05$, TBI/Veh/HB vs. TBI; $^{\#\#\#}p < 0.001$, TBI/CR8/HB vs. TBI/Veh/HB. *Scale bar* = 50 μm

substrates that promote transcription of other cyclins and progression through the cycle. During the first phase of the cell cycle, Gap 1 (G1), levels of cyclin D increase. Cyclin D binds to CDK4, promoting phosphorylation of the retinoblastoma (Rb) family of proteins. Phosphorylated Rb proteins dissociate from E2F transcription factors, which translocate to the cell nucleus and induce the transcription of other cyclins. Proteins involved in the G1 phase of the cell cycle have been identified as part of a pro-apoptotic pathway in post-mitotic neurons [9, 10]. Activation of CDK4 by cyclin D1 has been found to be necessary for apoptosis in neurons that re-enter the cell cycle [39, 41]. Furthermore, reduction of CDK4 expression is protective against apoptosis in primary neuronal cell cultures and ablation of the cyclin D1 gene limits lesion development and improves functional outcomes following TBI [42, 43].

Treatment with cell cycle inhibitors increases neuronal survival and reduces glial proliferation/activation in several CNS injury models, including rat and mouse TBI models [11–15, 21, 25–29]. After fluid percussion injury, administration of the pan-CDK inhibitor flavopiridol reduced cyclin D1 expression in neurons and glia in the cortex and hippocampus; treatment also decreased neuronal cell death, lesion volume, astroglial scar formation, and microglial activation and improved motor and cognitive recovery [11]. Central administration of another CDK inhibitor, roscovitine, 30 min after fluid percussion-induced brain injury, significantly decreased lesion volume, as well as improving motor and cognitive recovery [12]. Roscovitine also attenuated neuronal death and inhibited activation of CCA in neurons, as well as decreasing microglial activation and astrogliosis. In primary cortical microglial and neuronal cultures, roscovitine treatment attenuated neuronal cell death and decreased microglial activation as well as microglial-dependent neurotoxicity [12]. Central administration of CR8, a selective and highly potent CDK inhibitor structurally related to roscovitine, attenuated CCA pathways, and reduced post-traumatic apoptotic cell death at 24 h post-TBI [14, 15]. Administration of CR8 at 3 h post-injury limited CCA, reduced microglial activation and lesion volume, and improved behavioral outcomes in both mouse and rat models of experimental TBI [14, 15].

In the present study, the cell cycle markers cyclin D1, PCNA, and CDK4 were significantly increased following TBI/HB at 24 h and 30 days compared to TBI alone. It is well known that the upregulation of cell cycle proteins occurs in both post-mitotic cells (neurons, mature

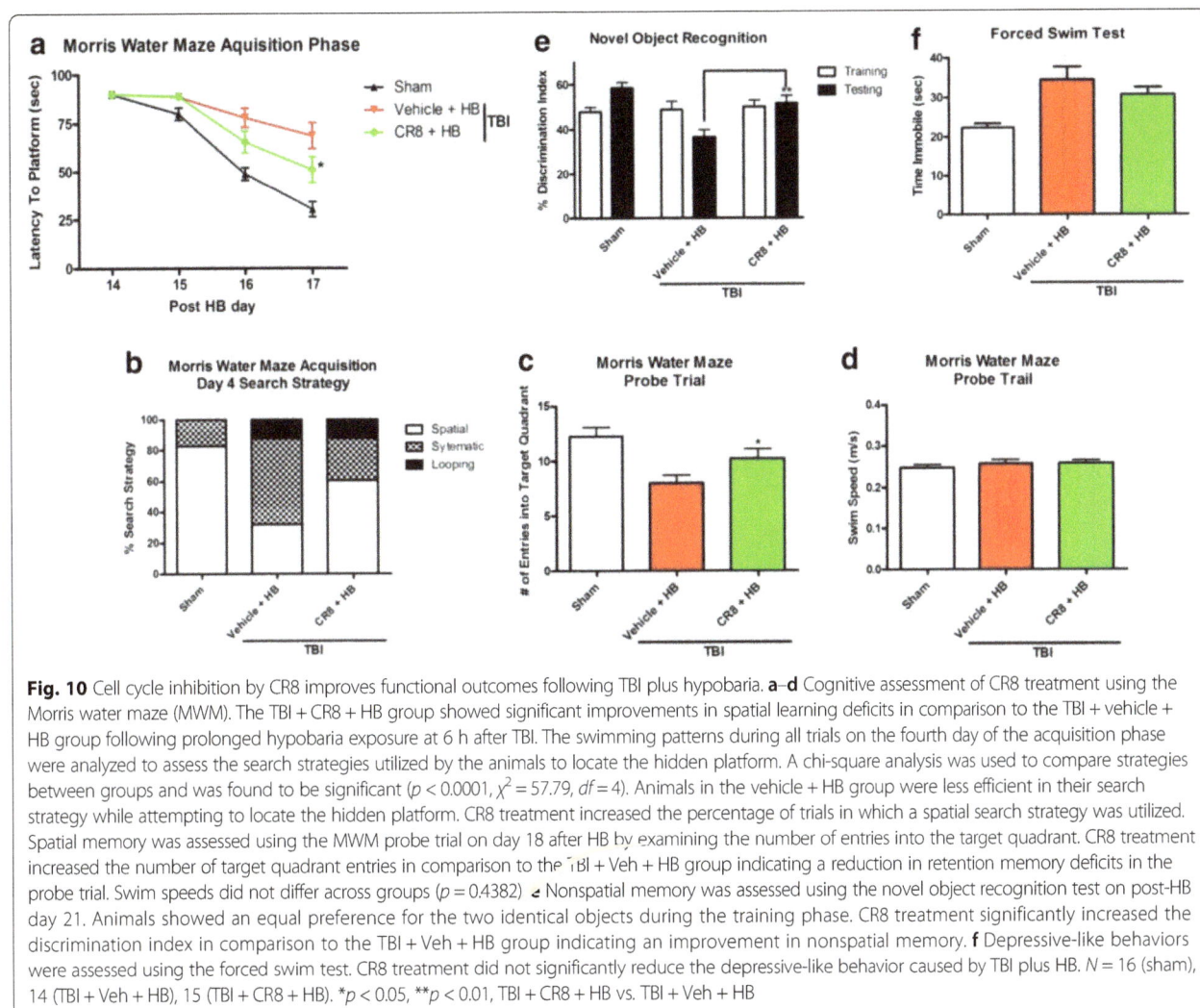

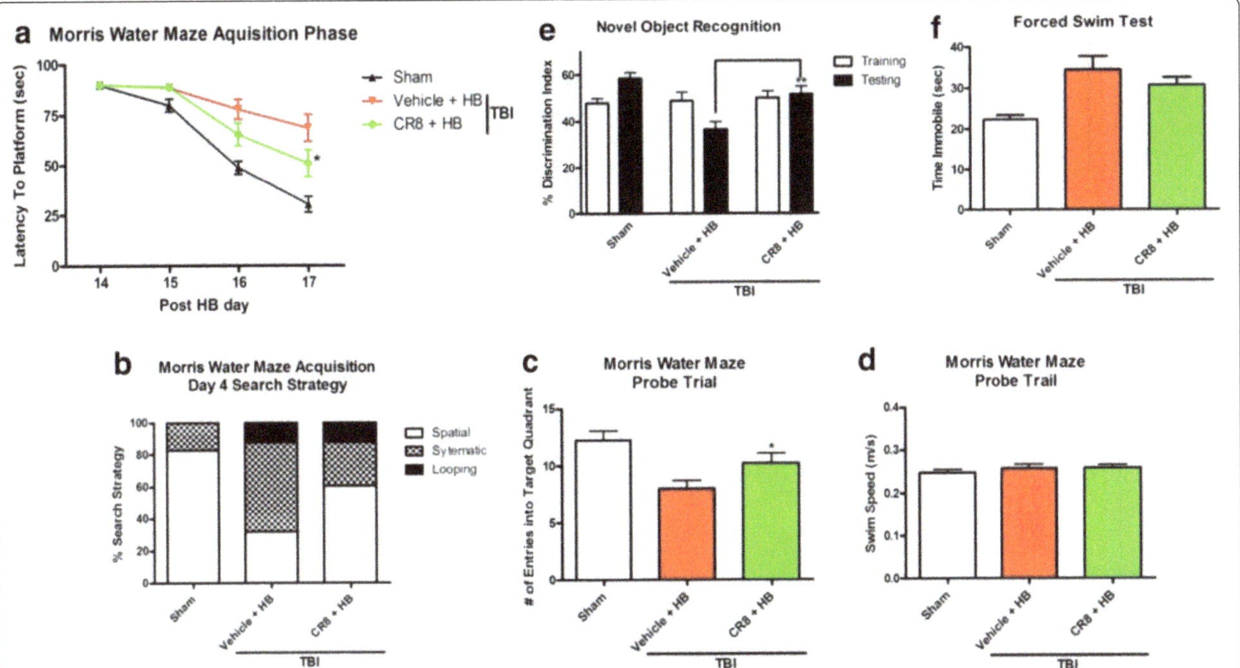

Fig. 10 Cell cycle inhibition by CR8 improves functional outcomes following TBI plus hypobaria. **a**–**d** Cognitive assessment of CR8 treatment using the Morris water maze (MWM). The TBI + CR8 + HB group showed significant improvements in spatial learning deficits in comparison to the TBI + vehicle + HB group following prolonged hypobaria exposure at 6 h after TBI. The swimming patterns during all trials on the fourth day of the acquisition phase were analyzed to assess the search strategies utilized by the animals to locate the hidden platform. A chi-square analysis was used to compare strategies between groups and was found to be significant ($p < 0.0001$, $\chi^2 = 57.79$, $df = 4$). Animals in the vehicle + HB group were less efficient in their search strategy while attempting to locate the hidden platform. CR8 treatment increased the percentage of trials in which a spatial search strategy was utilized. Spatial memory was assessed using the MWM probe trial on day 18 after HB by examining the number of entries into the target quadrant. CR8 treatment increased the number of target quadrant entries in comparison to the TBI + Veh + HB group indicating a reduction in retention memory deficits in the probe trial. Swim speeds did not differ across groups ($p = 0.4382$) **e** Nonspatial memory was assessed using the novel object recognition test on post-HB day 21. Animals showed an equal preference for the two identical objects during the training phase. CR8 treatment significantly increased the discrimination index in comparison to the TBI + Veh + HB group indicating an improvement in nonspatial memory. **f** Depressive-like behaviors were assessed using the forced swim test. CR8 treatment did not significantly reduce the depressive-like behavior caused by TBI plus HB. $N = 16$ (sham), 14 (TBI + Veh + HB), 15 (TBI + CR8 + HB). *$p < 0.05$, **$p < 0.01$, TBI + CR8 + HB vs. TBI + Veh + HB

oligodendroglia) and proliferating cell types including microglia and astrocytes after TBI. In addition to neurons, microglia, and astrocytes that are predominant cell types in the brain, mature oligodendrocytes also undergo apoptotic cell death at acute phase post-injury (e.g., d1, d3 post-injury). We demonstrate changes across brain cell types [11]. We have shown that CCA inhibitors (flavopiridol, CR8) significantly decrease oligodendroglial apoptosis in the injured spinal cord at 1 day post-injury [24, 26]. Whether or not hypobaria (HB) in TBI animals increases CCA expression in oligodendrocytes is intriguing, that merits further research. In addition, expression levels of the microglial/macrophage markers Iba-1 and gp91^{phox} and the astroglial marker GFAP were significantly higher in the TBI/HB group than in TBI animals without HB. Treatment with CR8 prior to HB exposure significantly reduced the expression of cell cycle, microglia/macrophage, and astrocytes markers in comparison to the vehicle-treated TBI/HB group. CR8 significantly reduced deficits in spatial learning and retention memory function caused by HB exposure plus TBI, as reflected by the MWM and novel object recognition tests. However, CR8 treatment did not reduce depressive-like behavioral changes associated with TBI + HB exposure. Chronic microglial activation at 30 days after TBI/HB was also attenuated by CR8 treatment. There was no significant difference between TBI/HB/CR8 and TBI-alone groups in any of the assays performed. Although CR8 treatment at current dose and timing of administration did not completely reverse CDK4 signaling in the injured cortex ($p < 0.05$, TBI/HB/CR8 vs. sham) at both acute and chronic time points post-injury, the other CCA components tested (cyclin D1, PCNA) as well as markers for inflammation (Iba-1, gp91) and astrogliosis (GFAP) were significantly reduced by CR8 treatment to close to a basal level. There was no significant difference between TBI/HB/CR8 and sham groups in the ipsilateral cortex and hippocampus at day 1 or days 28 post-injury. Thus, CR8-mediated reduction of CCA and neuroinflammation are associated with

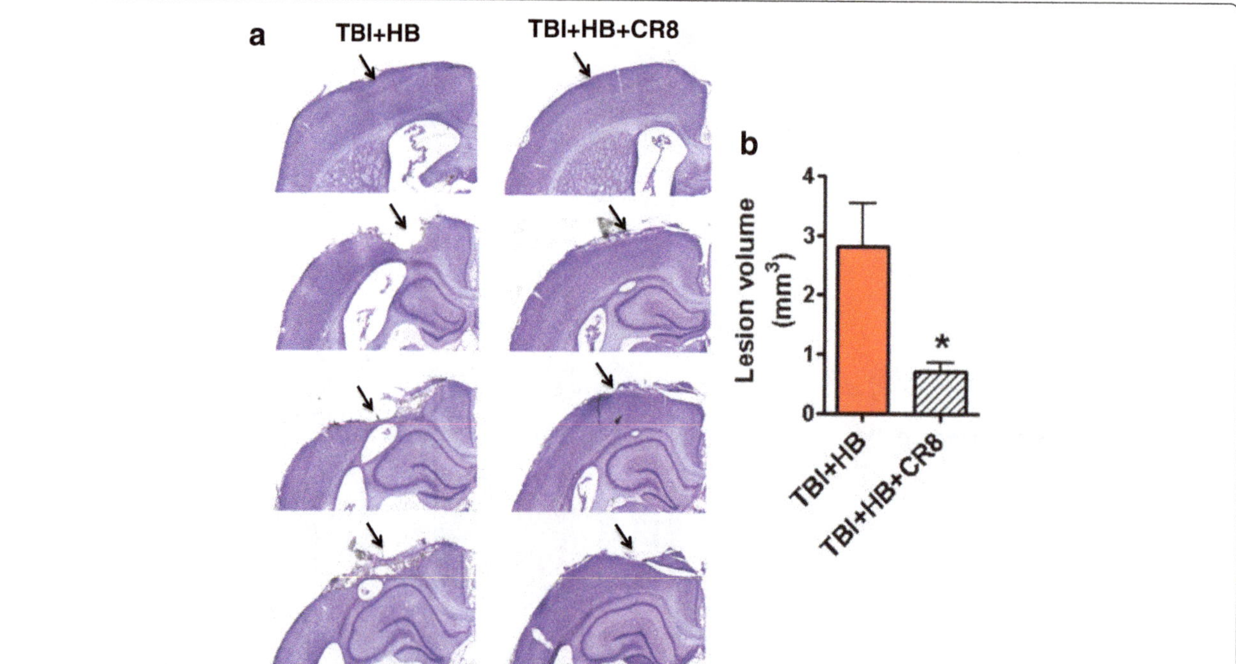

Fig. 11 CR8 treatment reduces lesion volume induced by hypobaria exposure following TBI. Stereological assessment of lesion volume was performed at 30 days post-injury. **a** Representative images from each group are shown. Lesion cavities are marked by *arrows*. **b** There was a significant reduction in lesion volume in the TBI + CR8 + HB group when compared with the TBI + Veh + HB group. $N = 5$/group. *$p < 0.05$, TBI + CR8 + HB vs. TBI + Veh + HB

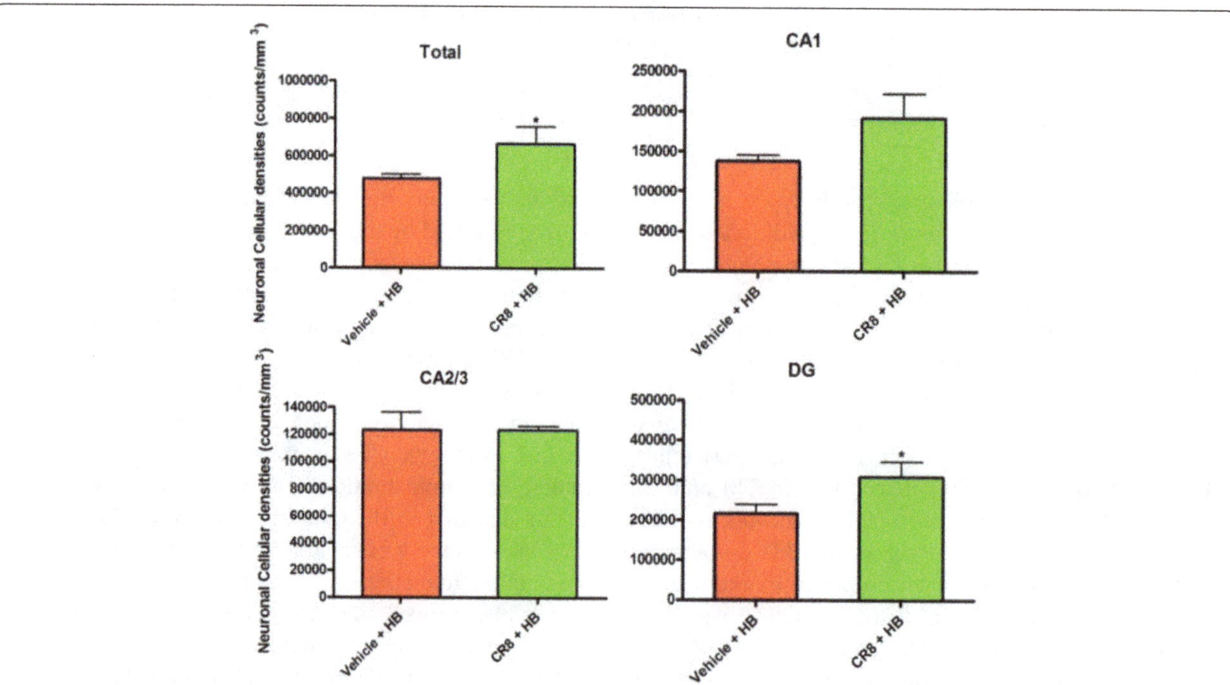

Fig. 12 Effect of CR8 treatment following TBI plus hypobaria on neuronal cell loss in the hippocampus. Total neuronal cell numbers in the hippocampus ipsilateral to the site of injury were evaluated at 30 days post-injury. Unbiased stereological quantifications show that treatment with CR8 increased total neuronal density in the hippocampus and in the DG subregion compared with the TBI + Veh + HB group. $N = 5$ (TBI/Veh + HB), 5 (TBI/CR8/HB). * $p < 0.05$ TBI + CR8 + HB vs. TBI + Veh + HB

improved functional outcome after HB exposure in TBI animals. In the present study, CR8 dose and timing of administration were based on previous studies using this compound in experimental animal models of TBI—which have shown neuroprotection by limiting microglial activation, astrocytosis, and neuronal loss. However, optimizing CR8 treatment condition is intriguing which merits further research. Collectively, these results suggest that increases in CCA activation caused by HB exposure following TBI result in neuronal cell death and neurotoxic microglial activation, which likely contribute to the exacerbation of cognitive dysfunction. CR8 treatment attenuated CCA and neuroinflammatory responses that were intensified by HB exposure following TBI. Given that changes in AE procedures and timing may not be possible because of the need to rapidly transport critically ill patients to definitive treatment sites, use of cell cycle inhibitors—previously examined in late human phase cancer treatment studies—should be explored as a way of limiting the negative consequences of AE in TBI patients.

Conclusions

Wartime casualties with traumatic brain injuries may be exposed to prolonged periods of hypobaria during aeromedical evacuation. As hypobaria exposure following TBI has been shown to worsen pathophysiological and cognitive outcomes, treatments to mitigate these effects must be identified. This study evaluated the effects of prolonged hypobaria in rats subjected to traumatic brain injury on cell cycle and neuroinflammatory pathways and examined the ability of the cell cycle inhibitor CR8 to alleviate the associated effects. Hypobaria exposure following TBI significantly increased markers of cell cycle activation and microglial activation. These changes were limited by treatment with the cell cycle inhibitor CR8 at 3 h post-injury. CR8 treatment also significantly reduced cognitive deficits associated with hypobaria exposure following injury.

Abbreviations

AD: Alzheimer's disease; AE: aeromedical evacuation; CA1, CA2, CA3: cornus ammonis 1, 2, 3; CCA: cell cycle activation; D.I.: discrimination index; DAPI: 4′,6-diamidino-2-phenylindole; DG: dentate gyrus; FP: fluid percussion; HB: hypobaria; HRP: horseradish peroxidase; Iba-1: ionized calcium-binding adapter molecule 1; MWM: Morris water maze; PCNA: proliferating cell nuclear antigen; Rb: retinoblastoma; RIPA: radioimmunoprecipitation assay; ROS: reactive oxygen species; SDS: sodium dodecyl sulfate; TBI: traumatic brain injury

Acknowledgements

This material is based on a research sponsored by the 711 HPW/XPT under Cooperative Agreement number FA8650-11-2-6D04. The US Government is authorized to reproduce and distribute reprints for governmental purposes notwithstanding any copyright notation thereon. The authors thank Shuxin Zhao and Katherine Cardiff for their expert technical assistance and Dr. Hegang Chen for expert statistical consultation.

The views expressed in this article are those of the authors and do not necessarily reflect the official policy or position of the Air Force, the Department of Defense, or the US Government.

Funding

This study was supported by the 711 HPW/XPT under Cooperative Agreement number FA8650-11-2-6D04. The funder had no role in the study design, data collection, and analysis, decision to publish, or preparation of the manuscript.

Authors' contributions

JWS contributed to the design of the studies, analysis, and interpretation of data; carried out the TBI surgery and behavioral test; and wrote and revised the manuscript. JW contributed to the design of the studies; performed the WB, data analysis, and interpretation; and wrote and revised the manuscript. JM, AK, MH, and SK performed the behavioral tests, IHC, data analysis, and tissue processing. AIF conceived the research, participated in interpretation of the data, and revised the manuscript. RF assisted with the grant proposal supporting this work, as well as in the review and editing. All authors read and approved the final manuscript.

Competing interests

Dr. Skovira was a participant in the Department of Defense Science, Mathematics and Research for Transformation (SMART) Scholarship for Service Program, and this manuscript represents a portion of his work in the completion of a Ph.D. from the University of Maryland, Baltimore. The other authors declare that they have no competing interests.

Consent for publication

Not applicable.

Author details

[1]Department of Anesthesiology and Center for Shock, Trauma and Anesthesiology Research (STAR), University of Maryland School of Medicine, Baltimore, MD 21201, USA. [2]Research Division Pharmacology Branch, United States Army Medical Research Institute of Chemical Defense, Aberdeen Proving Ground, Aberdeen, MD 21010, USA. [3]Program in Trauma, Center for the Sustainment of Trauma and Readiness Skills (C-STARS), University of Maryland School of Medicine, Baltimore, MD 21201, USA.

References

1. Faul M, Xu L, Waid MM, Coronado VG. Traumatic brain injury in the United States: emergency department visits. Hospitalizations and deaths 2002–2006. Atlanta: Centers for Disease Control and Prevention, National Center for Injury Prevention and Control; 2010.
2. Defense and Veterans Brain Injury Center. DOD TBI worldwide numbers since 2000. In: DOD TBI Worldwide Numbers. 2016. http://dvbic.dcoe.mil/sites/default/files/uploads/Worldwide%20Totals%202000-2014Q1.pdf. Accessed 15 June 2016
3. Reno J. Military aeromedical evacuation, with special emphasis on craniospinal trauma. Neurosurg Focus. 2010;28(5):E12.
4. Fang R, Dorlac G, Allan P, Dorlac W. Intercontinental aeromedical evacuation of patients with traumatic brain injuries during operations Iraqi Freedom and Enduring Freedom. Neurosurg Focus. 2010;28(5):E11.
5. Skovira JW, Kabadi SV, Wu J, Zhao Z, DuBose J, Rosenthal R, Fiskum G, Faden AI. Simulated aeromedical evacuation exacerbates experimental brain injury. J Neurotrauma. 2016. doi:10.1089/neu.2015.4189.
6. Goodman MD, Makley AT, Huber NL, Clarke CN, Friend LA, Schuster RM, Bailey SR, Barnes SL, Dorlac WC, Johannigman JA, Lentsch AB, Pritts TA. Hypobaric hypoxia exacerbates the neuroinflammatory response to traumatic brain injury. J Surg Res. 2011;165(1):30–7.
7. Faden AI. Microglial activation and traumatic brain injury. Ann Neurol. 2011;70(3):345.

8. Cernak I, Stoica B, Byrnes KR, Di Giovanni S, Faden AI. Role of the cell cycle in the pathobiology of central nervous system trauma. Cell Cycle. 2005;4(9): 1286–93.
9. Byrnes KR, Faden AI. Role of cell cycle proteins in CNS injury. Neurochem Res. 2007;32(10):1799–807.
10. Stoica BA, Byrnes KR, Faden AI. Cell cycle activation and CNS injury. Neurotox Res. 2009;16(3):221–37.
11. Di Giovanni S, Movseyan V, Ahmed F, Cernak I, Schinelli S, Stoica B. Cell cycle inhibition provides neuroprotection and reduces glial proliferation and scar formation after traumatic brain injury. PNAS. 2005;102(23):8333–8.
12. Hilton GD, Stoica BA, Byrnes KR, Faden AI. Roscovitine reduces neuronal loss, glial activation, and neurologic deficits after brain trauma. J Cereb Blood Flow Metab. 2008;11:1845–59.
13. Kabadi SV, Stoica BA, Byrnes KR, Hanscom M, Loane DJ, Faden AI. Selective CDK inhibitor limits neuroinflammation and progressive neurodegeneration after brain trauma. J Cereb Blood Flow Metab. 2012;32(1):137–49.
14. Kabadi SV, Stoica BA, Hanscom M, Loane DJ, Kharebava G, Murray Ii MG, Cabatbat RM, Faden AI. CR8, a selective and potent CDK inhibitor, provides neuroprotection in experimental traumatic brain injury. Neurotherapeutics. 2012;9(2):405–21.
15. Kabadi SV, Stoica BA, Loane DJ, Luo T, Faden AI. CR8, a novel inhibitor of CDK, limits microglial activation, astrocytosis, neuronal loss, and neurologic dysfunction after experimental traumatic brain injury. J Cereb Blood Flow Metab. 2014;34(3):502–13.
16. Dardiotis E, Karanikas V, Paterakis K, Fountas K, Hadjigeorgiou GM. Traumatic brain injury and inflammation: emerging role of innate and adaptive immunity. In: Agrawal A, editor. Brain injury—pathogenesis, monitoring, recovery and management. ISBN: 978-953-51-0265-6, InTech, March 2012
17. Colton C. Heterogeneity of microglial activation in the innate immune response in the brain. J Neuroimmume Pharmacol. 2009;4:399–418.
18. Loane DJ, Byrnes KR. Role of microglia in neurotrauma. Neurotherapeutics. 2010;7(4):366–77.
19. Ramlackhansingh AF, Brooks DJ, Greenwood RJ, Bose SK, Turkheimer FE, Kinnunen KM, Gentleman S, Heckemann RA, Gunanayagam K, Gelosa G. Sharp inflammation after trauma: microglial activation and traumatic brain injury. J Ann Neurol. 2011;70(3):374–83.
20. Kabadi SV, Hilton GD, Stoica BA, Zapple DN, Faden AI. Fluid-percussion-induced traumatic brain injury model in rats. Nat Protoc. 2010;5(9):1552–63.
21. Wu J, Zhao Z, Sabirzhanov B, Stoica BA, Kumar A, Luo T, Skovira J, Faden AI. Spinal cord injury causes brain inflammation associated with cognitive and affective changes: role of cell cycle pathways. J Neurosci. 2014;34(33):10989–1006.
22. Sarkara C, Zhaoa Z, Aungst S, Sabirzhanova B, Faden AI, Lipinski MM. Impaired autophagy flux is associated with neuronal cell death after traumatic brain injury. Autophagy. 2014;10(12):2208–22.
23. Liu S, Sarkar C, Dinizo M, Faden AI, Koh EY, Lipinski MM, Wu J. Disrupted autophagy after spinal cord injury is associated with ER stress and neuronal cell death. Cell Death Dis. 2015;6(1):e1582. doi:10.1038/cddis.2014.527.
24. Byrnes KR, Stoica BA, Fricke S, Di Giovanni S, Faden AI. Cell cycle activation contributes to post-mitotic cell death and secondary damage after spinal cord injury. Brain. 2007;130(Pt 11):2977–92.
25. Tian DS, Xie MJ, Yu ZY, Zhang Q, Wang YH, Chen B, Chen C, Wang W. Cell cycle inhibition attenuates microglia induced inflammatory response and alleviates neuronal cell death after spinal cord injury in rats. Brain Res. 2007; 1135(1):177–85.
26. Wu J, Stoica BA, Dinizo M, Pajoohesh-Ganji A, Piao C, Faden AI. Delayed cell cycle pathway modulation facilitates recovery after spinal cord injury. Cell Cycle. 2012;11(9):1782–95. doi:10.4161/cc.20153.
27. Wu J, Pajoohesh-Ganji A, Stoica BA, Dinizo M, Guanciale K, Faden AI. Delayed expression of cell cycle proteins contributes to astroglial scar formation and chronic inflammation after rat spinal cord contusion. J Neuroinflammation. 2012;9:169. doi:10.1186/1742-2094-9-169.
28. Wu J, Stoica BA, Luo T, Sabirzhanov B, Zhao Z, Guanciale K, Nayar SK, Foss CA, Pomper MG, Faden AI. Isolated spinal cord contusion in rats induces chronic brain neuroinflammation, neurodegeneration, and cognitive impairment. Involvement of cell cycle activation. Cell Cycle. 2014;13(15): 2446–58. doi:10.4161/cc.29420.
29. Wu J, Zhao Z, Zhu X, Renn CL, Dorsey SG, Faden AI. Cell cycle inhibition limits development and maintenance of neuropathic pain following spinal cord injury. Pain. 2016;157(2):488–503. doi:10.1097/j.pain.0000000000000393.
30. Rashidian J, Iyirhiaro GO, Park DS. Cell cycle machinery and stroke. Biochim Biophys Acta. 2007;1772(4):484–93.
31. Osuga H, Osuga S, Wang F, Fetni R, Hogan MJ, Slack RS, Hakim AM, Ikeda JE, Park DS. Cyclin-dependent kinases as a therapeutic target for stroke. Proc Natl Acad Sci U S A. 2000;97(18):10254–9.
32. Sanphui P, Pramanik SK, Chatterjee N, Moorthi P, Banerji B, Biswas SC. Efficacy of cyclin dependent kinase 4 inhibitors as potent neuroprotective agents against insults relevant to Alzheimer's disease. PLoS One. 2013;8(11): e78842. doi:10.1371/journal.pone.0078842.
33. Seward ME, Swanson E, Norambuena A, Reimann A, Cochran JN, Li R, Roberson ED, Bloom GS. Amyloid-β signals through tau to drive ectopic neuronal cell cycle re-entry in Alzheimer's disease. J Cell Sci. 2013;126(Pt 5): 1278–86. doi:10.1242/jcs.1125880.
34. Arendt T. Cell cycle activation and aneuploid neurons in Alzheimer's disease. Mol Neurobiol. 2012;46(1):125–35. doi:10.1007/s12035-012-8262-0.
35. Neve RL, McPhie DL. The cell cycle as a therapeutic target for Alzheimer's disease. Pharmacol Ther. 2006;111(1):99–113.
36. Katsel P, Tan W, Fam P, Purohit DP, Haroutunian V. Cell cycle checkpoint abnormalities during dementia: a plausible association with the loss of protection against oxidative stress in Alzheimer's disease. PLoS One. 2013; 8(7):e68361. doi:10.1371/journal.pone.0068361.
37. Kim H, Kwon Y-A, Ahn IS, Kim S, Kim S, Ahn Jo S, Kim DK. Overexpression of cell cycle proteins of peripheral lymphocytes in patients with Alzheimer's disease. Psychiatry Investig. 2016;13(1):127–34.
38. Silver J, Miller JH. Regeneration beyond the glial scar. Nat Rev Neurosci. 2004;5:146–56.
39. Kranenburg O, van der Eb AJ, Zantema A. Cyclin D1 is an essential mediator of apoptotic neuronal cell death. EMBO J. 1996;15:46–54.
40. Herrup K, Yang Y. Cell cycle regulation in the postmitotic neuron: oxymoron or new biology? Nat Rev Neurosci. 2007;8(5):368–78.
41. Shan B, Lee WH. Deregulated expression of E2F-1 induces S-phase entry and leads to apoptosis. Mol Cell Biol. 1994;14(12):8166–73.
42. Rashidian J, Iyirhiaro G, Aleyasin H, Rios M, Vincent I, Callaghan S, Bland RJ, Slack RS, During MJ, Park DS. Multiple cyclin-dependent kinases signals are critical mediators of ischemia/hypoxic neuronal death in vitro and in vivo. Proc Natl Acad Sci U S A. 2005;102(39):14080–5.
43. Kabadi SV, Stoica BA, Loane DJ, Byrnes KR, Hanscom M, Cabatbat RM, Tan MT, Faden AI. Cyclin D1 gene ablation confers neuroprotection in traumatic brain injury. J Neurotrauma. 2012;29(5):813–27.

5

Microglial-derived microparticles mediate neuroinflammation after traumatic brain injury

Alok Kumar[1,2], Bogdan A. Stoica[1,2], David J. Loane[1,2], Ming Yang[3], Gelareh Abulwerdi[1,2], Niaz Khan[1,2], Asit Kumar[1,2], Stephen R. Thom[3] and Alan I. Faden[1,2*]

Abstract

Background: Local and systemic inflammatory responses are initiated early after traumatic brain injury (TBI), and may play a key role in the secondary injury processes resulting in neuronal loss and neurological deficits. However, the mechanisms responsible for the rapid expansion of neuroinflammation and its long-term progression have yet to be elucidated. Here, we investigate the role of microparticles (MP), a member of the extracellular vesicle family, in the exchange of pro-inflammatory molecules between brain immune cells, as well as their transfer to the systemic circulation, as key pathways of inflammation propagation following brain trauma.

Methods: Adult male C57BL/6 mice were subjected to controlled cortical impact TBI for 24 h, and enriched MP were isolated in the blood, while neuroinflammation was assessed in the TBI cortex. MP were characterized by flow cytometry, and MP content was assayed using gene and protein markers for pro-inflammatory mediators. Enriched MP co-cultured with BV2 or primary microglial cells were used for immune propagation assays. Enriched MP from BV2 microglia or CD11b-positive microglia from the TBI brain were stereotactically injected into the cortex of uninjured mice to evaluate MP-related seeding of neuroinflammation in vivo.

Results: As the neuroinflammatory response is developing in the brain after TBI, microglial-derived MP are released into the circulation. Circulating enriched MP from the TBI animals can activate microglia in vitro. Lipopolysaccharide stimulation increases MP release from microglia in vitro and enhances their content of pro-inflammatory mediators, interleukin-1β and microRNA-155. Enriched MP from activated microglia in vitro or CD11b-isolated microglia/macrophage from the TBI brain ex vivo are sufficient to initiate neuroinflammation following their injection into the cortex of naïve (uninjured) animals.

Conclusions: These data provide further insights into the mechanisms underlying the development and dissemination of neuroinflammation after TBI. MP loaded with pro-inflammatory molecules initially released by microglia following trauma can activate additional microglia that may contribute to progressive neuroinflammatory response in the injured brain, as well as stimulate systemic immune responses. Due to their ability to independently initiate inflammatory responses, MP derived from activated microglia may provide a potential therapeutic target for other neurological disorders in which neuroinflammation may be a contributing factor.

Keywords: Microparticles, Microglia, Neuroinflammation, Traumatic brain injury, Interleukin-1β, miR-155

* Correspondence: afaden@anes.umm.edu
[1]Department of Anesthesiology, University of Maryland School of Medicine, Baltimore, MD, USA
[2]Shock, Trauma and Anesthesiology Research (STAR) Center, University of Maryland School of Medicine, Health Sciences Facility II (HSFII), #S247 20 Penn Street, Baltimore, MD 21201, USA
Full list of author information is available at the end of the article

Background

Microparticles (MP; also called microvesicles), a type of extracellular vesicle, are small membrane-bound bodies shed from the plasma membrane and released by cells during activation or cell death [1]. They are composed of the plasma membrane along with a limited amount of cytoplasm and measure 100 to 1000 nm in diameter [2]. MP are enriched in the lipid microdomains, where cholesterol, phospholipids, and receptors are clustered [3], and are distinguished from other extracellular vesicles such as exosomes (30–100 nm; endosomal origin) and apoptotic bodies (1000–2000 nm) [1]. MP can be released from virtually all cell types in the brain and contain molecular signals in the form of non-secreted proteins and DNA/RNA/microRNA (miR) molecules that may be involved in cell-to-cell communication during neurodevelopment and synaptic physiology [4]. MP and other extracellular vesicles have also been implicated in the development and progression of various neurological diseases [4]. For example, in transmissible spongiform encephalopathy accumulation and cell-to-cell transmission of infectious prion proteins (PrP^{sc}), extracellular vesicles are a key mechanism of prion disease propagation [5, 6]. In amyotrophic lateral sclerosis, accumulating evidence indicates that a mechanism for the progressive accumulation of misfolded mutant form of superoxide dismutase 1 (SOD1) is cell-to-cell propagation of SOD1 within the brain via extracellular vesicles that extend the range and toxicity during disease [7, 8]. Similar mechanisms are thought to contribute to neurotoxic amyloid-β formation in Alzheimer's disease models [9–11]; however, these data are more controversial given that other studies have shown that exosome-associated amyloid-β are neuroprotective [12, 13].

Traumatic brain injury (TBI) causes cell death and neurologic dysfunction through secondary injury mechanisms characterized by edema, neuronal cell death, glial activation, and infiltration of peripheral immune cells, among others [14]. The inflammatory response to TBI is highly complex and includes rapid proliferation and migration of resident microglia to the site of injury in response to damage-associated molecular patterns (DAMPs) and other factors released by injured tissue [15], as well as by infiltration of neutrophils and inflammatory monocyte subsets that contribute to the injury milieu [16]. If the immune response is unable to resolve effectively, or becomes dysregulated after TBI, it can contribute to chronic neurodegeneration, due to chronic activation of neurotoxic microglia [17]. Elevated levels of MP have been reported in the cerebrospinal fluid of TBI patients [18], and circulating MP derived from endothelial cells, platelets, and leukocytes have been measured acutely after severe isolated TBI [19]. These include cerebral endothelium-derived MP release following focal contusion injury [20] as well as neuronal- and astroglial-derived MP release following mixed contusion and diffuse axonal injury [21].

Given the increasingly recognized role for neuroinflammation in tissue damage after TBI, we examined whether posttraumatic circulating MP released after injury could be derived from microglia, as well as potential mechanisms of microglial MP involvement in cell-to-cell communication in the brain following trauma. We hypothesized that MP released by microglia contain pro-inflammatory molecules that contribute to the spread of brain inflammation. We used flow cytometry to identify the origin of brain-specific immune-related MP in the circulation following controlled cortical impact in mice. To investigate immunogenic properties of microglial-derived MP, we used BV2 microglia and primary microglial cell culture models. Finally, to demonstrate cell-to-cell propagation of neuroinflammatory mechanisms within the brain, we injected enriched MP derived from microglia isolated from TBI cortex or lipopolysaccharide (LPS)-stimulated microglia into the cortex of uninjured mice.

Methods

Animals

Studies were performed using C57BL/6 adult male mice (10–12 weeks old, 22–26 g). The mice were housed in the Animal Care facility at the University of Maryland School of Medicine under a 12-h light-dark cycle with ad libitum access to food and water. All surgical procedures were carried out in accordance with protocols approved by the Institutional Animal Care and Use Committee (IACUC) at the University of Maryland School of Medicine.

Controlled cortical impact

Our custom-designed controlled cortical impact (CCI) TBI device consists of a microprocessor-controlled pneumatic impactor with a 3.5-mm diameter tip. Mice were anesthetized with isoflurane evaporated in a gas mixture containing 70% N_2O and 30% O_2 and administered through a nose mask (induction at 4% and maintenance at 2%). Depth of anesthesia was assessed by monitoring respiration rate and pedal withdrawal reflexes. Mice were placed on a heated pad, and core body temperature was maintained at 37 °C. The head was mounted in a stereotaxic frame, and the surgical site was clipped and cleaned with Nolvasan and ethanol scrubs. A 10-mm midline incision was made over the skull, the skin and fascia were reflected, and a 5-mm craniotomy was made on the central aspect of the left parietal bone. The impounder tip of the injury device was then extended to its full stroke distance (44 mm), positioned to the surface of the exposed dura, and reset to impact the cortical surface. Moderate-level TBI was induced using an impactor velocity of 6 m/s and deformation depth of

2 mm as previously described [22]. After injury, the incision was closed with interrupted 6-0 silk sutures, anesthesia was terminated, and the animal was placed into a heated cage to maintain normal core temperature for 45 min post-injury. Sham animals underwent the same procedure as TBI mice except for the impact.

Study 1

Sham ($n = 6$) and TBI ($n = 6$) of C57BL/6J mice were anesthetized (100 mg/kg sodium pentobarbital, I.P.) at 24 h post-injury, and blood was collected in heparinized syringes by aortic puncture for blood MP analysis. Ipsilateral cortical tissue was rapidly dissected and snap-frozen on liquid nitrogen for RNA extraction

Study 2

Sham ($n = 5$) and TBI ($n = 5$) of C57BL/6J mice were anesthetized (100 mg/kg sodium pentobarbital, I.P.) at 7 days post-injury and transcardially perfused with ice-cold 0.9% saline (100 ml). Ipsilateral cortical and hippocampal tissues were rapidly dissected and processed for CD11b-positive selection and MP isolation.

Enriched MP isolation and analysis

Mice were anesthetized (100 mg/kg sodium pentobarbital, I.P.), and blood was collected in heparinized syringes by aortic puncture. Blood was immediately combined with fixative (100 μl/ml Caltag Reagent A fixation medium, Invitrogen, Carlsbad, CA) to diminish ex vivo microparticle (MP) aggregation. All reagents and solutions used for MP analysis were sterile and filtered (0.1-μm filter). Heparinized blood was centrifuged for 5 min at 1500×*g*, and supernatant was centrifuged at 15,000×*g* for 30 min to pellet platelets and other cell debris [23]. Blood supernatants were used to collect total blood MP (~250 μl) that were purified by adding PBS (4 ml) and centrifuged at 100,000×*g* for 60 min at 4 °C as previously described [23–30]. In each experiment, flow cytometry in combination with microbead standards ranging in size from 300 to 3000 nm was used to characterize MP size. MP were distinguished from larger (apoptotic body; >1000 nm) and smaller (exosomes; <100 nm) vesicles based on size (SSC), and their phenotype was confirmed using the unique MP surface marker, annexin V (details below; see Fig. 1a). In parallel experiments, equal numbers of circulating MP from sham and TBI mice (8×10^5 MP) were resuspended in 100 μl serum-free DMEM media and co-cultured with BV2 microglia (2×10^4 cells/well) for 24 h at 37 °C and at 5% CO_2 prior to cell extraction for markers of microglial activation. The enriched MP population obtained using this protocol may also contain other types of extracellular vesicles such as exosomes.

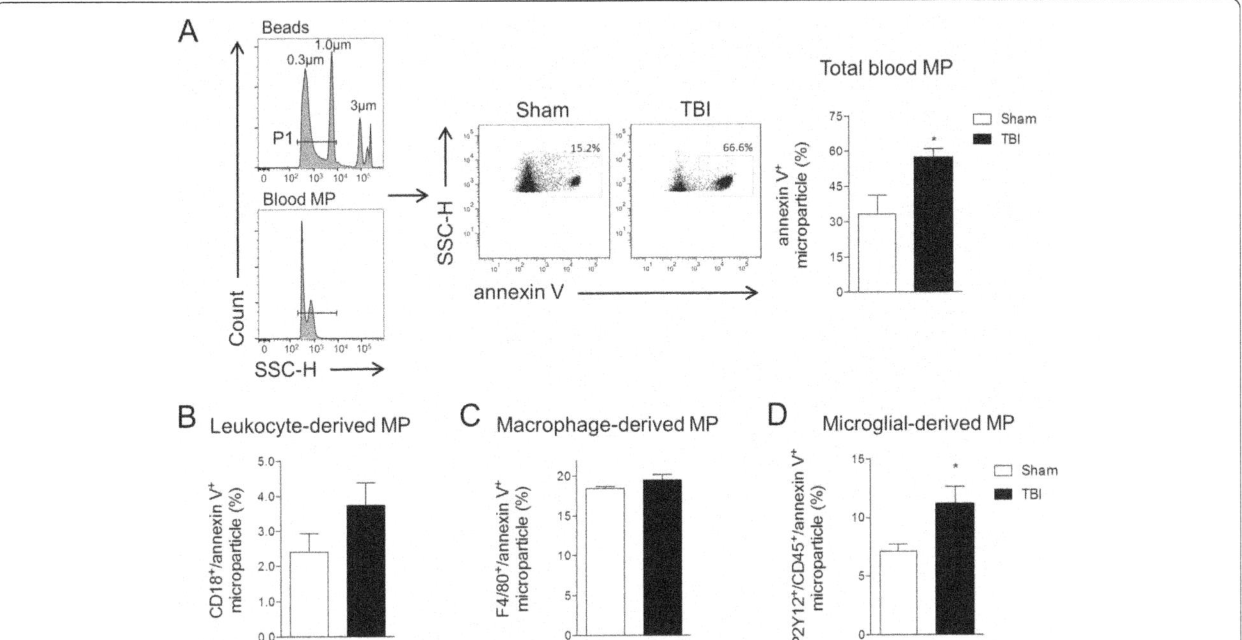

Fig. 1 Microglial-derived MP are increased in the blood following TBI. Flow cytometry analysis of enriched MP in the blood from sham and TBI mice at 24 h post-injury. **a** Representation of gating strategy used to characterize MP using SSC-H and standard microbeads (300- to 1000-nm diameter). Standard microbeads (P1 gated population) were used as an internal control to determine the size of MP in the blood, and annexin V staining confirmed MP characteristics. At 24 h post-injury, total blood MP is increased in TBI mice compared with sham-injured mice. **b** Measurements of leukocyte-derived (CD18), macrophage-derived (F4/80), and microglial-derived (P2Y12/CD45) MP in the blood from sham and TBI mice at 24 h post-injury. Microglial-derived MP are significantly increased in TBI mice when compared with sham-injured mice (*$p < 0.5$ vs sham; Student's *t* test; $n = 6$/group). *Bars* represent mean ± standard error of the mean (S.E.M.). Data represent results of three independent experiments

Total and cell-derived MP were identified by flow cytometry using an eight-color, triple-laser MACSQuant Analyzer (Miltenyi Biotec, Auburn, CA). MACSQuant was calibrated every other day with calibration beads (Miltenyi Biotec, Auburn, CA), and forward and side scatters were set at logarithmic gain. Photomultiplier tube voltage and triggers were optimized to detect submicron-sized particles. Microbeads of different diameters (0.3 μm (Sigma; LB3), 1.09 μm (Spherotech, Lake Forest, IL; BCP-10-5), and 3.0 μm (Spherotech, Lake Forest, IL; BP-30-5)) were used to set initial parameters and to confirm MP characteristics in each experiment. To reduce small particle contaminants, all reagents and solutions used for MP analysis were sterile and filtered (0.1-μm filter; EMD Millipore, Billerica, MA) before use. The expression of phosphatidylserine (PS) on MP was detected using an anti-annexin V (FITC or APC) (1:50, BD Biosciences PharMingen, catalog no: 556419) in annexin buffer (5 mM KCl, 1 mM $MgCl_2$, 136 mM NaCl, 2 mM $CaCl_2$, 1% BSA; pH 7.4). MP were incubated with antibodies for 30 min at room temperature (RT) in the dark. Annexin buffer (150 μl) was added to each sample prior to MACSQuant analysis. True-negative controls were established by a fluorescence-minus-one analysis and using isotype-matched irrelevant antibodies at the same concentration and under the same conditions. Annexin V-positive particles with diameters from 300 to 1000 nm were defined as MP. Blood MP were further characterized by double labeling with specific cell-specific antibodies: leukocytes (anti-CD18 (PE); 1:50, Biolegend; catalog no: 101408) and monocyte/macrophages (anti-F4/80 (APC); 1:50, Thermo Fisher, catalog no: MF48005). Microglial staining was performed using anti-P2Y12 (1:1000, AnaSpec Inc., Fremont, CA) and anti-CD45-PerCP (1:10, Miltenyi Biotec, Auburn, CA) as follows: MP were incubated with anti-P2Y12 in annexin buffer for 1 h at RT, washed and incubated with Alexa Fluor 488 goat anti-rabbit secondary antibodies (1:500; Life Technologies) for 30 min, washed and further incubated with pre-conjugated anti-CD45 for 30 min at RT, and washed in annexin buffer prior to analysis by flow cytometry. FlowJo software (Vx; Tree Star, Inc., Ashland, OR) was used for analysis, and data are presented as percent of annexin V-positive MP in the MP gate as set by microbeads, unless otherwise specified.

In vitro MP analysis

BV2 microglia (murine microglial cell line) were cultured in DMEM (Invitrogen, Carlsbad, CA) supplemented with 10% fetal equine serum (HyClone, Logan, UT), and 1% penicillin and streptomycin (Invitrogen) at 37 °C with 5% CO_2. DMEM media was filtered using 0.1-μm filters. BV2 microglia were seeded at a density of 0.6×10^6 in 60-mm dishes and stimulated with lipopolysaccharide (LPS, 20 ng/ml; Sigma-Aldrich) or control media for 24 h. MP released into conditioned BV2 microglial media were characterized using a MACSQuant flow cytometer (Miltenyi Biotec, San Diego, CA) analysis as described before. In parallel experiments, MP in conditioned media were pelleted by centrifugation as described before and MP-enriched pellets were either resuspended in RIPA buffer (Teknova, Hollister, CA) for Western blotting or extracted using TRIzol reagent (Invitrogen) for RNA analysis. In another experiment, BV2 microglia cells were stained with 1 μM calcein AM (Invitrogen) in DMEM for 30 min at 37 °C and then stimulated with LPS (20 ng/ml) for 24 h. Calcein AM-labeled MP were isolated from conditioned media by centrifugation at 100,000×*g* for 60 min at 4 °C [23–30] and were stained with anti-annexin V (APC) (1:50, BD Biosciences PharMingen, catalog no: 550474) for MP characterization by flow cytometry as described before.

Levels of endotoxin (LPS) in pelleted MP from control and LPS-stimulated BV2 microglia were determined using a LAL Chromogenic Endotoxin assay (Thermo Fisher Scientific, MA, USA) as per manufacturer's instructions. A standard curve was used to determine the concentration of endotoxin in each sample. Endotoxin levels are expressed as endotoxin unit per milliliter (EU/ml).

MP co-culture studies

BV2 microglia were seeded at a density of 0.6×10^6 in 60-mm dishes and stimulated with LPS (20 ng/ml) or control media for 24 h. MP released into conditioned BV2 microglial media were isolated by centrifugation as described before. Control and LPS-stimulated MP (total 8×10^5 MP) were co-cultured with BV2 microglia (2×10^4/96 well) or primary microglia (1×10^5/96 well) that were obtained from postnatal day 1 C57BL/6 mouse pups as previously described [31] for 24 h at 37 °C and at 5% CO_2 prior to cell extraction using TRIzol reagent (Invitrogen) to assess markers of microglial activation.

MP isolation from CD11b-positive cells from the sham and TBI cortex

Magnetic bead-conjugated anti-CD11b and MACS separation technology (Miltenyi Biotec, Auburn, CA) was used to isolate microglia/macrophages from sham and TBI brain tissue of C57BL/6J mice at 7 days post-injury ($n = 5$/group; study 2 above). Briefly, ipsilateral cortical and hippocampal tissues were rapidly microdissected, and a single cell suspension was prepared using enzymatic digestion (Neural Tissue Dissociation Kit; Miltenyi Biotec) in combination with a gentle MACS dissociator. Myelin was removed using Myelin Removal Beads II and LS columns (Miltenyi Biotec), and the cells were incubated with anti-CD11b microbeads (Miltenyi Biotec) and loaded onto MS columns (Miltenyi Biotec) placed in the magnetic field of a MACS separator. The negative fraction (flow through) was collected, and the column was washed three times with MACS buffer (Miltenyi Biotech). CD11b-positive cells were eluted by removing the magnetic field, resulting in the isolation of approximately 93% viable CD11b-positive cells from sham and TBI mice [32]. Expression level of CD11b-positive selected cells (MFI) was quantified by flow cytometry using anti-CD11b (APC) (1:50; Miltenyi Biotech, catalog no: 130-091-241). CD11b-positive cells were subsequently seeded at 1×10^5 cells/well in a 96-well plate in DMEM-F12 containing 10% fetal calf serum and incubated at 37 °C under 5% CO_2 for 24 h. Ex vivo-secreted MP from sham and TBI CD11b-positive cells were collected from condition media by ultra centrifugation as described before.

Intracortical injection of enriched MP

Study 1

Enriched MP were isolated from conditioned media of control and LPS (20 ng/ml)-stimulated BV2 microglia as described before. To neutralize the effects of MP, additional groups of control and LPS-stimulated MP were incubated with polyethylene glycol telomere B (PEG-TB; 6 µl per 100 µl media) for 1 h at RT as previously described [25]. MP were resuspended in 100 µl artificial CSF (Na 150, K 3.0, Ca 1.4, Mg 0.8, P 1.0, Cl 155 (mM); Harvard Apparatus, Holliston, MA, catalog no: 59-7316), and 1 µl (total 8×10^3 MP) was injected intracortically into C57BL/6 mice ($n = 6$) at stereotactic coordinates of 2.0 mm anteroposterior, 1.0 mm mediolateral to the bregma, and 1.0 mm below the pia using a 33-gauge sharp needle attached to a 10-µl Hamilton syringe (Hamilton Medical, Reno, NV, USA) and an injection rate of 1 µl/10 min. The needle remained in situ for 5 min to prevent backflow before being withdrawn slowly over 10 min. Twenty-four hours later, the mice were euthanized and cortical tissue was collected using TRIzol reagent (Invitrogen) to assess markers of cortical neuroinflammation.

Study 2

MP were isolated from conditioned media of control and LPS (20 ng/ml)-stimulated BV2 microglia as described before, and 1 µl MP (total 8×10^3 MP) were injected intracortically into C57BL/6 mice ($n = 4$) as described in study 1 above. Seven days later, mice were euthanized and the brains were removed to assess markers of microglial activation using histology.

Study 3

MP isolated from culture media of CD11b-positive cells from sham and TBI brain as described above were resuspended in 100 µl artificial CSF (Harvard Apparatus), and 1 µl MP (total 8×10^3 MP) were injected intracortically into C57BL/6 mice ($n = 4$) as described above. Twenty-four hours later, the mice were euthanized and cortical tissue was collected using TRIzol reagent (Invitrogen) to assess markers of cortical neuroinflammation.

Real-time PCR

Total RNA including miR was extracted from snap-frozen tissue, cells, or enriched MP, using a miRNeasy mini isolation kit (Qiagen, Valencia, CA). Complementary DNA (cDNA) synthesis was performed on 1 µg of total RNA using a Verso cDNA RT kit (Thermo Scientific, Pittsburg, PA), as per manufacturer's instructions. For messenger RNA (mRNA) analysis, real-time PCR was performed using TaqMan gene expression assays on an ABI 7900 HT FAST Real-Time PCR machine (Applied Biosystems). Gene expression was calculated relative to the endogenous control sample (GAPDH) to determine relative expression values ($2^{-\Delta\Delta Ct}$, where Ct is the threshold cycle). For miR analysis, a total of 10 ng of total RNA was reverse transcribed using TaqMan miRNA Reverse Transcription Kit (Applied Biosystems) with miR-specific primer of miR-155 and control U6. Reverse transcription reaction products (1.5 µl) were used for qPCR as described above. Following real-time PCR, miR expression was calculated relative to the endogenous control sample (U6) to determine relative expression values ($2^{-\Delta\Delta Ct}$, where Ct is the threshold cycle).

Western blotting

Proteins were extracted using RIPA buffer (Teknova, Hollister, CA), equalized, and loaded equally onto 5–20% gradient gels for SDS PAGE (Bio-Rad; Hercules, CA). Proteins were transferred onto nitrocellulose membranes and blocked overnight in 5% milk in 1x PBS containing 0.01% Tween-20 (PBS-T). The membrane was incubated in rabbit anti-interleukin-1β (anti-IL-1β) (1:1000; Cell Signaling, catalog no: sc-7884) and mouse anti-β-actin (1:20,000; Sigma, catalog no: A1978) overnight at 4 °C, then washed three times in PBS-T for 5 min, and incubated in appropriate HRP-conjugated secondary antibodies (Jackson Immuno Research Laboratories, West Grove, PA) for 1 h at RT. Membranes were washed three times in PBS-T, and proteins were visualized using Super Signal West Dura Extended Duration Substrate (Thermo Scientific, Rockford, IL). Chemiluminescence was captured using ChemiDoc TM XRS+ System (Bio-Rad; Hercules, CA), and protein bands were quantified by densitometric analysis using Image J (NIH, Bethesda, MD). The data reflects the intensity of the target protein band normalized based on the intensity of the endogenous control for each sample (expressed in arbitrary units).

Protein from cells was normalized to β-actin, and protein from MP was normalized to Ponceau-S.

Immunofluorescence imaging

Twenty-micrometer coronal brain sections from −1.70 mm from the bregma were selected, and standard immunostaining techniques were employed. Briefly, 20-μm sections were washed three times with 1x PBS, blocked for 1 h in goat serum containing 0.4% Triton X-100, and incubated overnight at 4 °C with primary antibody (rabbit anti-P2Y12 (1:1000, AnaSpec Inc., Fremont, CA; catalog no: AS-55043A), rabbit anti-Iba-1 (1:200; Wako Chemicals, Richmond, VA; catalog no: 019-197)). Sections were washed three times with 1x PBS and incubated with appropriate Alexa Fluor-conjugated secondary antibodies (Life Technologies) for 2 h at RT. Sections were washed three times with 1x PBS, counterstained with 4′,6-diamidino-2-phenylindole (DAPI; 1 μg/ml, Sigma), and mounted with glass cover slips using Hydromount solution (National Diagnostics, Atlanta, GA). Images were acquired using a fluorescent Nikon Ti-E inverted microscope, at ×10 (Plan Apo 10× NA 0.45) or ×20 (Plan APO 20× NA 0.75) magnification. Exposure times were kept constant for all sections in each experiment. All images were quantified using Nikon ND-Elements Software (AR 4.20.01). 6000–10,000 positive areas were quantified per mouse per experiment, and expression levels were expressed as binary area per region of interest (ROI) × 10^6.

Assessment of microglial morphology

Neurolucida software (MBF Biosciences, Williston, VT) was used to quantify cell body area and ramification length of P2Y12-positive microglia in the cortex, hippocampus, and thalamus of enriched MP intracortical injected mice as previously described [33]. Immunostained microglia were outlined using the live image setting so that the width of the ramified branches could be traced while focusing on the section. Cell bodies were outlined using the contour tool followed by tracing of the individual ramification using the dendrite line tool. Microglial ramification length is expressed in micrometers,, and cell body area is expressed in square millimeters.

Statistical analysis

Randomization and blinding protocols were employed, and individuals performing in vitro and in vivo analysis were blinded to isolated MP groups. Quantitative data were expressed as mean ± standard errors of the mean (S.E.M.). qPCR and flow cytometry data were analyzed by one-way ANOVA, followed by post hoc adjustments using a Student-Newman-Keuls test. Remaining data were analyzed using Student's t test. Statistical analyses were performed using GraphPad Prism Program, Version 3.02 for Windows (GraphPad Software, San Diego, CA, USA). A $p < 0.05$ was considered statistically significant.

Results

Microglia-derived microparticles are released into circulation following TBI

C57BL/6 male mice were subjected to TBI (moderate-level CCI) or sham surgery, and 24 h later, animals were euthanized and blood was collected for MP isolation and characterization. Ipsilateral cortical tissue was also collected to assess markers of brain inflammation. MP in blood were measured by flow cytometry for annexin V, which binds the externalized phosphatidylserine (PS) present on the surface of MP. To exclude the presence of annexin V-positive apoptotic bodies (>1000 nm) and smaller exosomes (<100 nm) in the sample, microbead standards (300, 1000, and 3000 nm) were used to gate on MP (MP gate set between 300 and 1000 nm) (Fig. 1a). There was a significant increase in annexin V-positive MP in the blood of TBI mice when compared to sham-injured controls ($p < 0.05$; Fig. 1a).

We next evaluated the origin of the circulating MP based on unique markers derived from parental cells. P2Y12/CD45-positive MP (microglial derived) were significantly increased in the circulation when compared to sham-injured control levels ($p < 0.05$; Fig. 1b). The CD18-positive MP (leukocyte derived) increase after TBI did not reach statistical significance, and TBI did not increase levels of F4/80-positive MP (monocyte derived) in the circulation at 24 h post-injury. These data indicate that microglial-derived MP are released into the circulation after moderate-level TBI.

Assessment of injured cortical tissue revealed a robust neuroinflammatory response to TBI, with increased mRNA expression of markers of microglial activation and the induction of pro-inflammatory cytokines and chemokines. Specifically, TBI resulted in a significant increase in mRNA for CD11b ($p < 0.01$), nitric oxide synthase 2 (NOS2, $p < 0.01$), interleukin-1β (IL-1β, $p < 0.05$), tumor necrosis factor-alpha (TNF-α, $p < 0.001$), C-C motif chemokine ligand 2 (CCL2, $p < 0.01$), interleukin-6 (IL-6, $p < 0.001$), pro-inflammatory microRNA-155 (miR-155, $p < 0.05$), and the purinergic receptor P2X7 ($p < 0.05$) when compared to the sham-injured group (Fig. 2a). Histological assessment of P2Y12 expression on microglia in the ipsilateral cortex revealed that the following moderate TBI P2Y12-positive microglia transform from a ramified morphological state to an activated state that withdrew branched processes to form thick bundles around highly enlarged cell bodies (Fig. 2b). Further, Neurolucida reconstruction analysis of P2Y12-positive cells demonstrated that ramification length was significantly decreased ($p < 0.01$) and cell body area was

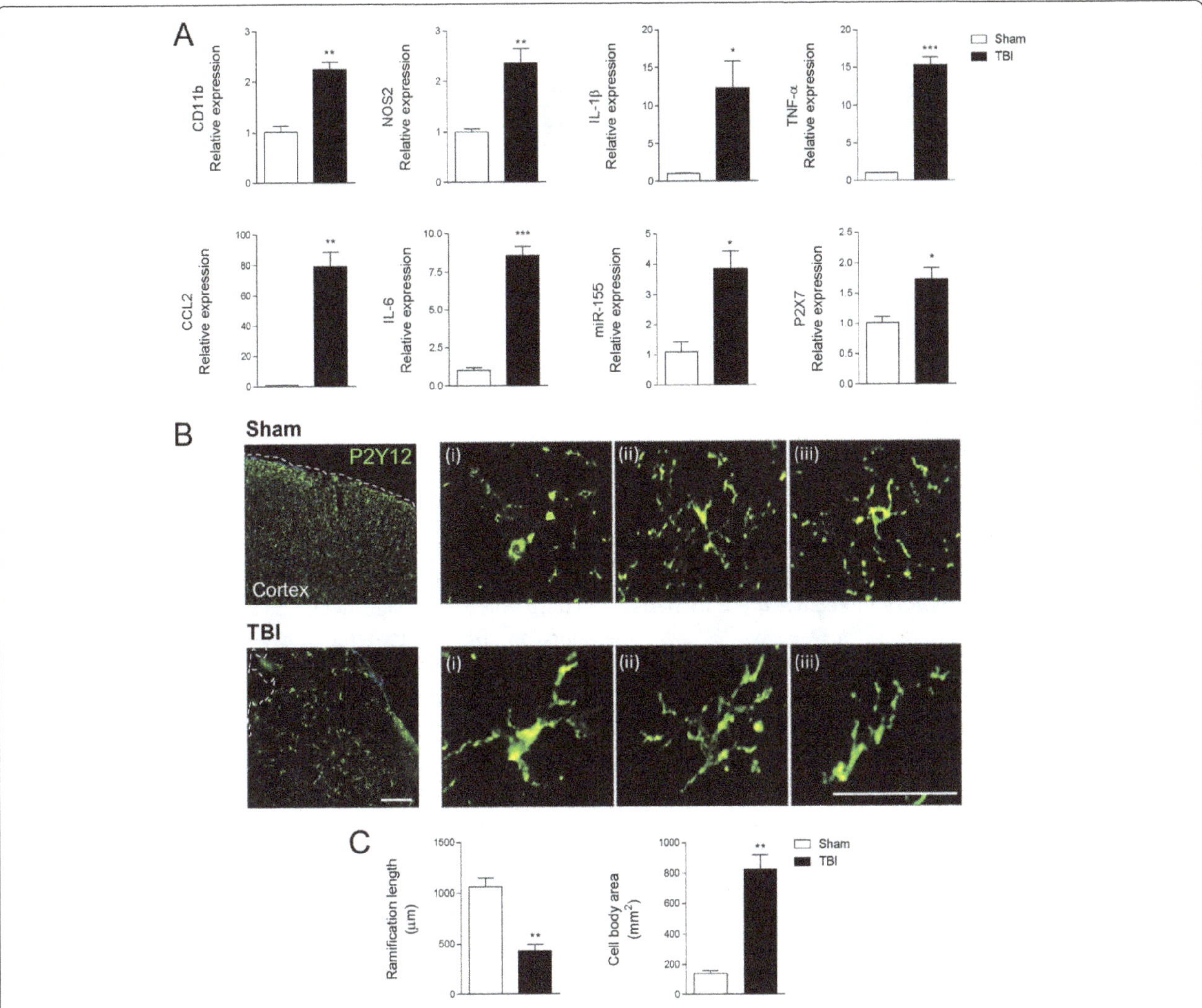

Fig. 2 Microglial activation in the TBI brain at 24 h post-injury. **a** Gene expression analysis of microglia activation in the cortex of sham and TBI mice at 24 h post-injury. Microglial receptors (CD11b, P2X7) and pro-inflammatory mediators (NOS2, IL-1β, TNF-α, CCL2, IL-6, and miR-155) were significantly increased in the injured cortex at 24 h post-injury (*$p < 0.05$, **$p < 0.01$, and ***$p < 0.001$ vs sham-injured; Student's *t* test; $n = 6$/group). **b** Immunofluorescence imaging for P2Y12-positive microglia in the cortex of sham and TBI mice at 24 h post-injury. Following TBI P2Y12-positive microglia transformed from a ramified morphology in sham to activated morphology displaying enlarged cell body, and thicker, and shorter, projections. Representative images taken at −2.06 mm from the bregma. *Scale bar* = 50 µm. **c** Morphological analysis of P2Y12-positive microglia using 3D-reconstruction Neurolucida software. When compared to sham-injured controls, P2Y12-positive microglia in the TBI cortex had reduced ramification length (**$p < 0.01$; Student's *t* test) and an enlarged cell body area (**$p < 0.01$; Student's *t* test; $n = 6$/group). *Bars* represent mean ± S.E.M.

significantly increased ($p < 0.01$) in microglia in the TBI cortex as compared to sham-injured cortex (Fig. 2c).

TBI-induced circulating microparticles activate microglia in vitro

To examine if circulating MP released after TBI could promote inflammation, we co-cultured BV2 microglia in the presence or absence of enriched MP from the blood of sham-injured and TBI mice (Fig. 3). Equal number of circulating enriched MP from sham and TBI blood (total 8×10^5) were incubated with naive BV2 microglia for 24 h, and subsequent activation was assessed by mRNA expression of selected microglial activation markers. When compared to BV2 microglia treated with sham circulating enriched MP, there was a significant increase in IL-1β ($p < 0.01$) and CCL2 ($p < 0.05$) in recipient microglia co-cultured with TBI circulating enriched MP (Fig. 3) and a trend towards increased in IL-6 and NOS2 expression in this group. There was also a significant increase in P2X7 ($p < 0.05$) in recipient microglia treated with TBI circulating enriched MP when compared to naïve microglia. There was no difference in expression of other pro-inflammatory molecules such as TNF-α and miR-155.

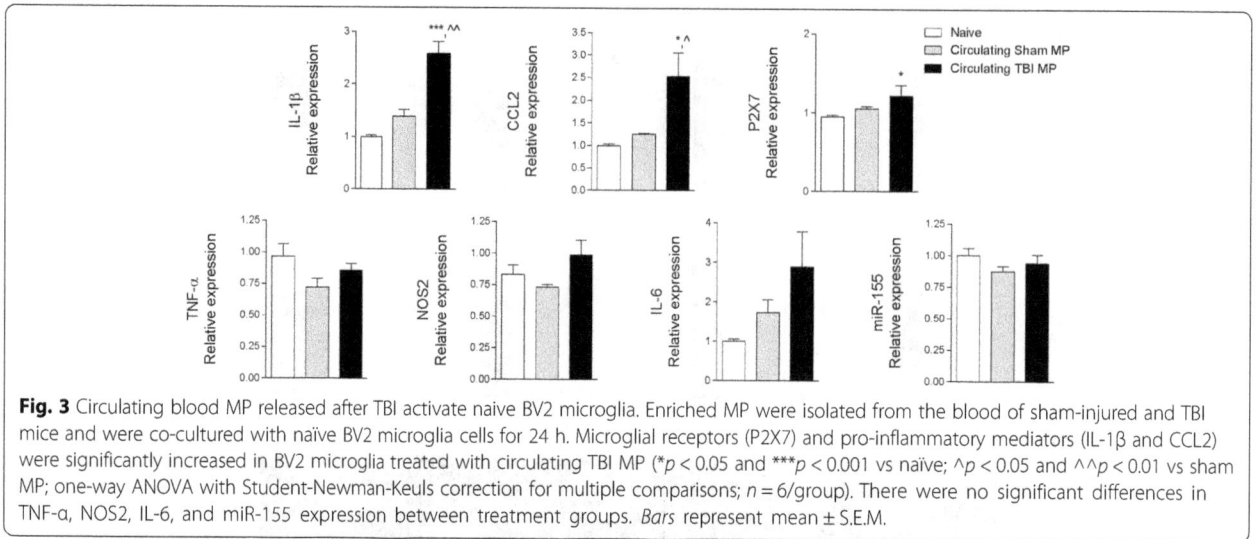

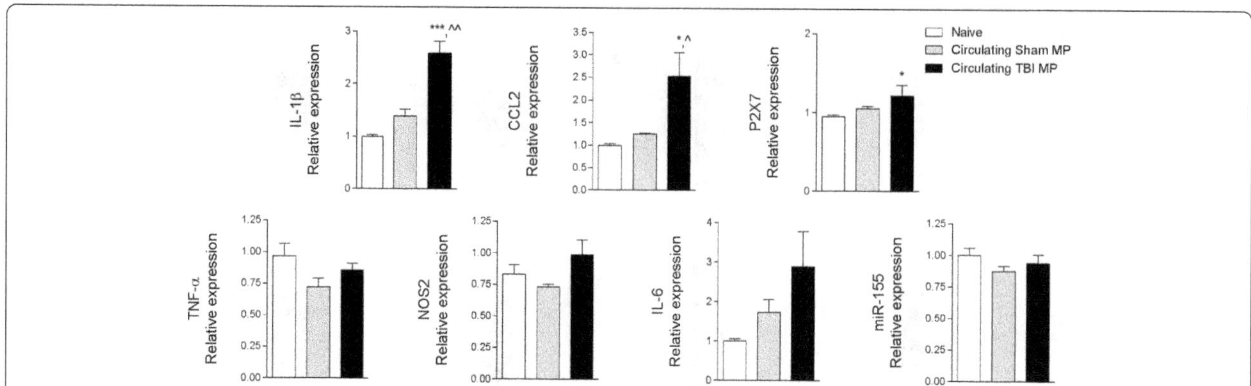

Fig. 3 Circulating blood MP released after TBI activate naive BV2 microglia. Enriched MP were isolated from the blood of sham-injured and TBI mice and were co-cultured with naïve BV2 microglia cells for 24 h. Microglial receptors (P2X7) and pro-inflammatory mediators (IL-1β and CCL2) were significantly increased in BV2 microglia treated with circulating TBI MP (*$p < 0.05$ and ***$p < 0.001$ vs naïve; ^$p < 0.05$ and ^^$p < 0.01$ vs sham MP; one-way ANOVA with Student-Newman-Keuls correction for multiple comparisons; $n = 6$/group). There were no significant differences in TNF-α, NOS2, IL-6, and miR-155 expression between treatment groups. *Bars* represent mean ± S.E.M.

LPS stimulation increases microparticle release in BV2 microglia, and pro-inflammatory molecules are enriched in microparticles

We performed a MP release assay in BV2 microglia following LPS stimulation (20 ng/ml) for 24 h. MP release was quantified by flow cytometry using Calcein AM-stained BV2 microglia that were co-stained with the MP marker annexin V. When compared to MP levels in control BV2 microglia, LPS stimulation significantly increased the number of annexin V/calcein AM-positive MP ($p < 0.001$ vs control; Fig. 4a). We next measured IL-1β and miR-155 in BV2 microglial cells and isolated enriched MP from the conditioned media to determine the relative expression of pro-inflammatory mediators in MP vs cellular compartments. Following LPS stimulation, IL-1β protein was not detected in the cells, but it was significantly increased in LPS-stimulated enriched MP ($p < 0.001$ vs LPS-stimulated cells; Fig. 4b). In addition, following LPS stimulation, miR-155 was significantly increased in BV2 microglial cells ($p < 0.05$ vs control cells; Fig. 4c). Notably, miR-155 was even more highly enriched in LPS-stimulated MP ($p < 0.01$ vs LPS-stimulated cells), indicating that enriched MP contain elevated concentrations of pro-inflammatory molecules IL-1β and miR-155 following activation.

LPS-stimulated microparticles activate microglia in vitro

To test the hypothesis that enriched MP from activated microglia can seed neuroinflammation, we isolated MP from control and LPS-stimulated BV2 microglia and co-cultured them with naïve BV2 or primary microglia for 24 h prior to assessing cellular markers of activation by qPCR. When compared to control enriched-MP-treated recipient BV2 microglia, there was a significant increase in IL-1β ($p < 0.001$), TNF-α ($p < 0.001$), CCL2 ($p < 0.001$), IL-6 ($p < 0.01$), and NOS2 ($p < 0.001$) mRNA in recipient BV2 microglia treated with LPS enriched MP (Fig. 5a). There was also a significant increase in miR-155 expression in BV2 microglia ($p < 0.001$) treated with LPS enriched MP when compared to cells treated with control MP (Fig. 5a).

To demonstrate the specific activity of microglial-derived enriched MP in activating microglia in these experiments, we neutralized MP by co-incubating them with polyethylene glycol telomere B (PEG-TB), a surfactant that depletes MP without activating blood immune cells [25]. To establish the dose of PEG-TB required to neutralize microglial-derived MP, we performed a dose response study in control and LPS-stimulated enriched MP derived from BV2 microglia and incubated them with increasing concentrations of PEG-TB for 1 h prior to MP characterization by flow cytometry. We determined that 6 μl PEG-TB/100 μl significantly depleted MP levels under both conditions (Fig. 5b), and this concentration was employed to neutralize microglial-derived MP activity in in vitro studies. Next, we determined that when LPS enriched MP were neutralized by PEG-TB and co-cultured with naïve BV2 microglia for 24 h, markers of microglial activation were significantly reduced. Specifically, recipient BV2 microglia incubated with LPS MP + PEG-TB had significantly reduced expression of IL-1β ($p < 0.001$) and TNF-α ($p < 0.001$) when compared to the LPS MP group (Fig. 5c). We confirmed the effects of LPS-stimulated enriched MP on primary cortical microglia. There was a significant increase in IL-1β ($p < 0.01$), TNF-α ($p < 0.01$), and IL-6 ($p < 0.05$) mRNA in recipient primary microglia treated with LPS enriched MP when compared to control MP-treated cells (Fig. 6). There was also a significant increase in miR-155 expression in primary microglia ($p < 0.01$) treated with LPS enriched MP when compared to cells treated with control MP (Fig. 6).

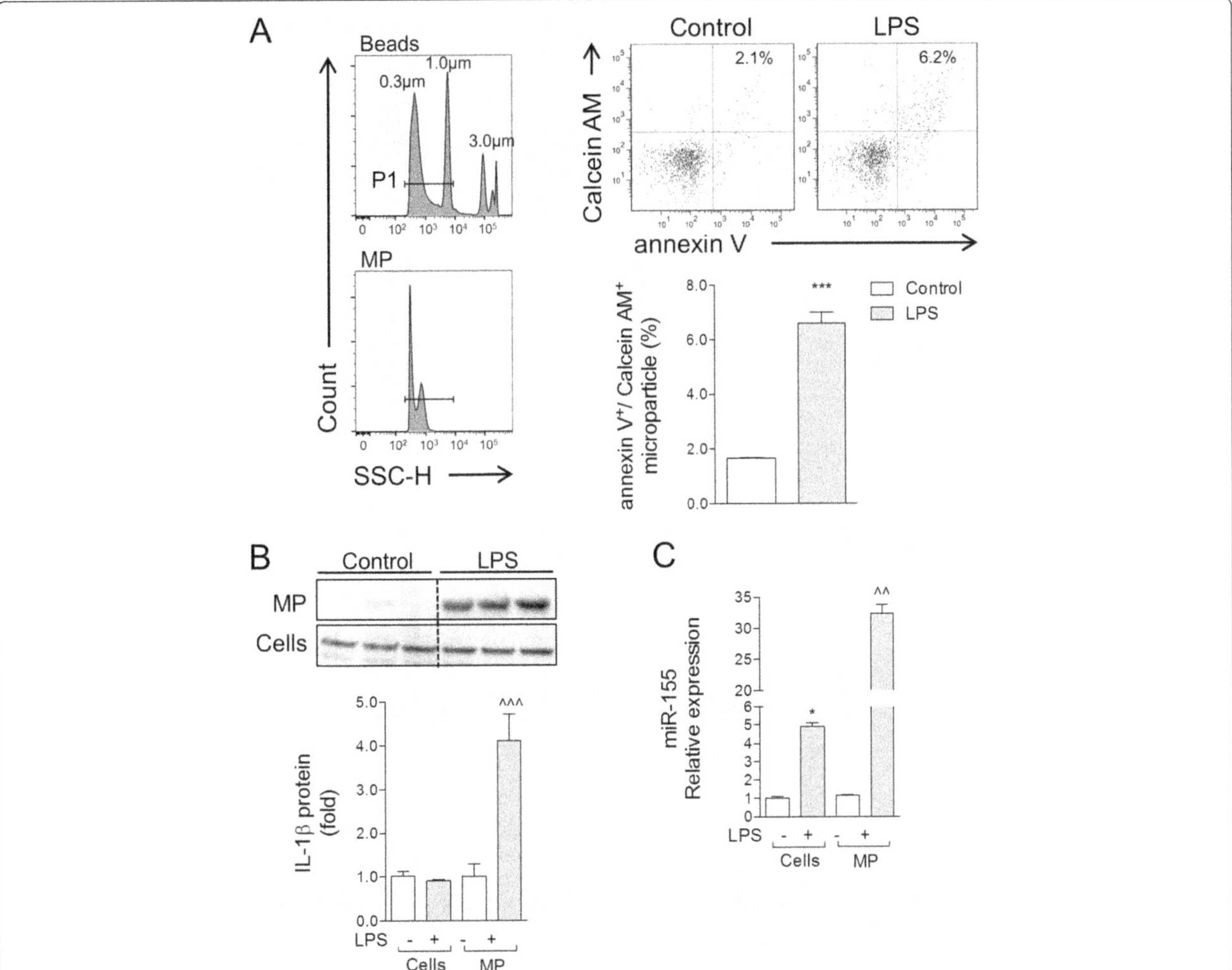

Fig. 4 Pro-inflammatory mediators are enriched in MP following lipopolysaccharide stimulation of BV2 microglia. **a** Calcein AM-stained BV2 microglia were stimulated with LPS (20 ng/ml) for 24 h, and MP were isolated by differential centrifugation and stained with anti-annexin V, prior to characterization by flow cytometry. When compared to MP levels in control BV2 microglia, LPS stimulation significantly increased the number of annexin V/calcein AM-positive MP (***$p < 0.001$ vs control; Student's *t* test; $n = 4$/group). **b** IL-1β protein expression in enriched MP vs cell lysates of control and LPS-stimulated BV2 microglia. Western blot analysis demonstrated that IL-1β protein was significantly increased in enriched MP following LPS stimulation (^^^$p < 0.001$ vs control MP; one-way ANOVA with Student-Newman-Keuls correction for multiple comparisons; $n = 3$/group). Lanes 1, 2, and 3 in both control and LPS refer to sample replicates. **c** miR-155 expression in enriched MP vs cell lysates of control and LPS-stimulated BV2 microglia. miR-155 was significantly increased in cell lysates of BV2 microglia following LPS stimulation (*$p < 0.05$ vs control cells), and its expression was elevated further in enriched MP (^^$p < 0.01$ vs control MP; one-way ANOVA with Student-Newman-Keuls correction for multiple comparisons; $n = 4$/group). *Bars* represent mean ± S.E.M. Data represent results of three independent experiments

Finally, we confirmed that the effects of LPS enriched MP on microglial activation were not due to LPS cross-over. We measured LPS levels in the LPS enriched MP samples using a limulus amebocyte lysate (LAL) assay and determined that the LPS concentration was negligible (0.081 ± 0.009 EU/ml (<0.1 ng)) and well below LPS concentrations previously shown to transfer LPS activity in enriched MP [34].

Microglial-derived microparticles can seed brain inflammation in vivo

To determine whether microglial-derived enriched MP could seed neuroinflammation in the uninjured brain, we isolated enriched MP from control and LPS-stimulated BV2 microglia and stereotactically injected them into the cortex of adult male C57BL/6 mice. As a control to demonstrate the specific activity of microglial-derived enriched MP in promoting brain inflammation, we neutralized enriched MP by co-incubating them with PEG-TB as described before. After 24 h, cortical tissue was collected and markers of brain inflammation were assessed. When LPS enriched MP were injected into the uninjured cortex, they produced a robust neuroinflammatory response resulting in a significant increase in IL-1β ($p < 0.01$), NOS2 ($p < 0.01$), TNF-α ($p < 0.001$), IL-6 ($p < 0.05$), and miR-155 ($p < 0.01$) when compared to the

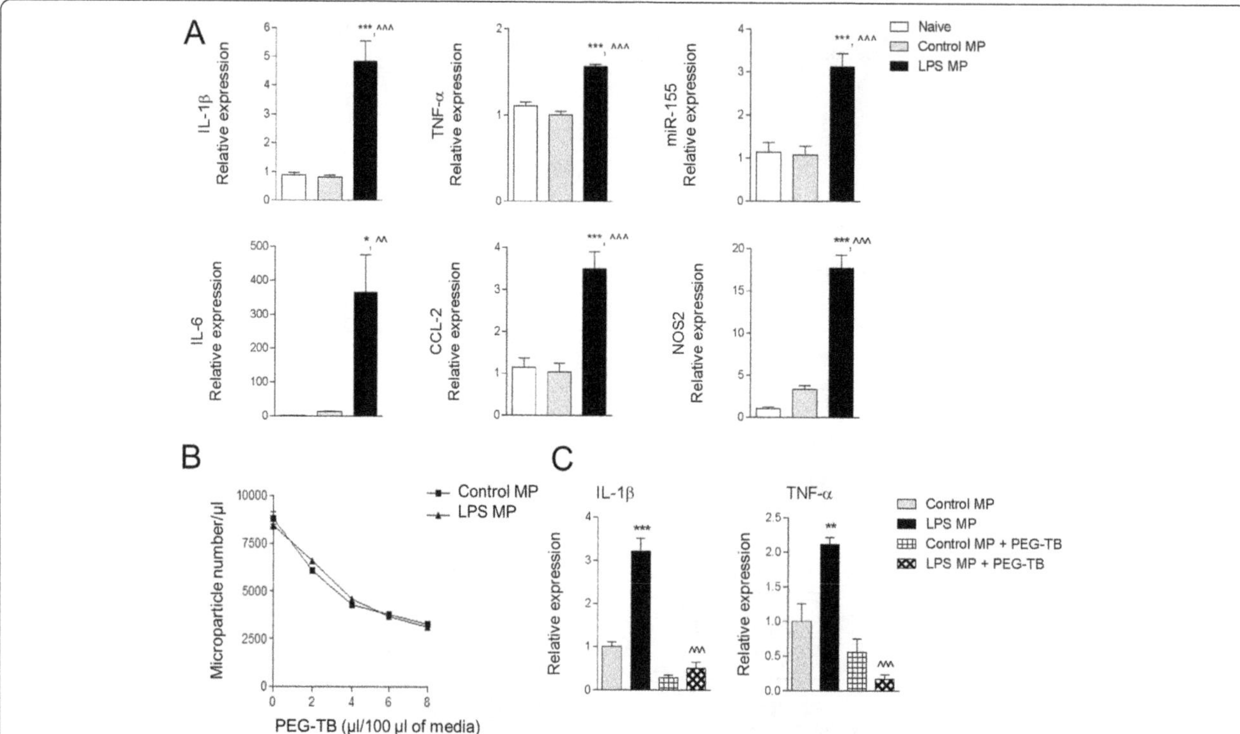

Fig. 5 Lipopolysaccharide-stimulated MP activate BV2 microglia. **a** Enriched MP were isolated from control and LPS-stimulated BV2 microglia and were co-cultured with naïve BV2 microglia for 24 h. Pro-inflammatory mediators (IL-1β, TNF-α, miR-155, IL-6, CCL2, and NOS2) were significantly increased in BV2 microglia treated with LPS MP (*$p < 0.05$ and ***$p < 0.001$ vs naïve; ^^$p < 0.01$ and ^^^$p < 0.001$ vs control MP; one-way ANOVA with Student-Newman-Keuls correction for multiple comparisons; $n = 4$/group). Data represent results of three independent experiments. **b** MP neutralization using PEG-TB. Enriched MP from control and LPS-stimulated BV2 microglia were incubated with increasing concentrations of PEG-TB for 1 h, and number of MP were quantified by flow cytometry. 6 µl PEG-TB/100 µl resulted in significant depletion of MP under both conditions. **c** Naïve BV2 microglia were co-cultured with control or LPS-stimulated MP ± PEG-TB (6 µl/100 µl) for 24 h. LPS MP treatment increased IL-1β and TNF-α in BV2 microglia (**$p < 0.01$ and ***$p < 0.001$ vs control MP), whereas co-treatment with PEG-TBI resulted in a significant decrease in IL-1β and TNF-α expression (^^^$p < 0.001$ vs LPS MP; one-way ANOVA with Student-Newman-Keuls correction for multiple comparisons; $n = 6$/group). *Bars* represent mean ± S.E.M.

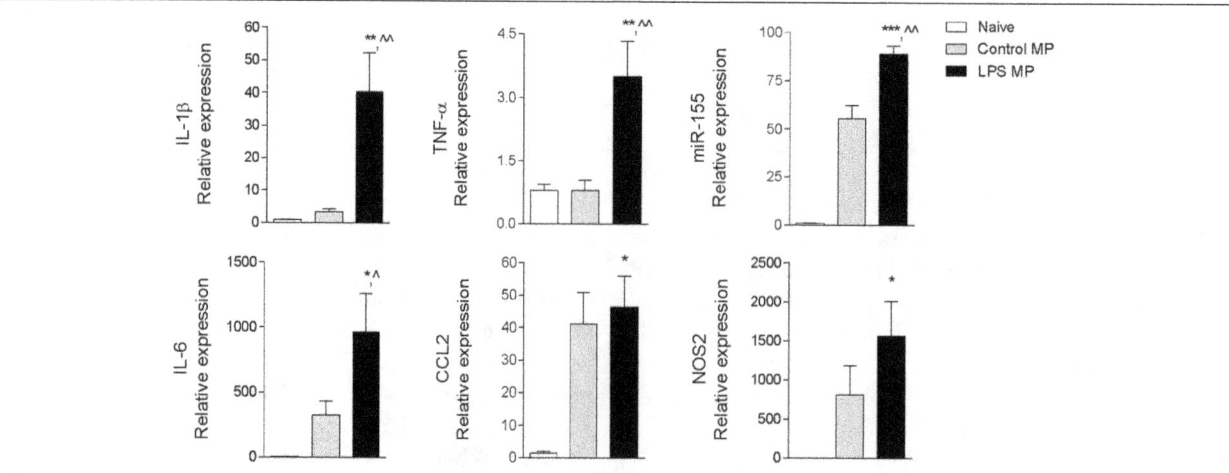

Fig. 6 Lipopolysaccharide-stimulated MP activate primary cortical microglia. Enriched MP were isolated from control and LPS-stimulated BV2 microglia and were co-cultured with primary cortical microglia for 24 h. Pro-inflammatory mediators (IL-1β, TNF-α, miR-155, IL-6, CCL2, and NOS2) were significantly increased in primary microglia treated with LPS MP (*$p < 0.05$, **$p < 0.001$, and ***$p < 0.001$ vs naïve; ^$p < 0.05$ and ^^$p < 0.01$ vs control MP; one-way ANOVA with Student-Newman-Keuls correction for multiple comparisons; $n = 5$/group). *Bars* represent mean ± S.E.M.

control MP-injected group (Fig. 7). Notably, when LPS enriched MP were neutralized by PEG-TB and injected into the uninjured cortex, the cortical neuroinflammatory response was attenuated, such that the LPS enriched MP + PEG-TB group had significantly reduced expression of IL-1β ($p < 0.001$), NOS2 ($p < 0.001$), TNF-α ($p < 0.001$), IL-6 ($p < 0.05$), and miR-155 ($p < 0.01$) when compared to the LPS enriched MP group (Fig. 7). Intracortical injection with control MP, control MP + PEG-TB, or PEG-TB alone did not promote a neuroinflammatory response in the cortex.

In a separate study, control and LPS enriched MP were stereotactically injected into the cortex of uninjured C57BL/6 mice. At 7 days post-surgery, mice were euthanized and brain tissue was saline perfused and fixed for immunohistochemical analysis of microglial activation in the cortex, hippocampus, and thalamus using Iba-1 and P2Y12 immunostaining. There was a significant increase in Iba-1 staining in the ipsilateral cortex, hippocampus, and thalamus of C57BL/6 injected with LPS enriched MP ($p < 0.001$) when compared to mice injected with control MP or sham mice (Fig. 8a–c). Further morphological analysis of P2Y12-positive microglia using Neurolucida reconstruction software revealed that C57BL/6 mice injected with LPS enriched MP resulted in increased microglial activation. Specifically, microglial ramifications were significantly reduced in length in the cortex and hippocampus of the LPS enriched-MP-injected cortex ($p < 0.01$ for both vs control MP), and the microglial cell body area was significantly increased in the cortex ($p < 0.001$), hippocampus ($p < 0.01$), and thalamus ($p < 0.01$ vs control MP; Fig. 9a–c). These data indicate that enriched MP derived from LPS-stimulated microglia produce a robust neuroinflammatory response when injected into the cortex of uninjured mice.

Microparticles produced by microglia/macrophage isolated from the TBI brain induce neuroinflammation in non-injured mice

To relate MP-mediated seeding of neuroinflammation to secondary injury mechanisms in the TBI brain, we subjected adult male C57BL/6 mice to sham or moderate-level TBI and isolated microglia/macrophages from the ipsilateral cortex at 7 days post-injury using MACS CD11b magnetic beads. We then cultured CD11b-positive cells for 24 h and collected microglia/macrophage-derived enriched MP from sham and TBI samples. Equal numbers of enriched MP (total 8×10^3 MP) were stereotactically injected into the cortex of uninjured adult male C57BL/6 mice, and cortical tissue was collected 24 h later to assess markers of neuroinflammation. Injection of sham MP significantly increased IL-1β ($p < 0.001$) and TNF-α ($p < 0.001$) expression, but not miR-155 expression, when compared to the naïve control group (Fig. 10). Furthermore, injection of TBI enriched MP significantly increased IL-1β ($p < 0.001$), TNF-α ($p < 0.05$), and miR-155 ($p < 0.01$) expression in the cortex when compared to the sham MP-injected group. Although there was a modest increase in IL-6 and NOS2 expression in sham MP and TBI enriched MP-injected groups when compared to the naïve control group, these changes did not reach statistical significance. These data indicate that enriched MP derived from the microglia/macrophages

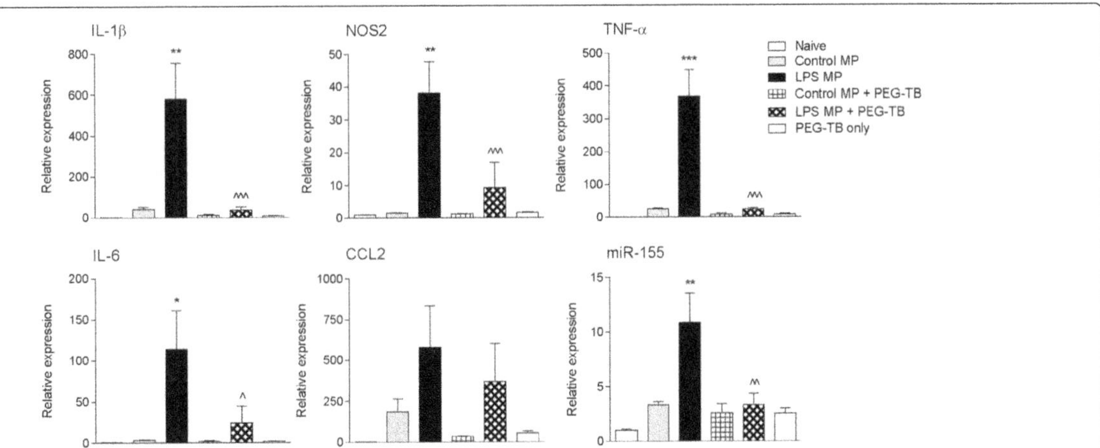

Fig. 7 Lipopolysaccharide-stimulated MP increase neuroinflammation in the cortex of uninjured mice. Enriched MP were isolated from control and LPS-stimulated BV2 microglia and were treated ± PEG-TB (6 μl/100 μl) prior to being stereotactically injected into the cortex of adult male C57BL/6 mice. Markers of cortical neuroinflammation were measured at 24 h postinjection. There was a significant increase in pro-inflammatory mediators (IL-1β, TNF-α, miR-155, IL-6, and NOS2) in the cortex of LPS MP-injected mice (**$p < 0.01$, ***$p < 0.001$ vs control MP-injected group). Neutralization of LPS MP prior to injection resulted in a significant decrease in each pro-inflammatory mediator (^$p < 0.05$, ^^$p < 0.01$, ^^^$p < 0.001$ vs LPS MP-injected group; one-way ANOVA with Student-Newman-Keuls correction for multiple comparisons; $n = 6$/group). *Bars* represent mean ± S.E.M.

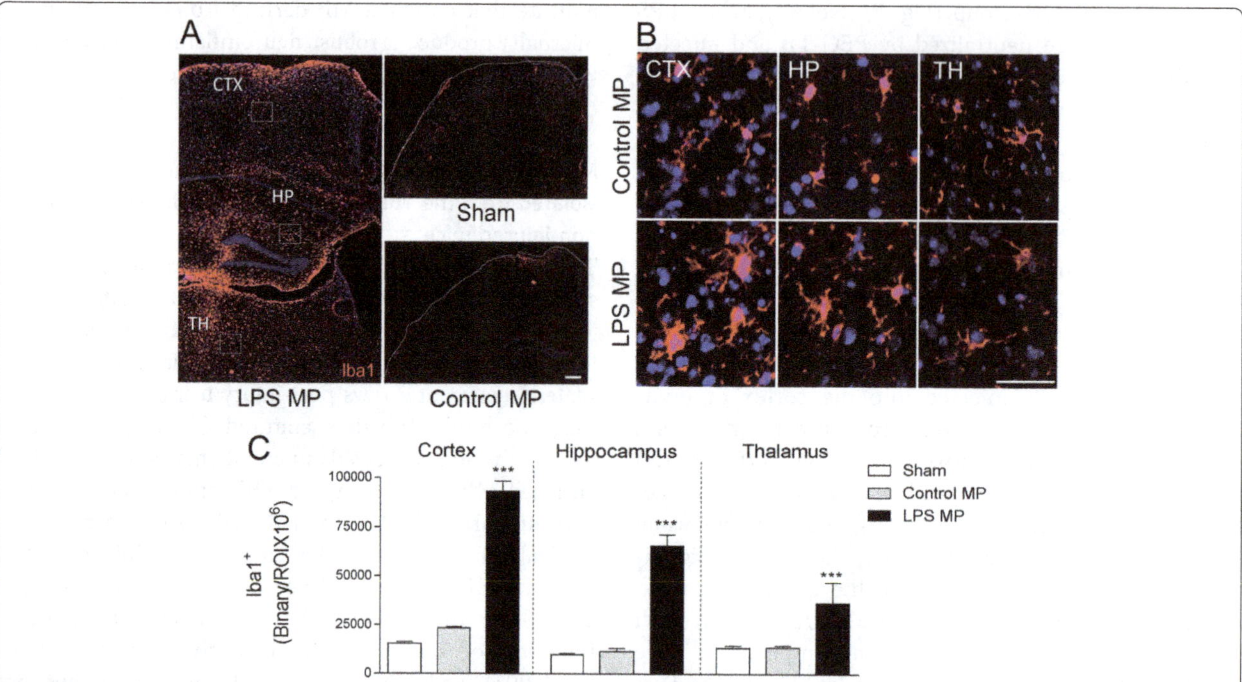

Fig. 8 Lipopolysaccharide-stimulated MP increase microglial activation in the cortex of uninjured mice. Enriched MP were isolated from control and LPS-stimulated BV2 microglia and were stereotactically injected into the cortex of adult male C57BL/6 mice. Iba-1 immunocytochemistry was performed at 7 days postinjection. **a** Representative Iba-1 staining (*red*) in the cortex (*CTX*), hippocampus (*HP*), and thalamus (*TH*). Images taken at −2.06 mm from the bregma; *scale bar* = 50 μm. **b** High-magnification images in control MP- and LPS MP-injected mice in the *CTX*, *HP*, and *TH*. LPS MP-injected Iba-1-positive microglia had enlarged cell body and thicker projection indicative of increased activation status. *Scale bar* = 100 μm. **c** Quantification of Iba-1 staining in the cortex, hippocampus, and thalamus at 7 days postinjection. There was a significant increase in Iba-1 immunoreactivity in the LPS MP-injected group when compared to the control MP-treated group (***$p < 0.001$ vs control MP; one-way ANOVA with Student-Newman-Keuls correction for multiple comparisons; $n = 4$/group). *Bars* represent mean ± S.E.M.

isolated from the TBI brain produce a robust neuroinflammatory response when injected into the uninjured cortex.

Discussion

TBI initiates complex local and systemic immune responses. However, the precise nature of posttraumatic neuroinflammation, its regulatory mechanisms, and role in secondary injury remain to be elucidated [35]. Recent studies have offered intriguing evidence regarding the potential role played by extracellular vesicles in cell-cell communication between immune cells and their targets [36, 37]. In the present study, we examined the release of microparticles (MP), a special class of extracellular vesicles, from the injured brain and their contribution to mechanisms of microglial activation and related neuroinflammation.

Although high levels of MP have been detected in the blood of TBI patients [18, 19], their cellular origins are not well defined. Clinical studies indicate that MP in the blood are primarily derived from platelets, with much smaller fractions released from erythrocytes, granulocytes, monocytes, lymphocytes, and endothelial cells [18, 19, 21, 38, 39]. Recent studies have highlighted the potential systemic pathological effects of MP following brain injury, including brain-trauma-associated coagulopathy [21]. MP released from neurons (NSE-positive MP) and astrocytes (GFAP-positive MP) accumulated in the circulation within 3 h of experimental TBI and were associated with microvascular fibrin deposition in the heart, kidney, and lung [21]. We observed a significant increase in total circulating MP at 24 h post-injury. Furthermore, an evaluation of the origin of circulating MP based on the presence of unique markers derived from parental cells revealed that microglial MP displayed the greatest increase (approximately twofold) following TBI, accounting for nearly 15% of total circulating MP. Although P2Y12 is also expressed on platelets [40], the detected P2Y12-positive MP were co-stained with CD45, a unique myeloid cell marker that is not expressed on platelets [41, 42], indicating that the P2Y12-positive MP enriched in the circulation following TBI were not derived from platelets. These data indicate that microglial-derived MP are released by the TBI brain and reach the systemic circulation. Importantly, we observed robust neuroinflammatory responses in the injured brain—with activation of P2Y12-positive microglia in the cortex, hippocampus, and thalamus—associated with upregulated expression of classical pro-inflammatory mediators (IL-1β, TNF-α, CCL2, IL-6, NOS2, and miR-155) in the injured cortex.

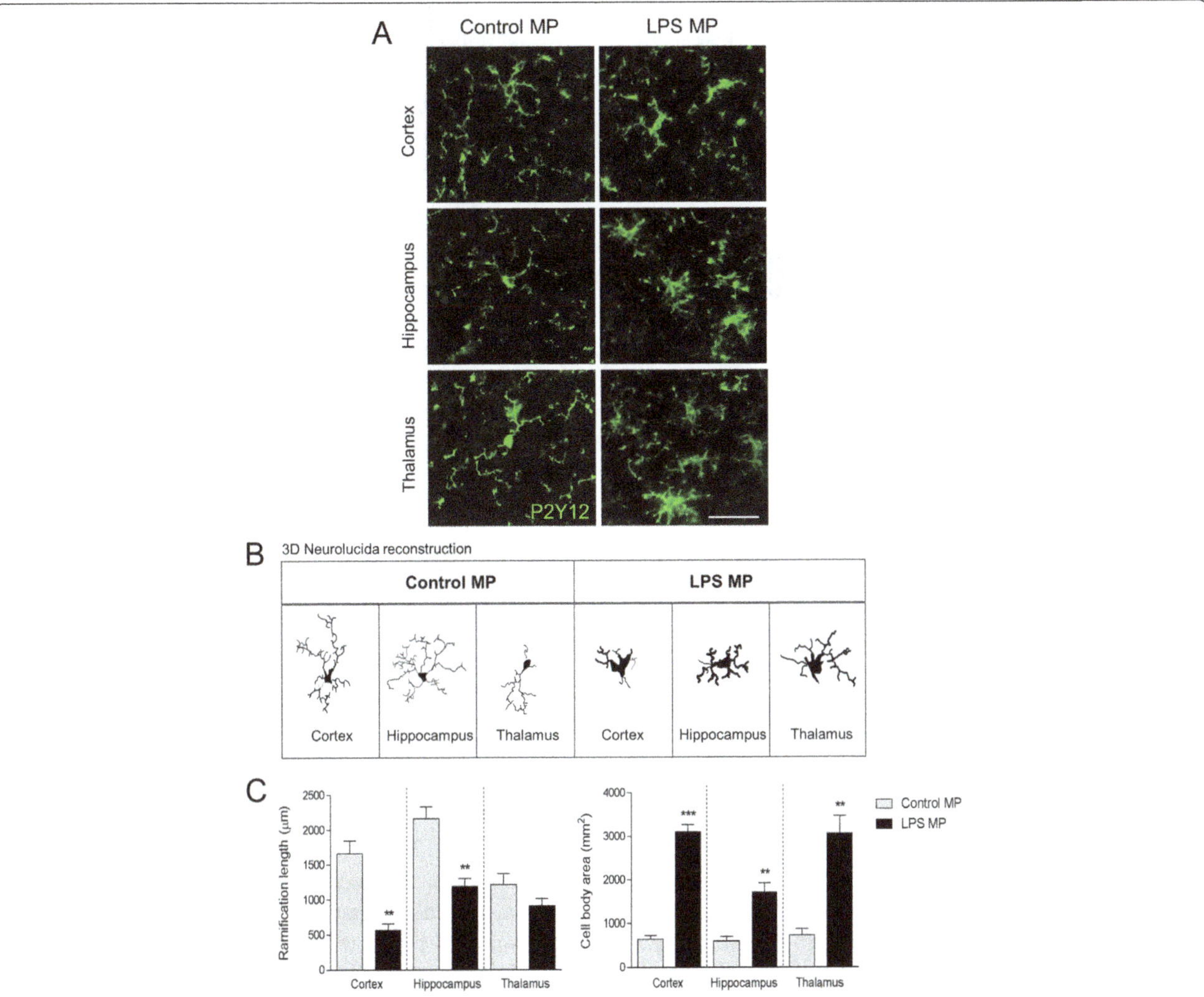

Fig. 9 Lipopolysaccharide-stimulated MP alter P2Y12 microglial morphology of the cortex of uninjured mice. Enriched MP were isolated from control and LPS-stimulated BV2 microglia and were stereotactically injected into the cortex of adult male C57BL/6 mice. P2Y12 immunocytochemistry was performed at 7 days postinjection. **a** High-magnification images of P2Y12-positive microglia (*green*) in control MP- and LPS MP-injected mice in the cortex (CTX), hippocampus (HP), and thalamus (TH). LPS MP-injected P2Y12-positive microglia have enlarged cell body and thicker projection indicative of increased activation status. *Scale bar* = 100 µm. **b** P2Y12-positive microglia in the CTX, HP, and TH of control MP- and LPS MP-injected mice. **c** Morphological analysis of P2Y12-positive microglia using 3D-reconstruction Neurolucida software. When compared to the control MP-injected group, P2Y12-positive microglia in the LPS MP-injected group had reduced ramification length in the cortex and hippocampus ($^{**}p < 0.01$; Student's *t* test), but not in the thalamus. In addition, the LPS MP-injected group had enlarged cell body area in each region ($^{**}p < 0.01$ and $^{***}p < 0.001$ vs control MP; Student's *t* test; $n = 4$/group). *Bars* represent mean ± S.E.M.

Previous studies indicated that microglia and other myeloid cells in vitro can shed MP, which store and release pro-inflammatory molecules such as IL-1β [43], inflammasome components, and MHCII protein [44]. These data suggest that MP produced by reactive myeloid cells, such as microglia, may propagate inflammation and the rapid dissemination and presentation of antigens. A major finding of our study was that circulating enriched MP from TBI mice significantly activated recipient microglia in vitro and up-regulated pro-inflammatory signaling molecules such as IL-1β and CCL2.

Similarly, MP from LPS-stimulated BV2 microglia significantly increased IL-1β, TNF-α, CCL2, IL-6, NOS2, and miR-155 expression in recipient BV2 or primary microglia, confirming the ability of MP to act as independent microglial activators. LPS stimulation of microglia is an established in vitro model for TBI neuroinflammation because LPS up-regulates key pro-inflammatory mediators in microglia (IL-1β, TNF-α, NOS2, CCL2) that are robustly up-regulated in microglia/macrophages in the injured cortex and hippocampus following TBI [31, 45, 46]. In the current study, we demonstrated that LPS-stimulated microglia release MP into conditioned media that can induce pro-inflammatory responses in non-activated recipient microglial cells. Importantly, MP depleted of their content by addition of

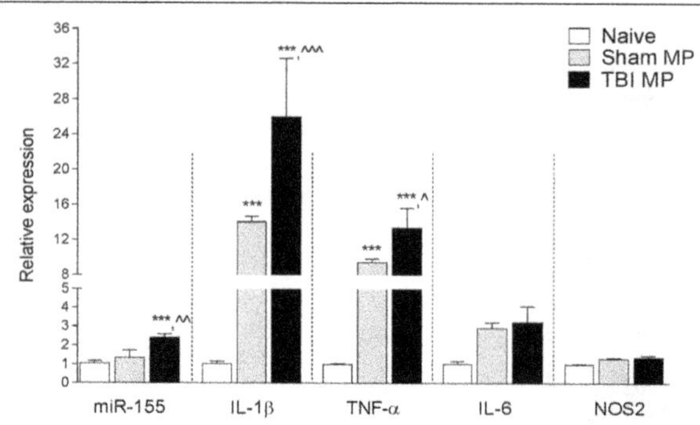

Fig. 10 MP isolated from CD11b-isolated microglia/macrophages following TBI increase neuroinflammation in the cortex of uninjured mice. CD11b-microglia/macrophages in the cortex of sham and TBI were isolated at 7 days post-injury and cultured for 24 h prior to collecting MP. Enriched MP were stereotactically injected into the cortex of adult male C57BL/6 mice and markers of cortical neuroinflammation were measured at 24 h postinjection. There was a significant increase in pro-inflammatory mediators (IL-1β and TNF-α) in the cortex of the control MP-injected group (***$p < 0.001$ vs naïve group). When compared to the control MP-injected group, there was a further significant increase in pro-inflammatory mediators (IL-1β, TNF-α, and miR-155) in the cortex of the TBI MP-injected group (^$p < 0.05$, ^^$p < 0.01$, ^^^$p < 0.001$ vs control MP-injected group; one-way ANOVA with Student-Newman-Keuls correction for multiple comparisons; $n = 5$/group). *Bars* represent mean ± S.E.M.

MP-neutralizing surfactant, PEG-TB, lost their ability to activate recipient cells, thus demonstrating the critical function of MP in promoting the pro-inflammatory response in the target cells.

We demonstrated that IL-1β and miR-155 were highly enriched in MP that can propagate a pro-inflammatory response in recipient cells. IL-1β does not contain an N-terminal signal sequence for secretion and therefore must be released from the cell through alternative mechanisms [47]. LPS stimulation increased IL-1β protein in enriched MP but not in microglia cells, where only IL-1β mRNA was elevated. Astrocyte-derived ATP has been shown to induce extracellular vesicle shedding and IL-1β release in microglia through a P2X7 receptor-dependent mechanism [43]. Notably, ATP is released following acute brain injury and promotes a powerful chemotactic response in microglia towards the site of injury [15]. In our study, the P2X7 receptor was significantly increased at sites of inflammation in the injured cortex; thus, P2X7 receptor-dependent mechanisms of MP release in microglia may be involved in the propagation of inflammation following TBI. Other mechanisms of MP release in microglia—such as MP fusion with the cell membrane, macropinocytosis [48], and direct release of their contents into the cytosol [37], as well as indirect mechanisms through binding of pattern-recognition receptors in the endosomal compartment (primarily Toll-like receptor 7/8—TLR7/8) [49]—may also contribute to the propagating neuroinflammation and warrant further investigation.

MP can also transfer miRs [50–53]. The levels of miR-155, a well-characterized pro-inflammatory miR in microglia [54], were highly enriched in microglial-derived MP. miR-155 has been shown to be a key regulator of the inflammatory response in experimental models of stroke, Parkinson's disease, amyotrophic lateral sclerosis, and multiple sclerosis [55–58]. We also demonstrated that miR-155 was significantly increased in the cortex of TBI mice, and its expression was significantly increased when LPS-stimulated MP from BV2 microglia or MP from CD11b-positive microglia/macrophages from the TBI brain were injected into the cortex of uninjured mice. Secreted miR-155 from adipocyte-derived MP in obese mice induces a pro-inflammatory activation state in macrophages that causes chronic inflammation and local insulin resistance [59]. Thus, secreted miR-155 from MP may be an important driver of neuroinflammation following TBI.

The pathogenic role of MP in the inflammatory response was demonstrated in vivo by showing that injection of microglial-derived MP induces neuroinflammation at the site of injection and at more distant sites. Cortical injection of enriched MP isolated from LPS-stimulated BV2 microglia significantly increased markers of microglial activation (Iba-1 and P2Y12 morphological transformation) in the ipsilateral cortex, hippocampus, and thalamus and upregulated pro-inflammatory markers in the cortex. These data support prior research that demonstrated that myeloid-derived microvesicles that are detected in the CSF of multiple-sclerosis patients and closely associate with disease course can propagate inflammation in vivo when injected locally [60]. Furthermore, cortical injections of enriched MP collected from ex vivo cultures of microglia/macrophages purified from TBI brain markedly induce expression of pro-inflammatory molecules miR-155, IL-1β, and TNF-α in the cortex of non-injured animals. To our knowledge, these latter observations describe the first use of purified brain microglia to demonstrate the transfer of the posttraumatic neuroinflammatory phenotype using MP as a vehicle.

It is important to recognize that the enriched MP population obtained using our experimental protocol may also contain other types of extracellular vesicles such as exosomes. In this study, we used established flow cytometry protocols to characterize MP properties [25], but this technique is limited to the identification of particles greater than 300 nm, preventing the detection of smaller microvesicles and all exosomes [61]. Electron microscopy can directly show that extracellular vesicles exist in a sample, but fixation processes involved in the technique can alter vesicle shape and size [62]. Other techniques such as dynamic light scattering and nanoparticle-tracking analyses have several limitations and introduce biases when characterizing extracellular vesicle properties [61, 63, 64]. The focus of the current study was the pathophysiological responses of microglial-derived MP rather than the nature of the enriched microvesicles. We determined that enriched MP derived from microglia could propagate neuroinflammation in vivo. We selectively depleted enriched MP by incubating them with PEG-TB, a drug that emulsifies MP without modifying circulating leukocyte activation [2, 25]. When we co-cultured depleted MP from LPS-stimulated BV2 microglia with recipient naïve BV2 microglia, or injected depleted MP into the cortex of uninjured mice, pro-inflammatory responses were significantly attenuated. These results support our hypothesis that it is the enriched MP component of purified extracellular vesicles derived from microglia that propagates neuroinflammation.

Conclusions

The major findings of these studies are that (1) microglial-derived MP are released after TBI, (2) circulating enriched MP from the TBI animals can activate microglia in vitro, (3) LPS activation increases MP release from microglia and elevates their content of pro-inflammatory mediators IL-1β and miR-155, and (4) enriched MP from activated microglia in vitro or CD11b-isolated microglia from the TBI brain ex vivo are sufficient to initiate neuroinflammation following intracortical injection in naïve animals. Given their ability to independently initiate pro-inflammatory responses, MP derived from activated microglia may provide a novel therapeutic target for TBI and other neurodegenerative disorders associated with neuroinflammation.

Abbreviations

CCI: Controlled cortical impact; CCL2: C-C motif chemokine ligand 2; IL-1β: Interleukin-1β; IL-6: Interleukin-6; miR-155: MicroRNA-155; MP: Microparticles; NOS2: Nitric oxide synthase 2; P2X7: P2X purinoceptor 7; PEG-TB: Polyethylene glycol telomere B; PS: Phosphatidylserine; SOD1: Superoxide dismutase 1; TBI: Traumatic brain injury; TNF-α: Tumor necrosis factor-alpha

Acknowledgements

We thank Dr. Boris Sabirzhanov and Dr. Junfang Wu for advice and expert technical support.
The views expressed in this article are those of the authors and do not necessarily reflect the official policy or position of the Air Force, the Department of Defense, or the US Government.

Funding

This study was supported by NIH grants R01NS037313 (A.I. Faden), R01 NS052568 (A.I. Faden), and R01NS082308 (D.J. Loane). This study was also supported by the 711 HPW/XPT under Cooperative Agreement number FA8650-15-2-6606. The funder had no role in the study design, data collection, and analysis, decision to publish, or preparation of the manuscript.

Authors' contributions

AK, BAS, DJL, SRT, and AIF designed research; AK, YM, GA, NK, and AK performed the research; AK and YM analyzed the data; AK, BAS, DJL, and AIF wrote the paper. All authors read and approved the final manuscript.

Competing interests

The authors declare that they have no competing interests.

Consent for publication

Consent for publication is not applicable for this manuscript.

Author details

[1]Department of Anesthesiology, University of Maryland School of Medicine, Baltimore, MD, USA. [2]Shock, Trauma and Anesthesiology Research (STAR) Center, University of Maryland School of Medicine, Health Sciences Facility II (HSFII), #S247 20 Penn Street, Baltimore, MD 21201, USA. [3]Department of Emergency Medicine, University of Maryland School of Medicine, Baltimore, MD, USA.

References

1. Burnier L, Fontana P, Kwak BR, Angelillo-Scherrer A. Cell-derived microparticles in haemostasis and vascular medicine. Thromb Haemost. 2009;101:439–51.
2. Bohman LE, Riley J, Milovanova TN, Sanborn MR, Thom SR, Armstead WM. Microparticles impair hypotensive cerebrovasodilation and cause hippocampal neuronal cell injury after traumatic brain injury. J Neurotrauma. 2016;33:168–74.
3. Davizon P, Munday AD, Lopez JA. Tissue factor, lipid rafts, and microparticles. Semin Thromb Hemost. 2010;36:857–64.
4. Zappulli V, Friis KP, Fitzpatrick Z, Maguire CA, Breakefield XO. Extracellular vesicles and intercellular communication within the nervous system. J Clin Invest. 2016;126:1198–207.
5. Castro-Seoane R, Hummerich H, Sweeting T, Tattum MH, Linehan JM, Fernandez de Marco M, Brandner S, Collinge J, Klohn PC. Plasmacytoid dendritic cells sequester high prion titres at early stages of prion infection. PLoS Pathog. 2012;8:e1002538.
6. Klohn PC, Castro-Seoane R, Collinge J. Exosome release from infected dendritic cells: a clue for a fast spread of prions in the periphery? J Infect. 2013;67:359–68.
7. Grad LI, Fernando SM, Cashman NR. From molecule to molecule and cell to cell: prion-like mechanisms in amyotrophic lateral sclerosis. Neurobiol Dis. 2015;77:257–65.
8. Basso M, Pozzi S, Tortarolo M, Fiordaliso F, Bisighini C, Pasetto L, Spaltro G, Lidonnici D, Gensano F, Battaglia E, et al. Mutant copper-zinc superoxide dismutase (SOD1) induces protein secretion pathway alterations and exosome release in astrocytes: implications for disease spreading and motor neuron pathology in amyotrophic lateral sclerosis. J Biol Chem. 2013;288: 15699–711.
9. Rajendran L, Honsho M, Zahn TR, Keller P, Geiger KD, Verkade P, Simons K. Alzheimer's disease beta-amyloid peptides are released in association with exosomes. Proc Natl Acad Sci U S A. 2006;103:11172–7.
10. Dinkins MB, Dasgupta S, Wang G, Zhu G, Bieberich E. Exosome reduction in vivo is associated with lower amyloid plaque load in the 5XFAD mouse model of Alzheimer's disease. Neurobiol Aging. 2014;35:1792–800.
11. Asai H, Ikezu S, Tsunoda S, Medalla M, Luebke J, Haydar T, Wolozin B, Butovsky O, Kugler S, Ikezu T. Depletion of microglia and inhibition of exosome synthesis halt tau propagation. Nat Neurosci. 2015;18:1584–93.
12. Yuyama K, Sun H, Sakai S, Mitsutake S, Okada M, Tahara H, Furukawa J, Fujitani N, Shinohara Y, Igarashi Y. Decreased amyloid-beta pathologies by intracerebral loading of glycosphingolipid-enriched exosomes in Alzheimer model mice. J Biol Chem. 2014;289:24488–98.

13. An K, Klyubin I, Kim Y, Jung JH, Mably AJ, O'Dowd ST, Lynch T, Kanmert D, Lemere CA, Finan GM, et al. Exosomes neutralize synaptic-plasticity-disrupting activity of Aβ assemblies in vivo. Mol Brain. 2013;6:47.
14. Loane DJ, Faden AI. Neuroprotection for traumatic brain injury: translational challenges and emerging therapeutic strategies. Trends Pharmacol Sci. 2010;31:596–604.
15. Davalos D, Grutzendler J, Yang G, Kim JV, Zuo Y, Jung S, Littman DR, Dustin ML, Gan WB. ATP mediates rapid microglial response to local brain injury in vivo. Nat Neurosci. 2005;8:752–8.
16. Kumar A, Loane DJ. Neuroinflammation after traumatic brain injury: opportunities for therapeutic intervention. Brain Behav Immun. 2012;26:1191–201.
17. Loane DJ, Kumar A, Stoica BA, Cabatbat R, Faden AI. Progressive neurodegeneration after experimental brain trauma: association with chronic microglial activation. J Neuropathol Exp Neurol. 2014;73:14–29.
18. Morel N, Morel O, Petit L, Hugel B, Cochard JF, Freyssinet JM, Sztark F, Dabadie P. Generation of procoagulant microparticles in cerebrospinal fluid and peripheral blood after traumatic brain injury. J Trauma. 2008;64:698–704.
19. Nekludov M, Mobarrez F, Gryth D, Bellander BM, Wallen H. Formation of microparticles in the injured brain of patients with severe isolated traumatic brain injury. J Neurotrauma. 2014;31:1927–33.
20. Andrews AM, Lutton EM, Merkel SF, Razmpour R, Ramirez SH. Mechanical injury induces brain endothelial-derived microvesicle release: implications for cerebral vascular injury during traumatic brain injury. Front Cell Neurosci. 2016;10:43.
21. Tian Y, Salsbery B, Wang M, Yuan H, Yang J, Zhao Z, Wu X, Zhang Y, Konkle BA, Thiagarajan P, et al. Brain-derived microparticles induce systemic coagulation in a murine model of traumatic brain injury. Blood. 2015;125:2151–9.
22. Loane DJ, Pocivavsek A, Moussa CE, Thompson R, Matsuoka Y, Faden AI, Rebeck GW, Burns MP. Amyloid precursor protein secretases as therapeutic targets for traumatic brain injury. Nat Med. 2009;15:377–9.
23. Yang M, Bhopale VM, Thom SR. Separating the roles of nitrogen and oxygen in high pressure-induced blood-borne microparticle elevations, neutrophil activation, and vascular injury in mice. J Appl Physiol (1985). 2015;119:219–22.
24. Thom SR, Yang M, Bhopale VM, Milovanova TN, Bogush M, Buerk DG. Intramicroparticle nitrogen dioxide is a bubble nucleation site leading to decompression-induced neutrophil activation and vascular injury. J Appl Physiol (1985). 2013;114:550–8.
25. Thom SR, Yang M, Bhopale VM, Huang S, Milovanova TN. Microparticles initiate decompression-induced neutrophil activation and subsequent vascular injuries. J Appl Physiol (1985). 2011;110:340–51.
26. Yang M, Kosterin P, Salzberg BM, Milovanova TN, Bhopale VM, Thom SR. Microparticles generated by decompression stress cause central nervous system injury manifested as neurohypophysial terminal action potential broadening. J Appl Physiol (1985). 2013;115:1481–6.
27. Xu J, Yang M, Kosterin P, Salzberg BM, Milovanova TN, Bhopale VM, Thom SR. Carbon monoxide inhalation increases microparticles causing vascular and CNS dysfunction. Toxicol Appl Pharmacol. 2013;273:410–7.
28. Thom SR, Bhopale VM, Yang M. Neutrophils generate microparticles during exposure to inert gases due to cytoskeletal oxidative stress. J Biol Chem. 2014;289:18831–45.
29. Yang M, Bhopale VM, Thom SR. Ascorbic acid abrogates microparticle generation and vascular injuries associated with high-pressure exposure. J Appl Physiol (1985). 2015;119:77–82.
30. Bhullar J, Bhopale VM, Yang M, Sethuraman K, Thom SR. Microparticle formation by platelets exposed to high gas pressures—an oxidative stress response. Free Radic Biol Med. 2016;101:154–62.
31. Loane DJ, Stoica BA, Tchantchou F, Kumar A, Barrett JP, Akintola T, Xue F, Conn PJ, Faden AI. Novel mGluR5 positive allosteric modulator improves functional recovery, attenuates neurodegeneration, and alters microglial polarization after experimental traumatic brain injury. Neurotherapeutics. 2014;11:857–69.
32. Kumar A, Barrett JP, Alvarez-Croda DM, Stoica BA, Faden AI, Loane DJ. NOX2 drives M1-like microglial/macrophage activation and neurodegeneration following experimental traumatic brain injury. Brain Behav Immun. 2016;58:291–309.
33. Kabadi SV, Stoica BA, Loane DJ, Byrnes KR, Hanscom M, Cabatbat RM, Tan MT, Faden AI. Cyclin D1 gene ablation confers neuroprotection in traumatic brain injury. J Neurotrauma. 2012;29:813–27.
34. Porro C, Di Gioia S, Trotta T, Lepore S, Panaro MA, Battaglino A, Ratclif L, Castellani S, Bufo P, Martinez MC, Conese M. Pro-inflammatory effect of cystic fibrosis sputum microparticles in the murine lung. J Cyst Fibros. 2013;12:721–8.
35. Loane DJ, Kumar A. Microglia in the TBI brain: the good, the bad, and the dysregulated. Exp Neurol. 2016;275(Pt 3):316–27.
36. Tkach M, Thery C. Communication by extracellular vesicles: where we are and where we need to go. Cell. 2016;164:1226–32.
37. Valadi H, Ekstrom K, Bossios A, Sjostrand M, Lee JJ, Lotvall JO. Exosome-mediated transfer of mRNAs and microRNAs is a novel mechanism of genetic exchange between cells. Nat Cell Biol. 2007;9:654–9.
38. Takeshita J, Mohler ER, Krishnamoorthy P, Moore J, Rogers WT, Zhang L, Gelfand JM, Mehta NN. Endothelial cell-, platelet-, and monocyte/macrophage-derived microparticles are elevated in psoriasis beyond cardiometabolic risk factors. J Am Heart Assoc. 2014;3:e000507.
39. Nie DM, Wu QL, Zheng P, Chen P, Zhang R, Li BB, Fang J, Xia LH, Hong M. Endothelial microparticles carrying hedgehog-interacting protein induce continuous endothelial damage in the pathogenesis of acute graft-versus-host disease. Am J Physiol Cell Physiol. 2016;310:C821–835.
40. Gachet C. P2Y(12) receptors in platelets and other hematopoietic and non-hematopoietic cells. Purinergic Signal. 2012;8:609–19.
41. French SL, Paramitha AC, Moon MJ, Dickins RA, Hamilton JR. Humanizing the protease-activated receptor (PAR) expression profile in mouse platelets by knocking PAR1 into the Par3 locus reveals PAR1 expression is not tolerated in mouse platelets. PLoS One. 2016;11:e0165565.
42. Chan HC, Ke LY, Chu CS, Lee AS, Shen MY, Cruz MA, Hsu JF, Cheng KH, Chan HC, Lu J, et al. Highly electronegative LDL from patients with ST-elevation myocardial infarction triggers platelet activation and aggregation. Blood. 2013;122:3632–41.
43. Bianco F, Pravettoni E, Colombo A, Schenk U, Moller T, Matteoli M, Verderio C. Astrocyte-derived ATP induces vesicle shedding and IL-1 beta release from microglia. J Immunol. 2005;174:7268–77.
44. Qu Y, Ramachandra L, Mohr S, Franchi L, Harding CV, Nunez G, Dubyak GR. P2X7 receptor-stimulated secretion of MHC class II-containing exosomes requires the ASC/NLRP3 inflammasome but is independent of caspase-1. J Immunol. 2009;182:5052–62.
45. Loane DJ, Stoica BA, Byrnes KR, Jeong W, Faden AI. Activation of mGluR5 and inhibition of NADPH oxidase improves functional recovery after traumatic brain injury. J Neurotrauma. 2013;30:403–12.
46. Stoica BA, Loane DJ, Zhao Z, Kabadi SV, Hanscom M, Byrnes KR, Faden AI. PARP-1 inhibition attenuates neuronal loss, microglia activation and neurological deficits after traumatic brain injury. J Neurotrauma. 2014;31:758–72.
47. MacKenzie A, Wilson HL, Kiss-Toth E, Dower SK, North RA, Surprenant A. Rapid secretion of interleukin-1beta by microvesicle shedding. Immunity. 2001;15:825–35.
48. Mulcahy LA, Pink RC, Carter DR. Routes and mechanisms of extracellular vesicle uptake. J Extracell Vesicles. 2014;3. doi:10.3402/jev.v3.24641. eCollection 2014.
49. Fabbri M, Paone A, Calore F, Galli R, Gaudio E, Santhanam R, Lovat F, Fadda P, Mao C, Nuovo GJ, et al. MicroRNAs bind to Toll-like receptors to induce prometastatic inflammatory response. Proc Natl Acad Sci U S A. 2012;109: E2110–2116.
50. Rozmyslowicz T, Majka M, Kijowski J, Murphy SL, Conover DO, Poncz M, Ratajczak J, Gaulton GN, Ratajczak MZ. Platelet- and megakaryocyte-derived microparticles transfer CXCR4 receptor to CXCR4-null cells and make them susceptible to infection by X4-HIV. Aids. 2003;17:33–42.
51. Mack M, Kleinschmidt A, Bruhl H, Klier C, Nelson PJ, Cihak J, Plachy J, Stangassinger M, Erfle V, Schlondorff D. Transfer of the chemokine receptor CCR5 between cells by membrane-derived microparticles: a mechanism for cellular human immunodeficiency virus 1 infection. Nat Med. 2000;6:769–75.
52. Mause SF, Ritzel E, Liehn EA, Hristov M, Bidzhekov K, Muller-Newen G, Soehnlein O, Weber C. Platelet microparticles enhance the vasoregenerative potential of angiogenic early outgrowth cells after vascular injury. Circulation. 2010;122:495–506.
53. Harrison EB, Hochfelder CG, Lamberty BG, Meays BM, Morsey BM, Kelso ML, Fox HS, Yelamanchili SV. Traumatic brain injury increases levels of miR-21 in extracellular vesicles: implications for neuroinflammation. FEBS Open Bio. 2016;6:835–46.
54. Su W, Aloi MS, Garden GA. MicroRNAs mediating CNS inflammation: small regulators with powerful potential. Brain Behav Immun. 2016;52:1–8.
55. Moore CS, Rao VT, Durafourt BA, Bedell BJ, Ludwin SK, Bar-Or A, Antel JP. miR-155 as a multiple sclerosis-relevant regulator of myeloid cell polarization. Ann Neurol. 2013;74:709–20.
56. Butovsky O, Jedrychowski MP, Cialic R, Krasemann S, Murugaiyan G, Fanek Z, Greco DJ, Wu PM, Doykan CE, Kiner O, et al. Targeting miR-155 restores

abnormal microglia and attenuates disease in SOD1 mice. Ann Neurol. 2015;77:75–99.

57. Thome AD, Harms AS, Volpicelli-Daley LA, Standaert DG. microRNA-155 regulates alpha-synuclein-induced inflammatory responses in models of Parkinson disease. J Neurosci. 2016;36:2383–90.
58. Pena-Philippides JC, Caballero-Garrido E, Lordkipanidze T, Roitbak T. In vivo inhibition of miR-155 significantly alters post-stroke inflammatory response. J Neuroinflammation. 2016;13:287.
59. Zhang Y, Mei H, Chang X, Chen F, Zhu Y, Han X. Adipocyte-derived microvesicles from obese mice induce M1 macrophage phenotype through secreted miR-155. J Mol Cell Biol. 2016;8:505–17.
60. Verderio C, Muzio L, Turola E, Bergami A, Novellino L, Ruffini F, Riganti L, Corradini I, Francolini M, Garzetti L, et al. Myeloid microvesicles are a marker and therapeutic target for neuroinflammation. Ann Neurol. 2012;72:610–24.
61. Perez-Pujol S, Marker PH, Key NS. Platelet microparticles are heterogeneous and highly dependent on the activation mechanism: studies using a new digital flow cytometer. Cytometry A. 2007;71:38–45.
62. Dragovic RA, Gardiner C, Brooks AS, Tannetta DS, Ferguson DJ, Hole P, Carr B, Redman CW, Harris AL, Dobson PJ, et al. Sizing and phenotyping of cellular vesicles using nanoparticle tracking analysis. Nanomedicine. 2011;7:780–8.
63. Lawrie AS, Albanyan A, Cardigan RA, Mackie IJ, Harrison P. Microparticle sizing by dynamic light scattering in fresh-frozen plasma. Vox Sang. 2009;96:206–12.
64. Oosthuyzen W, Sime NE, Ivy JR, Turtle EJ, Street JM, Pound J, Bath LE, Webb DJ, Gregory CD, Bailey MA, Dear JW. Quantification of human urinary exosomes by nanoparticle tracking analysis. J Physiol. 2013;591:5833–42.

6

Microglia processes associate with diffusely injured axons following mild traumatic brain injury in the micro pig

Audrey D. Lafrenaye[1*], Masaki Todani[1,2], Susan A. Walker[1] and John T. Povlishock[1]

Abstract

Background: Mild traumatic brain injury (mTBI) is an all too common occurrence that exacts significant personal and societal costs. The pathophysiology of mTBI is complex, with reports routinely correlating diffuse axonal injury (DAI) with prolonged morbidity. Progressive chronic neuroinflammation has also recently been correlated to morbidity, however, the potential association between neuroinflammatory microglia and DAI is not well understood. The majority of studies exploring neuroinflammatory responses to TBI have focused on more chronic phases of injury involving phagocytosis associated with Wallerian change. Little, however, is known regarding the neuroinflammatory response seen acutely following diffuse mTBI and its potential relationship to early DAI. Additionally, while inflammation is drastically different in rodents compared to humans, pigs and humans share very similar inflammatory profiles and responses.

Methods: In the current study, we employed a modified central fluid percussion model in micro pigs. Using this model of diffuse mTBI, paired with various immunohistological endpoints, we assessed the potential association between acute thalamic DAI and neuroinflammation 6 h following injury.

Results: Injured micro pigs displayed substantial axonal damage reflected in the presence of APP+ proximal axonal swellings, which were particularly prominent in the thalamus. In companion, the same thalamic sites displayed extensive neuroinflammation, which was observed using Iba-1 immunohistochemistry. The physical relationship between microglia and DAI, assessed via confocal 3D analysis, revealed a dramatic increase in the number of Iba-1+ microglial processes that contacted APP+ proximal axonal swellings compared to uninjured myelinated thalamic axons in sham animals.

Conclusions: In aggregate, these studies reveal acute microglial process convergence on proximal axonal swellings undergoing DAI, an interaction not previously recognized in the literature. These findings transform our understanding of acute neuroinflammation following mTBI and may suggest its potential as a diagnostic and/or a therapeutic target.

Keywords: Mild traumatic brain injury, Diffuse axonal injury, Neuroinflammation, Microglia, Micro pig

* Correspondence: forrestad@vcu.edu
[1]Department of Anatomy and Neurobiology, Virginia Commonwealth University Medical Center, P.O. Box 980709, Richmond, VA 23298, USA
Full list of author information is available at the end of the article

Background

Mild traumatic brain injury (mTBI) is a common insult that exacts devastating personal and social costs [1–4]. Diffuse mTBI is typically caused by acceleration-deceleration forces, such as those encountered during a motor vehicle accident or sports-related event. The forces generated by the rapid movement of the brain within the cranial vault lead to a multitude of complex metabolic, physiologic, and pathologic responses [5–9]. One pathology that frequently follows mTBI is diffuse axonal injury (DAI), in which force-induced stress results in discrete areas of scattered axonal disruption that ultimately progress to disconnection. This results in a proximal axonal segment that remains connected to the neuronal soma and a distal segment that progresses to Wallerian degeneration [10–13]. Advanced neuroimaging and histological studies have firmly established a positive correlation between DAI and TBI-induced morbidity both clinically and experimentally [10, 14–18].

In addition to DAI, progressive chronic neuroinflammation has been observed following TBI with the suggestion that this pathology is also associated to morbidity [19–24]. Neuroinflammation involves the activation of resident brain microglia and later includes systemic infiltrating macrophages in injuries that involve blood–brain barrier disruption. Upon activation/reactivation, resident microglia undergo morphological changes associated with activation, transforming from highly ramified "resting" or "surveying" phenotypes to activated microglia, with truncated processes, larger cell bodies, and less complex process networks and/or amoeboid morphologies [25–27]. Activated microglia are associated with a variety of detrimental as well as regenerative functions, including phagocytosis, cytokine secretion, and/or neurotrophin secretion [28–34]. To date, the majority of studies exploring neuroinflammatory responses to TBI, including our own, have focused on the phagocytic role of microglia in clearing Wallerian debris days following injury [29, 35–39]. Knowledge is, however, greatly lacking regarding any potential association between microglia and the proximal segment of axons undergoing DAI, independent of the degenerating distal axonal segment and/or Wallerian change.

Previously, our lab reported that while highly activated phagocytic microglia were commonly seen associated with distal degenerating axonal segments, little association was found between activated microglia and proximal axonal segments undergoing DAI [36, 39]. These studies, however, were not designed to address the aforementioned issue in that our previous studies were confined primarily to sub-acute and chronic post-injury time points. Thus, these studies provided no information regarding more acute neuroinflammatory changes or any potential relation to early DAI. Further, while our previous study utilizing transgenic mice allowed for the precise discrimination between proximal and distal axonal segments undergoing DAI, analysis was restricted to the optic nerve [36], a unique white matter region containing a homogeneous axonal population with potentially distinctive microglial responses to injury [40–42]. Lastly, as with the majority of published work in this area, our previous studies explored TBI-related neuroinflammation in rodents, whose systemic inflammatory responses are known to differ from humans [43–46]. In consideration of the fact that pig inflammatory profiles are much more human-like [47, 48], we revisited the issue of microglial response to DAI acutely following injury in a micro pig model of mTBI.

Using an adapted central fluid percussion injury (cFPI) model of diffuse mTBI, we evaluated the extent of acute neuroinflammation and its relation to axons undergoing DAI in the micro pig 6 h following injury. Large amyloid precursor protein (APP) containing swellings, indicative of the proximal segments of axons undergoing DAI, were found diffusely scattered throughout the brain, with consistent involvement of the thalamus, an area commonly affected in human TBI [49–54]. Acute neuroinflammation accompanied these axonal changes and mapped to the same sites within the thalamus. Importantly, activated microglial processes converged on proximal axonal swellings undergoing DAI to form increased numbers of physical contacts as compared to the number of contacts made between microglia and uninjured axons in sham animals.

Methods

Animals

Experiments were conducted in accordance with the Virginia Commonwealth University institutional guidelines concerning the care and use of laboratory animals (Institutional Animal Care and Use Committee), which adhere to regulations including, but not limited to, those set forth in the "Guide for the Care and Use of Laboratory Animals: 8th Edition" (National Research Council). Twenty-one adult male Yukatan micro pigs, weighing 15–25 kg (~6 months of age), were used for this study. Animals were housed in environmentally controlled pens in pairs on a 12-h light–dark cycle, with free access to food and water.

Surgical preparation and injury induction

Micro pigs were initially anesthetized with an intramuscular injection of 100 mg/ml xylazine (2.2 mg/kg; AnaSed Injection, Shenandoah, IA, USA) and 100 mg/ml Telazol (2.0 mg/kg; tiletamine HCL and zolazepam HCL; Pfizer, New York, NY, USA) followed by intravenous administration of sodium pentobarbital (60 mg/kg; Sigma-Aldrich, St. Louis, MO, USA). Once the absence of a corneal reflex was verified, the micro pig was intubated and ventilated with 1–2 % isoflurane mixed in 100 % oxygen throughout the experiment. Ophthalmic lubricant (Dechra, Overland Park, KS, USA) was applied to avoid damage or drying of the eye. Body temperature was monitored with a rectal thermometer and maintained at 37 °C with a heating pad. Catheters were placed in the right femoral artery and vein for continuous monitoring of mean arterial blood pressure (MABP), assessment of blood gases, and infusion of Lactated Ringer's (Hospira, Lake Forest, IL, USA) to maintain hydration. A midline incision was made from the supraorbital process to the nuchal crest and a 14-mm-diameter circular craniotomy was trephined along the sagittal suture, positioning the center of the craniotomy 15 mm anterior to lambda, which is on the nuchal crest, and leaving the dura intact. A stainless steal custom threaded hub (Custom Design and Fabrication, Richmond, VA, USA) was screwed into the craniotomy site to a depth of ~4 mm. Screws were then placed directly posterior and anterior-lateral to the craniotomy, and dental acrylic (methyl-methacrylate; Hygenic Corp., Akron, OH, USA) was applied around the hub and screws to insure hub stability. The procedures used to induce cFPI in the micro pig were consistent with those described previously in the rodent [55]. This injury is induced by releasing a pendulum to impact a fluid-filled cylinder that generates a fluid pulse. The fluid pressure wave is transduced through the injury hub to the surface of the dura and ultimately to the cerebral spinal fluid and brain. Briefly, anesthetized micro pigs were connected to a central fluid percussion device retrofitted with a L-shaped stainless steal adaptor that allowed for a sealed connection to the injury hub. Micro pigs were then injured at a magnitude of 1.68 ± 0.4 atm with a pressure pulse measured by a transducer affixed to the injury device and displayed on an oscilloscope (Tektronix, Beaverton, OR, USA). Immediately after injury induction, animals were disconnected from the injury device, the screws and hub were removed from the bone, and the dental acrylic, hub, and screws were removed en bloc. This injury did not result in any breach of the dura mater. Gel foam was placed over the craniotomy/injury site, to alleviate minute bone bleeding, and the scalp was sutured. Animals were maintained under anesthetic for the duration of the 6-h post-injury monitoring period. Identical surgical procedures were followed for sham-injured animals, without the release of the pendulum to induce the injury.

Physiological assessment

To preclude the possibility that observed pathology was associated with TBI-induced systemic abnormalities, detailed physiological assessments were performed throughout the 6-h post-injury monitoring period. Heart rate, arterial blood pressure, rectal temperature, and hemoglobin oxygen saturation were monitored and recorded throughout the experiment via a Cardell® MAX-12HD (Sharn Veterinary, Inc., Chicago, IL, USA). The femoral artery was cannulated for continuous monitoring of MABP and for blood sampling to determine arterial oxygen tension (PaO_2), arterial carbon dioxide pressure ($PaCO_2$), and pH values using a Stat Profile pHOx (NOVA Biomedical, Waltham, MA, USA). The resting $PaCO_2$ level was maintained between 35 and 40 mmHg by adjusting the rate and/or tidal volume of the respirator. All animals maintained physiological homeostasis (i.e., 60 mmHg < MABP < 90 mmHg, hemoglobin oxygen saturation >90 %, 90 BPM < heart rate < 140 BPM; Table 1).

Tissue processing

At 6-h post-sham or cFPI, micro pigs were overdosed with 3-ml euthasol euthanasia-III solution (Henry Schein, Dublin, OH, USA) transcardially perfused with 0.9 % saline followed by 4 % paraformaldehyde/0.2 % glutaraldehyde in Millonig's buffer (136 mM sodium phosphate monobasic/109 mM sodium hydroxide) for immunohistochemical analysis. After transcardial perfusion, the brains were removed and post-fixed in 4 % paraformaldehyde/0.2 % glutaraldehyde/Millonig's buffer for 36–48 h. Post-fixed brains were blocked into 5-mm coronal segments throughout the rostral-caudal extent using a tissue slicer (Zivic Instruments, Pittsburgh, PA, USA). In our hands, cFPI in the micro pig produced symmetrical bilateral microscopic pathology, which involved multiple brain loci. The burden of DAI, however,

Table 1 Systemic physiology was within normal ranges throughout the 6-h post-injury monitoring period

Variable	Group	Pre-injury	Post-injury
Weight	Sham	19.13 ± 4.72	
	TBI	20.12 ± 3.37	
pH	Sham	7.47 ± 0.03	7.48 ± 0.03
	TBI	7.49 ± 0.03	7.52 ± 0.02*
$paCO_2$ mmHg	Sham	39.23 ± 4.20	37.92 ± 1.37
	TBI	40.83 ± 2.81	37.61 ± 1.11
paO_2 mmHg	Sham	585.25 ± 53.92	359.74 ± 187.80
	TBI	558.50 ± 41.42	492.18 ± 116.09
MABP mmHg	Sham	94.29 ± 14.94	86.13 ± 20.19
	TBI	89.53 ± 8.83	79.90 ± 8.24
Hemoglobin O_2 (%)	Sham	$99.90 \pm 1.74 \times 10^{-14}$	99.19 ± 0.61
	TBI	99.83 ± 0.167	99.50 ± 0.58

TBI traumatic brain injury, *MABP* mean arterial blood pressure
*Significant difference compared with sham values at same measurement point $p < 0.05$. Values are mean ± standard deviation of the mean

was particularly consistent within the thalamus, leading us to focus on this region for the current communication. Segments containing the thalamus were bisected at the midline and the left side was analyzed. The 5-mm coronal segments containing the thalamus were coronally sectioned in 0.1 M phosphate buffer with a vibratome (Leica, Bannockburn, IL, USA) at a thickness of 40 µm. Sections were collected serially in six-well plates (240 µm between sections in each well) and stored in Millonig's buffer at 4 °C. For the quantification of both axonal injury and microglial activation, a random well (1–6) was selected using a random number generator and six sections representing the rostral-caudal axis contained within the selected well were analyzed. All histological analyses were restricted to the thalamus using anatomical landmarks and were performed by an investigator blinded to animal injury (sham or mTBI).

Detection and assessment of axonal injury

To visualize the breakdown of axonal transport within the axonal segment proximal to its neuronal soma, a process indicative of DAI, immunofluorescence targeting the normally expressed and anterogradely transported amyloid precursor protein (APP) was performed.

For the preliminary assessment of DAI in the micro pig brain following cFPI sections from various brain regions throughout the rostra-caudal extent were blocked and permeabilized in 1.5 % Triton/10 % NGS/PBS followed by overnight incubation with the primary rabbit antibody against the C-terminus of β-APP (1:700; Cat.# 51–2700, Life Technologies, Carlsbad, CA, USA) in 10 % NGS/PBS at 4 °C. A biotinylated goat anti-rabbit IgG (1:1000; Cat.# BA-1000, Vector Laboratories, Burlingame, CA, USA) secondary antibody was used. The sections were then incubated in avidin biotinylated enzyme complex using the Vectastain ABC kit (Vector Laboratories, Burlingame, CA, USA) followed by visualization with 0.05 % diaminobenzidine/0.01 % H_2O_2/0.3 % imidazole/PBS. The tissue was mounted, dehydrated, and cover-slipped. Visualization of APP-labeled axonal swellings was performed using a Nikon Eclipse 800 microscope (Nikon, Tokyo, Japan) equipped with an Olympus DP71 camera (Olympus, Center Valley, PA, USA).

To quantify the degree of thalamic DAI, immunofluorescence was used, in order to differentiate between the axonal swellings that contain a large amount of APP and the neuronal soma that contain lower amounts of APP. Briefly, six thalamic sections per animal (as detailed above) were blocked and permeabilized in 10 % normal goat serum and 1.5 % Triton followed by overnight incubation with a primary rabbit antibody against the C-terminus of β-APP (1:700; Cat.# 51–2700, Life Technologies, Carlsbad, CA, USA) at 4 °C. Secondary antibody, Alexa Fluor 568-conjugated goat anti-rabbit IgG (1:500; Cat.# A-11011, Life Technologies, Carlsbad, CA, USA) was then incubated and the tissue was mounted using Vectashield hardset mounting medium with Dapi (Cat.# H-1500; Vector Laboratories, Burlingame, CA, USA). Tissue from all animals was processed concomitantly to obviate variability in staining intensity. Visualization of APP-labeled axonal swellings was performed using a Nikon Eclipse 800 microscope (Nikon, Tokyo, Japan) equipped with an Olympus DP71 camera (Olympus, Center Valley, PA, USA). Image acquisition settings were held constant for all animals. Images (60 images per animal; 10 images in each of the 6 sections assessed) were taken by a blinded investigator at 10× magnification (0.72-mm^2 field) in a systematically random fashion starting at the dorsal lateral aspect of the thalamus. Dapi signal was used for field advancement and to verify focus as well as restriction within the thalamus. A fluorescent intensity threshold was set for all images to eliminate any neuronal somatic expression of APP from the assessment. The number of APP$^+$ axonal swellings was analyzed using the particle analysis function in ImageJ software (NIH, Bethesda, MD, USA). The number of APP$^+$ swellings per unit area was quantified for each image and averaged for each animal.

Detection and semi-quantification of microglia activation

To identify microglia, immunohistochemistry against the calcium binding protein, Iba-1 (1:1000; Cat.# 51–2700, Life Technologies, Carlsbad, CA, USA), was done. Briefly, six sections per animal (as explicated above) were blocked and permeabilized in 1.5 % Triton/10 % NGS/PBS followed by overnight incubation with the primary antibody in 10 % NGS/PBS at 4 °C. A biotinylated goat anti-rabbit IgG (1:1000; Cat.# BA-1000, Vector Laboratories, Burlingame, CA, USA) secondary antibody was used. The sections were then incubated in avidin biotinylated enzyme complex using the Vectastain ABC kit (Vector Laboratories, Burlingame, CA, USA) followed by visualization with 0.05 % diaminobenzidine/0.01 % H_2O_2/0.3 % imidazole/PBS. The tissue was mounted, dehydrated, and cover-slipped. Tissue from all animals was processed concomitantly to reduce variability between animals. The diffuse nature of the microscopic pathology, as well as the extensive area of the micro pig thalamus, precluded the use of traditional stereological quantification. Therefore, the entire thalamus was assessed for each of the six sections selected for each animal. Visualization of Iba-1-labeled microglia was performed using a Nikon Eclipse 800 microscope (Nikon, Tokyo, Japan). Identification of microglia activation was based on specific morphological criteria. Microglia with highly ramified fine process networks that were lightly labeled with Iba-1 were considered non-reactive, while microglia with thicker, shorter, or absent processes and darker Iba-1 labeling were identified as active/reactive [25–27]. The degree of microglia activation was assessed using a graded scale from 0 to 5 (0 = no microglial activation observed, 1 = ramified microglia with thicker processes and darker Iba-1 labeling observed in ~5 % of the thalamus, 2 = activated microglia observed in ~5–10 % of the thalamus, 3 = activated microglia observed in ~10 < 25 % of the thalamus, 4 = activated microglia observed in ~25 < 50 % of the thalamus, and 5 = activated microglia observed in >50 % of the thalamus). Two blinded investigators analyzed all sections independently and their scores were averaged for each animal.

Tissue processing for microglia morphology and process contact analyses

A subset of tissue sections taken from 9 injured and 3 sham animals were triple labeled with the following antibodies: rabbit anti β-APP (1:700; Cat.# 51–2700, Life Technologies, Carlsbad, CA, USA), rabbit anti Iba-1 (1:1000; Cat.# 019-19741, Wako, Osaka, Japan), and rat anti-myelin basic protein (1:1000; Cat#NB600-717, Novus Biologicals, Littleton, CO, USA). To reduce the amount of lipid within the tissue and enhance antibody penetration, the sections were dehydrated then rehydrated through varying percentages of ethanol, with the tissue beginning and ending in PBS. The tissue was blocked and permeabilized with 10 % NGS/1.5 % Triton/PBS followed by incubation with the rabbit anti-APP antibody over night at 4 °C followed by incubation with Alexa Fluor 488-conjugated goat anti-rabbit secondary antibody (1:500; Cat.# A11034, Life Technologies, Carlsbad, CA, USA). Tyramide amplification of the APP signal (primary antibody diluted to 1:5000) was performed on the majority of sections to further reduce the risk of cross-reaction with the Iba-1 antibody, using a rabbit Alexa-488 conjugated Tyramide amplification kit (Cat.# T20922, Life Technologies, Carlsbad, CA, USA) according to the manufacturer's instructions. Following APP immunolabeling, the tissue was blocked once again with 10 % NGS then incubated with the rabbit anti-Iba-1 and rat anti-MBP antibodies. Alexa Fluor 568-conjugated goat anti-rat IgG (1:500; Cat.# A11077, Life Technologies, Carlsbad, CA, USA) and Alexa Fluor 633-conjugated goat anti-rabbit IgG (1:500; Cat.# A21071, Life Technologies, Carlsbad, CA, USA) were used for the visualization of MBP and Iba-1, respectively. Controls to assess cross-reactivity among all antibodies were performed using the following antibody combinations: no primary/rabbit Alexa-488 (or rabbit Alexa-488 tyramide amplification), rat Alexa-568, rabbit Alexa-633; rat anti-MBP primary/rabbit Alexa-633 secondary; rabbit anti-Iba-1 primary/rat Alexa-568 secondary; rabbit anti-APP primary (either 1:700 or 1:5000 followed by second blocking step/rabbit Alexa-633 secondary). For all controls, any cross-reactivity was below background detection limits (data not shown). Tissue was mounted using Vectashield hardset mounting medium with Dapi (Cat.# H-1500; Vector Laboratories, Burlingame, CA, USA) and *z*-stacked images (10–25-μm-thick stacks; 0.32 μm between steps; sham = 6 *z*-stacks, injured = 19 *z*-stacks) were captured on a Zeiss LSM 710 confocal microscope (Carol Zeiss, Oberkochen, Germany). Regions for imaging were selected based on the APP profile for injured animals and the penetration of MBP for the sham animals. Three-dimensional reconstructions of the *z*-stacks were made using Velocity software (PerkinElmer, Waltham, MA, USA).

Microglia morphology analysis

For the morphological analysis of microglia, 2D representations of the Iba-1-labeled Alexa 633 channel 3D reconstructions (sham = 1 reconstruction from each of 3 animals; injured = 1 reconstruction from each of 9 animals) were used. Each individual cell with an identifiable soma and process network within the reconstruction was assessed. The soma size, the total number of processes (with each new branch point designating the origin of a new process), the average process length, the number of primary processes that directly originate from the soma, and the number of terminal process endpoints/tips for each microglial cell were quantified manually using ImageJ software (NIH, Bethesda, MD, USA). These morphological features and particularly the assessment of total number of processes and the number of terminal process endpoints provide detailed data indicating the complexity/ramification of the process network of individual microglia.

Microglia process contact analyses

Triple-labeled 3D reconstructions performed using Velocity software were used for the analysis of microglia process contacts with DAI in injured micro pigs or intact axonal segments in sham animals. All APP+ axonal swellings contained within each 3D image were assessed in injured animals and 10 myelinated fibers per 3D image, chosen via random-number generator determined *x*, *y* coordinates, were assessed for sham animals. The length of the proximal axonal swelling (from APP+ axonal stem to the disconnected base of APP+ swelling) or the intact myelinated MBP+ axonal segment for sham animals was measured using Velocity software. Microglia process contacts were identified manually on 3D images and confirmed by stepping through the *z*-stacks. All microglial contacts within the delineated axonal segments were included in the analysis.

Electron microscopy

To evaluate the ultrastructural characteristics of DAI in the micro pig thalamus while verifying microglia process contacts on these axonal swellings, a subset of tissue was immunolabeled with either rabbit anti β-APP (1:700; Cat.# 51–2700, Life Technologies, Carlsbad, CA, USA) or rabbit anti Iba-1 (1:1000; Cat.# 019–19741, Wako, Osaka, Japan), followed by incubation with biotinylated goat anti-rabbit IgG (1:1000; Cat.# BA-1000, Vector Laboratories, Burlingame, CA, USA) secondary antibody. The reaction product was visualized with 0.05 % diaminobenzidine/0.01 % hydrogen peroxide/ 0.3 % imidazole in 0.1 M phosphate buffer and the tissue was prepared for EM analysis. In this approach, tissue sections were osmicated, dehydrated, and embedded in epoxy resin on plastic slides. After resin curing, the slides were studied with routine light microscopy to identify the precise thalamic areas for excision. Once identified, these sites were removed, mounted on plastic studs, and 70-nm sections were cut serially and mounted on Formvar-coated slotted grids. The grids were stained in 5 % uranyl acetate in 50 % methanol and 0.5 % lead citrate. Ultrastructural qualitative analysis was performed using a JEOL JEM 1230 transmission electron microscope (JEOL-USA, Peabody, MA, USA) equipped with Ultrascan 4000SP CCD and Orius SC1000 CCD cameras (Gatan, Pleasanton, CA, USA).

Statistical analysis

Data was tested for normality using a Shapiro-Wilk analysis. Normally distributed data was analyzed via one-way analysis of variance (ANOVA). Non-parametric data were analyzed using a Mann–Whitney *U* test. Statistical significance was set at a p value <0.05. Data are presented as mean ± standard error of the mean (SEM).

Results

Mild diffuse traumatic brain injury does not generate physiologic or macroscopic pathology in the pig

The cFPI used in this study has been successfully employed in rodents for decades to mimic the movement of the brain within the cranial vault following non-contusive diffuse mTBI with high efficacy and consistency [55]. This injury generated virtually no macroscopic pathology in the micro pig brain (Fig. 1). While limited subarachnoid bleeding, particularly overlying the occipital cortex and cerebellum, was observed, macroscopic hemorrhage within the brain parenchyma was not detected. Isolated petechial hemorrhage was observed in a few injured animals, however, this did not interfere with any of the analyses performed. Additionally, these injuries were not accompanied by contusion, hematoma formation, ventricular enlargement, or tissue loss throughout the rostral-caudal extent of the micro pig brain. Collectively, these features speak to the mild diffuse nature of the injury employed.

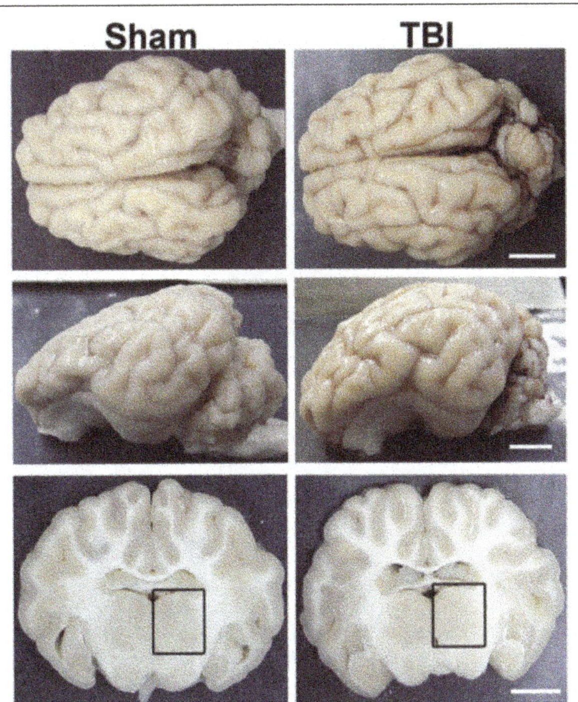

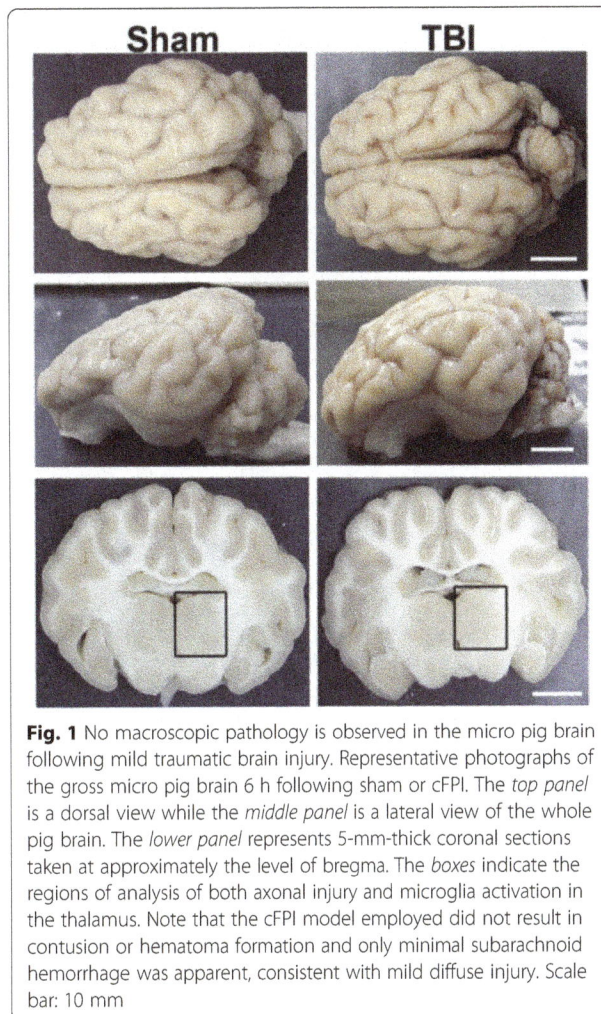

Fig. 1 No macroscopic pathology is observed in the micro pig brain following mild traumatic brain injury. Representative photographs of the gross micro pig brain 6 h following sham or cFPI. The *top panel* is a dorsal view while the *middle panel* is a lateral view of the whole pig brain. The *lower panel* represents 5-mm-thick coronal sections taken at approximately the level of bregma. The *boxes* indicate the regions of analysis of both axonal injury and microglia activation in the thalamus. Note that the cFPI model employed did not result in contusion or hematoma formation and only minimal subarachnoid hemorrhage was apparent, consistent with mild diffuse injury. Scale bar: 10 mm

To evaluate the possibility of confounding systemically induced change in this model, each animal's systemic physiology was closely monitored for the duration of the experiment, both prior to the induction of injury and for the entire 6-h post-sham or injury period. Core temperature was also monitored and maintained at 37 °C to negate the possibility of protection due to hypothermia. As depicted in Table 1, averages of the pre- and post-injury physiologic values, taken throughout the 6-h post-injury monitoring period, were primarily consistent with sham-injured control animals (one-way ANOVA, weight $F_{1,19} = 0.199$, $p = 0.661$; pre-injury pH $F_{1,19} = 2.169$, $p = 0.157$; pre-injury $paCO_2$ $F_{1,19} = 0.732$, $p = 0.403$; post-injury $paCO_2$ $F_{1,19} = 0.199$, $p = 0.660$; pre-injury paO_2 $F_{1,19} = 1.000$, $p = 0.330$; post-injury paO_2 $F_{1,19} = 2.860$, $p = 0.107$; pre-MABP $F_{1,15} = 0.150$, $p = 0.704$; post-injury MABP $F_{1,15} = 0.115$, $p = 0.739$; pre-injury hemoglobin O_2 $F_{1,19} = 0.435$, $p = 0.518$; post-injury hemoglobin O_2 $F_{1,19} = 0.739$, $p = 0.401$; sham $n = 3$,

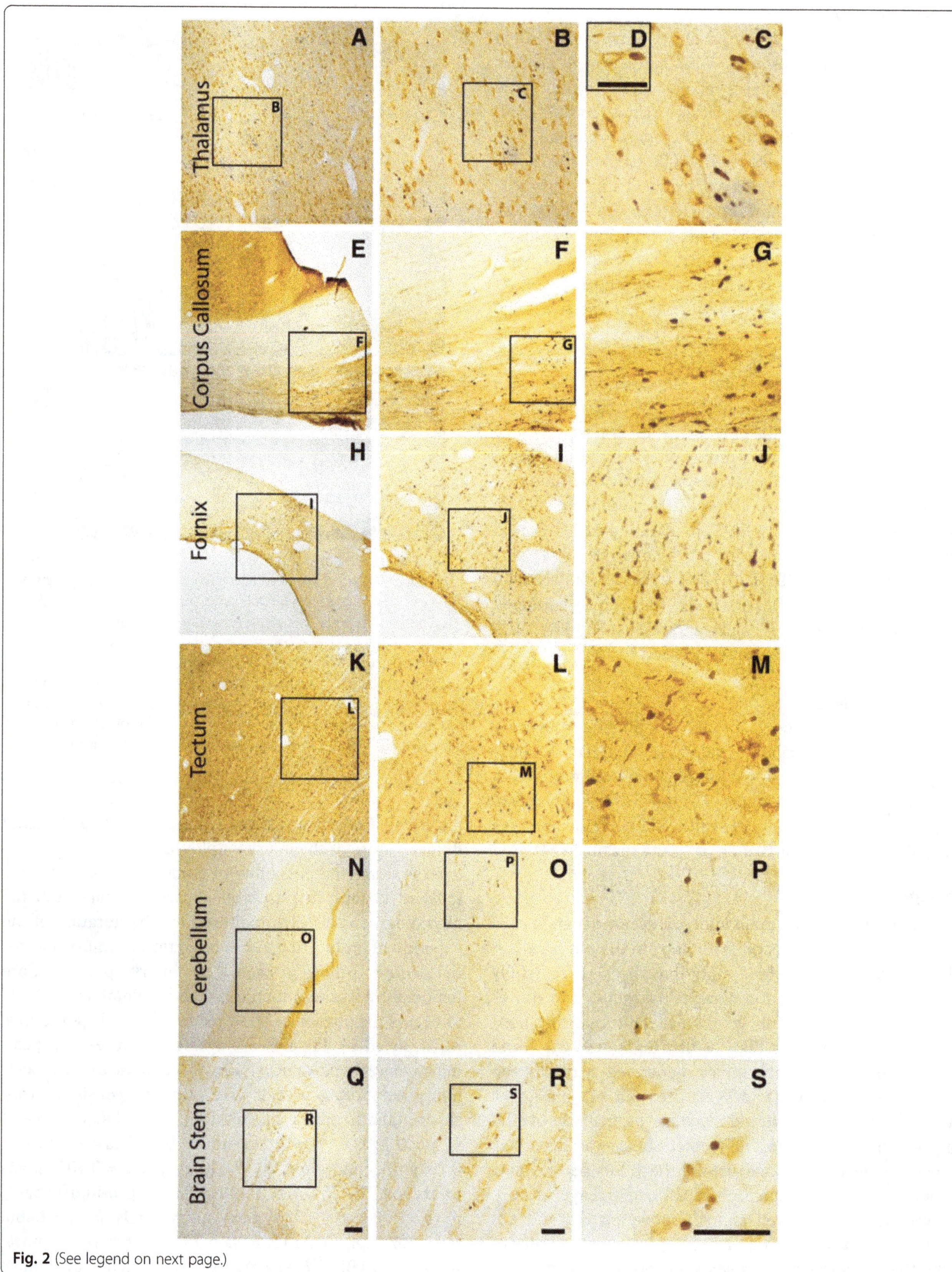

Fig. 2 (See legend on next page.)

(See figure on previous page.)
Fig. 2 Axonal injury is observed in various regions throughout the micro pig brain following cFPI. Representative photomicrographs of APP immunohistochemistry in regions of the micro pig brain that demonstrated DAI in animals sustaining cFPI. Images in the *middle panel* (**b**, **f**, **i**, **l**, **o**, **r**) are magnified regions indicated in the images of the *left panel* (**a**, **e**, **h**, **k**, **n**, **q**) and images in the *right panel* (**c**, **g**, **j**, **m**, **p**, **s**) are magnified regions indicated in the *middle panel* (**b**, **f**, **i**, **l**, **o**, **r**), respectively. Note that DAI within the thalamus and tectum was diffusely distributed throughout the domain, while DAI within the other regions was more localized. Also note that while not common, APP+ proximal axonal swellings in continuity with the neuronal soma (**d**) were observed in the thalamus. Scale bar in **q**: 200 μm; **r** and **s**: 100 μm; **d**: 50 μm

mTBI $n = 18$). Post-injury pH, however, was slightly higher than sham ($F_{1,19} = 6.174$, $p = 0.022$). Importantly, these values were all within normal ranges throughout the experiment (Table 1). The paO_2, both prior to and following injury, was higher than typically reported due to our use of 100 % O_2. While these values are higher than are typically observed, the paO_2 remained well below the lower limit for oxygen toxicity [56, 57]. Importantly, since all physiologic parameters evaluated were within normal ranges, pathology observed could be attributed to the mTBI and not to additional systemic physiological changes.

Extensive DAI is apparent in the thalamus following mTBI

Since axonal injury is a pathological hallmark associated with much of the morbidity following TBI [10, 11, 14–18], the extent of DAI was qualitatively assessed in various regions of the micro pig brain 6 h following sham or cFPI. This time point was chosen, based on our initial observations in this model, which revealed robust DAI by 6-h post-injury in the micro pig brain (unpublished findings). Pronounced DAI, identified as APP+ proximal axonal swellings, indicative of impaired protein transport in the proximal axonal segment remaining attached to the neuronal soma following disconnection [53, 54, 58, 59], was observed in the thalamus, corpus callosum, fornix, tectum of the midbrain, cerebellum, and brainstem (Fig. 2). While, in some animals, other brain regions displayed more densely localized DAI, diffuse thalamic DAI was the most consistent finding across animals. As thalamic damage is also a common occurrence in human TBI [49–52], we concentrated our quantitative histological analysis on this anatomical region (one-way ANOVA $F_{1,19} = 6.677$, $p = 0.018$; sham $n = 3$, TBI $n = 18$; Fig. 3). Consistent with previous studies examining DAI via APP accumulation, no APP+ axonal swellings were observed in sham-injured micro pigs (Fig. 3a). Following cFPI, however, substantial APP+ proximal axonal swellings were apparent throughout the thalamic domain (Fig. 3). DAI within the micro pig thalamus appeared as large (~5 μm in diameter) APP+ spheroids diffusely distributed in patches throughout the dorsal-ventral and rostral-caudal extent of the thalamus.

To explore the subcellular pathology of DAI in the micro pig thalamus 6 h following diffuse mTBI, the ultrastructure of these APP+ proximal axonal swellings was assessed (Fig. 4). The majority of proximal axonal swellings, as identified by immunoelectron microscopy against APP, demonstrated ultrastructural alterations consistent with axonal damage. Disordered and clumped neurofilaments were commonly observed within APP containing axonal swellings, with some cases displaying a neurofilamentous core surrounded by organelles (Fig. 4c). Other proximal swellings exhibited predominant organelle accumulation. These findings were consistent with ultrastructural descriptions of human TBI-induced acute axonal pathology [60]. These subcellular changes in the proximal axonal swellings were not, however, consistent with the initiation of Wallerian degeneration [12, 58], which was observed in distal axonal swellings that lacked APP immunoreactivity

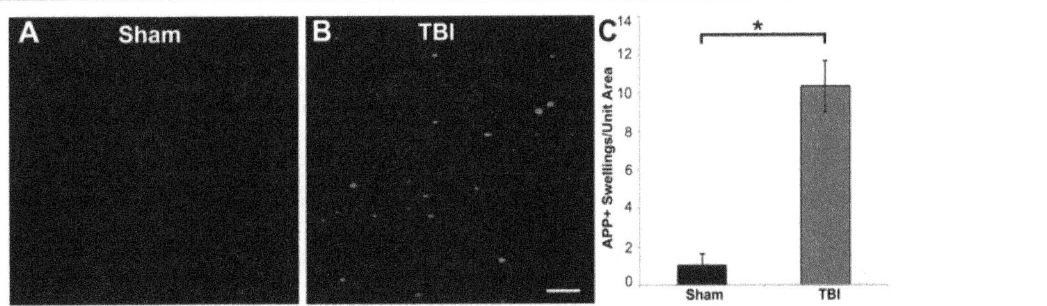

Fig. 3 Abundant DAI is readily apparent 6 h following cFPI in the micro pig thalamus. Representative photomicrographs of APP immunofluorescence in the thalamus of animals sustaining sham (**a**) or cFPI (**b**). While sham-injured animals had little to no APP labeling, prevalent APP+ axonal swellings, indicative of DAI, were apparent following injury. **c** Bar graph depicting the average number of APP labeled axonal swellings/ 0.72 mm^2 of thalamic tissue. Graph depicts mean ± standard error of the mean. *$p < 0.05$. Scale bar: 50 μm

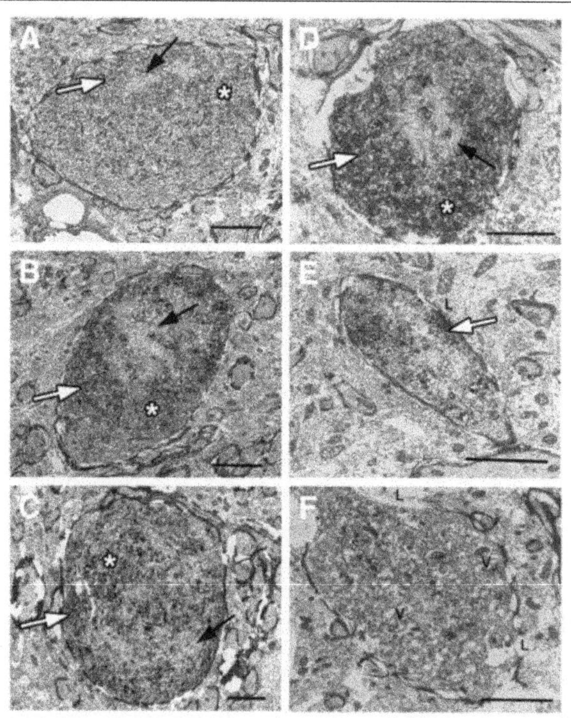

Fig. 4 Ultrastructural characteristics of acute DAI within the micro pig thalamus are consistent with human DAI. Representative electron micrographs of axonal swellings labeled with (**a**–**e**) or without (**f**) APP (*white arrows*). **a**–**e** Consistent with ultrastructural axonal pathology in humans, APP+ proximal axonal swellings in the pig following central fluid percussion injury display clumped disordered neurofilaments (*black arrows*) and areas of organelle accumulation (*asterisks*). **f** Distal axonal swellings, lacking APP labeling, demonstrate characteristics consistent with Wallerian degeneration, including, vacuolization (V) and lucent zones surrounding aspects of the swelling indicating axolemmal or myelin disruption (L). Scale bar **b**–**e**: 2 μm

(Fig. 4f). These APP− distal axonal swellings displayed vacuolization and/or increase cytoplasmic electron density consistent with Wallerian change. Distal, APP−, axonal swellings also displayed areas of axolemmal or myelin disruption, reflected in lucent zones surrounding aspects of the swelling (Fig. 4f).

Acute thalamic microglia activation following mTBI occurs in areas sustaining DAI

Neuroinflammation, as identified by Iba-1+ microglia with activated morphologies, within the micro pig thalamus was assessed using a graded scale from 0 to 5 (0 = no observed microglial activation and 5 = activated microglia observed in >50 % of the coronal thalamic section; sham $n = 3$, TBI $n = 18$). While the microglia within the sham thalami were evenly distributed and primarily non-reactive, with spindly ramified process networks that were lightly labeled with Iba-1, some isolated microglia demonstrated thicker, shorter processes with more substantial Iba-1 labeling (Fig. 5a–d). Following cFPI, however, microglia activation was pervasive, with pockets of morphologically active microglia, exhibiting heavy Iba-1 labeling, thicker processes, and less complex process networks, dispersed throughout the micro pig thalamus (Mann–Whitney U test, $p = 0.006$; Fig. 5e–h).

The process network of individual microglial cells was analyzed in either sham or injured thalami to verify the morphological alterations observed using the above semi-quantitative assessment (Mann–Whitney U test: soma size $p = 0.613$, process length $p = 0.994$, total process number $p = 0.001$, primary process number $p = 0.059$, process endpoints $p = 0.001$; sham $n = 30$ cells, TBI $n = 70$ cells). The microglia in sham-injured micro pigs had ramified/complex process networks, reflected primarily by the total process number and the number of terminal process endpoints per cell (Fig. 5). Microglia within the thalamus of micro pigs sustaining mTBI-induced DAI, however, had fewer overall processes and less terminal process endpoints, indicative of a less complex and/or ramified process network (Fig. 5i, l, n). While the soma size, number of primary processes, and the average process length remained comparable between sham microglia and microglia following mTBI, the drastic reduction in the complexity/ramification of the microglial process network with injury confirms morphological alterations consistent with resident microglial activation [25–27, 61, 62] .

Interestingly, the degree of microglial activation within the thalamus, as assessed via the microglial activation score, was significantly correlated to the amount of DAI observed in each animal (Spearman's rho correlation coefficient = 0.763, $p = 0.000$; $n = 21$). Additionally, the areas of dense microglial activation appeared consistent with the thalamic sites that demonstrated the highest degree of DAI. Therefore, the spatial relationship between activated Iba-1+ microglia and DAI within the injured thalamus was assessed. As depicted in Fig. 6, regions that contained DAI also contained a plethora of morphologically activated microglia, whereas, areas in the injured thalamus that did not sustain DAI primarily contained non-reactive, ramified microglia.

Microglia processes preferentially contact DAI proximal axonal swellings acutely post-injury

To investigate the possibility that activated microglial processes converge on proximal axonal swellings sustaining mTBI-induced DAI in the micro pig thalamus, the number of microglia processes that contacted APP+ axonal swellings in injured animals or normal myelinated axons in sham animals was assessed (Mann–Whitney U test $p = 0.018$; sham $n = 60$ axonal segments, TBI $n = 60$ axonal swellings). Following sham injury, microglia processes made contact with myelinated axons, however, these contacts were sparse (Fig. 7a) and

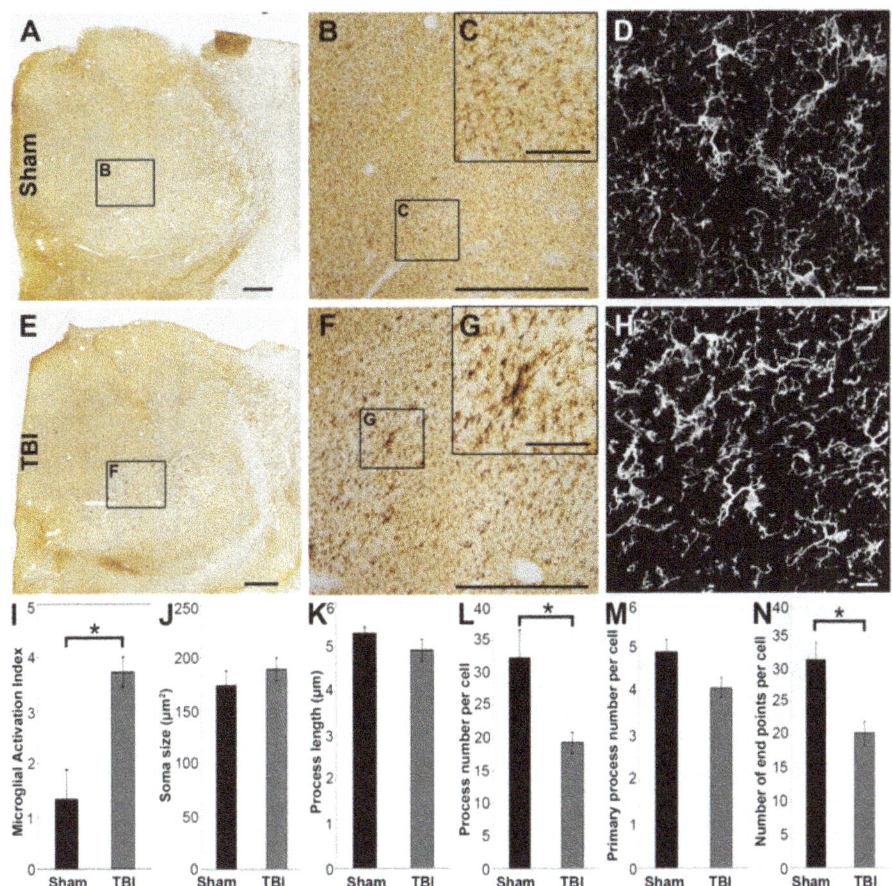

Fig. 5 Extensive microglial activation is observed in the micro pig thalamus 6 h following diffuse mTBI. Representative photomicrographs of the microglial marker Iba-1 in the thalamus of sham-injured (**a**–**d**) or central fluid percussion injured (**e**–**h**) micro pigs. **b** and **f** are magnified regions indicated in **a** and **e**, and **c** and **d** are magnified regions indicated in **b** and **f**, respectively. **d** and **h** are two-dimensional flattened images of three-dimensional stacks through microglia in the sham (**d**) or injured thalamus (**h**). Note that the microglia appear ramified in sham-injured animals, indicating a quiescent state. While ramified microglia are present in brain-injured pigs, a large proportion of microglia have retracted, amoeboid or stellate morphologies, indicating activation. Bar graphs illustrating the degree of microglial activation in the thalamus (**i**) as well as the average soma size (**j**), average process length (**k**), average process number (**l**), average number of primary processes (**m**), and average number of end points (**n**) per Iba-1+ cell. Scale bar **a** and **e** = 1 mm, **b** and **f** = 200 µm, **c** and **g** = 40 µm, **d** and **h** = 10 µm. Graph depicts the mean ± standard error of the mean. $*p < 0.05$

primarily consisted of microglia processes passing by and/or crossing over myelinated axons (sham = 63.39 % of total contacts, TBI = 25.23 % of total contacts). This is shown in more detail in an additional movie file (Additional file 1). Conversely, nearly double the number of microglia processes contacted APP+ proximal axonal swellings following diffuse mTBI (Fig. 7). The majority of these contacts were bulbous end processes (TBI = 58.16 % of total contacts, sham = 36.61 % of total contacts) as apposed to processes passing over axons, which were common in the sham. An additional movie file represents these finding in more detail (Additional file 2). The percentage of microglial processes that appeared to cradle or "cup" the axon were also increased when contacting APP+ swellings compared to sham myelinated axons (TBI = 16.60 % of total contacts, sham = 6.09 % of total contacts).

To further evaluate the increase in microglial process convergence on proximal segments of axons sustaining DAI, qualitative ultrastructural analysis of microglia morphology and process contacts were performed utilizing immunoelectron microscopy targeting Iba-1 (Fig. 8). Microglial cell bodies were easily recognized in sham thalami, however microglial processes were fine and widely dispersed with few processes directly associating with axons (Fig. 8a, b). Following diffuse mTBI, both the Iba-1+ microglial processes and soma were more prominent. As previously described, microglia with myelin and other cellular debris, indicative of active phagocytosis, were present in areas of Wallerian degeneration

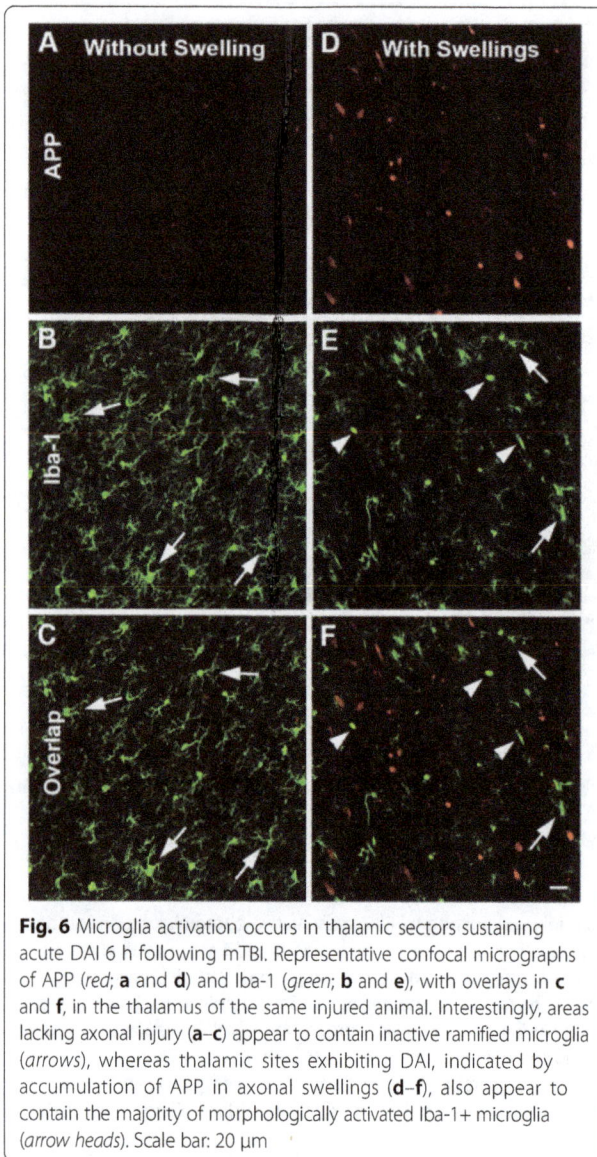

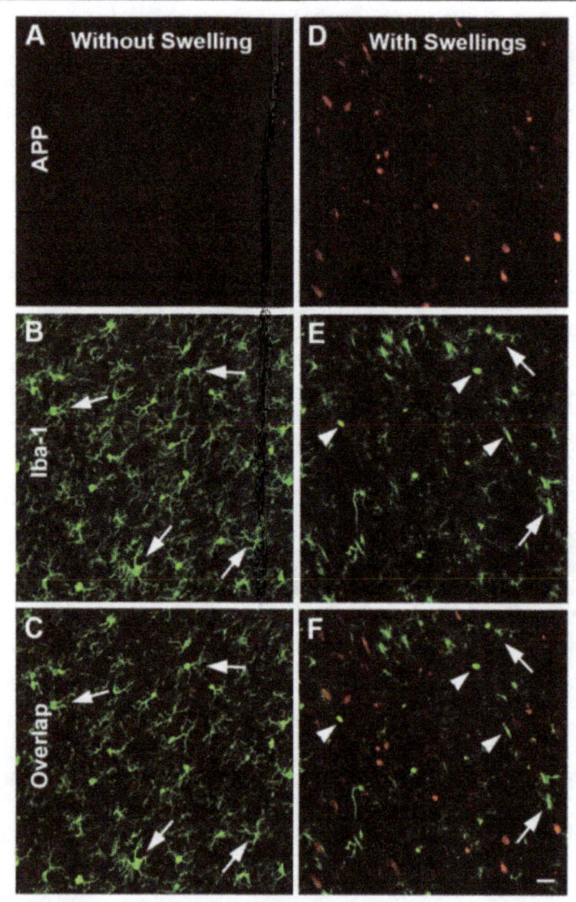

Fig. 6 Microglia activation occurs in thalamic sectors sustaining acute DAI 6 h following mTBI. Representative confocal micrographs of APP (*red*; **a** and **d**) and Iba-1 (*green*; **b** and **e**), with overlays in **c** and **f**, in the thalamus of the same injured animal. Interestingly, areas lacking axonal injury (**a**–**c**) appear to contain inactive ramified microglia (*arrows*), whereas thalamic sites exhibiting DAI, indicated by accumulation of APP in axonal swellings (**d**–**f**), also appear to contain the majority of morphologically activated Iba-1+ microglia (*arrow heads*). Scale bar: 20 μm

(Fig. 8c). In the presence of proximal axonal swellings, as ultrastructurally identified using the common features observed and displayed in Fig. 4, however, microglia did not display sub-cellular alterations consistent with phagocytosis. Rather, small Iba-1+ points of contact were observed (Fig. 8d, e). In some cases, the microglial processes could be traced from the site of axonal contact back to the microglia soma, however, the majority of processes passed out of the plane of section (Fig. 8e, f). These data suggest that while microglia do phagocytize debris from the degenerating distal axon, they do not participate in phagocytosis of the proximal axonal swelling acutely post-mTBI, rather microglial processes appear to preferentially contact and/or converge on proximal axonal swellings.

Discussion

The current study demonstrates acute microglial process convergence on proximal swellings of axons sustaining acute DAI in the micro pig thalamus, an association not previously recognized in the literature. Throughout this study, we employed a cFPI model in adult micro pigs to evaluate the diffuse pathology associated with mTBI in a higher order gyrencephalic animal more comparable to humans [47, 48]. This cFPI model, which has been successfully employed in rodents for decades, involves the transmission of a fluid pressure pulse to the brain and CSF through the intact dura mater, mimicking the movement of the brain following non-contusive diffuse mTBI in a reproducible fashion [55, 58, 63]. Using this model of cFPI, we demonstrated that diffuse mTBI in the micro pig produced substantial DAI, particularly within the thalamus, an area commonly affected in human TBI [49–52], without concomitant contusion or hematoma formation. Importantly, micro pig DAI was shown to be ultrastructurally consistent with that seen in humans [60] indicating that this model replicates human-like features of mTBI-associated diffuse pathology.

In concert with this axonal damage, extensive neuroinflammation, as identified by morphological alterations, indicative of microglial activation [25–27], was observed in the thalamus of micro pigs acutely following mTBI. Neuroinflammation is common following CNS injury in a variety of disease states and has been observed years following TBI in the human population [37, 51, 62, 64–69]. This chronic neuroinflammatory response has recently been observed in rodent models of trauma as well and is thought to be associated with negative outcomes both clinically and experimentally [19–23]. For a decade, it has been accepted that microglia react to CNS injury within minutes [70], however, little is known regarding acute neuroinflammation occurring minutes to hours following diffuse mTBI.

Previous studies, including our own, have focused on the phagocytic activity of microglia sub-acutely (days) following injury in rodents [29, 35–37, 39]. Specifically, we and others have identified an association between microglia phagocytosis and injured axons undergoing Wallerian degeneration days following injury in the rodent. Sub-acute phagocytosis has also been observed following demyelination and axonal injury in models of multiple sclerosis and leukodystrophy as well as during synaptic pruning during normal development [30, 62, 65, 71, 72]. It is possible, due to the fact that the current study only assess microglia at one acute time-point post-mTBI, that the observed process convergence on proximal axonal swellings is an early indication of microglial progression to phagocytic reactivity. Microglia, however, have non-phagocytic functions that are less well understood [28–33]. In healthy brain, endogenous microglia

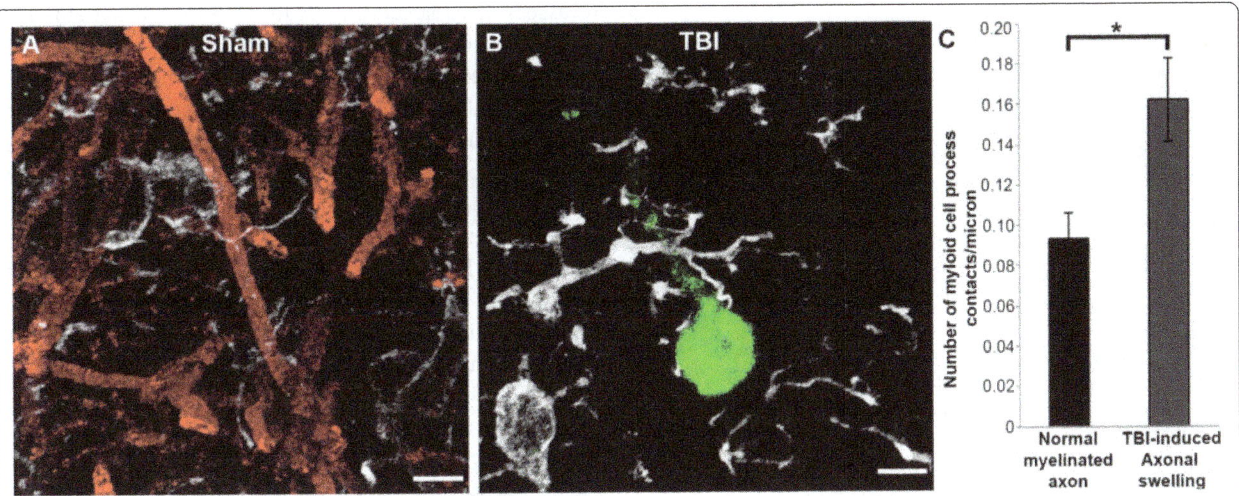

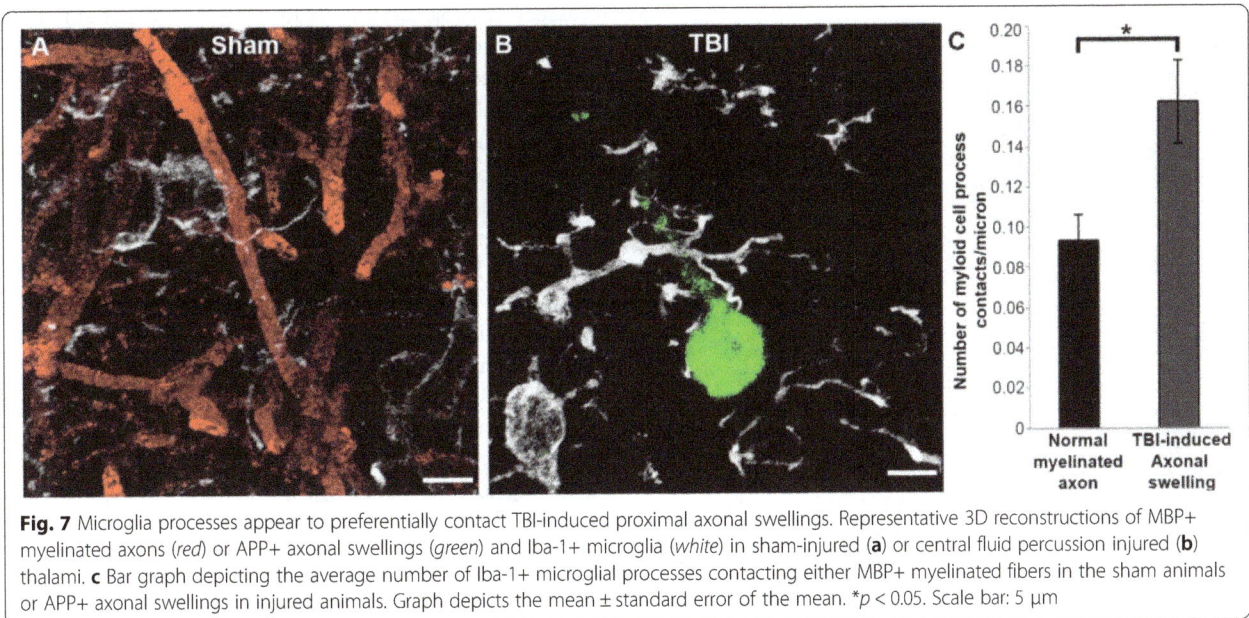

Fig. 7 Microglia processes appear to preferentially contact TBI-induced proximal axonal swellings. Representative 3D reconstructions of MBP+ myelinated axons (*red*) or APP+ axonal swellings (*green*) and Iba-1+ microglia (*white*) in sham-injured (**a**) or central fluid percussion injured (**b**) thalami. **c** Bar graph depicting the average number of Iba-1+ microglial processes contacting either MBP+ myelinated fibers in the sham animals or APP+ axonal swellings in injured animals. Graph depicts the mean ± standard error of the mean. *$p < 0.05$. Scale bar: 5 μm

have been shown to survey the parenchyma by extending highly dynamic processes that interact with the other cells of the CNS [73, 74]. This dynamic microglial process remodeling is altered under the influence of neuronal signals [27, 70, 75–77]. Additionally, a low calcium environment can activate microglial process convergence on neurons [78]. Microglial processes have also recently been shown to preferentially contact and functionally alter neurons with specific electrophysiological characteristics [61, 79].

While our study did not explore dynamic process remodeling, rather it assessed a snapshot of process dynamics acutely following mTBI, our findings indicate that non-phagocytic microglia processes preferentially interact with and/or converge on the proximal aspects of diffusely injured axons. Our previous studies and clinical observation indicate that the proximal axonal segments of neurons sustaining DAI do not immediately progress to cell death. Rather, they plastically adapt and remodel [14, 80–82], precluding the likelihood of acute phagocytosis. Calcium influx, however, has been well documented to occur acutely in axons sustaining DAI [83, 84]. This influx might alter the calcium concentration in the extracellular space immediately surrounding the proximal axonal swelling, which could act as a signal for microglial process convergence. Additionally, diffusely injured axons display acute electrophysiological alterations [85–87] which could modulate microglial responses.

Activated microglia are typically categorized into different subgroups of M1, inflammatory microglia, or alternatively activated/anti-inflammatory M2 microglia. These sub-groups, which have been observed in rodents, humans, and pigs, express either pro- (M1) or anti- (M2) inflammatory cytokines and are activated via different signaling pathways [29, 47, 88–91]. The specific functions of M2-activated microglia following mTBI are not well understood, however, it is speculated that M2 microglia are neuroprotective [22, 92, 93]. It is possible that the M2-activated microglia population is preferentially associated with the proximal swellings undergoing DAI, however, due to the limited study of neuroinflammation in pig, further investigation would be required to verify this potential phenomenon.

Conclusions

In summary, we demonstrated that central fluid percussion injury in adult micro pigs precipitated substantial acute axonal injury in the thalamus that is ultrastructurally similar to acute DAI in humans. Extensive microglial activation was also observed in the same thalamic sites, which directly correlated to the burden of thalamic axonal injury. The physical relationship between activated microglial processes and the proximal swelling of axons sustaining acute DAI was dramatically increased compared to uninjured myelinated thalamic axons in sham animals. In aggregate, these studies reveal acute microglial process convergence on proximal axonal swellings undergoing DAI, an interaction not previously recognized in the literature.

Current clinical techniques have emerged that allow for the visualization of neuroinflammation in the human population via PET imaging [51, 64, 94]. Our current finding that early microglial activation is directly associated with acute DAI in the micro pig, paired with the similarities between pig and human inflammatory

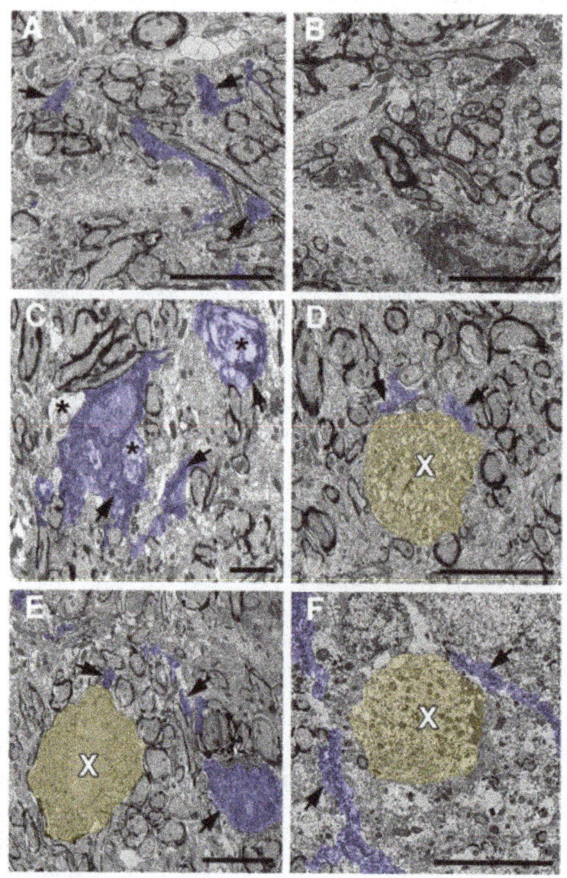

Fig. 8 Ultrastructural evidence of non-phagocytic microglial processes directly contacting proximal axonal swellings undergoing acute DAI. Representative electron micrographs of Iba-1 immuno-electron-microscope-labeled microglia in the thalamus of sham (**a** and **b**) and injured (**c–f**) animals. Iba-1-labeled structures in **a** and **c–f** are *pseudo-colored blue* for clarity. Note that, microglia processes containing Iba-1 (*arrows*) within the thalamus of sham-injured animals (**a** and **b**) are widely dispersed with no apparent association with axonal segments. Following cFPI, however, Iba-1+ microglial processes are much more prevalent. Some phagocytic microglia (**c**), containing material consistent with Wallerian degeneration (*asterisks*), are present following injury. These phagocytic microglia are primarily localized to areas of axonal damage/Wallerian degeneration. **d–f** Microglial processes (*pseudo-colored blue*) associating with axonal swellings (*pseudo-colored yellow*), as identified using the common ultrastructural features observed previously for diffuse axonal injury, appeared most frequently as **d** Iba-1 immunolabeled (*arrows*) puncta adjacent to the axonal swelling (*white X*), however, some cases **e** and **f** allowed for the tracing of microglia processes over short distances. Importantly, the Iba-1+ microglia processes found associated with axonal swellings did not reveal ultrastructural changes consistent with phagocytosis. Scale bar: 5 μm

profiles and responses [47, 48], suggests that this association could be exploited in humans early in the post-traumatic period. Recent observations indicating similar associations between DAI and neuroinflammation in humans weeks to years following injury lend credence to this possibility [69]. Techniques utilizing PET imaging to visualize human neuroinflammation could be employed to assess areas sustaining acute DAI in TBI patients in a way never before possible. Additionally, alterations in neuroinflammatory biomarkers within the serum following TBI could also be used in conjunction with these imaging techniques to estimate the total burden of diffuse injury and better tailor treatment in the human population. Future studies exploring the temporal relationship between neuroinflammation and the pathological progression of DAI through to sub-acute and even chronic time points in this higher order micro pig model could prove invaluable in understanding the interplay between DAI and neuroinflammation in the gyrencephalic brain.

Additional files

Additional file 1: Processes of ramified microglia primarily pass over normal myelinated fibers in the sham thalamus. Movie representing 3D reconstructions of confocal *z*-stacks of thalamic sites from sham-injured animals, in which Dapi-labeled nuclei are in *blue*, MBP+ myelinated axons are in *red*, and Iba-1+ microglia are in *white*. *Purple circles* highlight contacts between microglial processes and normal myelinated fibers. Notice that while only a few microglial processes come in direct apposition with normal myelinated fibers, the majority of microglial processes that do contact myelinated fibers do not terminate at the axon; rather pass over the myelinated fiber. Scale bar: 10 μm.

Additional file 2: Processes of activated microglia terminate on proximal swellings of axons sustaining acute DAI. Movie representing 3D reconstructions of confocal *z*-stacks of thalamic sites from cFPI animals, in which Dapi-labeled nuclei are in *blue*, MBP+ myelinated axons are in *red*, APP+ proximal axonal swellings are in *green*, and Iba-1+ microglia are in *white*. *Purple circles* highlight contacts between microglial processes and APP+ proximal axonal swellings. Note that the majority of microglial processes that come into contact with APP+ axonal swellings terminate on the proximal swelling, indicating process convergence. Scale bar: 10 μm.

Abbreviations

ANOVA: analysis of variance; APP: amyloid precursor protein; cFPI: central fluid percussion injury; DAI: diffuse axonal injury; MABP: mean arterial blood pressure; mTBI: mild traumatic brain injury; PaO_2: arterial oxygen tension; $PaCO_2$: arterial carbon dioxide pressure.

Competing interests

The authors declare that they have no competing interests.

Authors' contributions

ADL carried out the microscopic and ultrastructural analyses, conceived, designed, and coordinated the study, and wrote the manuscript. MT carried out the micro pig surgeries and physiological monitoring/analysis and participated in the microglial activation analysis. SAW participated in the micro pig surgeries and the design of the microscopic and ultrastructural studies. JTP participated in the micro pig surgeries and the ultrastructural analyses, conceived of the study and participated in its design, and wrote the manuscript. All authors read and approved the final manuscript.

Acknowledgements

The authors would like to thank Dr. Scott Henderson for his expertise in microscopy and image analysis, Dr. Robert Hamm for his biostatistical assistance and knowledge as well as Drs. David Loane, Kevin Wang, Patrick Kochanek, and Michelle Block for invigorating scientific discussions and suggestions. We would also like to recognize Lynn Davis, Jesse Sims, Karen Gorse, Judy Williamson, Frances White, and Dr. Thomas Taetzsch for invaluable technical assistance. This work was performed as a component of the Operation Brain Trauma Therapy consortium, which is supported by U.S. Army grants W81XWH-10-1-0623 and WH81XWH-14-2-0018. Microscopy was performed at the VCU Department of Anatomy and Neurobiology Microscopy Facility, supported, in part, with funding from NIH-NINDS Center core grant 5P30NS047463.

Author details

[1]Department of Anatomy and Neurobiology, Virginia Commonwealth University Medical Center, P.O. Box 980709, Richmond, VA 23298, USA. [2]Advanced Medical Emergency and Critical Care Center, Yamaguchi University Hospital, Yamaguchi, Japan.

References

1. Langlois JA, Rutland-Brown W, Wald MM. The epidemiology and impact of traumatic brain injury: a brief overview. J Head Trauma Rehabil. 2006;21:375–8.
2. Coronado VG, Xu L, Basavaraju SV, McGuire LC, Wald MM, Faul MD, et al. Surveillance for traumatic brain injury-related deaths—United States, 1997–2007. MMWR Surveill Summ. 2011;60:1–32.
3. Koskinen S, Alaranta H. Traumatic brain injury in Finland 1991–2005: a nationwide register study of hospitalized and fatal TBI. Brain Inj. 2008;22:205–14.
4. Feigin VL, Theadom A, Barker-Collo S, Starkey NJ, McPherson K, Kahan M, et al. Incidence of traumatic brain injury in New Zealand: a population-based study. Lancet Neurol. 2013;12:53–64.
5. Barkhoudarian G, Hovda DA, Giza CC. The molecular pathophysiology of concussive brain injury. Clin Sports Med. 2011;30:33–48. vii–iii.
6. Farkas O, Povlishock JT. Cellular and subcellular change evoked by diffuse traumatic brain injury: a complex web of change extending far beyond focal damage. Prog Brain Res. 2007;161:43–59.
7. McGinn M, Povlishock J. Cellular and molecular mechanisms of injury and spontaneous recovery. In: Handbook of clinical neurology. 2015;127:67–87.
8. Hemphill MA, Dauth S, Yu CJ, Dabiri BE, Parker KK. Review traumatic brain injury and the neuronal microenvironment : a potential role for neuropathological mechanotransduction. Neuron. 2015;85:1177–92.
9. Greve MW, Zink BJ. Pathophysiology of traumatic brain injury. Mt Sinai J Med. 2009;76:97–104.
10. Gennarelli TA, Thibault LE, Adams JH, Graham DI, Thompson CJ, Marcincin RP. Diffuse axonal injury and traumatic coma in the primate. Ann Neurol. 1982;12:564–74.
11. Povlishock JT. Pathobiology of traumatically induced axonal injury in animals and man. Ann Emerg Med. 1993;22:980–6.
12. Kelley BJ, Farkas O, Lifshitz J, Povlishock JT. Traumatic axonal injury in the perisomatic domain triggers ultrarapid secondary axotomy and Wallerian degeneration. Exp Neurol. 2006;198:350–60.
13. Smith DH, Meaney DF. Axonal damage in traumatic brain injury. Neurosci. 2000;6:483–95.
14. Adams JH, Graham DI, Murray LS, Scott G. Diffuse axonal injury due to nonmissile head injury in humans: an analysis of 45 cases. Ann Neurol. 1982;12:557–63.
15. Kraus MF, Susmaras T, Caughlin BP, Walker CJ, Sweeney JA, Little DM. White matter integrity and cognition in chronic traumatic brain injury: a diffusion tensor imaging study. Brain. 2007;130(Pt 10):2508–19.
16. Browne KD, Chen X-H, Meaney DF, Smith DH. Mild traumatic brain injury and diffuse axonal injury in swine. J Neurotrauma. 2011;28:1747–55.
17. Johnson VE, Stewart W, Smith DH. Axonal pathology in traumatic brain injury. Exp Neurol. 2013;246:35–43.
18. Scheid R, Walther K, Guthke T, Preul C, von Cramon DY. Cognitive sequelae of diffuse axonal injury. Arch Neurol. 2006;63:418–24.
19. Johnson VE, Stewart JE, Begbie FD, Trojanowski JQ, Smith DH, Stewart W. Inflammation and white matter degeneration persist for years after a single traumatic brain injury. Brain. 2013;136:28–42.
20. Loane DJ, Kumar A, Stoica B, Cabatbat R, Faden AI. Progressive neurodegeneration after experimental brain trauma: association with chronic microglial activation. J Neuropathol Exp Neurol. 2013;73:14–29.
21. Kumar A, Loane DJ. Neuroinflammation after traumatic brain injury: opportunities for therapeutic intervention. Brain Behav Immun. 2012;26:1191–201.
22. Kumar A, Stoica B, Sabirzhanov B, Burns MP, Faden AI, Loane DJ. Traumatic brain injury in aged animals increases lesion size and chronically alters microglial/macrophage classical and alternative activation states. Neurobiol Aging. 2013;34:1397–411.
23. Hinson HE, Rowell S, Schreiber M. Clinical evidence of inflammation driving secondary brain injury. J Trauma Acute Care Surg. 2015;78:184–91.
24. Bell MJ, Kochanek PM, Doughty L, Carcillo J, Adelson PD, Clark RSB, et al. Interleukin-6 and interleukin-10 in cerebrospinal fluid after severe traumatic brain injury in children. J Neurotrauma. 1997;14:451–7.
25. Taetzsch T, Levesque S, McGraw C, Brookins S, Luqa R, Bonini MG, et al. Redox regulation of NF-κB p50 and M1 polarization in microglia. Glia. 2015;63:423–40.
26. Byrnes KR, Loane DJ, Stoica B, Zhang J, Faden AI. Delayed mGluR5 activation limits neuroinflammation and neurodegeneration after traumatic brain injury. J Neuroinflammation. 2012;9:43.
27. Haynes SE, Hollopeter G, Yang G, Kurpius D, Dailey ME, Gan W-B, et al. The P2Y12 receptor regulates microglial activation by extracellular nucleotides. Nat Neurosci. 2006;9:1512–9.
28. Kyritsis N, Kizil C, Zocher S, Kroehne V, Kaslin J, Freudenreich D, et al. Acute inflammation initiates the regenerative response in the adult zebrafish brain. Science. 2012;338:1353–6.
29. Aguzzi A, Barres B, Bennett ML. Microglia: scapegoat, saboteur or something else ? Inflammation. 2013;339:156–62.
30. Parkhurst CN, Yang G, Ninan I, Savas JN, Yates JR, Lafaille JJ, et al. Microglia promote learning-dependent synapse formation through brain-derived neurotrophic factor. Cell. 2013;155:1596–609.
31. Miyamoto A, Wake H, Moorhouse AJ, Nabekura J. Microglia and synapse interactions: fine tuning neural circuits and candidate molecules. Front Cell Neurosci. 2013;7(May):70.
32. Batchelor PE, Porritt MJ, Martinello P, Parish CL, Liberatore GT, Donnan G, et al. Macrophages and microglia produce local trophic gradients that stimulate axonal sprouting toward but not beyond the wound edge. Mol Cell Neurosci. 2002;21:436–53.
33. Venkatesan C, Chrzaszcz M, Choi N, Wainwright MS. Chronic upregulation of activated microglia immunoreactive for galectin-3/Mac-2 and nerve growth factor following diffuse axonal injury. J Neuroinflammation. 2010;7:32.
34. Jebelli J, Su W, Hopkins S, Pocock J, Garden GA. Glia: guardians, gluttons, or guides for the maintenance of neuronal connectivity? Ann N Y Acad Sci. 2015;1351:1–10.
35. Shitaka Y, Tran HT, Bennett RE, Sanchez L, Levy M, Dikranian K, et al. Repetitive closed-skull traumatic brain injury in mice causes persistent multifocal axonal injury and microglial reactivity. J Neuropathol Exp Neurol. 2012;70:551–67.
36. Wang J, Fox MA, Povlishock JT. Diffuse traumatic axonal injury in the optic nerve does not elicit retinal ganglion cell loss. J Neuropathol Exp Neurol. 2013;72:768–81.
37. Oehmichen M, Theuerkauf I, Meißner C. Is traumatic axonal injury (AI) associated with an early microglial activation? Application of a double-labeling technique for simultaneous detection of microglia and AI. Acta Neuropathol. 1999;97:491–4.
38. Gyoneva S, Ransohoff RM. Inflammatory reaction after traumatic brain injury: therapeutic potential of targeting cell–cell communication by chemokines. Trends Pharmacol Sci. 2015;1–10.
39. Kelley BJ, Lifshitz J, Povlishock JT. Neuroinflammatory responses after experimental diffuse traumatic brain injury. J Neuropathol Exp Neurol. 2007;66:989–1001.
40. Lawson L, Perry V, Gordon S. Heterogeneity in the distribution and morphology of microglia in the normal adult mouse brain. Neuroscience. 1990;39:151–70.
41. McKay SM, Brooks DJ, Hu P, McLachlan EM. Distinct types of microglial activation in white and grey matter of rat lumbosacral cord after mid-thoracic spinal transection. J Neuropathol Exp Neurol. 2007;66:698–710.
42. Ogura K, Ogawa M, Yoshida M. Effects of ageing on microglia in the normal rat brain: immunohistochemical observations. Neuroreport. 1994;5:1224–6.
43. Seok J, Warren HS, Cuenca AG, Mindrinos MN, Baker HV, Xu W, et al. Genomic responses in mouse models poorly mimic human inflammatory diseases. Proc Natl Acad Sci U S A. 2013;110:3507–12.
44. Heinz S, Haehnel V, Karaghiosoff M, Schwarzfischer L, Müller M, Krause SW, et al. Species-specific regulation of toll-like receptor 3 genes in men and mice. J Biol Chem. 2003;278:21502–9.
45. Roshick C, Wood H, Caldwell HD, McClarty G. Comparison of gamma interferon-mediated antichlamydial defense mechanisms in human and mouse cells. Infect Immun. 2006;74:225–38.

46. Mikaberidze A. Molecular mimicry and the generation of host defense protein diversity. Cell. 1993;72:823–6.
47. Fairbairn L, Kapetanovic R, Sester DP, Hume D. The mononuclear phagocyte system of the pig as a model for understanding human innate immunity and disease. J Leukoc Biol. 2011;89:855–71.
48. Wernersson R, Schierup MH, Jørgensen FG, Gorodkin J, Panitz F, Staerfeldt H-H, et al. Pigs in sequence space: a 0.66X coverage pig genome survey based on shotgun sequencing. BMC Genomics. 2005;6:70.
49. Anderson CV, Wood DM, Bigler ED, Blatter DD. Lesion volume, injury severity, and thalamic integrity following head injury. J Neurotrauma. 1996;13:59–65.
50. Schiff ND, Giacino JT, Kalmar K, Victor JD, Baker K, Gerber M, et al. Behavioural improvements with thalamic stimulation after severe traumatic brain injury. Nature. 2007;448:600–3.
51. Ramlackhansingh AF, Brooks DJ, Greenwood RJ, Bose SK, Turkheimer FE, Kinnunen KM, et al. Inflammation after trauma: microglial activation and traumatic brain injury. Ann Neurol. 2011;70:374–83.
52. Ross DT, Graham DI, Adams JH. Selective loss of neurons from the thalamic reticular nucleus following severe human head injury. J Neurotrauma. 1993;10:151–65.
53. Sherriff FE, Bridges LR, Sivaloganathan S. Early detection of axonal injury after human head trauma using immunocytochemistry for beta-amyloid precursor protein. Acta Neuropathol. 1994;87:55–62.
54. Gentleman SM, Nash MJ, Sweeting CJ, Graham DI, Roberts GW. Beta-amyloid precursor protein (beta APP) as a marker for axonal injury after head injury. Neurosci Lett. 1993;160:139–44.
55. Dixon CE, Lyeth BG, Povlishock JT, Findling RL, Hamm RJ, Marmarou A, et al. A fluid percussion model of experimental brain injury in the rat. J Neurosurg. 1987;67:110–9.
56. Bove A. Diving medicine. Am J Respir Crit Care Med. 2014;189:1479–86.
57. Thomson L, Paton J. Oxygen toxicity. Paediatr Respir Rev. 2014;15:120–3.
58. Hånell A, Greer JE, McGinn MJ, Povlishock JT. Traumatic brain injury-induced axonal phenotypes react differently to treatment. Acta Neuropathol. 2014;129:317–32.
59. Wang J, Hamm RJ, Povlishock JT. Traumatic axonal injury in the optic nerve: evidence for axonal swelling, disconnection, dieback, and reorganization. J Neurotrauma. 2011;28:1185–98.
60. Christman CW, Grady MS, Walker SA, Holloway KL, Povlishock JT. Ultrastructural studies of diffuse axonal injury in humans. J Neurotrauma. 1994;11:173–86.
61. Eyo UB, Peng J, Swiatkowski P, Mukherjee A, Bispo A, Wu L-J. Neuronal hyperactivity recruits microglial processes via neuronal NMDA receptors and microglial P2Y12 receptors after status epilepticus. J Neurosci. 2014;34:10528–40.
62. Yamasaki R, Lu H, Butovsky O, Ohno N, Rietsch AM, Cialic R, et al. Differential roles of microglia and monocytes in the inflamed central nervous system. J Exp Med. 2014;211:1533–49.
63. Lafrenaye AD, Krahe TE, Povlishock JT. Moderately elevated intracranial pressure after diffuse traumatic brain injury is associated with exacerbated neuronal pathology and behavioral morbidity in the rat. J Cereb Blood Flow Metab. 2014;34:1628–36.
64. Coughlin JM, Wang Y, Munro C, Ma S, Yue C, Chen S, et al. Neuroinflammation and brain atrophy in former NFL players: an in vivo multimodal imaging pilot study. Neurobiol Dis. 2015;74:58–65.
65. Kondo Y, Adams JM, Vanier MT, Duncan ID. Macrophages counteract demyelination in a mouse model of globoid cell leukodystrophy. J Neurosci. 2011;31:3610–24.
66. Tönges L, Günther R, Suhr M, Jansen J, Balck A, Saal KA, et al. Rho kinase inhibition modulates microglia activation and improves survival in a model of amyotrophic lateral sclerosis. Glia. 2014;62:217–32.
67. Nemeth CL, Reddy R, Bekhbat M, Bailey J, Neigh GN. Microglial activation occurs in the absence of anxiety-like behavior following microembolic stroke in female, but not male, rats. J Neuroinflammation. 2014;11:174.
68. Howell OW, Rundle JL, Garg A, Komada M, Brophy PJ, Reynolds R. Activated microglia mediate axoglial disruption that contributes to axonal injury in multiple sclerosis. J Neuropathol Exp Neurol. 2010;69:1017–33.
69. Ryu J, Horkayne-Szakaly I, Xu L, Pletnikova O, Leri F, Eberhart C, et al. The problem of axonal injury in the brains of veterans with histories of blast exposure. Acta Neuropathol Commun. 2014;2:1–14.
70. Davalos D, Grutzendler J, Yang G, Kim JV, Zuo Y, Jung S, et al. ATP mediates rapid microglial response to local brain injury in vivo. Nat Neurosci. 2005;8:752–8.
71. Schafer DP, Lehrman EK, Stevens B. The "quad-partite" synapse: microglia-synapse interactions in the developing and mature CNS. Glia. 2013;61:24–36.
72. Neumann H, Kotter MR, Franklin RJM. Debris clearance by microglia: an essential link between degeneration and regeneration. Brain. 2009;132(Pt 2):288–95.
73. Baalman K, Marin M, Ho TS-Y, Godoy M, Cherian L, Robertson C, et al. Axon initial segment-associated microglia. J Neurosci. 2015;35:2283–92.
74. Nimmerjahn A, Kirchhoff F, Helmchen F. Resting microglial cells are highly dynamic surveillants of brain parenchyma in vivo—supporting online material. Science. 2005;308:1314–9.
75. Damani MR, Zhao L, Fontainhas AM, Amaral J, Fariss RN, Wong WT. Age-related alterations in the dynamic behavior of microglia. Aging Cell. 2011;10:263–76.
76. Wake H, Moorhouse AJ, Miyamoto A, Nabekura J. Microglia: actively surveying and shaping neuronal circuit structure and function. Trends Neurosci. 2013;36:209–17.
77. Krabbe G, Matyash V, Pannasch U, Mamer L, Boddeke HWGM, Kettenmann H. Activation of serotonin receptors promotes microglial injury-induced motility but attenuates phagocytic activity. Brain Behav Immun. 2012;26:419–28.
78. Eyo UB, Gu N, De S, Dong H, Richardson JR, Wu L-J. Modulation of microglial process convergence toward neuronal dendrites by extracellular calcium. J Neurosci. 2015;35:2417–22.
79. Chen Z, Jalabi W, Hu W, Park H-J, Gale JT, Kidd GJ, et al. Microglial displacement of inhibitory synapses provides neuroprotection in the adult brain. Nat Commun. 2014;5(July):4486–98.
80. Lifshitz J, Kelley BJ, Povlishock JT. Perisomatic thalamic axotomy after diffuse traumatic brain injury is associated with atrophy rather than cell death. J Neuropathol Exp Neurol. 2007;66:218–29.
81. Greer JE, McGinn MJ, Povlishock JT. Diffuse traumatic axonal injury in the mouse induces atrophy, c-Jun activation, and axonal outgrowth in the axotomized neuronal population. J Neurosci. 2011;31:5089–105.
82. Grady MS, McLaughlin MR, Christman CW, Valadka AB, Fligner CL, Povlishock JT. The use of antibodies targeted against the neurofilament subunits for the detection of diffuse axonal injury in humans. J Neuropathol Exp Neurol. 1993;52:143–52.
83. Wolf JA, Stys PK, Lusardi T, Meaney D, Smith DH. Traumatic axonal injury induces calcium influx modulated by tetrodotoxin-sensitive sodium channels. J Neurosci. 2001;21:1923–30.
84. LoPachin RM, Lehning EJ. Mechanism of calcium entry during axon injury and degeneration. Toxicol Appl Pharmacol. 1997;143:233–44.
85. Cohen AS, Pfister BJ, Schwarzbach E, Grady MS, Goforth PB, Satin LS. Injury-induced alterations in CNS electrophysiology. Prog Brain Res. 2007;161:143–69.
86. Greer JE, Povlishock JT, Jacobs KM. Electrophysiological abnormalities in both axotomized and nonaxotomized pyramidal neurons following mild traumatic brain injury. J Neurosci. 2012;32:6682–7.
87. Reeves TM, Phillips LL, Povlishock JT. Myelinated and unmyelinated axons of the corpus callosum differ in vulnerability and functional recovery following traumatic brain injury. Exp Neurol. 2005;196:126–37.
88. Girard S, Brough D, Lopez-Castejon G, Giles J, Rothwell NJ, Allan SM. Microglia and macrophages differentially modulate cell death after brain injury caused by oxygen-glucose deprivation in organotypic brain slices. Glia. 2013;61:813–24.
89. Tang Y, Le W. Differential roles of M1 and M2 microglia in neurodegenerative diseases. Mol Neurobiol 2015. Epub ahead of print.
90. Tam WY, Ma CHE. Bipolar/rod-shaped microglia are proliferating microglia with distinct M1/M2 phenotypes. Sci Rep. 2014;4:7279.
91. Martinez FO, Helming L, Milde R, Varin A, Melgert BN, Draijer C, et al. Genetic programs expressed in resting and IL-4 alternatively activated mouse and human macrophages: Similarities and differences. Blood. 2013;121:57–69.
92. Karve IP, Taylor JM, Crack PJ. The contribution of astrocytes and microglia to traumatic brain injury. Br J Pharmacol 2015. Epub ahead of print.
93. Wang G, Shi Y, Jiang X, Leak RK, Hu X, Wu Y, et al. HDAC inhibition prevents white matter injury by modulating microglia/macrophage polarization through the GSK3β/PTEN/Akt axis. PNAS. 2015;112:2853–58.
94. Banati RB. Visualising microglial activation in vivo. Glia. 2002;40:206–17.

7

Impact of nutrition on inflammation, tauopathy, and behavioral outcomes from chronic traumatic encephalopathy

Jin Yu[1], Hong Zhu[1], Saeid Taheri[1], William Mondy[1], Stephen Perry[2] and Mark S. Kindy[1,3,4,5*]

Abstract

Background: Repetitive mild traumatic brain injuries (rmTBI) are associated with cognitive deficits, inflammation, and stress-related events. We tested the effect of nutrient intake on the impact of rmTBI in an animal model of chronic traumatic encephalopathy (CTE) to study the pathophysiological mechanisms underlying this model. We used a between group design rmTBI closed head injuries in mice, compared to a control and nutrient-treated groups.

Methods: Our model allows for controlled, repetitive closed head impacts to mice. Briefly, 24-week-old mice were divided into five groups: control, rmTBI, and rmTBI with nutrients (2% of NF-216, NF-316 and NF-416). rmTBI mice received four concussive impacts over 7 days. Mice were treated with NutriFusion diets for 2 months prior to the rmTBI and until euthanasia (6 months). Mice were then subsequently euthanized for macro- and micro-histopathologic analysis for various times up to 6 months after the last TBI received. Animals were examined behaviorally, and brain sections were immunostained for glial fibrillary acidic protein (GFAP) for astrocytes, iba-1 for activated microglia, and AT8 for phosphorylated tau protein.

Results: Animals on nutrient diets showed attenuated behavioral changes. The brains from all mice lacked macroscopic tissue damage at all time points. The rmTBI resulted in a marked neuroinflammatory response, with persistent and widespread astrogliosis and microglial activation, as well as significantly elevated phospho-tau immunoreactivity to 6 months. Mice treated with diets had significantly reduced inflammation and phospho-tau staining.

Conclusions: The neuropathological findings in the rmTBI mice showed histopathological hallmarks of CTE, including increased astrogliosis, microglial activation, and hyperphosphorylated tau protein accumulation, while mice treated with diets had attenuated disease process. These studies demonstrate that consumption of nutrient-rich diets reduced disease progression.

Keywords: Animal model, Chronic traumatic encephalopathy, Concussion, Pathophysiology, Repetitive, Diet, Inflammation, Neurodegeneration, Behavior

Background

Mild traumatic brain injury (mTBI) is a result of concussive head traumas that are considered a growing issue, with millions of sports-, military-, and recreation-related concussions occurring each year [1, 2]. In the USA alone, over four million concussions occur each year, which is a considerable problem [3, 4]. Evidence from various studies on the physical properties, neuroimaging, neuropathology, and basic science experiments has determined that these concussive injuries and related subconcussive impacts have led to the development of both acute and chronic post-traumatic sequelae [5, 6]. Recently, the discovery of chronic traumatic encephalopathy (CTE) following "repetitive head injuries" has been seen in the majority of sports programs including football, soccer, hockey, and boxing, and is a serious problem [7–10].

Much of the information we have about CTE has been derived from data collected from autopsies and retrospective

* Correspondence: kindym@health.usf.edu
[1]Department of Pharmaceutical Sciences, College of Pharmacy, University of South Florida, 12901 Bruce B. Downs Blvd., MDC 30, Tampa, FL 33612, USA
[3]Departments of Molecular Medicine, Molecular Pharmacology, Physiology and Pathology and Cell Biology, and Neurology, College of Medicine, University of South Florida, Tampa, FL, USA

and population studies [11]. Because of the nature of the disorder, the incidence and prevalence are difficult to determine [12]. The risk factors associated with the development and progression of CTE are not well known, yet we understand that repetitive blunt force trauma to the head and body, blast impacts, and acceleration-deceleration influences can trigger the processes [13]. CTE has a myriad of clinical presentations that include impairments in cognition, behavior, and mood, and in some cases, chronic headache and motor and cerebellar dysfunction [14]. Behavioral changes such as irritability, judgment issues, increased risk-taking, and depression are characteristic and prominent early in the disease course. Unfortunately, the only way to diagnose the disease is through histological and immunohistochemical analyses that show the presence of hyperphosphorylated tau as multifocal or diffuse cortical and subcortical regions within the brain [15, 16]. In addition, the presence of inflammation during CTE is accompanied by the activation of astrocytes and microglial cells [17].

The mechanisms associated with the pathophysiological changes seen in CTE are still not well documented. Because of this, researchers have attempted to generate paradigms that best define the clinical evidence [18–20]. Various models of CTE have been developed including closed head repetitive mild traumatic brain injury (rmTBI) to mimic the pathological outcomes [21]. CTE may be a compilation of co-morbidities, normal or accelerated aging, or other factors that contribute to the symptomology [22]. Based on current data, following a TBI (or multiple TBIs), neurodegenerative conditions set in years afterwards, which is why accumulation of information takes a significant time to understand the potential mechanisms involved [23]. Over the years, experimental models that are representative of CTE and the neurological sequelae such as post-concussion syndrome (PCS), post-traumatic stress disorder (PTSD), and mild cognitive impairment (MCI) may be well represented by repetitive brain injury [24]. The behavioral patterns observed in CTE patients include cognitive deficits, increased risk-taking, depression-like behavior, and sleep disturbances [25, 26]. Therefore, rmTBI models result in the histopathological hallmarks of CTE, including increased astrogliosis, microglial activation, and phosphorylated tau immunoreactivity.

In the current study, our goal was to determine the influence of diets rich in vegetables and fruits on the outcomes associated with rmTBI or CTE. Mice were fed diets enriched in fruits and vegetables for 2 months and then subjected to rmTBI. The results demonstrated that diets high in phytonutrients were able to attenuate the "CTE-like" pathology provoked by the rmTBI. Behavioral changes, inflammation, and tau pathology were examined in mice chronically exposed to the diets. The results suggest that supplementation of mice with the enhanced diets limited the extent of the CTE, reduced inflammation, and altered pathways typical of CTE. These data suggest that these diets may be beneficial in altering the presentation of CTE seen in models of rmTBI and improve outcome.

Methods

Animal care and maintenance

All animals used in this study were treated in accordance with the National Institutes of Health Guidelines for the Care and Use of Laboratory Animals, and all procedures were performed under the approval of the Institutional Animal Care and Use Committee at the University of South Florida. Adult male, human Tau mice (hTau, Taconic, Hudson, NY) were purchased and housed with five mice per cage. Animals were 24 weeks of age at the start of the experiment and were maintained on a 12-h light/dark cycle (lights on at 7:00 a.m.). All animals were randomized to the various groups. Prior to TBI, animals were fed for 2 months a normal diet or a normal diet with ~2% supplementation of the different materials NF-216 (GrandFusion – Fruit and Veggie #1 Blend), NF-316 (GrandFusion – Fruit #2 Blend), and NF-416 (GrandFusion – Vegetable #3 Blend) [27]. See Table 1 for composition of supplementation. In addition to the vitamins, through the isolation/extraction process, the phytonutrients in the fruits and vegetables are maintained and non-oxidized. Animals were gavaged with the supplements on a daily basis, once per day. GrandFusion supplements were prepared by NutriFusion, LLC (www.nutrifusion.com). Average food intake was 3.81 ± 0.08 g/day/mouse, and the average consumption of diets was 0.09 ± 0.006 g/day/mouse.

TBI injury

The rmTBI mouse model was used to deliver a controlled, consistent injury to all animals [28]. Adult mice were anesthetized with ketamine (60–90 mg/kg) and xylazine (6–9 mg/kg) or isoflurane (5% induction, 1–2% maintenance). The degree of anesthesia was assessed by testing of interdigital pinch withdrawal reflex. Lacrilube ophthalmic ointment was applied to both eyes to prevent drying. For the repetitive closed head injury, following anesthesia, the mouse was placed in the pneumatic impactor device (Precision Systems and Instrumentation, Fairfax Station, VA) and was subjected to a closed head injury of 4 m/s (speed), 3.8 mm (depth), and 200 ms (dwell time). The mouse was returned to its home cage and monitored until it is awake. The procedure was repeated up to three times (four total injuries), spaced 2–3 days apart (i.e., M, W, F, M). Animals were returned to their home cages after recovery from anesthesia and monitored daily for any signs of discomfort or other abnormal behavior. See diagram for outline of behavioral testing.

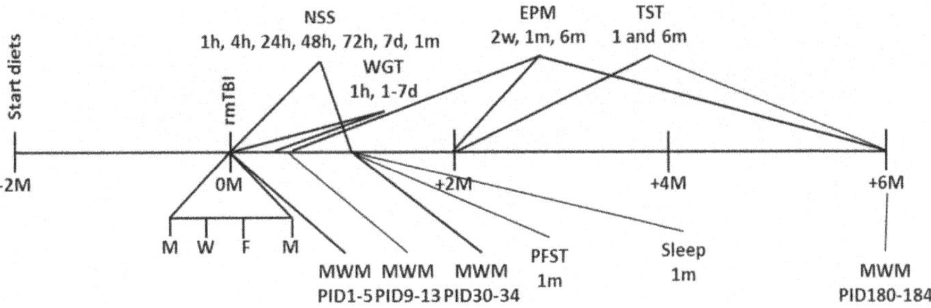

Neurological Severity Score

To characterize the effects of the nutritional diet on repetitive mTBI/CTE in this model, a Neurological Severity Score (NSS) was used to evaluate the neurological impairment, compared to uninjured controls, as previously described [29]. The NSS is a composite clinical score consisting of 10 individual clinical parameters, including tasks on motor function, alertness, and general physiological behavior (Table 2). Mice (10 per group) were tested at 1, 4, 24, 48, and 72 h post-injury, as well as at 7-day and 1-month time points. Severity of injury was defined by the initial NSS measured at 1 h post-TBI and is a reliable predictor of late outcome [29].

Assessment of motor function

Vestibulomotor function was determined by a wire grip test (WGT) 1 h after TBI and on post-injury days 1–7 [30]. Mice (10 per group) were picked up by the tail and placed on a metal wire suspended between two upright bars 30 cm above a padded floor. The mice were assessed for the time and manner they could hold onto the wire and were recorded and scored on a scale of 0–5. Mice were tested three consecutive times at each of the indicated time points. The score reported is the average of these individual trials by individuals blinded to the treatments. A composite group score was then calculated as the mean of these scores at each time point and then used for analysis.

Assessment of spatial learning and memory

Control and repetitive mTBI groups were tested in the Morris water maze (MWM) acutely (acquisition trials on post-injury days [PIDs] 1–5 and probe trial on PID 6), subacutely (acquisition trials on PIDs 9–13 and probe trial on PID 14), and chronically at 1 (acquisition trials on PIDs 30–34 and probe trial on PID 35) and 6 months (acquisition trials on PIDs 180–184 and probe trial on PID 185) after the final head impact. Mice had to locate an invisible platform submerged 5 mm below the water level in a circular pool (dimensions, 90 × 60 cm; temperature, 24 ± 3 °C), based on the spatial location of six strategic visual cues fixed at distinct positions around the pool. The water was made opaque by adding nontoxic, water-soluble tempera paint. Data were recorded with the help of video cameras (SMART video tracking system, San Diego Instruments, San Diego, CA).

For training days (acquisition phase), all mice (15 per group, per time point) were given a maximum test duration of 60 s to find the hidden platform. The latency to reach the platform was recorded by the video tracking system. Mice that failed to locate the platform within the time limit were guided to it and allowed to rest and orient themselves for 15 s. The acquisition phase testing was conducted over five consecutive days, with four trials on each day, with the goal of locating the submerged hidden platform from different starting points and orientations (north, south, east, and west). On day 6 of MWM testing, all animals were tested for visual acuity and swimming speed using a visible platform paradigm. None of the animals were excluded from further testing based on the visual acuity and motor evaluation tests. On day 6, all mice also underwent a probe trial (retention phase), where the platform was removed from the pool. Mice were given 30 s to swim, and time spent in the target quadrant (quadrant where the platform had been) versus the other quadrants was assessed as described previously.

Assessment of anxiety-related and risk-taking behaviors

Anxiety-related and risk-taking behavior of the mice was evaluated using the elevated plus maze (EPM) test. Mice (15 per group, per time point) were evaluated at 2 weeks, 1 month, and 6 months from the last head impact. The EPM consisted of two opposing open arms (35 × 5 cm) and two closed arms (35 × 5 × 15 cm) that extended from a central platform (5 × 5 cm) elevated 60 cm above the floor. A small raised lip (0.5 cm) around the edges of the open arms prevents animals from slipping off. Mice were placed individually on the central platform facing an open arm, away from the examiner, and were allowed to freely explore the maze for 5 min under even overhead fluorescent lighting. The behavior of each mouse was monitored using a SMART video tracking system (San Diego Instruments, San Diego, CA). Time spent in the open and closed arms was determined, and each mouse was only tested once in the maze.

Table 1 Composition of GrandFusion supplements

Blend #1: Fruit and Vegetable Blend (NF-216)

6 Essential Vitamins	Minimum Premix Claim Per 225.00 mg	
Nutrient	**% dv**	**Label Claim**
Vitamin A	50.00	2,500.000 IU
Vitamin C	50.00	30.000 mg
Vitamin D	50.00	200.000 IU
Vitamin E	50.00	15.000 IU
Vitamin B1	50.00	0.7500 mg
Vitamin B6	50.00	1.000 mg

Vegetable: Pwd Tomato, Broccoli, Carrot, Shitake Mushrooms
Fruit: Pwd Cranberry, Apple, Orange Made from 100% organic materials

Blend #2: Fruit Blend (NF-316)

6 Essential Vitamins	Minimum Premix Claim Per 225.00 mg	
Nutrient	**% dv**	**Label Claim**
Vitamin A	50.00	2,500.000 IU
Vitamin C	50.00	30.000 mg
Vitamin D	50.00	200.000 IU
Vitamin E	50.00	15.000 IU
Vitamin B1	50.00	0.7500 mg
Vitamin B6	50.00	1.000 mg

Fruit: Pwd Orange, Cranberry, Apple, Cherry, Blueberry, Strawberry, Shitake Mushrooms
Made from 100% organic materials

Blend #3: Vegetable Blend (NF-416)

6 Essential Vitamins	Minimum Premix Claim Per 225.00 mg	
Nutrient	**% dv**	**Label Claim**
Vitamin A	50.00	2,500.000 IU
Vitamin C	50.00	30.000 mg
Vitamin D	50.00	200.000 IU
Vitamin E	50.00	15.000 IU
Vitamin B1	50.00	0.7500 mg
Vitamin B6	50.00	1.000 mg

Vegetable: Pwd Spinach, Broccoli, Carrot, Tomato, Beet, Shitake Mushrooms
Made from 100% organic materials

Assessment of depression-like behavior

To determine the long-term effects of mTBI on depression-like behavior, mice (15 per group) were tested in the Porsolt forced swim test (PFST) and the tail suspension test (TST) at 1 month post-injury [31, 32].

Porsolt forced swim test

Mice were placed in an open glass cylinder (diameter 12 cm, height 24 cm, and water level 16 cm) containing water at 23–25 °C. The time for the test was 6 min, with the first 2 min for habituation and the last 4 min used

Table 2 Neurological Severity Score

Task	Description	Score (success/failure)
Exit circle	Ability and initiative to exit a circle of 30 cm in diameter within 3 min	
Monoparesis/hemiparesis	Assess paresis of upper and/or lower limb	0/1
Straight walk/gait	Initiative and motor ability to walk straight	
Startle reflex	Innate reflex assessment; mouse should bounce in response to a loud hand clap	0/1
Seeking behavior	Physiological behavior as a sign of "interest" in the environment	
Beam balancing	Ability to balance on a beam of 7 mm in width for at least 10 s	0/1
Round stick balancing	Ability to balance on a round stick of 5 mm in diameter for at least 10 s	
Beam walk: 3 cm	Ability to cross a 30-cm-long beam: 3-cm-wide beam	0/1
Beam walk: 2 cm	Ability to cross a 30-cm-long beam (increased difficulty): 2-cm-wide beam	
Beam walk: 1 cm	Ability to cross a 30-cm-long beam (increased difficulty): 1-cm-wide beam	0/1
Total score		Of 10

Adapted from [29]. One point is awarded for the lack of a tested reflex or for the inability to perform the tasks outlined in the table, and no point for succeeding. A maximal Neurological Severity Score (NSS) of 10 points thus indicates severe neurological dysfunction, with failure of all tasks, and a normal healthy mouse would get a score of a zero on the tasks above. Roughly, NSS score: 1–4, mild TBI; 5–7, moderate TBI; 8–10, severe TBI

for analysis. Two different experimenters were blinded to the groups of mice evaluated for behavior, manually. A mouse was judged to be immobile when it remained floating in the water, making only those movements necessary to keep its head above the water surface.

Tail suspension test

Briefly, mice were suspended by the tail to a bar elevated 40 cm above the surface of a table. The duration of the test was 6 min. Two different experimenters blinded to the groups of mice manually evaluated the behavior. The immobility time of the tail-suspended mice was measured and defined as the absence of limb movement. These tests were done at 2 and 6 months.

Assessment of sleep behavior

Electroencephalography (EEG) and electromyography (EMG) data were acquired in mice at 1 month post-injury (15 per group) using implantable telemetry devices (Data Sciences International, ST. Paul, MN) and the Dataquest A.R.T. system (Data Sciences International). The transmitter was implanted intraperitoneally through a mid-line abdominal incision. EEG lead implantation was performed by insertion of leads in small burr holes overlying the cortex. EMG leads EMG electrodes were implanted into the neck muscle. The EEG electrodes were secured with dental cement, and the EMG electrodes were secured with sutures. Mice were allowed to recover and were individually housed in a sound-attenuated and ventilated chamber on a standard light/dark cycle, with food and water available ad libitum. After a 7-day acclimation and recovery period, the telemetry EEG/EMG devices were activated and continuous recordings were obtained for a total of 24 h (6 PM to 6 PM) [33]. EEG and EMG data were analyzed in 1-min epochs using Neuroscore software devices (Data Sciences International). Using both manual scoring and automated software, EEG/EMG recordings were broken down into active wake, non-rapid eye movement (NREM) sleep, and REM sleep. Raw EMG signals were full-wave rectified, integrated, and quantified in arbitrary units. Active wake was classified as low-amplitude EEG with high EMG activity. NREM sleep was classified as high-amplitude EEG dominated by delta band components (0–4 Hz). REM sleep was classified as low-amplitude EEG with low EMG activity. In addition to total sleep/wake time, power band (i.e., delta, theta, alpha, and beta) and power spectral (frequency) analysis of sleep/wake states was further assessed to study the quality of NREM and REM sleep in each animal.

Immunohistochemistry

At the indicated times following rmTBI, the mice underwent transcardial perfusion with ice-cold 0.01 M phosphate-buffered saline (PBS) (pH 7.4), followed by fixation with 4% para-formaldehyde (PFA) in PBS. Brain tissue from all animals was dissected and post-fixed in 4% PFA for 24 h. Following fixation, the tissue underwent dehydration first in 30% sucrose for 24 h each. Tissue was placed in optimal cutting temperature (OCT) compound (Tissue-Tek) and was sliced on a cryostat (Microm HE 505E) into 30 μm coronal sections. Tissue sections were then floated in PBS. Six mice were included in each of the above groups. For each mouse, five representative coronal sections were selected for staining by collecting a single section every 1000 μm along a rostral–caudal axis beginning 1.1 mm anterior to and ending 2.5 mm posterior to bregma. The primary antibodies used included rabbit anti-mouse glial fibrillary acidic protein (GFAP) polyclonal IgG (Millipore, Billerica, MA, USA), mouse anti-human phospho-PHF-tau (pTau) monoclonal IgG (AT8, specific for pSer202/pThr205 tau phosphorylation sites) (Thermo Scientific, Rochester, Illinois, USA), and rabbit anti-mouse iba-1 (DAKO, Santa Clara, CA, USA) diluted to 1:1000.

The secondary antibodies used were all diluted to 1:20,000 and included donkey anti-rabbit (Jackson ImmunoResearch, West Grove, PA, USA). All sections were blocked in 0.01 M PBS (pH 7.4) and 7% normal donkey serum [NDS] (VectorLabs, Burlingame, CA). Primary and secondary agents were diluted in 0.1% Triton X-100/PBS and 1% normal donkey serum.

Image quantification

Immunohistochemical images were collected on a Nikon microscope, and image analyses were performed blinded to the experimental group. ImageJ software (http://rsbweb.nih.gov/ij/) was used to apply a standard threshold to the images.

Western blot analyses

Relative levels of tau, p-tau, GFAP, iba-1, cathepsin B, and actin in the supernatant fraction from the brain extract were determined by Western blot (polyclonal antibodies: Cathepsin B, sc-13985; β-actin, sc-130657; Santa Cruz Biotechnology, Santa Cruz, CA; tau, ThermoFisher, Rochester, IL; p-tau, ThermoFisher, Rochester, IL; iba-1, DAKO, Santa Clara, CA), as described previously [34]. Relative intensities of Western blot bands were assessed by densitometry in triplicate for each sample. Densitometric analysis was done using IQTL software (GE Life Sciences, Piscataway, NJ). For protein studies, the entire lesional area was harvested for Western blot analysis. In control or sham animals, a similar region was harvested.

ELISA analysis

For quantitative analysis of cytokines, an ELISA was used to measure the levels of tumor necrosis factor-α (TNF-α), interleukin-1β (IL-1β), or transforming growth factor-β (TGF-β) in the brain tissue [35]. Cytokines were extracted from mouse brains as follows: frozen hemibrains were placed in tissue homogenization buffer containing protease inhibitor cocktail (Sigma, St Louis, MO, USA) 1:1000 dilution immediately before use and homogenized using polytron. Tissue sample suspensions were distributed in aliquots and snap frozen in liquid nitrogen for later measurements. Invitrogen ELISA kits were then used, according to manufacturer directions (Carlsbad, CA, USA).

Statistical analysis

All statistical analyses were performed using SAS statistical software version 9.3. All tests were two-sided and conducted at 5% significance level. Continuous variables were summarized using sample means. All studies used 10 mice per group. All data are presented as means ± standard error of the mean (SEM). Ipsilateral and contralateral sides were compared to the corresponding sides between groups [i.e., repetitive ipsilateral vs. single ipsilateral vs. control ipsilateral (left side)]. Normalized GFAP, pTau, and iba-1 immunoreactive areas were evaluated with thresholded pixel areas analyzed using one-way analysis of variance (ANOVA) including injury group (control, single hit, and repeated hits) as the factor. Post hoc analyses based on Tukey's method to adjust for multiple comparisons were conducted to compare pairs of injury groups.

Results

Quantification of and immunolocalization of tau

In order to determine the impact of the nutritional diets on the development and progression of CTE, 24-week-old hTau mice were fed diets supplemented with GrandFusion diets (2%) for 2 months. The diets were as follows: group 3 received a 2% GrandFusion (GF1, NF-216—Fruit and Veggie #1 Blend), with the ND; group 4 received a 2% GrandFusion diet (GF2, NF-316—Fruit #2 Blend); and group 5 received a 2% GrandFusion diet (GF3, NF-416—Vegetable #3 Blend) (Table 1). The diets contain similar level of vitamins, phytochemicals, and phytonutrients that might impact the outcomes. These are same diets that were used in previous studies [27]. The animals were examined for food intake and body weight every week for the 24 weeks of feeding. The mice on all diets maintained a constant intake of food over the course of the study (data not shown). In addition, consistent with the food intake, all of the mice showed a similar gain in weight over the 8 months.

The mice were subjected to closed head rmTBI as described previously [28]. Mice were examined for phosphor-tau (p-tau) presence in the brain following rmTBI and the impact of the diets on altering p-tau expression. Figure 1 shows that control mice at 14 months of age show little p-tau pathology (Fig. 1a). Mice subjected to rmTBI showed a dramatic increase in p-tau pathology compared to the control animals (Fig. 1b). With the presence of the diets, there was a significant reduction in the p-tau pathology suggesting the diets had an effect on rmTBI-induced outcomes (Fig. 1c–e). Western blot analysis of the mice from the above studies shows the changes in p-tau versus tau in the brains of the mice with and without rmTBI and with and without GF diets (Fig. 1f, g). As seen in the figure, with rmTBI, the levels of p-tau are increased 5–10 fold compared to the control animals, while the mice on the GF diets showed an attenuation of p-tau expression.

RmTBI results in a transient Neurological Severity Score elevation and short-lived motor deficits that are ameliorated with diets

In NSS testing, severity of impact for rmTBI groups fell in the mild spectrum. We found that averaged NSS scores were statistically different between the injury and treated groups and that the effect of the diets on outcomes was significant. Figure 2a shows that rmTBI at 6 months post-injury, the NSS was significantly higher in the rmTBI

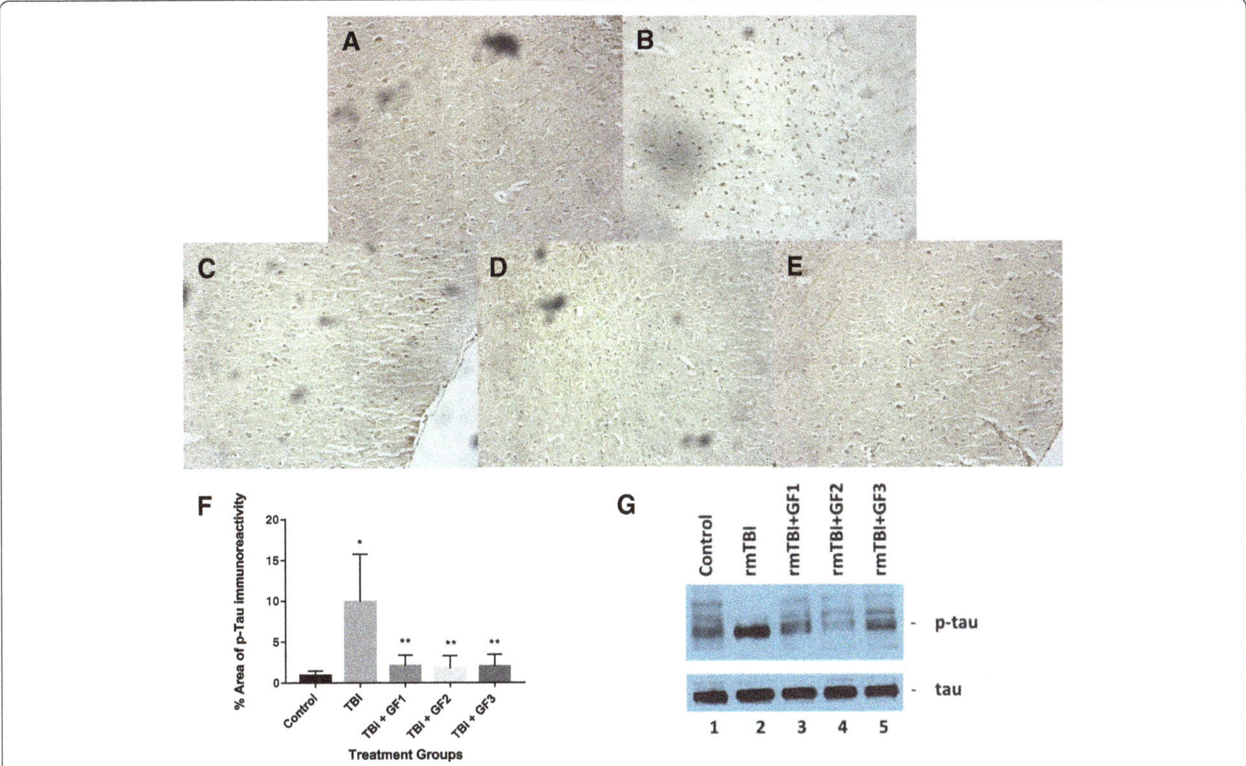

Fig. 1 Effects of GF diets on tau pathology. Control hTau mice (**a**), hTau mice + rmTBI (**b**), hTau mice + rmTBI plus NF-216 (**c**, GF1), hTau mice + rmTBI plus NF-316 (**d**, GF2), and hTau mice + rmTBI plus NF-416 (**e**, GF3). Mice were fed a normal diet or diets supplemented with 2% GF for 2 months prior to rmTBI and then for 4 months after rmTBI. Animals were euthanized and subjected to immunohistochemical analysis (**a**–**f**) or Western blot analysis (**g**). **f** Graphical representation of p-tau immunohistochemistry in **a**–**e**. Each group represents mean ± SD ($n = 10$ per group). *$p < 0.001$ compared to TBI group

group compared to the control group. In addition, the animals on the diets had an attenuation of the NSS following rmTBI.

Vestibulomotor function was assessed by WGT, and there were significant effects of injury group on performance. We found that averaged wire grip scores were statistically different between rmTBI group and the control group and that the effect of injury was significant at 1 h to day 7 post-injury, even after adjustment for multiple comparisons ($p_{adj} < 0.05$; Kruskal-Wallis). Post hoc analyses found significant difference at the 5% significance level, at 1 h to 7 days post-injury, with the rmTBI group statistically different from the control group. In addition, the GF groups all showed a significant difference compared to the rmTBI group. We also found that the performance on the WGT improved over time, with wire grip scores increasing over time in the repeat injury group (both groups, $p < 0.001$; Friedman).

Impact of rmTBI and diets on cytokine levels

To determine the impact of the diets on neuroinflammation in the mouse brain after rmTBI, mouse brains were examined for the expression of inflammatory markers. We evaluated the levels of the cytokines tumor necrosis factor-α (TNF-α), interleukin-1β (IL-1β), and transforming growth factor-β (TGF-β) at 6 months after rmTBI (Fig. 3). As seen in the figure, rmTBI that resulted in "CTE-like" effects elevated cytokine levels that were still increased at 6 months after injury. The GF diets significantly reduced or attenuated TNF-α, IL-1β, and TGF-β levels after injury. All the diets showed an effect reducing the above cytokine levels by 67% (TNF-α), 85% (IL-1β), and 80% (TGF-β).

Changes in cathepsin B levels following rmTBI and effect of diets

Our previous studies have shown that TBI results in an increase in cathepsin B protein and activity that can lead to inflammatory mediators such as IL-1β. To determine the impact of rmTBI on cathepsin B levels and diets associated with the alterations in inflammation (Fig. 4), we measured cathepsin B protein and activity at 4 months following injury. rmTBI increased cathepsin B levels in the brain, and the GF diets reduced or attenuated the increase (Fig. 4). These results suggest that reduction in inflammation occurring with treatments was partially the result of inhibition of cathepsin B activity.

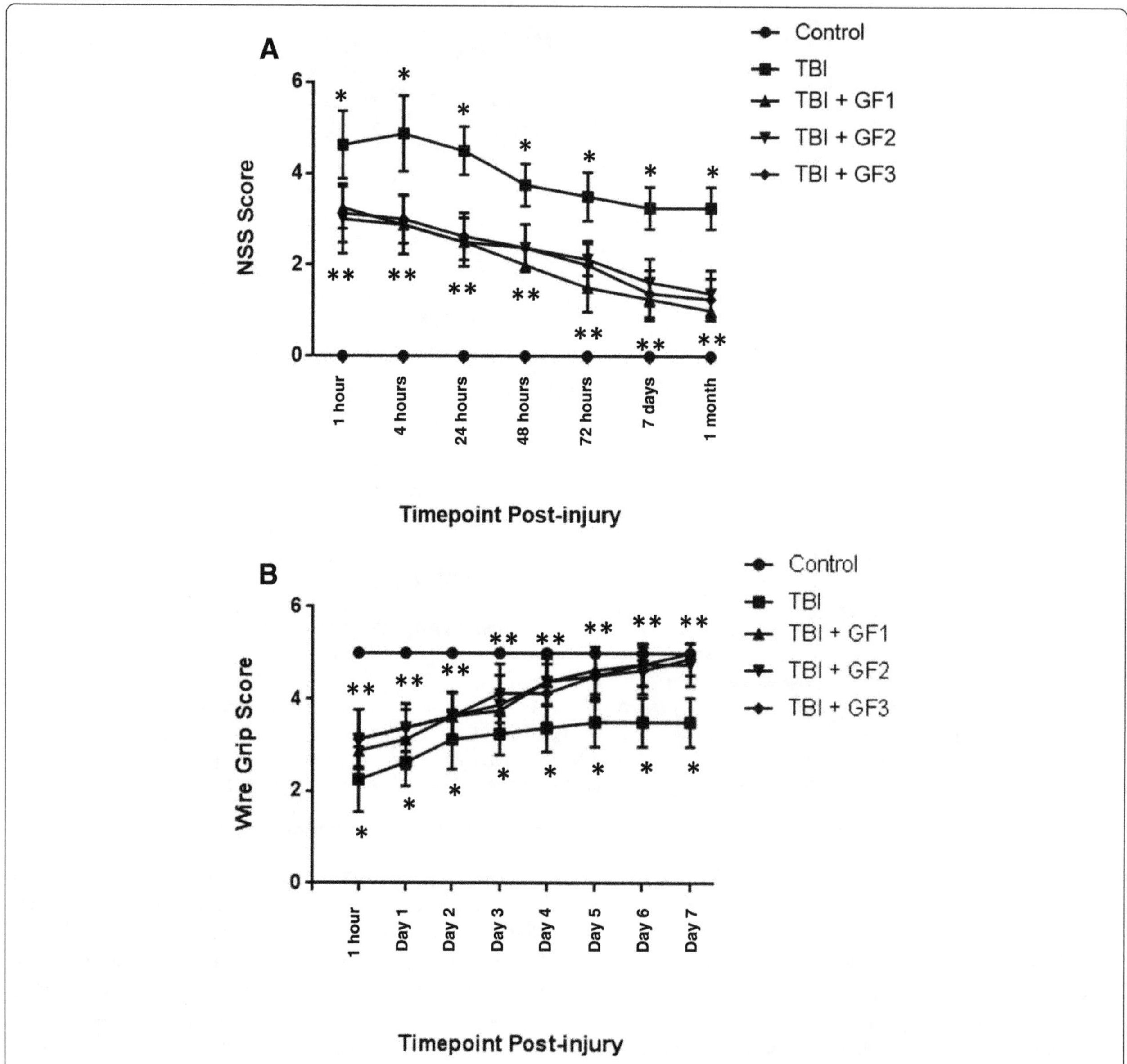

Fig. 2 Repetitive mild traumatic brain injury (rmTBI) results in elevated Neurological Severity Scores (NSS) and transient vestibulomotor deficits. **a** rmTBI mice +/− were assessed with an NSS at 1, 4, 24, 48, and 72 h post-injury, as well as at 7-day and 1-month time points. Repetitive mTBI mice exhibited significantly elevated scores, compared to control mice, and mice fed GF diets had reduced NSS score compared to rmTBI alone. **b** Mice underwent wire grip testing 1 h after TBI and on post-injury days 1–7. rmTBI resulted in short-lived vestibulomotor dysfunction, compared to controls, at 1 h to 7 days post-injury (Kruskal-Wallis). There were significant differences between rmTBI mice plus diets and rmTBI alone on post-injury days 1–7. *$p < 0.05$ versus control mice. **$p < 0.01$ versus rmTBI mice. Values are mean ± SD

Impact of rmTBI and diets on glial activation following rmTBI

To further analyze the impact of the diets on neuroinflammation in the mouse brain after rmTBI, brains were examined for the expression of glial inflammatory markers. We evaluated the levels of the astrocyte (GFAP) and microglial (iba-1) at 6 months after rmTBI (Figs. 5 and 6). As seen in the figures, rmTBI that resulted in "CTE-like" effects elevated both iba-1 (Fig. 5) and GFAP (Fig. 6) levels that were still increased at 6 months after injury. The GF diets significantly reduced or attenuated iba-1 and GFAP levels after injury. All the diets showed an effect reducing the above glial markers by 67% (iba-1) and 82% (GFAP).

Repetitive mild traumatic brain injury causes persistent deficits with spatial learning and memory

We next determined the hippocampal-dependent spatial learning and long-term memory in the rmTBI and rmTBI + GF diets mice using the MWM (Fig. 7). Animals from all groups showed daily improvements in their abilities to

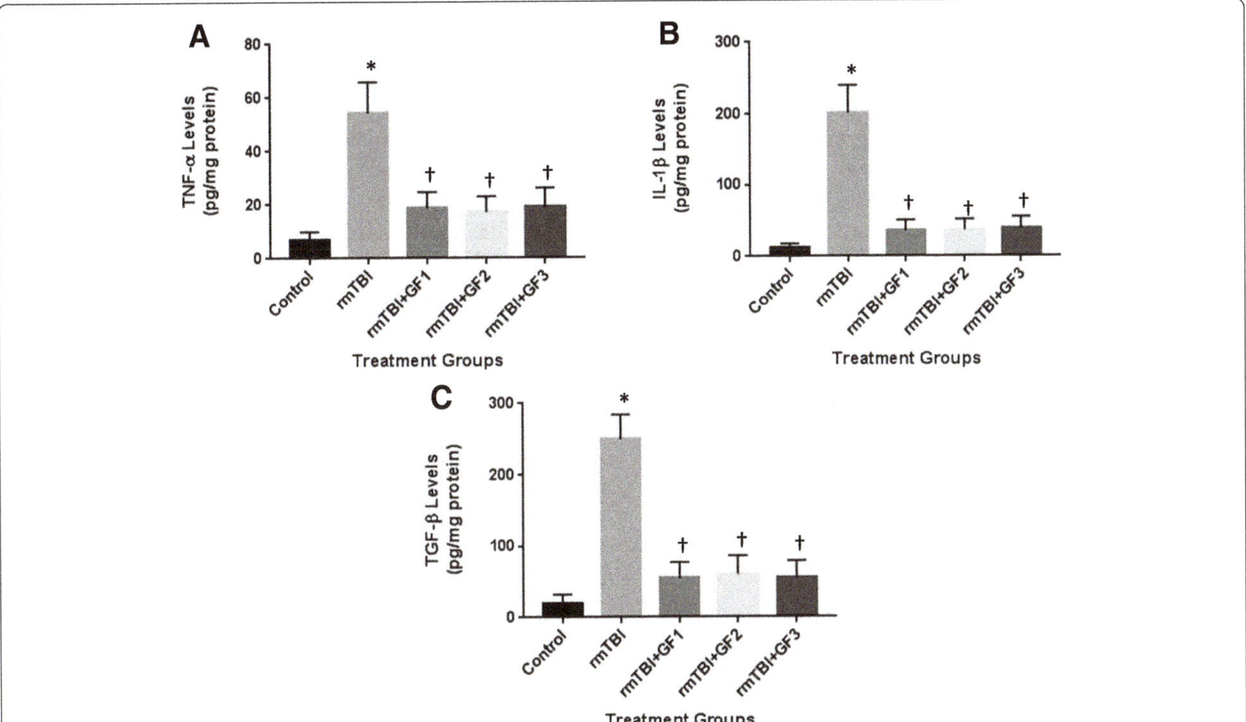

Fig. 3 Reduced inflammatory markers in the brain after rmTBI. Mice were grouped as control, rmTBI, or rmTBI subjected to various diets followed by 24 h of recovery. Quantitative analysis of TNF-α (**a**), IL-1β (**b**), and TGF-β (**c**) in the rmTBI brain was determined by ELISA. Brain homogenates were subjected to ELISA. The results are expressed as mean ± SD ($n = 10$, *$P < 0.001$ compared to the sham group; < 0.001 compared to the rmTBI group)

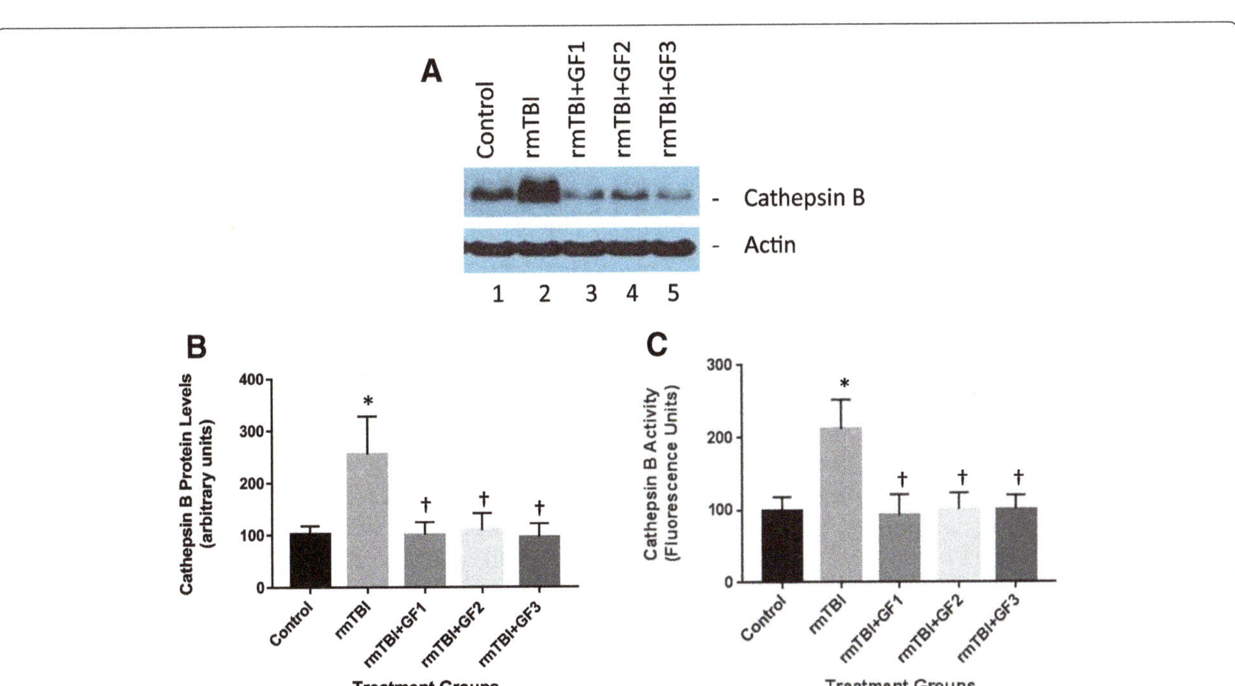

Fig. 4 The effect of GF diets on cathepsin protein levels and B activity. **a** Brain cathepsin B protein levels were determined 4 months following rmTBI. Western blot analysis of the cathepsin B levels in the brains of control, rmTBI, and rmTBI + GF diets. **b** Quantitative analysis of cathepsin B protein levels of the mice in **a**. **c** Brain cathepsin B activities were determined in the mice following 4 months after rmTBI in control, rmTBI, and rmTBI + GF diets. The results are expressed as mean ± SD ($n = 10$, *$p < 0.001$ compared to the control group; †$p < 0.01$ versus rmTBI group)

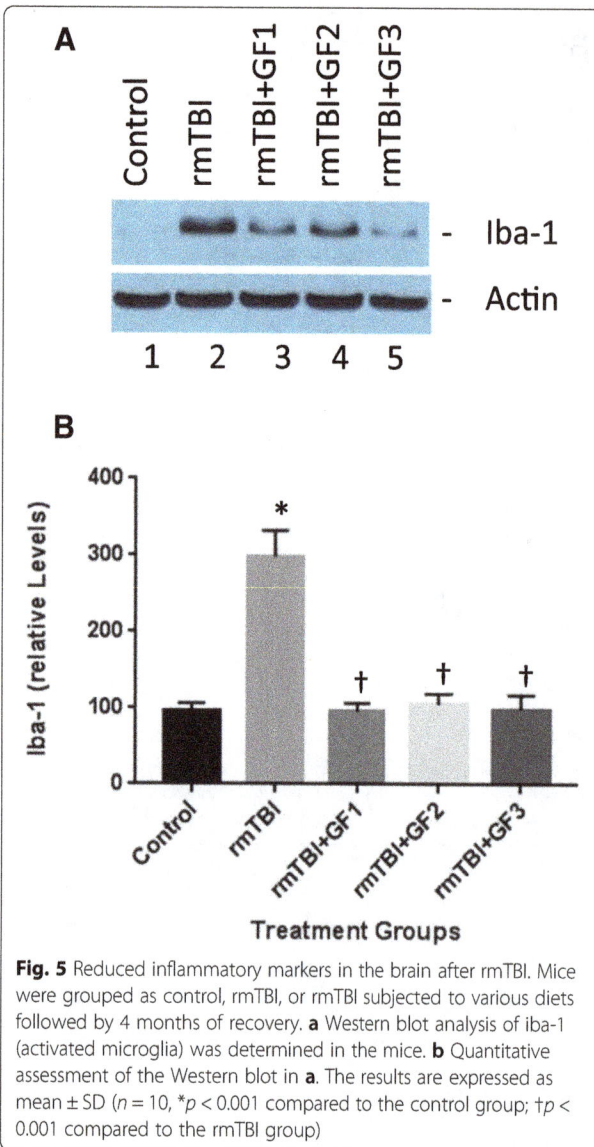

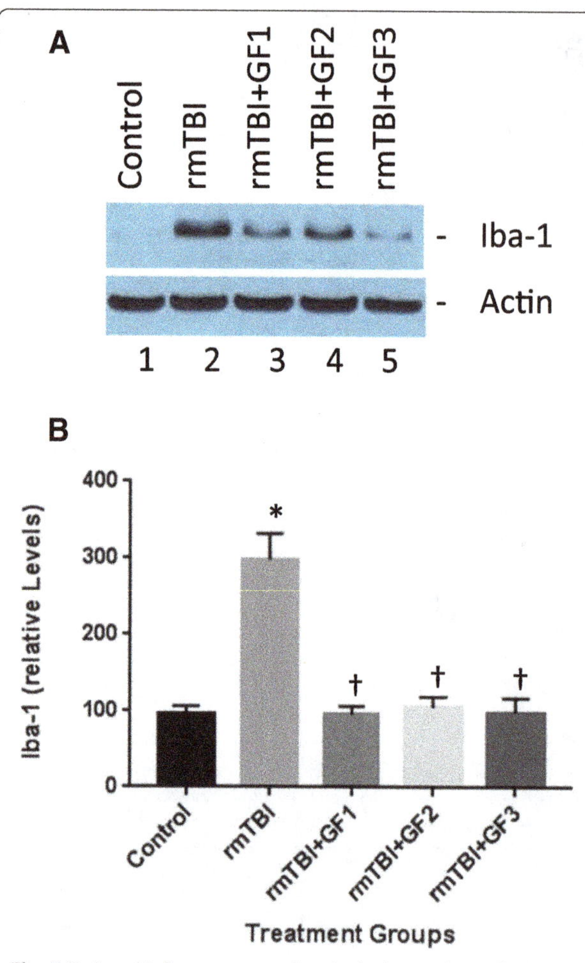

Fig. 5 Reduced inflammatory markers in the brain after rmTBI. Mice were grouped as control, rmTBI, or rmTBI subjected to various diets followed by 4 months of recovery. **a** Western blot analysis of iba-1 (activated microglia) was determined in the mice. **b** Quantitative assessment of the Western blot in **a**. The results are expressed as mean ± SD ($n = 10$, *$p < 0.001$ compared to the control group; †$p < 0.001$ compared to the rmTBI group)

locate the hidden platform during the acquisition phase of the MWM task; however, rmTBI mice demonstrated increased latencies. Mice maintained on the DF diets showed an attenuation of the changes and were similar to the control animals. At the acute and subacute time points, we found that the main effect of time, the main effect of injury group, and the interaction of time and injury group were statistically significant (Fig. 7a, b). At 1 month post-injury, the main effect of time and the main effect of injury group were statistically significant, and the GF diets were significantly different compared to the rmTBI group (Fig. 7c). At 6 months post-injury, we found that time and the interaction of time and injury group were significant and that the main effect of GF injury group was significant to the rmTBI group (Fig. 7d). Post hoc analyses found that, at the acute time point, all pairs of injury groups (control vs. repetitive mTBI) were statistically different at the 5% significance level. At the subacute time point, the analyses found statistically significant differences between the control and the repetitive mTBI groups. At 1 month post-injury, we found statistically significant differences when comparing control to repetitive mTBI groups. At 6 months, we found statistically significant differences when comparing control to repetitive mTBI groups. In addition, the diet-treated animals showed significant difference at all time points compared to the rmTBI group.

For the probe trial testing, analyses comparing the control groups found significant differences in the distribution pattern of the time that mice spent in the four quadrants at any of the time points. When comparing the rmTBI and the control injury group, we found significant differences in the distribution of the time that mice spent in the four quadrants. When analyzing within each time point, we found significant differences between the control and the repeat group at the acute time point. The difference was significant at both the subacute and 1-month time points and at 6 months. In addition, the diet-treated animals showed significant difference at all time points compared to the rmTBI group.

Subsequent analysis was performed to evaluate the preference for the target quadrant compared to the other three quadrants. Findings from the probe test indicate that mice from the uninjured control groups, at all time points, spent a significantly higher percentage of time in the target quadrant (the location that contained the platform during training), when compared to the other equivalent zones (Fig. 7e–h). We found that mice in the control group spent significantly more time in the target quadrant than in any of the other three quadrants at the acute, subacute, 1-month, and 6-month time points post-injury. In contrast, rmTBI mice exhibited impaired spatial memory, failing to show significant discrimination and preference for the target quadrant, compared to the other quadrants (Fig. 7e–h). We did not find that mice in the repetitive injury group spent significantly more time in the target quadrant than in any other quadrants at any of the post-injury times. Meanwhile, mice fed GF diets showed a significant increase in the time spent in the target quadrant and less time in any other quadrant (Fig. 7e–h).

rmTBI resulted in subacute anxiety leading to increased risk-taking activity which is attenuated in GF diets

We used the EPM to determine the effect of rmTBI on anxiety-related and risk-taking behaviors. One-way ANOVA revealed that the amount of time spent in the open arm differed significantly between the control and injury group +/− diets at 14 days, 1 month, and 6 months. At 2 weeks post-injury, mTBI mice exhibited increased anxiety-like behavior (Fig. 8a). Post hoc analyses found significant differences at the 5% significance level at 14 days post-injury between the control and the

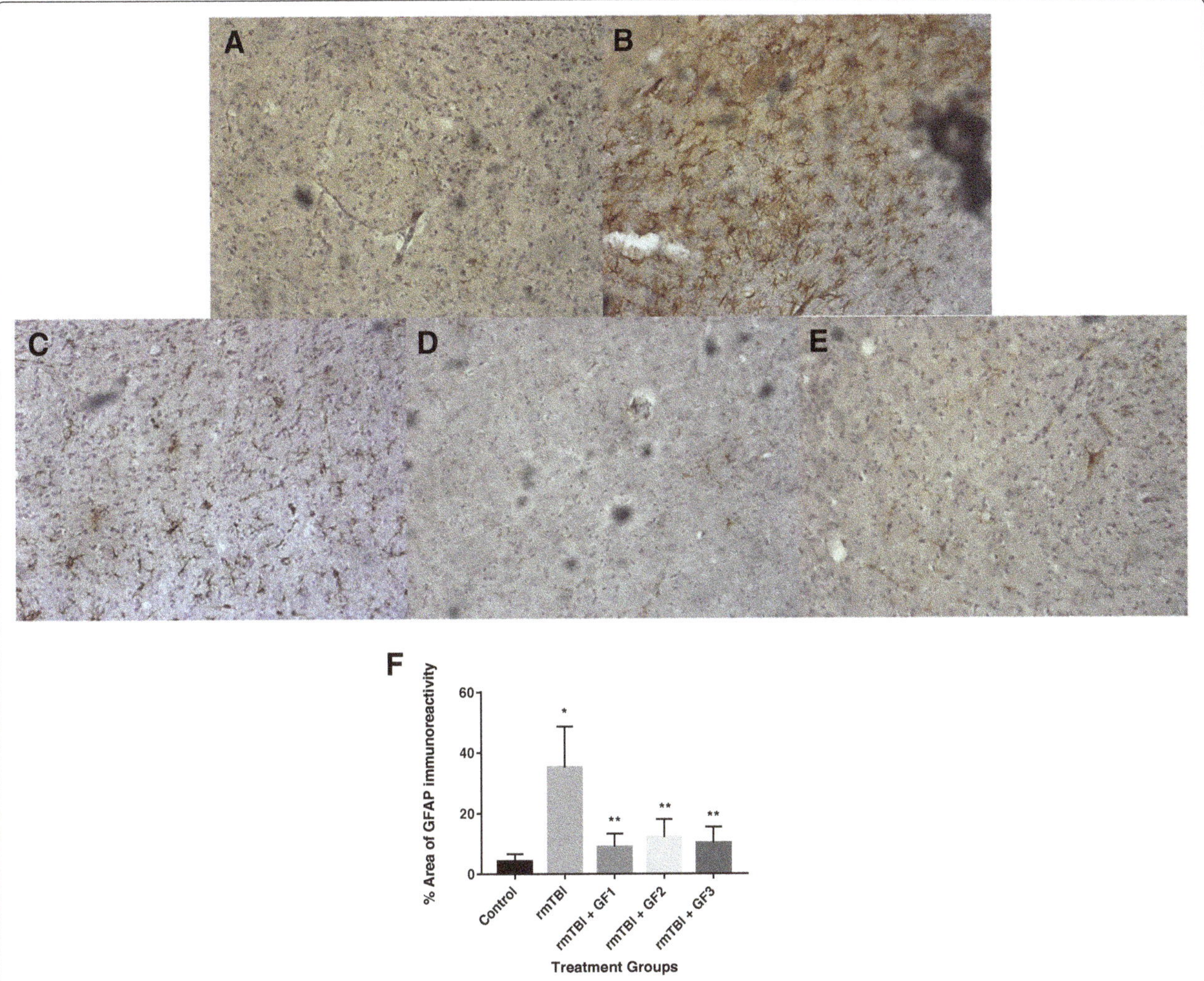

Fig. 6 Reduced inflammatory markers in the brain after rmTBI. Mice were control, rmTBI, or rmTBI subjected to various diets followed by 4 months of recovery. **a**–**e** Immunohistochemical analysis of GFAP (activated astrocytes) was determined in the mice. Control hTau mice (**a**), hTau mice + rmTBI (**b**), hTau mice + rmTBI plus NF-216 (**c**, GF1), hTau mice + rmTBI plus NF-316 (**d**, GF2), and hTau mice + rmTBI plus NF-416 (**e**, GF3). **f** Quantitative assessment of the western histology in **a**–**e**. The results are expressed as mean ± SD ($n = 10$, $^*p < 0.001$ compared to the control group; ** $p < 0.001$ compared to the rmTBI group)

repetitive injury groups. rmTBI resulted in significantly reduced time spent in the open arms of the maze, consistent with increased anxiety. At day 14 post-injury, the mice with GF diets showed an increased time in the open arms consistent with decreased anxiety.

At the 1- and 6-month time points, significant differences were found in post hoc analyses between the controls and repetitive injury group. Mice in the rmTBI group spent an increased amount of time on the open arms of the EPM, compared to control mice (Fig. 8b). Such increased exploratory activity in the open arms and reduced fearfulness are consistent with increased risk taking, as noted in other studies [36]. This increased risk taking persisted and progressed in the rmTBI mice out to 6 months (Fig. 8c). However, the GF diet-fed mice showed an attenuation of the presence in the open arm supports decreased risk-taking and a maintenance of normal activity.

Repetitive mild traumatic brain injury results in depression-like behavior at 1 month

At 1 month post-injury, in the Porsolt FST, there was a significant effect of injury severity on depression-like behavior. Data from the swim test indicated significant differences between groups. Post hoc analyses found significantly increased immobility time in the rmTBI group, compared to the control group (Fig. 8d). The TST revealed comparable effects of mTBI on depression-like behavior as the FST. Similar analyses carried out on data from the TST suggested that immobility times differed significantly between injury groups. rmTBI mice demonstrated significantly increased immobility time, compared to the control group

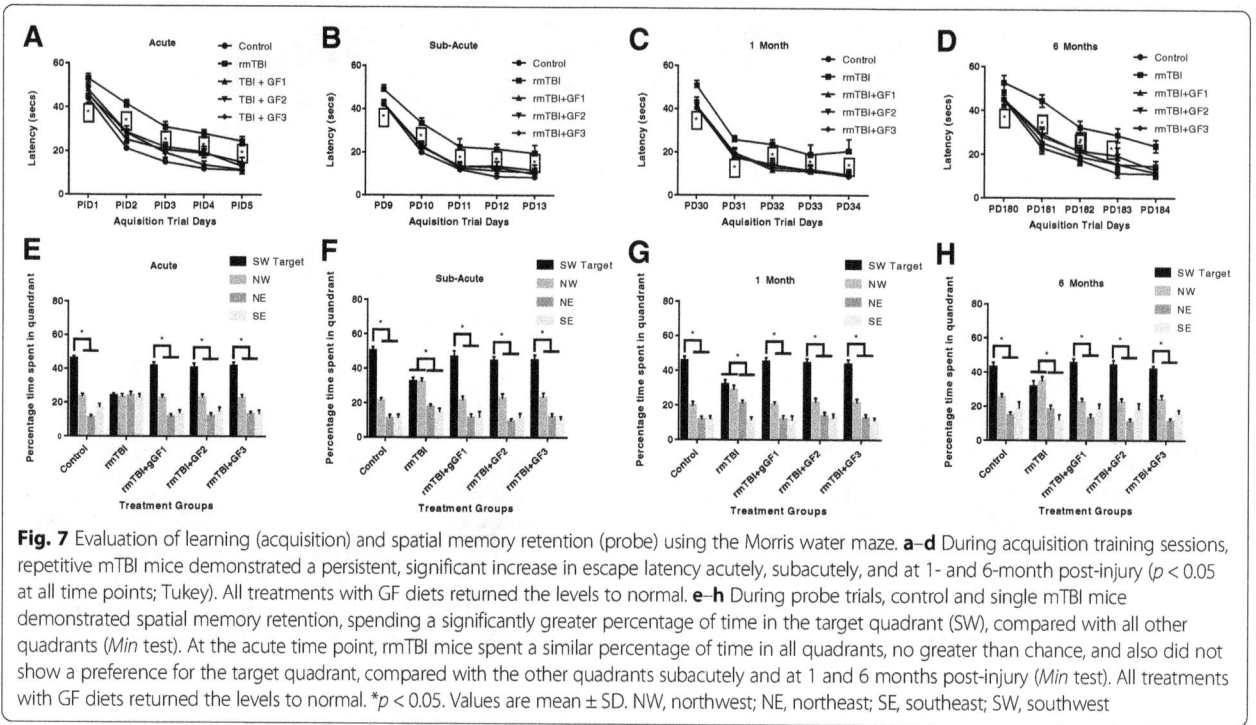

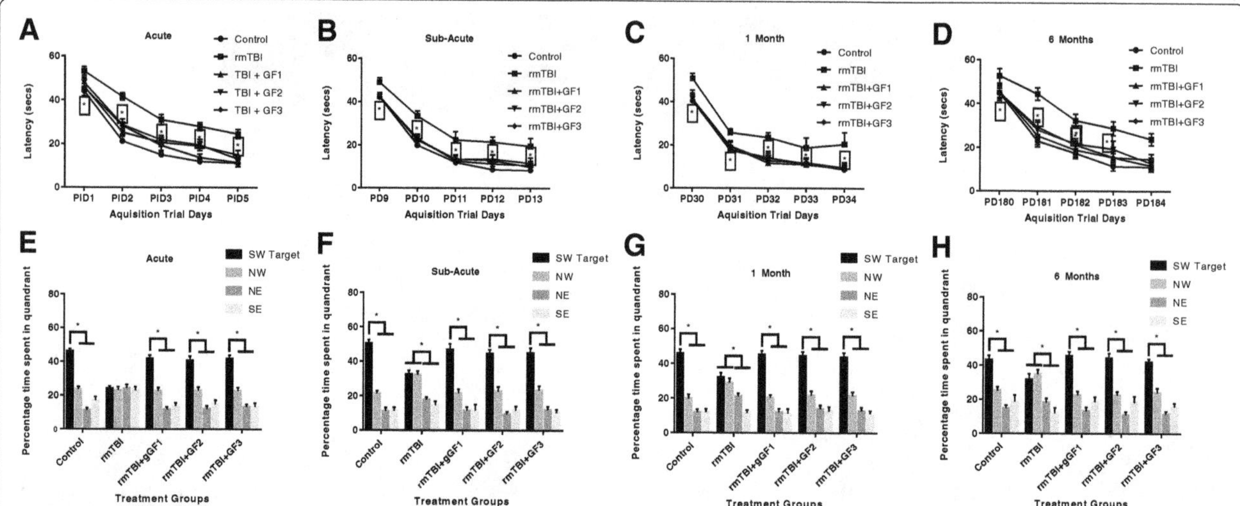

Fig. 7 Evaluation of learning (acquisition) and spatial memory retention (probe) using the Morris water maze. **a–d** During acquisition training sessions, repetitive mTBI mice demonstrated a persistent, significant increase in escape latency acutely, subacutely, and at 1- and 6-month post-injury ($p < 0.05$ at all time points; Tukey). All treatments with GF diets returned the levels to normal. **e–h** During probe trials, control and single mTBI mice demonstrated spatial memory retention, spending a significantly greater percentage of time in the target quadrant (SW), compared with all other quadrants (*Min* test). At the acute time point, rmTBI mice spent a similar percentage of time in all quadrants, no greater than chance, and also did not show a preference for the target quadrant, compared with the other quadrants subacutely and at 1 and 6 months post-injury (*Min* test). All treatments with GF diets returned the levels to normal. $*p < 0.05$. Values are mean ± SD. NW, northwest; NE, northeast; SE, southeast; SW, southwest

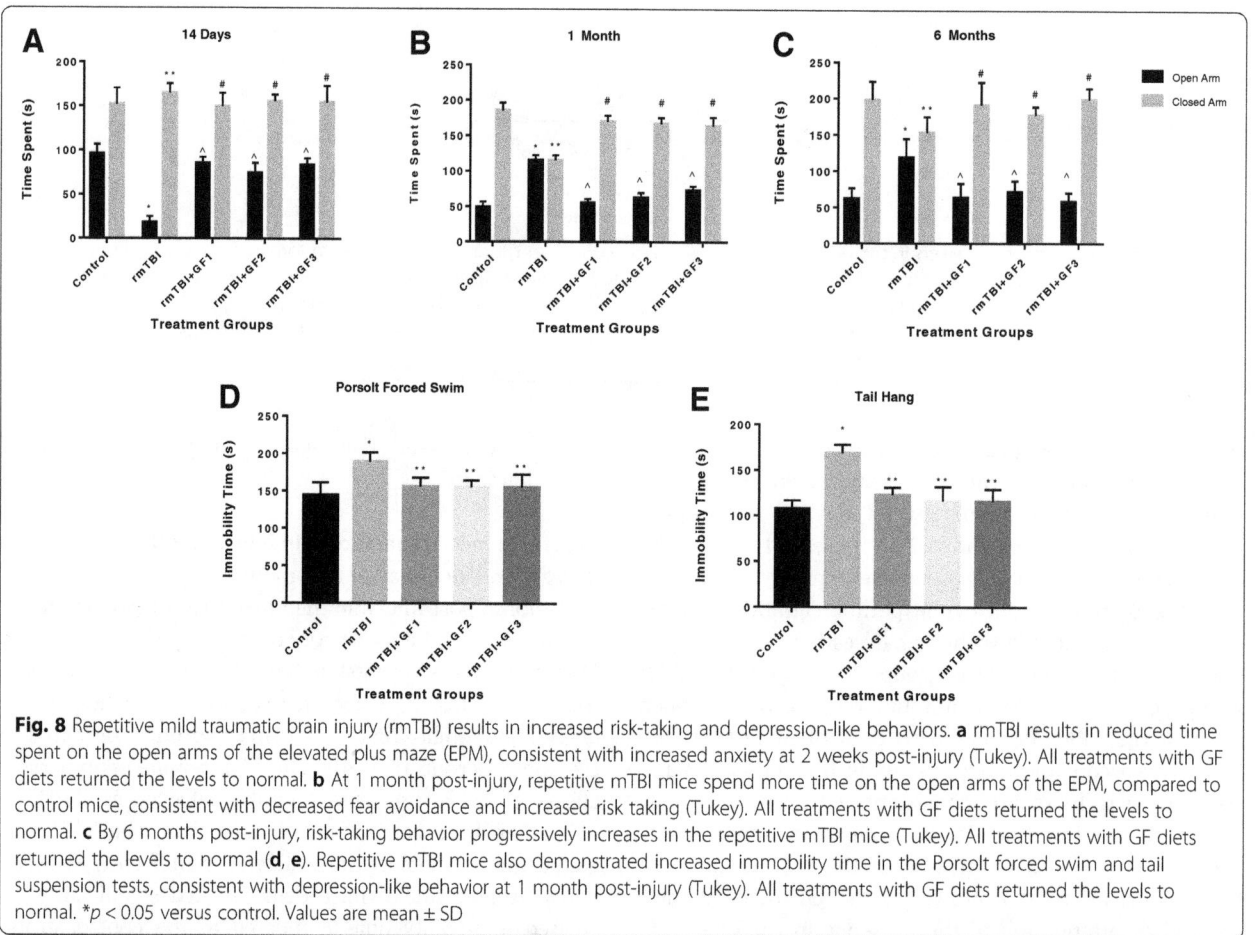

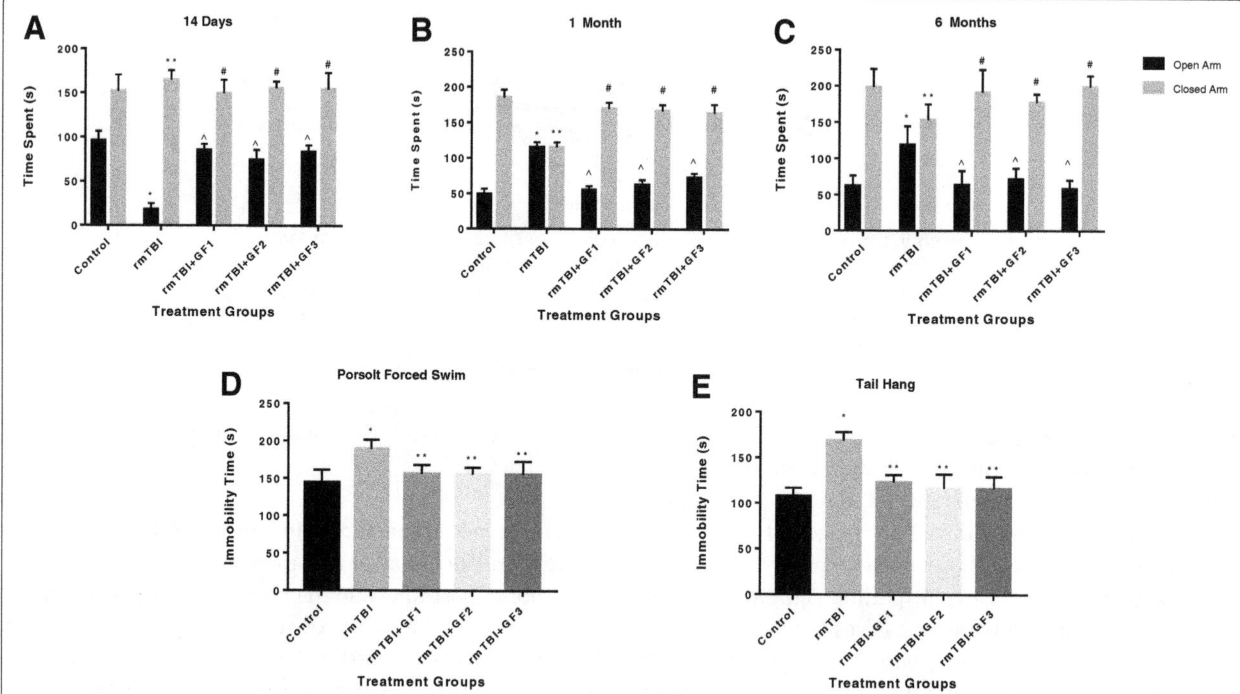

Fig. 8 Repetitive mild traumatic brain injury (rmTBI) results in increased risk-taking and depression-like behaviors. **a** rmTBI results in reduced time spent on the open arms of the elevated plus maze (EPM), consistent with increased anxiety at 2 weeks post-injury (Tukey). All treatments with GF diets returned the levels to normal. **b** At 1 month post-injury, repetitive mTBI mice spend more time on the open arms of the EPM, compared to control mice, consistent with decreased fear avoidance and increased risk taking (Tukey). All treatments with GF diets returned the levels to normal. **c** By 6 months post-injury, risk-taking behavior progressively increases in the repetitive mTBI mice (Tukey). All treatments with GF diets returned the levels to normal (**d**, **e**). Repetitive mTBI mice also demonstrated increased immobility time in the Porsolt forced swim and tail suspension tests, consistent with depression-like behavior at 1 month post-injury (Tukey). All treatments with GF diets returned the levels to normal. $*p < 0.05$ versus control. Values are mean ± SD

(Fig. 8e). The rmTBI mice on GF diets showed a return to control levels in both the FST and TST suggesting protective effects on the rmTBI. No differences were seen in the TST (data not shown).

Mild traumatic brain injury mice exhibit sleep disturbances at 1 month

To evaluate the long-term effect of rmTBI +/− diets on sleep-wake behavior, we used infrared videography and electrophysiological monitoring [37]. We determined that the effect of rmTBI on percent wake time was statistically significant (Fig. 9a). The percentage of wake time in the rmTBI group was significantly different from those recorded in the control group. With the significant increase in wake time, we found a concomitant reduction in NREM sleep in the rmTBI mice. We found that the effect of injury group on percent NREM time was statistically significant. The percentage of NREM time in the rmTBI group was significantly different from those recorded in the control group. We also found that the effect of the rmTBI on the percent REM time was not statistically significant. However, mice on the diets showed a decrease in wake time and an increase in NREM time (statistically significant).

We sought to further examine the quality of NREM and REM sleep in these mice. During NREM sleep, there was an increase in cortical activity with a significant shift toward higher frequencies (Fig. 9b). The prevalence was significantly different across levels of frequency, and the rmTBI group had a significant effect on prevalence through its interaction with frequency. Analyses found that the effect of rmTBI group on frequency prevalence was statistically significant at all frequency levels compared to the control group. In addition, we found significant difference between the rmTBI and the rmTBI + GF diets, suggesting that there was an impact by the diets on the NREM activity.

Repetitive mTBI also caused NREM sleep fragmentation as well (Fig. 9c, d). We found that the rmTBI group had a significant effect on both the number of episodes and

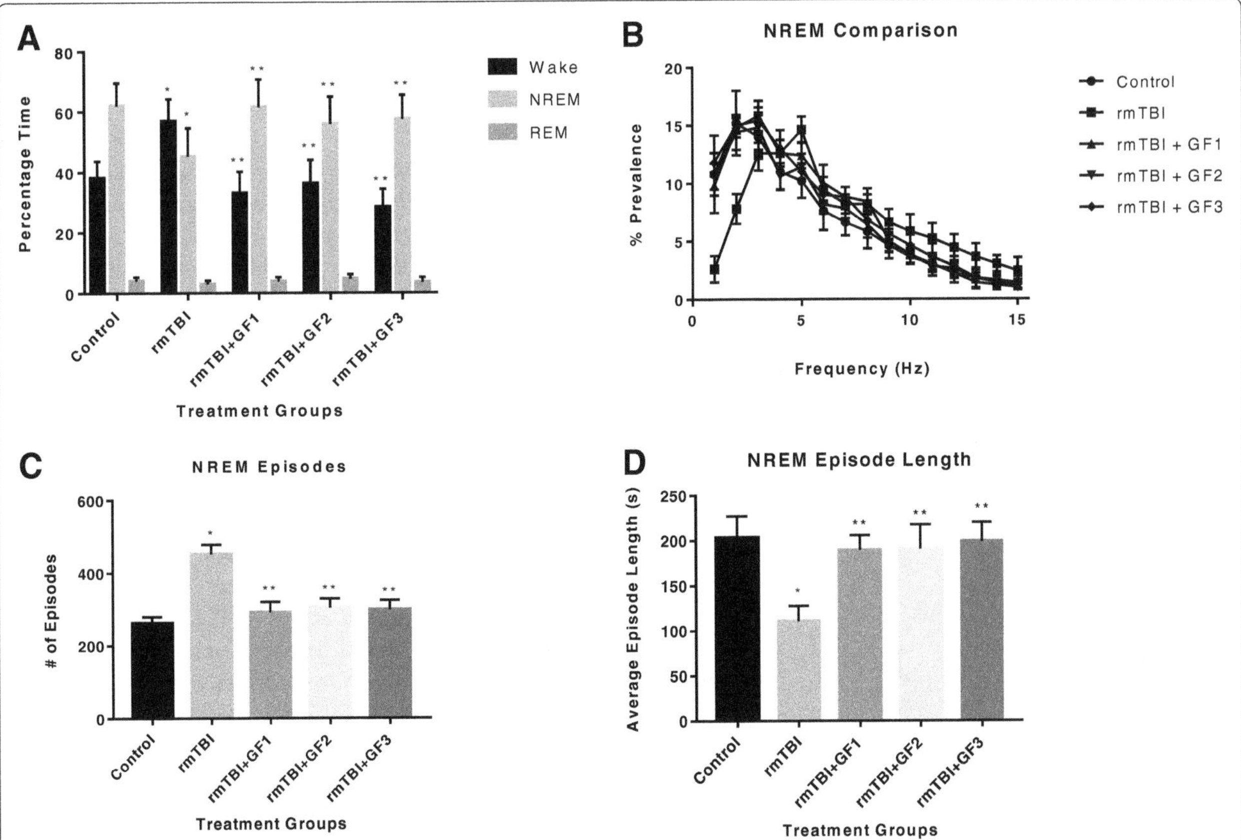

Fig. 9 Repetitive mild traumatic brain injury (rmTBI) results in sleep pattern disturbances (**a**). Mice repetitive rmTBI exhibit a significant reduction in NREM sleep as well as a significant increase in wake time over the course of 24 h (Tukey). $*p < 0.05$, compared to control mice. **b** Quality of NREM sleep is disrupted by rmTBI. Power spectral analysis demonstrated a significant rightward theta shift in rmTBI animals. Control animals displayed a significantly higher power spectrum for 1–2 Hz, compared to rmTBI groups. Single and repetitive rmTBI mice had a significantly higher frequency at 5 Hz, compared to age-matched controls (Tukey). Single rmTBI mice also had a significant difference at 12 and 13 Hz, compared to control mice (Tukey). $*p < 0.05$, repetitive rmTBI versus control mice; $^{\#}p < 0.05$, single rmTBI versus control mice. **c** Repetitive rmTBI mice exhibited a greater number of NREM episodes, compared to the single rmTBI and control groups, with **d** significantly reduced episode lengths (Tukey). $*p < 0.05$. Values are mean ± SD. NREM, non-rapid eye movement; REM, rapid eye movement

average episode length. The number of episodes in the rmTBI mice was significantly increased from those observed in the control group (Fig. 9c). The average episode length in the rmTBI mice was also significantly reduced, compared to control mice (Fig. 9d). Meanwhile, mice on the GF diets subjected to rmTBI had attenuated NREM episodes and increased NREM episode length, comparable to the control animals. Both were statistically significant compared to the rmTBI animals. Effect of injury was significant on REM EMG data. Analyses revealed that the rmTBI mice demonstrated significantly increased EMG activity, compared to controls, during REM sleep (Fig. 10). However, mice on the GF diets showed an attenuation of the REM EMG activity.

Discussion

In the present study, we examined the impact of diets rich in vegetables and/or fruits on outcomes and recovery/repair from rmTBI and the potential link to CTE. Our studies have shown that long-term intake of these diets for 2 months prior to rmTBI and 6 months subsequent to the injury improved behavioral outcomes, reduced inflammation, and diminished tauopathy in a mouse model of CTE.

A number of recent studies have implicated rTBI in the pathogenesis associated with CTE [38]. A chronic increase in phosphorylated tau (p-tau) immunostaining has been detected in the cortex, amygdalae, and the hippocampus of individuals subjected to rTBI. A number of models have been developed to study the mechanisms associated with rTBI and CTE [39]. For the lack of a better model, a rmTBI seems to be the most relevant approach to study the pathophysiology related to CTE [40]. In these models, p-tau staining was associated with increased GFAP-positive astrocytes and iba-1-positive microglial cells [41]. These markers are consistent with the appearance in reported cases of CTE and individuals that experience chronic mild repetitive head traumas [42]. The presence of the inflammation and glial markers is most likely due to several different parameters [43]. The microglial activation and reactive astrocytosis are probably the result of the primary injury, the repetitive mTBI, and the consequences of a progressive, chronic neuroinflammatory condition that contributes to secondary and potentially tertiary responses [44]. In addition, the presence of the p-tau and deposition may contribute to the continued inflammation, i.e., inflammation begets inflammation [45]. The resulting injury and inflammation contributes to glial activation and neuronal cell death that will give rise to more inflammation and glial activation and more cell death, etc. They may be one of the main issues related to CTE [46]. We continue to see inflammation at the 6-month time point in our model suggesting that chronic inflammation is critical to the disease process [47].

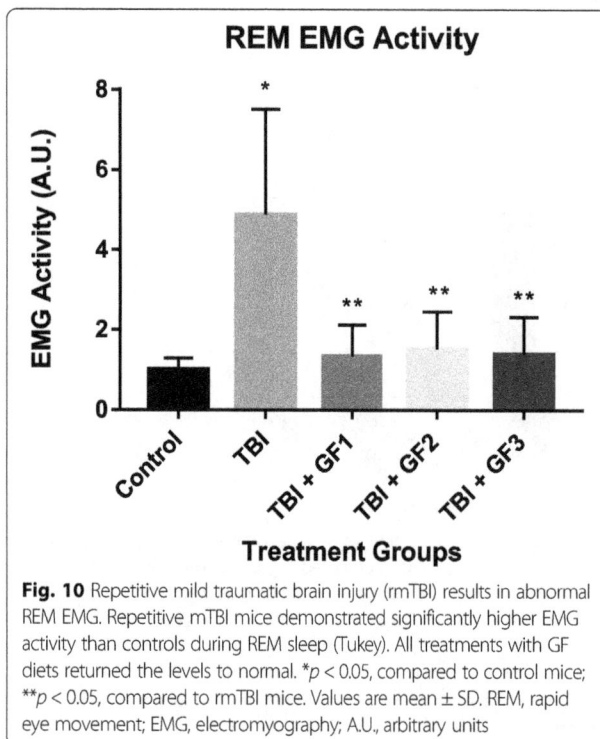

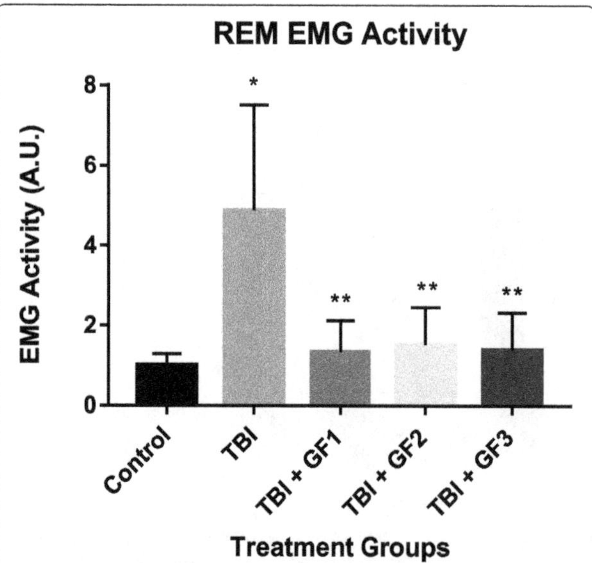

Fig. 10 Repetitive mild traumatic brain injury (rmTBI) results in abnormal REM EMG. Repetitive mTBI mice demonstrated significantly higher EMG activity than controls during REM sleep (Tukey). All treatments with GF diets returned the levels to normal. *$p < 0.05$, compared to control mice; **$p < 0.05$, compared to rmTBI mice. Values are mean ± SD. REM, rapid eye movement; EMG, electromyography; A.U., arbitrary units

Recent studies from our group have demonstrated that application of nutrient rich diets may alter the outcomes associated with neurological disorders, aging, and TBI [27, 34]. As shown previously, mice provided a diet enriched in fruits and vegetables help to attenuate the damage instigated by middle cerebral artery occlusion (MCAo) and maintain behavioral parameters [27]. These studies also further validated that phyto-nutriceuticals were capable of limiting inflammation and oxidative stress while stimulating neuronal proliferation. We also showed that when aged rats were provided the GF diets, there appeared to be an effect upon the aging process by a reduction in inflammatory markers, oxidative stress, and an increase in behavioral movement [34]. A recent related study showed that when mice were pre-exposed to these diets, there was a protection from the detrimental effects of TBI. When exposed to controlled cortical impact, the mice showed cortical damage, increased inflammation, and behavioral deficits. However, when exposed to GF diets, the mice had preserved neuronal function, reduced inflammatory markers, and improved or attenuated outcomes. As seen in the behavioral studies, most of the behavioral outcomes were suppressed but not completely obviated following TBI as seen in other studies, while the grip-strength showed a complete recovery. The grip strength test is not as selective as some of the other test; therefore, it needs to be taken within the complete context of the study. These data suggest that consumption of diets enriched in fruits and vegetables either naturally or through powdered form can provide protection from the detrimental effects of injury.

We describe the impact of long-term treatment of mice to diets enriched with vegetable and/or fruit concentrates in a model of repetitive mild TBI. Mice subjected to rmTBI showed chronic inflammatory responses and increased tau phosphorylation out to 6 months. The neuroinflammatory response with GFAP and iba-1 persisted out to the 6-month time point. The application of the GF diets to the mice, pre- and post-injury, reduced the neuroinflammation as apparent with both cytokine and glia activation. In addition, behavior and p-tau were both attenuated in the animal model suggesting an impact on the disease process. The studies further define the interplay between neuroinflammation and tau phosphorylation or vice versa, in the pathology and behavioral manifestations. They demonstrated that diets containing anti-oxidants, anti-inflammatory agents, and other compounds may have some interventional aspect in a mouse model of "CTE" and may provide a potential preventative/therapeutic approach. While in the context of a "real world" setting, predicting when and where TBI(s) might occur is not possible to preload with phytochemicals and phytonutrients. However, the studies suggest that using a diet like used in the study will help to attenuate the damage caused by TBIs.

Conclusion

Here, we show that treatment of mice with diets enriched in fruits and vegetables (phytochemicals) can alter the pathogenesis of CTE. Although treatment was started prior to the CTE, the indications are that the presence of these diets helped to attenuate the disease process, reduce inflammation, and improve outcomes. These data suggest that diets enriched in phytochemicals and other entities will help to limit the extent of injury following TBIs and reduce the potential progression to CTE in individuals.

Abbreviations

CTE: Chronic traumatic encephalopathy; GFAP: Glial fibrillary acidic protein; IL-1β: Interleukin-1beta; TBI: Traumatic brain injury

Acknowledgements

The authors wish to acknowledge NutriFusion, LLC for providing the GrandFusion® diets for the studies. We thank Mr. William Grand for reviewing the manuscript prior to submission. GrandFusion® is a patent pending product of NutriFusion, LLC.

Funding

This work was partially supported by grants from the National Institutes of Health (R01 ES016774-01, R21AG043718, 1P20GM109091, 2P20GM103444, and 5P30GM103342), VA Merit Award, a grant from the National Science Foundation (IIP-0903795), an AHA SFRN grant, and VA Merit Review (M.S.K.). Dr. Kindy is a Senior Research Career Scientist in the VA.

Authors' contributions

JY and MSK provided the study concept and the design. JY, HZ, ST, WM, and MSK acquired the data. SP and MSK provided the analysis and interpretation of the data. MSK drafted the manuscript. All authors critically reviewed the manuscript for important intellectual content. JY and MSK supervised the study. All authors read and approved the final manuscript.

Consent for publication

All authors consent to publication of the data.

Competing interests

Dr. Stephen Perry is a technical and science consultant for NutriFusion, LLC.

Author details

[1]Department of Pharmaceutical Sciences, College of Pharmacy, University of South Florida, 12901 Bruce B. Downs Blvd., MDC 30, Tampa, FL 33612, USA. [2]NutriFusion®, LLC, 10641 Airport Pulling Rd., Suite 31, Naples, FL 34109, USA. [3]Departments of Molecular Medicine, Molecular Pharmacology, Physiology and Pathology and Cell Biology, and Neurology, College of Medicine, University of South Florida, Tampa, FL, USA. [4]James A. Haley VA Medical Center, Tampa, FL, USA. [5]Shriners Hospital for Children, Tampa, FL, USA.

References

1. Petraglia AL, Maroon JC, Bailes JE. From the field of play to the field of combat: a review of the pharmacological management of concussion. Neurosurgery. 2012;70:1520–33.
2. Dashnaw ML, Petraglia AL, Bailes JE. An overview of the basic science of concussion and subconcussion: where we are and where we are going. Neurosurg Focus. 2012;33:1–9.
3. Langlois JA, Rutland-Brown W, Wald MM. The epidemiology and impact of traumatic brain injury: a brief overview. J Head Trauma Rehabil. 2006;21: 375–8.
4. Bailes JE, Petraglia AL, Omalu BI, Nauman E, Talavage T. Role of subconcussion in repetitive mild traumatic brain injury. J Neurosurg. 2013; 119:1235–45.
5. Turner RC, Lucke-Wold BP, Robson MJ, Omalu BI, Petraglia AL, Bailes JE. Repetitive traumatic brain injury and development of chronic traumatic encephalopathy: a potential role for biomarkers in diagnosis, prognosis, and treatment? Front Neurol. 2012;3:186.
6. McKee AC, Cantu RC, Nowinski CJ, Hedley-Whyte ET, Gavett BE, Budson AE, Santini VE, Lee HS, Kubilus CA, Stern RA. Chronic traumatic encephalopathy in athletes: progressive tauopathy after repetitive head injury. J Neuropathol Exp Neurol. 2009;68:709–35.
7. Omalu B, Bailes J, Hamilton RL, Kamboh MI, Hammers J, Case M, Fitzsimmons R. Emerging histomorphologic phenotypes of chronic traumatic encephalopathy in American athletes. Neurosurgery. 2001;69: 173–83.
8. Omalu BI, Bailes J, Hammers JL, Fitzsimmons RP. Chronic traumatic encephalopathy, suicides and parasuicides in professional American athletes: the role of the forensic pathologist. Am J Forensic Med Pathol. 2010;31:130–2.
9. Omalu BI, DeKosky ST, Minster RL, Kamboh MI, Hamilton RL, Wecht CH. Chronic traumatic encephalopathy in a National Football League player. Neurosurgery. 2005;57:128–34.
10. Stern RA, Daneshvar DH, Baugh CM, Seichepine DR, Montenigro PH, Riley DO, Fritts NG, Stamm JM, Robbins CA, McHale L, Simkin I, Stein TD, Alvarez VE, Goldstein LE, Budson AE, Kowall NW, Nowinski CJ, Cantu RC, McKee AC. Clinical presentation of chronic traumatic encephalopathy. Neurology. 2003; 81:1122–9.
11. McKee AC, Alosco ML, Huber BR. Repetitive Head Impacts and Chronic Traumatic Encephalopathy. Neurosurg Clin N Am. 2016;27:529–35.
12. Guskiewicz KM, Marshall SW, Bailes J, McCrea M, Harding HP Jr, Matthews A, et al. Recurrent concussion and risk of depression in retired professional football players. Med Sci Sports Exerc. 2007;39:903–9.
13. Zaloshnja E, Miller T, Langlois JA, Selassie AW. Prevalence of long-term disability from traumatic brain injury in the civilian population of the United States, 2005. J Head Trauma Rehabil. 2008;23(6):394–400.
14. McCrory P, Meeuwisse WH, Aubry M, Cantu B, Dvorak J, Echemendia RJ, et al. Consensus statement on concussion in sport: the 4th International

Conference on Concussion in Sport held in Zurich, November 2012. Br J Sports Med. 2013;47:250–8.

15. Huber BR, Alosco ML, Stein TD, McKee AC. Potential Long-Term Consequences of Concussive and Subconcussive Injury. Phys Med Rehabil Clin N Am. 2016;27:503–11.
16. Muller MB, Lucassen PJ, Yassouridis A, Hoogendijk WJ, Holsboer F, Swaab DF. Neither major depression nor glucocorticoid treatment affects the cellular integrity of the human hippocampus. Eur J Neurosci. 2001;14:1603–12.
17. Najjar S, Pearlman DM, Alper K, Najjar A, Devinsky O. Neuroinflammation and psychiatric illness. J Neuroinflammation. 2013;10:43.
18. Allen GV, Gerami D, Esser MJ. Conditioning effects of repetitive mild neurotrauma on motor function in an animal model of focal brain injury. Neuroscience. 2000;99:93–105.
19. Conte V, Uryu K, Fujimoto S, Yao Y, Rokach J, Longhi L, et al. Vitamin E reduces amyloidosis and improves cognitive function in Tg2576 mice following repetitive concussive brain injury. J Neurochem. 2004;90:758–64.
20. Creeley CE, Wozniak DF, Bayly PV, Olney JW, Lewis LM. Multiple episodes of mild traumatic brain injury result in impaired cognitive performance in mice. Acad Emerg Med. 2004;11:809–19.
21. Dewitt DS, Perez-Polo R, Hulsebosch CE, Dash PK, Robertson CS. Challenges in the development of rodent models of mild traumatic brain injury. J Neurotrauma. 2013;30:688–701.
22. Goldstein LE, Fisher AM, Tagge CA, Zhang XL, Velisek L, Sullivan JA, et al. Chronic traumatic encephalopathy in blast-exposed military veterans and a blast neurotrauma mouse model. Sci Transl Med. 2012;4:134ra160.
23. Hawkins BE, Krishnamurthy S, Castillo-Carranza DL, Sengupta U, Prough DS, Jackson GR, et al. Rapid accumulation of endogenous tau oligomers in a rat model of traumatic brain injury: possible link between traumatic brain injury and sporadic tauopathies. J Biol Chem. 2013;288:17042–50.
24. Kane MJ, Angoa-Perez M, Briggs DI, Viano DC, Kreipke CW, Kuhn DM. A mouse model of human repetitive mild traumatic brain injury. J Neurosci Methods. 2012;203:41–9.
25. Mouzon BC, Bachmeier C, Ferro A, Ojo JO, Crynen G, Acker CM, et al. Chronic neuropathological and neurobehavioral changes in a repetitive mTBI model. Ann Neurol. 2014;75:241–54.
26. Small GW, Kepe V, Siddarth P, Ercoli LM, Merrill DA, Donoghue N, Bookheimer SY, Martinez J, Omalu B, Bailes J, Barrio JR. PET scanning of brain tau in retired national football league players: preliminary findings. Am J Geriatr Psychiatry. 2012;21:138–44.
27. Yu J, Zhu H, Gattoni-Celli S, Taheri S, Kindy MS. Dietary supplementation of GrandFusion® mitigates cerebral ischemia-induced neuronal damage and attenuates inflammation. Nutr Neurosci. 2015;6:154–63.
28. Ojo JO, Mouzon B, Greenberg MB, Bachmeier C, Mullan M, Crawford F. Repetitive mild traumatic brain injury augments tau pathology and glial activation in aged hTau mice. J Neuropathol Exp Neurol. 2013;72:137–51.
29. Flierl MA, Stahel PF, Beauchamp KM, Morgan SJ, Smith WR, Shohami E. Mouse closed head injury model induced by a weight-drop device. Nat Protoc. 2009;4:1328–37.
30. Adelson PD, Dixon CE, Robichaud P, Kochanek PM. Motor and cognitive functional deficits following diffuse traumatic brain injury in the immature rat. J Neurotrauma. 1997;14:99–108.
31. Petit-Demouliere B, Chenu F, Bourin M. Forced swimming test in mice: a review of antidepressant activity. Psychopharmacology. 2005;177:245–55.
32. Porsolt RD, Le Pichon M, Jalfre M. Depression: a new animal model sensitive to antidepressant treatments. Nature. 1977;266:730–2.
33. Bilkei-Gorzo A, Racz I, Michel K, Zimmer A. Diminished anxiety- and depression-related behaviors in mice with selective deletion of the Tac1 gene. J Neurosci. 2002;22:10046–52.
34. Yu J, Zhu H, Perry S, Taheri S, Kindy MS. Daily supplementation with GrandFusion® improves memory and learning in aged rats. Aging (Albany NY). 2017;9:1041–54.
35. Hook GR, Yu J, Sipes N, Pierschbacher M, Hook V, Kindy M. The cysteine protease cathepsin B is an important drug target and cysteine protease inhibitors are potential therapeutics for traumatic brain injury. J Neurotrauma. 2014;31:515–29.
36. Tang X, Yang L, Sanford LD. Individual variation in sleep and motor activity in rats. Behav Brain Res. 2007;180:62–8.
37. Tang X, Sanford LD. Telemetric recording of sleep and home cage activity in mice. Sleep. 2002;25:691 9.
38. Johnson VE, Stewart W, Arena JD, Smith DH. Traumatic brain injury as a trigger of neurodegeneration. Adv Neurobiol. 2017;15:383–400.
39. Mouzon BC, Bachmeier C, Ojo JO, Acker CM, Ferguson S, Paris D, Ait-Ghezala G, Crynen G, Davies P, Mullan M, Stewart W, Crawford F. Lifelong behavioral and neuropathological consequences of repetitive mild traumatic brain injury. Ann Clin Transl Neurol. 2017;5(1):64–80.
40. Ferguson S, Mouzon B, Paris D, Aponte D, Abdullah L, Stewart W, Mullan M, Crawford F. Acute or delayed treatment with anatabine improves spatial memory and reduces pathological sequelae at late time-points after repetitive mild traumatic brain injury. J Neurotrauma. 2017;34(8):1676–91.
41. Robinson S, Berglass JB, Denson JL, Berkner J, Anstine CV, Winer JL, Maxwell JR, Qiu J, Yang Y, Sillerud LO, Meehan WP 3rd, Mannix R, Jantzie LL. Microstructural and microglial changes after repetitive mild traumatic brain injury in mice. J Neurosci Res. 2017;95(4):1025–35.
42. Ojo JO, Mouzon BC, Crawford F. Repetitive head trauma, chronic traumatic encephalopathy and tau: challenges in translating from mice to men. Exp Neurol. 2016;275(Pt 3):389–404.
43. Shitaka Y, Tran HT, Bennett RE, Sanchez L, Levy MA, Dikranian K, Brody DL. Repetitive closed-skull traumatic brain injury in mice causes persistent multifocal axonal injury and microglial reactivity. J Neuropathol Exp Neurol. 2011;70(7):551–67.
44. Yoshiyama Y, Uryu K, Higuchi M, Longhi L, Hoover R, Fujimoto S, McIntosh T, Lee VM, Trojanowski JQ. Enhanced neurofibrillary tangle formation, cerebral atrophy, and cognitive deficits induced by repetitive mild brain injury in a transgenic tauopathy mouse model. J Neurotrauma. 2005;22(10):1134–41.
45. Shih RH, Wang CY, Yang CM. NF-kappaB signaling pathways in neurological inflammation: a mini review. Front Mol Neurosci. 2015;8:77.
46. Lim S, Chun Y, Lee JS, Lee SJ. Neuroinflammation in synucleinopathies. Brain Pathol. 2016;26(3):404–9.
47. Stephenson J, Nutma E, van der Valk P, Amor S. Inflammation in CNS neurodegenerative diseases. Immunology. 2018;154:204–19.

8

Inflammation in epileptogenesis after traumatic brain injury

Kyria M. Webster[1], Mujun Sun[1], Peter Crack[2], Terence J. O'Brien[1], Sandy R. Shultz[1] and Bridgette D. Semple[1*]

Abstract

Background: Epilepsy is a common and debilitating consequence of traumatic brain injury (TBI). Seizures contribute to progressive neurodegeneration and poor functional and psychosocial outcomes for TBI survivors, and epilepsy after TBI is often resistant to existing anti-epileptic drugs. The development of post-traumatic epilepsy (PTE) occurs in a complex neurobiological environment characterized by ongoing TBI-induced secondary injury processes. Neuroinflammation is an important secondary injury process, though how it contributes to epileptogenesis, and the development of chronic, spontaneous seizure activity, remains poorly understood. A mechanistic understanding of how inflammation contributes to the development of epilepsy (epileptogenesis) after TBI is important to facilitate the identification of novel therapeutic strategies to reduce or prevent seizures.

Body: We reviewed previous clinical and pre-clinical data to evaluate the hypothesis that inflammation contributes to seizures and epilepsy after TBI. Increasing evidence indicates that neuroinflammation is a common consequence of epileptic seizure activity, and also contributes to epileptogenesis as well as seizure initiation (ictogenesis) and perpetuation. Three key signaling factors implicated in both seizure activity and TBI-induced secondary pathogenesis are highlighted in this review: high-mobility group box protein-1 interacting with toll-like receptors, interleukin-1β interacting with its receptors, and transforming growth factor-β signaling from extravascular albumin. Lastly, we consider age-dependent differences in seizure susceptibility and neuroinflammation as mechanisms which may contribute to a heightened vulnerability to epileptogenesis in young brain-injured patients.

Conclusion: Several inflammatory mediators exhibit epileptogenic and ictogenic properties, acting on glia and neurons both directly and indirectly influence neuronal excitability. Further research is required to establish causality between inflammatory signaling cascades and the development of epilepsy post-TBI, and to evaluate the therapeutic potential of pharmaceuticals targeting inflammatory pathways to prevent or mitigate the development of PTE.

Keywords: Inflammation, Traumatic brain injury, Epilepsy, Post-traumatic epilepsy, Seizures, Cytokine, Interleukin, Astrocytes

Background

Epilepsy is a common and debilitating consequence of traumatic brain injuries (TBI), with recurrent spontaneous seizures contributing to progressive neurodegeneration and greatly interfering with quality of life as well as increasing the risk of injury and death. Epileptogenesis, the neurobiological process by which epilepsy develops, occurs as part of the ongoing secondary injury events triggered by a brain insult, including neuroinflammation. Previous evidence from clinical and preclinical studies has suggested that aspects of the inflammatory response may also promote seizure activity itself (ictogenesis).

The aim of this review was to evaluate the published evidence regarding the role of inflammation in the development of post-traumatic epilepsy (PTE), drawing upon data from both clinical studies and experimental models. In particular, we summarize the current understanding of mechanisms by which neuroinflammatory mediators can influence neuronal excitability, either directly or indirectly. We focused in particular on three

* Correspondence: Bridgette.Semple@unimelb.edu.au
[1]Department of Medicine (The Royal Melbourne Hospital), The University of Melbourne, Kenneth Myer Building, Melbourne Brain Centre, Royal Parade, Parkville, VIC 3050, Australia

key signaling pathways which are known to be involved in TBI-induced secondary pathogenesis, and more recently, have been implicated in seizure activity and the process of epileptogenesis. Lastly, potential mechanisms underlying age-specific vulnerability to hyperexcitability and epileptogenesis are discussed. This review also acts to highlight knowledge gaps in the field, identifying key areas for future research. Ultimately, a mechanistic understanding of how neuroinflammation contributes to the development of epilepsy after brain injury may identify novel therapeutic targets, to reduce or prevent PTE for survivors of brain injuries.

Traumatic brain injury and epilepsy

TBI is a major global public health problem and a leading cause of mortality and morbidity [1, 2]. It is particularly prevalent in childhood and adolescence, as a result of falls, inflicted trauma, sports-related injuries, and motor vehicle accidents. An earlier review of 11 studies examining TBI incidence in Australia, North America, and Europe estimated a median of 691 injuries per 100,000 population under 20 years of age [2]. Of note, children under the age of 5 had the highest incidence of Emergency Department admissions for TBI [2].

TBI is any insult to the brain from an external mechanical force, including penetrative or blunt trauma [1, 3]. These can include focal injuries, such as lesions caused by contusions or hemorrhages, or diffuse injuries, such as with traumatic axonal injury [4]. TBI involves a primary insult, defined as the immediate structural damage caused by the external mechanical force. This is followed by a secondary injury, which includes a myriad of neuropathological processes including excitotoxicity, neuroinflammation, oxidative stress, and apoptosis [1, 3, 5]. These secondary processes commence within minutes after TBI, can persist for months to years, and are thought to contribute to the expansion of tissue damage [6, 7]. The manifestation and severity of secondary injury processes can differ depending on injury type, severity, and individual factors [8]. The biomechanics and biochemical components of the physiological response to TBI have been reviewed in detail elsewhere [7, 9].

PTE is a common consequence of TBI, defined as spontaneous, recurrent, and chronic seizures following a head injury [10, 11]. Clinical diagnosis is often based upon one or more unprovoked seizures occurring later than 1 week after a TBI, as an indicator that epileptogenesis is occurring [12]. Epileptogenesis is the process by which epilepsy develops; that is, when an otherwise normally functioning brain becomes biased towards abnormal recurrent electrical activity, increasing the propensity to develop spontaneous recurrent seizures [13, 14]. It is thought to develop through three phases: (1) the initial trigger; (2) the latency period, during which the changes initiated in phase one cause a transformational bias in the brain towards epileptic activity; and (3) the onset of spontaneous seizures and the establishment of chronic epilepsy (Fig. 1) [15–18]. After TBI, the

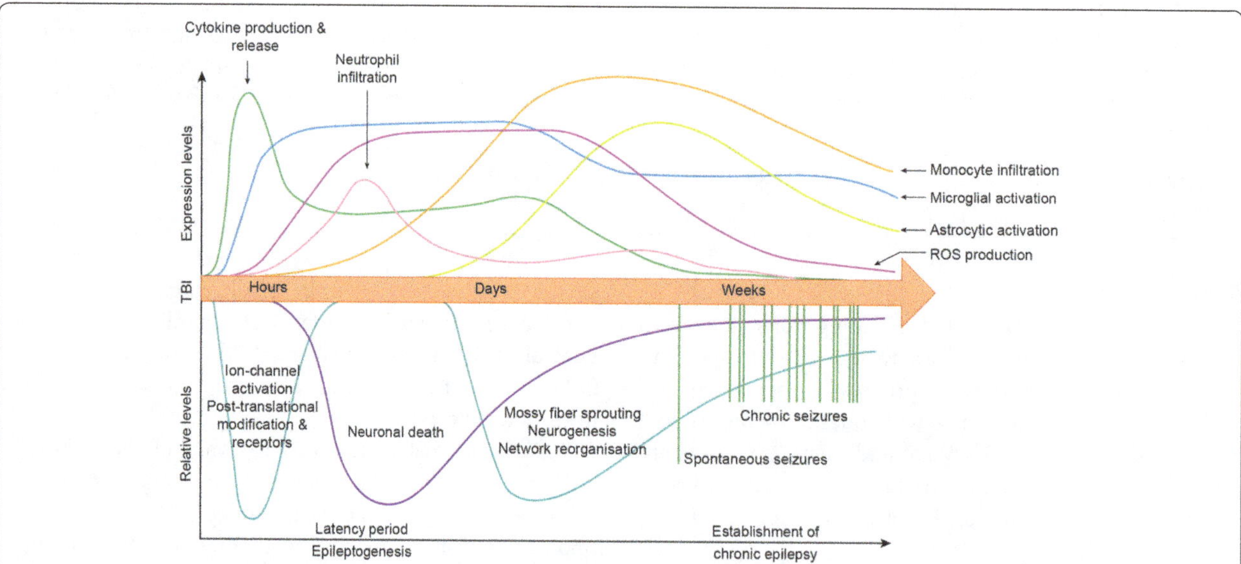

Fig. 1 Summary of the progression of inflammatory factors and epileptogenesis after TBI. After TBI, epileptogenesis occurs after a latent period of months to years. Within hours after the injury, a myriad of cytokines are released at high levels which can continue for days. This is concurrent with activation of ion-channels and post-translational modifications of various receptors associated with neuronal excitation and inhibition, which can occur as early as minutes after the injury. Local immune cells are activated, and peripheral immune cells are also recruited to the area within hours to days. Neuroinflammation can persist for weeks after the injury, coincidental with widespread neuronal loss. In the later phase of epileptogenesis, processes such as neurogenesis and mossy fiber sprouting in the hippocampus contribute to an increasingly excitable neuronal environment. It may be weeks, months, or years before spontaneous seizures and the establishment of chronic and persistent epilepsy manifests

latency period may be many years in duration, and epileptogenesis is associated with ongoing secondary injury processes which can bias towards hyperexcitability [14].

The reported incidence of developing epilepsy after TBI ranges from 4.4 to 53%, depending on the population studied [12]. There are several factors that have been associated with a greater risk of developing PTE, including higher injury severity and a lower age-at-insult [10, 19, 20]. It has been estimated that 10–20% of children with severe TBI develop PTE, although the risk after injury has been reported at up to 60%, with the wide range of estimates most likely due to the large variation in severity, heterogeneity of the initial insult, and difficulties in diagnosis and follow-up [10, 20]. Children under the age of 5 may be at highest risk for early post-traumatic seizure development [10, 12, 21], with one study finding that this age group were more likely to have a seizure within the first week after injury (17%), compared to patients over 5 years of age with similar injuries (2%) [22]. In adults, the presence of acute intracerebral hematoma has been consistently associated with a higher risk of developing PTE, as are penetrative insults and depressed skull fractures [12, 22, 23].

Several neuropathological hallmarks have been associated with the development of PTE. An early and persistent increase in hippocampal excitability has been observed in both patients and animal models [24]. This net increase in excitability is thought to result from the selective loss of vulnerable inhibitory interneurons concurrent with the reorganization of excitatory circuitry [25, 26]. Recurrent excitatory circuitry in the hippocampal dentate gyrus may manifest as mossy fiber sprouting, where the axons of dentate granule cells form abnormal connections with neighboring neurons in response to a loss of CA3 pyramidal cell targets and hilar interneurons [27, 28].

The onset of PTE is also commonly associated with hippocampal sclerosis, involving the loss of pyramidal neurons, and concurrent reactive gliosis, consistent with temporal lobe epilepsy (TLE) [29]. An estimated 35–62% of patients with PTE have seizures originating from the temporal lobe [30, 31]. However, overlaying cortical regions have also been implicated in post-TBI epileptogenesis, as these regions may also exhibit neuronal loss, chronic neuroinflammation, and network reorganization resulting in spontaneous epileptiform activity [26, 32].

Clinical management and treatment of PTE is challenging, as seizures are commonly resistant to existing anti-seizure drugs (ASDs) [10, 20, 33, 34]. Classical ASDs, such as phenytoin, carbamazepine, valproate benzodiazepines, are ineffective in reducing or preventing PTE [34–36]. While early post-injury prophylaxis with ASDs may reduce or prevent early post-injury seizures [37], there is little evidence to indicate that these treatments can be disease-modifying and prevent the development of PTE or spontaneous unprovoked seizures long-term [38]. Once a patient has developed seizures, polypharmacy is often employed in an attempt to control the seizures, yet a significant proportion of TBI patients who develop epilepsy will develop drug-resistance, defined as a failure to achieve seizure cessation after trialling more than two tolerated and appropriate ASD treatments [33, 34]. However, the use of multiple ASDs simultaneously could have unpredictable consequences due to potential interactions with various secondary processes and the reduced cerebral perfusion commonly present after TBI [20]. Seizures are particularly detrimental during periods of brain development as they can cause permanent adverse effects, including cognitive deficits [39, 40]. Due to increased susceptibility to post-traumatic seizures after an early age-of-insult, as well as inherent difficulties in controlling or treating PTE, further research is needed to understand the mechanisms that contribute to the generation of post-traumatic seizures, particularly in pediatric age groups.

Neuroinflammation after TBI

Inflammation is a central component of the secondary injury after TBI, and the subject of intense research as a promising target for treatment. In healthy tissue, inflammation typically acts to combat invading pathogens and preserve the health of the tissue [41]. However, in pathological conditions such as trauma, inflammation can also function as a reactionary system to either aggravate or ameliorate tissue damage [42, 43]. Increased neuroinflammation after TBI has been associated with poor outcomes and progression to various sequelae including neurodegenerative diseases [43–47].

The main hallmarks of the cerebral inflammatory response after TBI include blood-brain barrier (BBB) dysfunction, edema, microglial, and astrocytic activation and migration, the release of inflammatory factors such as cytokines and the recruitment of blood-derived leukocytes into brain parenchyma [48]. Neutrophils, recruited from the peripheral circulation within hours after TBI, mediate early pathogenesis by promoting edema and oxidative stress, and the production of inflammatory cytokines and neurotoxic proteases [49, 50]. Cytokines can be released rapidly after injury as they are synthesized and stored locally by neurons and glia [48].

Under physiological conditions, the BBB is a highly stringent barrier between vessels and brain tissue, which mediates the transport of blood components such as immune cells into the brain [51]. After TBI, this barrier can be compromised, allowing peripheral inflammatory cells into the brain and the injured area [52]. Chemoattractant cytokines, called chemokines, further facilitate the recruitment and transmigration of inflammatory leukocytes [53]. By their actions at the BBB as well as direct chemoattraction, chemokines including CXCL8 and CCL2 (also known as monocyte chemoattractant protein-1) are key mediators in the migration of neutrophils and monocytes, respectively, to the site of injury [54].

Once in the brain, these cells release a plethora of inflammatory cytokines, chemokines, and reactive oxygen species (ROS) to perpetuate inflammation and oxidative stress in the injured brain. Both clinical and experimental studies have demonstrated a pronounced elevation of many cytokines after TBI, including tumor necrosis factor (TNF-α), transforming growth factor-β (TGF-β), and interleukin-1β (IL-1β), -6, and -10, with downstream activation of intracellular signaling cascades involving nuclear factor Kappa-light-chain-enhancer of activated B cells (NF-κB) [1, 44, 48, 55–57]. Released cytokines in turn can recruit additional blood-borne neutrophils and monocytes into the injured tissue, propagating the inflammatory cascade.

Inflammation in the brain has a duality in function after injury, which manifests through the actions of many different cell types. For example, microglial activation is integral in tissue repair, surveillance of pathogenic factors and host defense [58]. However, activated microglia can also release cytotoxic factors such as ROS to induce oxidative stress [59–61]. Astrocytes can promote tissue repair in the central nervous system (CNS) through the release of insulin-like growth factor [47], but are also implicated in the perpetuation of inflammation by an over-production of cytokines such as IL-6 [62, 63], as well as modulation of the BBB and neuronal function to promote excitability and seizure production [64].

Cytokines themselves also have a complex role after TBI, as experimental studies have yielded conflicting findings of both deleterious contributions and participation in repair processes after CNS insult [48]. One cytokine that displays such paradox is TNF-α, which has been associated with increased neurological damage, including demyelination and BBB breakdown, in several experimental models of TBI [65, 66]. However, increased levels of TNF-α may conversely have a neuroprotective function in the late stages of inflammation post-TBI, at 2–4 weeks after the injury, as suggested from a mouse model of TBI [56]. The varied roles of inflammatory mediators in the pathological environment after TBI is likely dependent on many different factors, including timing of release, the location and cell types involved, the differing physics of protein-protein interactions of cytokines, and their relative amounts. The multifarious dynamics of this response may contribute to the progression of a chronic state of damage, leading to the myriad of secondary consequences of TBI, including PTE.

Inflammation in epileptogenesis

The long-standing concept that seizures result from an imbalance between reduced γ-aminobutyric acid (GABA)-ergic inhibition and enhanced glutamatergic excitation [67, 68], based upon the presence of large amplitude EEG discharges during the seizure event itself, is an over-simplified of a very complex network response. While excessive glutamatergic excitation has historically been considered of as the precipitating factor for a focal seizure, there is a lack of strong data to support this hypothesis. Instead, paradoxically, accumulating evidence indicates that increased synchronised GABAergic interneuronal activity is sufficient to disrupt neuronal networks and initiate the transition from interictal to ictal activity resulting in focal seizures [69]. The recruitment of neighboring neurons and subsequent seizure progression is then hypothesized to be mediated by an elevation in extracellular potassium [70]. Adding to the complexity of network-based activity, both excitatory and inhibitory roles of GABA and glutamatergic neurons have been reported, and a range of extrasynaptic as well as synaptic neurotransmitter receptors and ion channels have been implicated in seizures, in addition to those traditionally implicated, such as NMDA and $GABA_A$ receptors [71].

However, strong evidence also implicates a role for inflammation in seizure pathologies [45]. Seizure activity readily induces an inflammatory response, including the activation of microglia and production of pro-inflammatory cytokines [47, 63]. More importantly, experimental data has suggested that inflammatory mediators may initiate or trigger early seizures, preceding the onset of diagnosed epilepsy. For example, systemic inflammation by injection of bacterial lipopolysaccharide results in a lowered seizure threshold [72]. In the next sections, we will review clinical and experimental evidence suggesting an inherent link between inflammatory signaling, neuropathology, and seizure activity in the injured brain, as a likely mechanism of importance in the development and progression of PTE.

Seizures increase inflammation

Experimentally, induction of a seizure induces the rapid activation of glial cells in surrounding parenchyma, which respond by the production and release of inflammatory molecules [73]. Much of the research that has shown an increase in inflammation after seizures have used experimental models of status epilepticus. This involves the administration of a chemical or electrical pro-convulsant stimulus to create a sustained seizure event (the initial insult) followed by a latency period before the onset of spontaneous recurrent seizures to model epilepsy [74, 75]. In these experimental models, the inflammatory response displays a distinct temporal profile after induction, characterized by the early activation of astrocytes and microglia followed by BBB breakdown and neuronal activation [63, 76, 77]. In addition to the investigation of protein release, microarray analysis of gene transcripts have also demonstrated an upregulation of inflammatory genes [78]. Specific cell surface toll-like receptors (TLR's), which respond to a range of inflammatory cytokines and other stress-related factors, are highly upregulated after pilocarpine-induced seizures on forebrain microglia of adult mice [77]. Simultaneously, a robust increase in cytokine levels has been observed in both chemically and electrically induced experimental models of epilepsy in adult rodents [77, 79, 80]. For example, IL-1β is expressed at low levels in a healthy brain, but is robustly upregulated for up to 60 days after the induction of self-sustaining limbic status epilepticus in rodents, a model using hippocampal electrical stimulation [76]. TNF-α and IL-6 are also rapidly upregulated after status epilepticus, peaking within 30 min of seizure onset and remaining elevated for up to 72 h in rats that progressed to spontaneous seizures [76].

These experimental findings that seizures result in inflammation are confirmed by evidence in the clinical setting. Analysis of cerebrospinal fluid (CSF) from newly diagnosed adult patients with tonic-clonic seizures detected an upregulation of IL-6 and IL-1 receptors (IL-1Rs) [81, 82]. Matched serum samples revealed a higher levels of IL-6 compared to in the CSF, suggesting that these cytokines likely originated in the brain [82]. High levels of cytokines including IL-1β and high-mobility group box protein-1 (HMGB1) have also been identified in neurons and glia of surgically resected epileptic tissue [83]. Together, these findings indicate that neuroinflammation is a common consequence of seizure activity.

Inflammation contributing to seizures

Accumulating evidence suggests that neuroinflammation is also a contributor to epileptogenic pathology after TBI [45, 63, 84]. In particular, experimental models have demonstrated that glial cell activation and recruitment and the synthesis of inflammatory factors, may precede and/or occur concurrently with epileptogenic events [85, 86]. For example, in a rodent model of experimental TBI, a reduced threshold to electroconvulsive shock-induced seizures was reversed when minocycline, a tetracycline antibiotic known to inhibit brain infiltration of monocytes and microglia, was applied [87, 88], implicating both microglial activity and pro-inflammatory cytokines in post-traumatic seizure activity.

Much of the evidence for a role of inflammation in epileptogenesis has focused on the effect of cytokines in seizure susceptibility. Cytokines can act as classical neurotransmitters through receptor modulation and phosphorylation at the neuronal membrane [89]. Models of chronic inflammation, such as transgenic mice systemically overexpressing IL-6 or TNF-α, can reduce seizure threshold and predispose the brain to seizure induced-neuronal loss [90, 91]. Indeed, inflammatory signaling may promote the loss of GABAergic neurons in the hippocampus, resulting in an increased propensity for seizures due to a reduction in synaptic inhibition [92].

N-methyl-D-aspartate (NMDA) receptors play a critical role in the glutamatergic system to contribute to neuronal excitability, and previous evidence suggests both direct and indirect interactions between these receptors and cyokines [93]. Cytokines have been found to inhibit the uptake of glutamate by astrocytes in culture [94] and modulate excitatory neurotransmission in the brain through NMDA and alpha-amino-3-hydroxyl-5-methyl-4-isoxazole-propoinate (AMPA) receptors [95, 96]. For example, IL-1β produced by microglia can enhance NMDA-mediated Ca^{2+} currents through cell surface type 1 IL-1R (IL-1R1) co-localized on pyramidal cell dendrites [89]. Pre-synaptic NMDA receptors are agonists for Ca^{2+}-mediated glutamate release, and when activated by inflammatory factors such as IL-1β and HMGB1 can cause an excess of intracellular Ca^{2+} leading to an extracellular hyperexcitability and excitotoxicity [95]. Several other cytokines including TNF-α and IL-10 have also been associated with the regulation of seizure duration in experimental kindling models [97, 98]. Though these correlations have been seen in multiple studies with different models, the mechanisms underlying the relationship between the inflammatory environment and epileptogenesis, particularly in the context of brain injury, remain still poorly understood.

There is limited clinical data to confirm a cause-and-effect link between inflammation and the pathophysiology of epilepsy, however increasing evidence supports this hypothesis. Many studies have now demonstrated that early exposure of the brain to immune responses can have varied and persistent consequences on adult physiology [99–102]. Febrile seizures (FS) and febrile status epilepticus in children is a risk factor for developing epilepsy later in life [103], which may be induced by fever often associated with inflammation and infection [47]. Although the mechanisms underlying FS remains unclear, it is thought that cytokines play a key role in its development [104]. One study has reported specific polymorphisms in the promoter region of cytokine genes, including IL-1β, in children with FS compared to controls [105]. Such genetic variation may influence the production of IL-1β in both healthy tissue and after injury or stimulus [106], and similar polymorphisms have also been observed at a high frequency in patients with TLE [107].

Recently, the hypothesis of glial functions playing a pivotal role in biasing the neuronal network towards an epileptogenic environment has been gaining traction [108, 109]. In particular, interactions between neurons, glia, and the inflammatory mediators IL-1β, HMGB-1, and TGF-β, have been implicated in promoting seizure susceptibility, as described below. The main signaling pathways implicated in the proposed link between inflammation and epileptogenesis of these three mediators is summarized in Fig. 2.

IL-1β/IL-1R signaling in TBI and PTE

IL-1 is a family of pro-inflammatory cytokines that act as key mediators of the innate immune response [110]. The IL-1 family consists of 7 agonists (e.g., IL-1α and β) and 3 receptor antagonists [110], and amongst these the IL-1β isoform has been the most commonly studied in the brain injury and epilepsy settings. In the CNS, IL-1β can be produced by a range of cells including microglia, astrocytes, endothelial cells (EC), neurons, and peripheral leukocytes upon infiltrating into the brain [111–113]. IL-1β exerts its action on multiple cell types primarily via IL-1R1 [114–119]. This initiates intracellular signaling via NF-κB transcription factor, p38 mitogen-activated protein kinase (MAPK), or other factors [118, 120]. Several studies have demonstrated that IL-1β binding to IL-1R stimulates immune cell activation and induces the production of neurotoxic molecules [114, 115, 117–119].

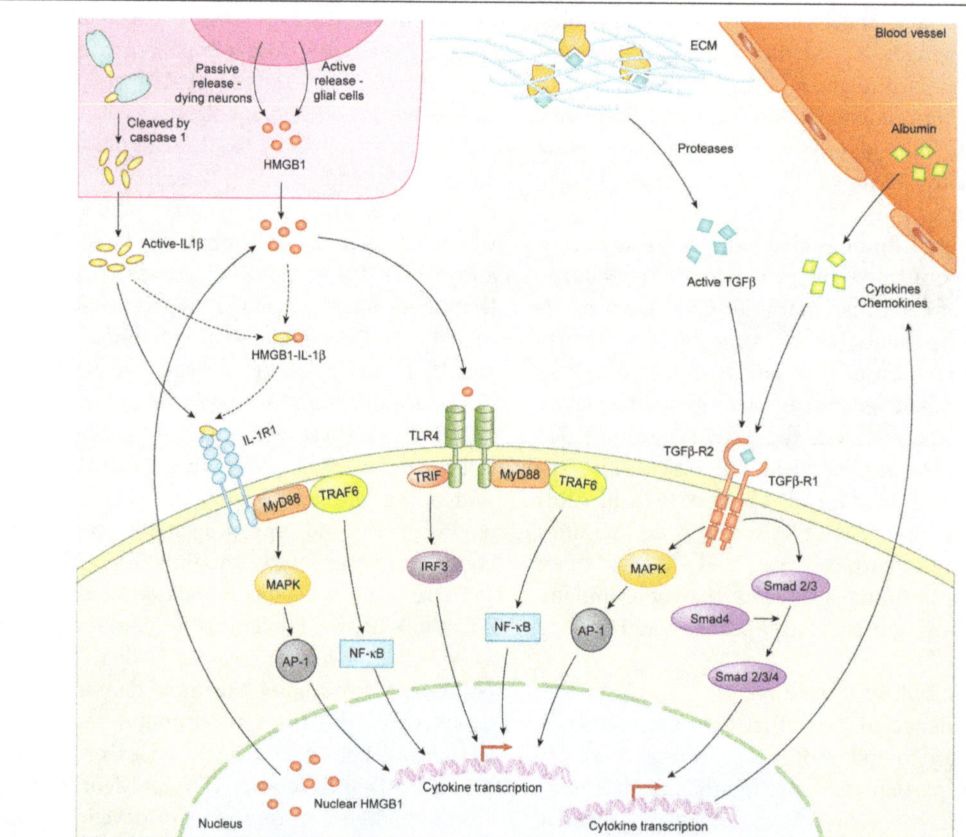

Fig. 2 Summary of three key signaling cascades that may mediate the link between inflammation and epileptogenesis. HMGB1, IL-1β, TGF-β, and serum albumin have varied release mechanisms from multiple cell types in order to activate their signaling pathways. After injury, HMGB1 may be passively released from necrotic neurons to the extracellular space, or released actively from activated microglia and astrocytes. HMGB1 can bind to multiple receptors on many different cell types, such as TLR4, which can activate MyD88 independent pathways such as the phosphorylation of interferon regulatory transcription factor 3 (IRF3) leading to the transcription and release of interferons-α and -β, as well as other interferon-induced genes. HMGB1-TLR4 can also activate NF-κB signaling both directly or via TNF receptor-associated factor 6 (TRAF6). This can lead to a rapid nuclear transcription of various immune-related processes, as reviewed elsewhere [250]. Caspase-1 mediates cleavage of inactive pro-IL-1β to active IL-1β, allowing for its relocation into the extracellular space, where IL-1β can bind to IL-1R1 either directly or in complex with HMGB1. The IL-1β/IL-1R1 complex can then induce NF-κB signaling via TRAF6 or activate MyD88-dependent MAPK signaling, which has been linked to the production of various neurotoxic molecules. TGF-β is released in an inactive form from cells and binds to the extracellular matrix. Proteases, released after injury, cleave the inactive protein to active TGF-β, which is able to bind to the two TGF-β receptors. Mechanical breakdown of the BBB allows serum albumin into the extracellular space, where it can also bind to TGF-β receptor1 and receptor2, which signal via Smad complex proteins or MAPK signaling pathways, respectively, to regulate the immune response. This pathway has also been implicated in post-translational changes to a variety of voltage-dependent ion channels implicated in changes to neuronal excitability [94]

There are several lines of evidence implicating IL-1β in the development of PTE. Firstly, IL-1β is rapidly and highly upregulated following experimental and clinical TBI. In rodent models, Il-1β expression is upregulated as early as 1 h post-TBI [121, 122] and peaks between 12 and 24 h [54, 123, 124]. This response may then persist for several months post-injury [125]. Consistent with experimental findings, analysis of protein, and gene expression in post-mortem brain tissue from TBI patients found that IL-1β was upregulated in individuals who died 6–122 h post-injury [126]. This is consistent with reports of elevated IL-1β in the CSF and serum of severe TBI patients [127, 128], correlated with poor outcomes in both children and adults [19, 129]. Thus IL-1β levels are elevated during the period of secondary injury after TBI, which has been postulated to also be an important time period for the epileptogenic process [130]. Notably, numerous studies indicate that modulating IL-1β signaling is broadly beneficial in experimental TBI models. Treatment with an IL-1β neutralizing antibody alleviated TBI-induced microglial activation, neutrophil infiltration, cerebral edema, and cognitive deficits in mouse models of TBI [131, 132]. In line with this finding, IL-1R1 deficient mice also showed decreased cerebral edema and leukocyte infiltration following TBI [133], and post-injury administration of an IL-1R1 antagonist attenuated neuronal cell death and cognitive dysfunction in rats [134]. A phase II clinical trial employing an IL-1R antagonist treatment (100 mg/day subcutaneously administered for 5 days) was recently conducted in patients with severe diffuse TBI, demonstrating safety penetration into the plasma and brain extracellular fluid, and an alteration of the immune profile [135].

One of the key clinical studies linking IL-1β with PTE was conducted by Diamond and colleagues, who examined whether genetic variation in the IL-1β gene and CSF/serum IL-1β ratios correlated with PTE development in a cohort of 256 patients with moderate to severe TBI [136]. Serum and CSF were collected from a portion of subjects within the first week post-injury, and IL-1β levels were assessed in relation to the later incidence of PTE. Further, IL-1β tagging and functional single nucleotide polymorphisms (SNPs) were genotyped to evaluate its association to PTE. Elevated CSF/serum IL-1β ratios were found to be associated with increased risk of PTE, and one of IL-1β SNPs, rs1143634, showed an association between the heterozygote genotype and increased PTE risk [136]. Further research is required to determine the contribution of genetic variability to IL-1β function and how this may influence the inflammatory response after TBI.

IL-1β has also been linked to other epilepsies in addition to PTE. For example, IL-1β may play a role in epileptogenesis that follows FS. Specifically, IL-1β levels were found to be acutely upregulated in rats after prolonged FS, and IL-1β levels remained elevated only in rats that developed spontaneous limbic seizures after prolonged FS [137]. In another study, IL-1R1 deficient mice were found to be resistant to experimental FS [138].

There are a number of possible mechanisms by which IL-1β may contribute to PTE. IL-1β can modulate neuronal hyperexcitability through Ca^{2+}, glutamatergic, and GABAergic pathways [139]. By acting on glia cells, IL-1β mediates astrocytes and microglia activation, formation of a glial scar, and the release of neurotoxic mediators to promote cell loss, features which are associated with epileptic foci in the brain [140]. Furthermore, IL-1β signaling may promote epileptogenesis by enhancing BBB permeability and enhancing the recruitment of peripheral leukocytes into the brain [141–144]. There are many proposed mechanisms of IL-1β signaling in areas that are still poorly understood, and future research into these may reveal the way in which they interact to increase the risk of epileptogenesis.

Although less commonly studied, other members of the IL-1 family have also been investigated in the context of TBI and epilepsy. For example, an upregulation of IL-1α has been reported in brain tissue following experimental TBI [145, 146]. In the clinical setting, peripheral blood mononuclear cells collected from epilepsy patients exhibited greater production of IL-1α in response to stimulation in vitro compared to cells from non-epileptic controls [147]. However, no association has been found between gene polymorphisms of IL-1α and TBI outcomes [148], nor IL-1α and seizure pathogenesis [149]. Taken together, there is much accumulating experimental and clinical evidence implicating IL-1 cytokines in epileptogenesis, however further studies are needed to delineate their precise roles and whether therapeutically targeting them can mitigate PTE.

HMGB1/TLR4 signaling in PTE

HMGB1 was originally identified as a ubiquitous, highly evolutionarily conserved, chromatin-binding protein, most often found in the cell nucleus of healthy tissues [150–152]. Discovered in 1973, and named due to its ability to migrate quickly during gel electrophoresis [153], HMGB1 participates in the formation of nucleosomes and is important in the regulation of gene transcription [151, 154, 155]. More recently, HMGB1 has been identified as a damage-associated molecular pattern (DAMP) [150], which are molecules that are able to initiate or perpetuate inflammation. Complete gene deficiency of HMGB1 is lethal during early postnatal life, indicating its essential role in transcriptional control [156]. A 98% homology between human HMGB1 and mouse HMGB1 enables clinically relevant experimental investigation through animal models [157].

HMGB1 has two modes of cellular release in injured tissue. Immediately after injury, necrosis allows a passive release of significant amounts of HMGB1 from the nucleus into the extracellular space [158]. HMGB1 may undergo post-translational oxidation and acetylation, resulting in its active release by immune cells in response to various cytokines including itself, allowing a powerful positive feedback loop during inflammation [157, 159–161]. In addition, HMGB1 may be released upon activation by a wide range of cells in the CNS including neurons, microglia, macrophages, monocytes, natural killer cells, dendritic cells, ECs, and platelets [162].

High levels of HMGB1 have been found in epileptogenic tissue resected during surgery [83, 163], implicating a role for this DAMP in neuronal hyperexcitability. Experimental evidence from an animal model of temporal lobe epilepsy suggests that HMGB1 contributes to seizure activity and epilepsy [164]. One previous study by Maroso and colleagues demonstrated that intracerebral injection of HMGB1 in wild type mice increased seizure activity in response to a stimulus [165]. This pro-convulsant effect of HMGB1 is most likely mediated through one of its key signaling receptors, TLR4, as a comparable increase in seizure susceptibility was not seen in non-functional TLR4 mutant mice [165]. TLR4 mutant mice were also found to be intrinsically resistant to seizures as compared to wild type mice [165]. Interfering with the binding of HMGB1 to TLR4 has been shown to reduce both seizure frequency and onset. For example, TLR4 antagonists and BoxA, a competitive antagonist to HMGB1 comprising of the BoxA domain of the protein, have been reported to reduce and even inhibit epileptic activity that is resistant to standard ASDs in an animal model of temporal lobe epilepsy [166].

In another recent study, the mechanism by which HMGB1 signaling promotes neuronal hyperexcitability and seizure activity was found to be through an increase in NMDA receptor function in TLR4-expressing hippocampal neurons [167]. This effect was dependent on the oxidation of HMGB1 characteristic of its active release from immune cells, and was associated with high levels of NMDA-induced excitotoxic cell death [167]. Because the inflammatory environment after TBI involves the rapid production of ROS and free radicals [168, 169], there is a physiological preference towards the extracellular oxidation of HMGB1, thus increasing TLR4-mediated augmentation of NMDA functionality and promoting seizure susceptibility [167].

Downstream of HMGB1, TLR4 mRNA expression is upregulated in response to brain insult [170], consistent with upregulation of this receptor during seizure activity in experimental models of epilepsy [165]. TLR4 is able to transmit signals via both myeloid differentiation primary response gene 88 (MyD88) dependent and independent pathways [171]. It is through the MyD88 dependent pathway that TLR4 is able to activate NF-κB, which may be responsible for increasing pro-inflammatory cytokine expression to augment the inflammatory response [172, 173]. This pathway has generated great interest recently, and with the potential to modulate epileptic activity, even in drug-resistant epilepsy, further research is needed to confirm the potential of this pathway as a target for therapeutic intervention in the development of PTE.

Previous research has also suggested that HMGB1 is able to enhance inflammation through forming a complex with different cytokines, including IL-1β [174]. HMGB1 bound to IL-1β has been isolated from cell cultures when co-incubated [174]. Studies of joint inflammation in animals have also shown that when HMGB1 is present with IL-1β there is an enhanced inflammatory response, most likely through action on with IL-1 receptor 1[175], Whilst this complex has yet to be identified in brain tissue, further research is needed into this pathway as it may play a vital role in extending a bias towards epileptogenesis.

By contributing to acute and chronic seizures, both directly and indirectly, the HMGB1-TLR4 axis is therefore a promising target for TLEs that are resistant to ASDs [165, 167]. This is important in the context of TBI, as seizure pathology can begin as early as the day of a brain injury [176]. Together, these data support a key role for HMGB1 in neuronal hyperexcitability and implicate the HMGB1-TLR4 signaling pathway as a potential therapeutic target to modulate post-traumatic epileptogenesis.

TGF-β/albumin involvement in PTE

Vascular dysfunction has been associated with many types of focal and acquired epilepsies, including PTE [177]. BBB dysfunction is also a common feature of TBI in both patients and experimental models [6, 178]. Vascular dysfunction after TBI, in particular the localized breakdown of the BBB surrounding focal regions of tissue damage, is hypothesized to trigger a series of epileptogenic processes [179]. For example, increased permeability of the BBB is evident by magnetic resonance imaging with gadolinium and co-localized with the focal epileptogenic region in patients with PTE [180, 181].

A proposed mechanism of BBB breakdown in this context is through the TGF-β/albumin-mediated signaling pathway. In the laboratory, experimental opening of the BBB in the rodent neocortex was found to trigger epileptogenesis, which was recapitulated by exposure of the brain to serum albumin [182]. Albumin has been shown to induce the production of excitatory synapses experimentally both in vitro and in vivo [183]. Serum albumin in the rodent brain has been shown to result in hypersynchronized responses to electrical stimulation [184], analogous to those observed in animal models of epilepsy [185, 186]. The formation of epileptiform activity after albumin exposure is delayed, suggesting that the mechanism of action is complex rather than a direct effect by albumin [184]. One possible mechanism which has been receiving scrutiny is the activation of astrocytes by serum albumin [109, 187], activating a TGF-β receptor-mediated signaling cascade [64, 182, 184].

TGF-β is a pleiotropic cytokine involved in various cellular processes, including cell growth, differentiation, morphogenesis, apoptosis, and immune responses through intercellular communication in many different cell types [188–190]. Signaling is mediated by binding of TGF-β to two serine threonine kinase receptors, which when activated cause the phosphorylation of the Smad protein complex and the p38 MAPK pathway [191]. A role for TGF-β has been implicated in many different CNS diseases, related to its upregulation in Alzheimer's disease, multiple sclerosis, ischemic brain injury, and TBI [192]. TGF-β is thought to have neuroprotective properties, and is associated with both microglial activation and the wound healing response [193]. Paradoxically, TGF-β also appears to contribute to excitotoxicity, adding to the dual role of inflammation which is dependent on the context and cell types involved [194]. Further research into the variation in response from this pathway is needed, as this may reveal insights into the dual role of inflammation and how to bias the brain towards neuroprotection rather than neurodegeneration.

The binding of albumin to TGF-β receptor has been characterized experimentally in rodent models of BBB disruption, resulting in the activation of TGF-β signaling [184]. The induction of experimental BBB dysfunction to induce epileptiform activity can be prevented through blockage of albumin binding to TGF-β receptors [184]. Much of the published literature has focused on albumin's interaction with the TGF-β signaling pathway in disease models, but there is some suggestion that TGF-β may also play a role in PTE from animal models with similar pathologies. In rodent models of epilepsy, TGF-β is reportedly upregulated in both neurons [195] and hippocampal astrocytes [196]. The action of TGF-β in astrocytes following exposure to albumin has also been shown to induce pro-ictogenic cytokine production, resulting in increased neuronal excitability in experimental models [197]. TGF-β has also been implicated experimentally in excitatory synaptogenesis in a post-injury epilepsy model [183]. As neuronal reorganization and synaptogenesis are hypothesized to be a potential mechanism underlying chronic seizures and are well-documented consequences of CNS trauma, this action of TGF-β may be critical for the progression of brain injury to epilepsy [183, 198, 199]. In summary, the actions of TGF-β in the injured and epileptic brain remain poorly understood, but the potentially paradoxical behavior of this cytokine warrants further investigation.

Age-specific vulnerability to PTE

Neuroinflammation is a key aspect of secondary injury that can vary according to the stage of brain development, which may underlie differences in clinical outcomes between patients who suffer a TBI during childhood and patients who suffer a TBI during adulthood [200]. Many studies now suggest that the early postnatal brain has an enhanced propensity for inflammation, described as a 'window of susceptibility' [200–202]. Early support for this hypothesis came from experimental evidence that 3-week old (juvenile) rats showed a higher susceptibility to IL-1β-induced BBB breakdown compared to adult rats [203, 204]. These observations are most likely not due to an immaturity of the BBB integrity at a younger age, as the tight junctions that maintain the BBB are fully developed from prenatal stages [205], but rather to a unique global chemokine expression profile that is distinctly different to the adult CNS [200]. In experimental autoimmune encephalomyelitis, a model of multiple sclerosis that shares some of the inflammatory processes of PTE, many chemokines involved in the recruitment of T cells and monocytes into the brain are robustly upregulated to 2–6-fold higher in juveniles compared to adults, including CCL2, CCL3, and CCL6 [200, 206–208]. There is also some evidence in the clinical context that the response of the immune system in the brain after a pathogenic challenge also differs between adults and children, with children presenting with higher production of IL-1 and IL-10 from peripheral blood monocytes after pathogenic stimulation [209]. Several cytokines have been detected at elevated levels in both CSF and serum of children after TBI, including IL-1α, IL-6, IL-12, and TNF-α, though how this response may correspond to the clinical differences at different ages after TBI are still relatively underinvestigated [210–212].

Microglia present differently within the immature brain compared to adults. During early postnatal development, their morphology is distinct, with fewer processes than those in the adult brain [213], and in an experimental pathogenic model, neonatal brain injury induced a markedly reduced activation compared to the robust activation seen in adult brain tissue [214]. Activated microglia typically adopt a phagocytic morphology and are associated with neuronal death, which is thought to be a critical aspect of normal brain development [201, 215]. There are also more circulating macrophages in the developing brain compared to adults under basal conditions associated with dying neurons and glia, particularly in the corpus callosum [213, 216]. Neutrophil infiltration into brain parenchyma after injury differs across ages, with a much higher level of infiltration detected experimentally in postnatal day 7 (p7) rats than in adults [214]. This neutrophil infiltration can persist 2–3 days after a pathogenic challenge and was found to be concurrent with damage to vasculature [203, 204, 214].

Increased seizure susceptibility in the immature brain may result from several contributing factors. Glutamate is the primary neurotransmitter in both the adult and developing brain [217], yet there is low expression of the glutamate type 1 transporter, therefore, clearance from the synaptic cleft is markedly slower compared that in the adult brain [218]. GABA receptor action is normally inhibitory in the adult brain, but is predominantly excitatory during early brain development due to high intracellular concentrations of chloride as a result of differential developmental expression of specific chloride ion transporters [219–221]. During early cortical development, experimental models have shown that GABA is predominantly depolarizing, progressing through childhood to the hyperpolarizing state found in the healthy adult brain [222, 223]. A recent study of experimental mesial temporal lobe epilepsy found a depolarizing role of GABA receptor, which was highly upregulated in surviving epileptic neurons [224], suggesting that the early neurodevelopmental environment may be more vulnerable to hyperexcitability after an insult. NMDA receptors are also more permeable to Ca^{2+} during development and desensitize more slowly [225]. In addition to a shorter post-ictal refractory period compared to the adult brain [226, 227], this inherently increased excitability of the pediatric brain may underlie an increased propensity for PTE after TBI during early childhood.

However, other studies have noted that the immature brain may conversely show resistance to seizure-related pathology; for example, chemical stimulation to experimentally induce sustained hyperexcitability is more difficult in the immature brain [39]. Infant brains may also be more resistant to excitotoxic-induced cell death than the adult brain [228]. Due to the apparent paradox of age-related differences, further study pertaining to the specific excitability of the developing environment is needed, particularly in the context of brain injury.

Inflammation in pediatric PTE

As a result of the abovementioned evidence of age-specific responses to both inflammatory stimuli and seizures, a potential link between neuroinflammation and seizure susceptibility particularly during early childhood is under intense scrutiny. Experimental studies have implicated a role for neuroinflammation in increased seizure susceptibility in the immature brain; for example, exposure to several chemoconvulsant challenges revealed a lower seizure threshold in immature rats compared to adults [102]. The authors attribute this response to increased TNF-α or IL-1β production by activated microglia in the hippocampus in immature rats, which was associated with cognitive deficits and widespread neuronal loss [102, 229]. Changes in seizure threshold caused by neuroinflammation in the pediatric brain are associated with long-term alterations in glutamate receptors in the hippocampus, and a resultant increase in neuronal network excitability [229, 230].

In addition to the younger brain having an increased propensity for an enhanced neuroinflammatory response, age-specific differences in important epileptogenic factors have been identified. One such difference is NMDA receptor density, which has been shown experimentally to peak at p28 at approximately 160% of adult levels [231]. NMDA receptors also have a different subunit composition in the developing brain compared to the adult brain, resulting in different functional properties [232, 233]. Due to these changes, NMDA receptors are able to depolarize more easily in the presence of glutamate, resulting in a longer duration of excitatory postsynaptic currents [218, 234].

Therapeutic targeting of post-traumatic inflammation to prevent PTE

TBI induces a neuroinflammatory cascade in the brain, leading to persistent and perpetuating neurodegeneration and likely contributing to an increased risk of initiating epileptogenesis, resulting in the development of PTE. In the context of the ongoing pursuit of novel therapeutic targets to prevent PTE, both clinical and experimental studies provide compelling evidence implicating IL-1β and HMGB1 as pivotal players in the cascade. Due to their early and varied role in the neuroinflammatory cascade after injury and emerging roles in the regulation of neuronal excitability, pharmacological targeting of these mechanisms may prove beneficial at reducing PTE. Further pre-clinical studies are needed to elucidate the exact mechanisms by which these and other inflammatory mediators initiate or perpetuate the process of epileptogenesis.

Several different animal models of PTE have been well studied over the past decade [235]. These experimental models have demonstrated that TBI results in both acute and chronic changes to the neuronal environment that likely contribute to epileptogenesis, such as hyperexcitable recurrent circuitry in the dentate gyrus of the hippocampus [235–237]. Whilst these models allow for the investigation of various mechanisms and testing of potential therapeutics, rodent models of PTE are not without limitations. Some models can produce a high level of epileptiform activity when measured with electroencephalogram, but most models are limited in the amount of spontaneous seizure activity they induce, leading to the need for higher animal numbers [11, 238]. One study that used a controlled cortical impact model of PTE, found that only 20–36% of animals given a severe TBI developed spontaneous behavioral seizures [239]. Though this presents logistical challenges, this incidence is only slightly higher than the estimated incidence in the clinical setting, which one study found to be 16.7% for severe TBI [240]. Animal models are also notoriously time-consuming as the latency to spontaneous seizure onset can be weeks to months after the initial injury [238, 241]. To increase the number of animals that can be investigated in relation to epileptogenesis and combat time restraints, some studies incorporate the administration of a pro-convulsant agent, such as pentylenetetrazol (PTZ), to unveil changes to seizure threshold as a surrogate marker of seizure susceptibility [235, 238, 241]. Many neuropathological processes that occur following TBI, including the neuroinflammatory response, can also differ greatly due to the developmental state of the brain at the time of impact [1]. This confound should be taken into account when investigating both the underlying mechanisms of epileptogenesis and piloting novel therapeutic interventions. Despite these limitations, these models show high clinical relevance and are useful tools with which to study PTE, and they are continually being improved upon.

Much investigation of neuroinflammatory intervention as a therapeutic option after TBI has focused on broad-target agents, such as minocycline, erythropoietin, and progesterone. All of these treatments were proposed to reduce neuroinflammation after TBI, generating promising results in pre-clinical research but failing to produce short-term improvement after TBI during clinical trials, as reviewed elsewhere [242]. However, these treatments, which are both pleiotropic in nature and relatively safe for long-term use, may have more success in relation to the chronic outcomes such as PTE as many of the effects of neuroinflammation persist long after the offending insult, yet few studies have considered the potential effects of anti-inflammatory treatments on long-term epileptogenesis after injury. Hypothermia is another broad-target treatment for neuroinflammation that has had some success in providing neuroprotection in the context of TBI and spinal cord injuries, with some evidence suggesting that it may also prevent epileptogenesis [243–245]. The potential to prevent or reduce PTE by targeting other inflammatory mediators in the post-injury neural environment, such as serum albumin and TGF-β, have not yet been explored. Additional potential targets include TNF-α, which has been shown to influence neurotransmission by altering excitatory post-synaptic currents and decreasing GABA-mediated inhibitory synaptic strength in hippocampal neurons [246]; the prostaglandin receptor EP2, which mediates COX-2 inflammatory signaling and appears to promote seizures by aggravating neuronal injury [247]; as well as factors involved in regeneration and regrowth such as fibroblast growth factor, tropomyosin receptor kinase B, and insulin-like growth factor-1. [248, 249]

Conclusion

This review of the published literature has found that several inflammatory mediators, including IL-1β and HMGB1, exhibit epileptogenic and ictogenic properties, acting on glia and neurons both directly and indirectly to influence neuronal excitability. As neuroinflammation is a central component of the neuropathology after TBI, comparable mechanisms are likely to be involved in the process of epileptogenesis leading to PTE. An increased understanding of how inflammation influences epileptogenesis may reveal novel therapeutic targets and strategies to prevent or reduce seizures after TBI. As PTE is often resistant to existing pharmaceutical treatments [33, 34, 36], there is an urgent need for further research to develop preventative treatments to improve both the quality and longevity of life for TBI survivors.

Abbreviations

ASDs: Anti-seizure drugs; AMPA: Alpha-amino-3-hydroxy-5-methyl-4-isoxazole-propoinate; BBB: Blood-brain barrier; CA3: Region III of hippocampus proper; CCL2: Chemokine (C-C Motif) ligand 2; CCL3: Chemokine (C-C Motif) ligand 3; CCL6: Chemokine (C-C Motif) ligand 6; CNS: Central nervous system; COX-2: Cyclooxygenase-2; CSF: Cerebrospinal fluid; CXCL8: Chemokine (C-X-C motif) ligand 8; DAMP: Damage associated molecular pattern; EC: Endothelial cells; EP2: Receptor for prostaglandin E2; FS: Febrile seizures; GABA: γ-aminobutyric acid; HMGB1: High mobility group box 1 protein; IL-1R: IL-1 receptor; IL-1R1: Cell surface type 1 IL-1 receptor; IL-1α: Interleukin-1α; IL-1β: Interleukin-1β; IL-6: Interleukin-6; IL-10: Interleukin-10; IL-12: Interleukin-12; IRF3: Interferon regulatory transcription factor 3; MAPK: Mitogen-activated protein kinase; MyD88: Myeloid differentiation primary response gene 88; NF-κB: Nuclear factor Kappa-light-chain-enhancer of activated B cells; NMDA: N-methyl-d-aspartate; p7: Postnatal day 7; p28: Postnatal day 28; PTE: Post-traumatic epilepsy; PTZ: Pentylenetetrazol; ROS: Reactive oxygen species; SNPs: Single nucleotide polymorphisms; TBI: Traumatic brain injury; TGF-β: Transforming growth factor-β; TLE: Temporal lobe epilepsy; TLR: Toll-like receptor; TNF-α: Tumor necrosis factor- α; TRAF6: TNF receptor associated factor 6

Acknowledgements

Figures were prepared by Elsevier Illustration Services.

Funding

BDS and SRS are supported by fellowships from the National Health and Medical Research Council of Australia. This manuscript was written with support from the Rebecca L Cooper Medical Research Foundation.

Authors' contributions

KMW and BDS conceptualized and designed the manuscript; KMW, MS, and BDS drafted the manuscript; PC, TJO'B, and SRS provided critical revisions and intellectual input. All authors read and approved the final manuscript.

Competing interests
The authors declare that they have no competing interests.

Consent for publication
Not Applicable.

Author details
[1]Department of Medicine (The Royal Melbourne Hospital), The University of Melbourne, Kenneth Myer Building, Melbourne Brain Centre, Royal Parade, Parkville, VIC 3050, Australia. [2]Department of Pharmacology and Therapeutics, The University of Melbourne, Parkville, VIC 3050, Australia.

References
1. Potts MB, Koh S-E, Whetstone WD, Walker BA, Yoneyama T, Claus CP, et al. Traumatic injury to the immature brain: inflammation, oxidative injury, and iron-mediated damage as potential therapeutic targets. NeuroRx. 2006;3(2): 143–53.
2. Thurman DJ. The epidemiology of traumatic brain injury in children and youths: a review of research since 1990. J Child Neurol. 2016;31(1):20–7.
3. Maas AIR, Stocchetti N, Bullock R. Moderate and severe traumatic brain injury in adults. Lancet Neurol. 2008;7(8):728–41.
4. Khoshyomn S, Tranmer BI. Diagnosis and management of pediatric closed head injury. Semin Pediatr Surg. 2004;13(2):80–6.
5. Schouten JW. Neuroprotection in traumatic brain injury: a complex struggle against the biology of nature. Curr Opin Crit Care. 2007;13(2):134–42.
6. Hinson HE, Rowell S, Schreiber M. Clinical evidence of inflammation driving secondary brain injury: a systematic review. J Trauma Acute Care Surg. 2015;78(1):184–91.
7. Dashnaw ML, Petraglia AL, Bailes JE. An overview of the basic science of concussion and subconcussion: where we are and where we are going. Neurosurg Focus. 2012;33(6):1–9.
8. Prins ML, Hovda DA. Developing experimental models to address traumatic brain injury in children. J Neurotrauma. 2003;20(2):123–37.
9. Blennow K, Hardy J, Zetterberg H. The neuropathology and neurobiology of traumatic brain injury. Neuron. 2012;76(5):886–99.
10. Appleton RE, Demellweek C. Post-traumatic epilepsy in children requiring inpatient rehabilitation following head injury. J Neurol Neurosurg Psychiatry. 2002;72(5):669–72.
11. Statler KD, Scheerlinck P, Pouliot W, Hamilton M, White HS, Dudek FE. A potential model of pediatric posttraumatic epilepsy. Epilepsy Res. 2009;86(2-3):221–3.
12. Frey LC. Epidemiology of posttraumatic epilepsy: a critical review. Epilepsia. 2003;44:11–7.
13. Fisher RS, Boas WV, Blume W, Elger C, Genton P, Lee P, et al. Epileptic seizures and epilepsy: definitions proposed by the International League against Epilepsy (ILAE) and the International Bureau for Epilepsy (IBE). Epilepsia. 2005;46(4):470–2.
14. Pitkanen A, Immonen R. Epilepsy related to traumatic brain injury. Neurotherapeutics. 2014;11(2):286–96.
15. DeLorenzo RJ, Sun DA, Deshpande LS. Cellular mechanisms underlying acquired epilepsy: the calcium hypothesis of the induction and maintenance of epilepsy (vol 105, pg 229, 2005). Pharmacol Ther. 2006;111(1):287–325.
16. Goldberg EM, Coulter DA. Mechanisms of epileptogenesis: a convergence on neural circuit dysfunction. Nat Rev Neurosci. 2013;14(5):337–49.
17. Temkin NR. Preventing and treating posttraumatic seizures: the human experience. Epilepsia. 2009;50:10–3.
18. Walker MC, White HS, Sander J. Disease modification in partial epilepsy. Brain. 2002;125:1937–50.
19. Chiaretti A, De Benedictis R, Polidori G, Piastra M, Iannelli A, Di Rocco C. Early post-traumatic seizures in children with head injury. Childs Nerv Syst. 2000;16(12):862–6.
20. Barlow KM, Spowart JJ, Minns RA. Early posttraumatic seizures in non-accidental head injury: relation to outcome. Dev Med Child Neurol. 2000;42(9):591–4.
21. Hahn YS, Fuchs S, Flannery AM, Barthel MJ, McLone DG. Factors influencing posttraumatic seizures in children. Neurosurgery. 1988;22(5):864 7.
22. Jennett B. Trauma as a cause of epilepsy in childhood. Dev Med Child Neurol. 1973;15(1):56–62.
23. Desai BT, Whitman S, Coonleyhoganson R, Coleman TE, Gabriel G, Dell J. Seizures and civilian head-injuries. Epilepsia. 1983;24(3):289–96.
24. Li H, McDonald W, Parada I, Faria L, Graber K, Takahashi DK, et al. Targets for preventing epilepsy following cortical injury. Neurosci Lett. 2011;497(3):172–6.
25. Santhakumar V, Ratzliff ADH, Jeng J, Toth Z, Soltesz I. Long-term hyperexcitability in the hippocampus after experimental head trauma. Ann Neurol. 2001;50(6):708–17.
26. Cantu D, Walker K, Andresen L, Taylor-Weiner A, Hampton D, Tesco G, et al. Traumatic brain injury increases cortical glutamate network activity by compromising GABAergic control. Cereb Cortex. 2015;25(8):2306–20.
27. Santhakumar V, Bender R, Frotscher M, Ross ST, Hollrigel GS, Toth Z, et al. Granule cell hyperexcitability in the early post-traumatic rat dentate gyrus: the 'irritable mossy cell' hypothesis. J Physiol London. 2000;524(1):117–34.
28. Santhakumar V, Aradi I, Soltesz I. Role of mossy fiber sprouting and mossy cell loss in hyperexcitability: a network model of the dentate gyrus incorporating cell types and axonal topography. J Neurophysiol. 2005;93(1):437–53.
29. Lowenstein DH, Thomas MJ, Smith DH, McIntosh TK. Selective vulnerability of dentate hilar neurons following traumatic brain injury - a potential mechanistic link between head trauma and disorders of the hippocampus. Neurology. 1992;42(7):1427.
30. Diaz-Arrastia R, Agostini MA, Frol AB, Mickey B, Fleckenstein J, Van Ness PC. Neurophysiologic and neuroradiologic features of intractable epilepsy after traumatic brain injury in adults. Arch Neurol. 2000;57(11):1611–6.
31. Hudak AM, Trivedi K, Harper CR, Booker K, Caesar RR, Agostini M, et al. Evaluation of seizure-like episodes in survivors of moderate and severe traumatic brain injury. J Head Trauma Rehab. 2004;19(4):290–5.
32. Yang L, Afroz S, Michelson HB, Goodman JH, Valsamis HA, Ling DSF. Spontaneous epileptiform activity in rat neocortex after controlled cortical impact Injury. J Neurotrauma. 2010;27(8):1541–8.
33. Semah F, Picot MC, Adam C, Broglin D, Arzimanoglou A, Bazin B, et al. Is the underlying cause of epilepsy a major prognostic factor for recurrence? Neurology. 1998;51(5):1256–62.
34. Larkin M, Meyer RM, Szuflita NS, Severson MA, Levine ZT. Post-traumatic, drug-resistant epilepsy and review of seizure control outcomes from blinded, randomized controlled trials of brain stimulation treatments for drug-resistant epilepsy. Cureus. 2016;8(8):e744.
35. Temkin NR. Antiepileptogenesis and seizure prevention trials with antiepileptic drugs: meta-analysis of controlled trials. Epilepsia. 2001;42(4):515–24.
36. Beghi E. Overview of studies to prevent posttraumatic epilepsy. Epilepsia. 2003;44:21–6.
37. Torbic H, Forni AA, Anger KE, Degrado JR, Greenwood BC. Use of antiepileptics for seizure prophylaxis after traumatic brain injury. Am J Health Syst Pharm. 2013;70(9):759–66.
38. Kirmani BF, Robinson DM, Fonkem E, Graf K, Huang JH. Role of anticonvulsants in the management of posttraumatic epilepsy. Front Neurol. 2016;7:32.
39. Kubova H, Mares P, Suchomelova L, Brozek G, Druga R, Pitkanen A. Status epilepticus in immature rats leads to behavioural and cognitive impairment and epileptogenesis. Eur J Neurosci. 2004;19(12):3255–65.
40. Statler KD. Pediatric posttraumatic seizures: epidemiology, putative mechanisms of epileptogenesis and promising investigational progress. Dev Neurosci. 2006;28(4-5):354–63.
41. Hickey WF. Basic principles of immunological surveillance of the normal central nervous system. Glia. 2001;36(2):118–24.
42. Auffray C, Sieweke MH, Geissmann F. Blood monocytes: development, heterogeneity, and relationship with dendritic cells. Annu Rev Immunol. 2009;27:669–92.
43. Cederberg D, Siesjo P. What has inflammation to do with traumatic brain injury? Childs Nerv Syst. 2010;26(2):221–6.
44. DeKosky ST, Blennow K, Ikonomovic MD, Gandy S. Acute and chronic traumatic encephalopathies: pathogenesis and biomarkers. Nat Rev Neurol. 2013;9(4):192–200.
45. Riazi K, Galic MA, Pittman QJ. Contributions of peripheral inflammation to seizure susceptibility: cytokines and brain excitability. Epilepsy Res. 2010;89(1):34–42.
46. Utagawa A, Truettner JS, Dietrich WD, Bramlett HM. Systemic inflammation exacerbates behavioral and histopathological consequences of isolated traumatic brain injury in rats. Exp Neurol. 2008;211(1):283–91.

47. Vezzani A, Granata T. Brain inflammation in epilepsy: experimental and clinical evidence. Epilepsia. 2005;46(11):1724–43.
48. Morganti-Kossmann MC, Rancan M, Stahel PF, Kossmann T. Inflammatory response in acute traumatic brain injury: a double-edged sword. Curr Opin Crit Care. 2002;8(2):101–5.
49. Hudome S, Palmer C, Roberts RL, Mauger D, Housman C, Towfighi J. The role of neutrophils in the production of hypoxic-ischemic brain injury in the neonatal rat. Pediatr Res. 1997;41(5):607–16.
50. Owen CA, Campbell EJ. The cell biology of leukocyte-mediated proteolysis. J Leukoc Biol. 1999;65(2):137–50.
51. Chodobski A, Zink BJ, Szmydynger-Chodobska J. Blood-brain barrier pathophysiology in traumatic brain injury. Transl Stroke Res. 2011;2(4):492–516.
52. Dempsey RJ, Baskaya MK, Dogan A. Attenuation of brain edema, blood-brain barrier breakdown, and injury volume by ifenprodil, a polyamine-site N-methyl-D-aspartate receptor antagonist, after experimental traumatic brain injury in rats. Neurosurgery. 2000;47(2):399–404.
53. Ransohoff RM, Tani M. Do chemokines mediate leukocyte recruitment in post-traumatic CNS inflammation? Trends Neurosci. 1998;21(4):154–9.
54. Semple BD, Bye N, Rancan M, Ziebell JM, Morganti-Kossmann MC. Role of CCL2 (MCP-1) in traumatic brain injury (TBI): evidence from severe TBI patients and CCL2-/- mice. J Cereb Blood Flow Metab. 2010;30(4):769–82.
55. Nonaka M, Chen XH, Pierce JES, Leoni MJ, McIntosh TK, Wolf JA, et al. Prolonged activation of NF-kappa B following traumatic brain injury in rats. J Neurotrauma. 1999;16(11):1023–34.
56. Scherbel U, Raghupathi R, Nakamura M, Saatman KE, Trojanowski JQ, Neugebauer E, et al. Differential acute and chronic responses of tumor necrosis factor-deficient mice to experimental brain injury. Proc Natl Acad Sci U S A. 1999;96(15):8721–6.
57. Sherwood ER, Prough DS. Interleukin-8, neuroinflammation, and secondary brain injury. Crit Care Med. 2000;28(4):1221–3.
58. Kreutzberg GW. Microglia: a sensor for pathological events in the CNS. Trends Neurosci. 1996;19(8):312–8.
59. Braughler JM, Hall ED. Central nervous system trauma and stroke. I. Biochemical considerations for oxygen radical formation and lipid peroxidation. Free Radic Biol Med. 1989;6(3):289–301.
60. Hall ED, Braughler JM. Central nervous system trauma and stroke. II. Physiological and pharmacological evidence for involvement of oxygen radicals and lipid peroxidation. Free Radic Biol Med. 1989;6(3):303–13.
61. Smith SL, Andrus PK, Zhang JR, Hall ED. Direct measurement of hydroxyl radicals, lipid peroxidation, and blood-brain barrier disruption following unilateral cortical impact head injury in the rat. J Neurotrauma. 1994;11(4):393–404.
62. Campbell IL, Abraham CR, Masliah E, Kemper P, Inglis JD, Oldstone MB, et al. Neurologic disease induced in transgenic mice by cerebral overexpression of interleukin 6. Proc Natl Acad Sci U S A. 1993;90(21):10061–5.
63. Ravizza T, Balosso S, Vezzani A. Inflammation and prevention of epileptogenesis. Neurosci Lett. 2011;497(3):223–30.
64. David Y, Cacheaux LP, Ivens S, Lapilover E, Heinemann U, Kaufer D, et al. Astrocytic dysfunction in epileptogenesis: consequence of altered potassium and glutamate homeostasis? J Neurosci. 2009;29(34):10588–99.
65. Tchelingerian JL, Monge M, Lesaux F, Zalc B, Jacque C. Differential oligodendroglial expression of the tumor-necrosis-factor receptors in-vivo and in-vitro. J Neurochem. 1995;65(5):2377–80.
66. Shohami E, Ginis I, Hallenbeck JM. Dual role of tumor necrosis factor alpha in brain injury. Cytokine Growth Factor Rev. 1999;10(2):119–30.
67. Matsumoto H, Marsan CA. Cortical cellular phenomena in experimental epilepsy: ictal manifestations. Exp Neurol. 1964;9:305–26.
68. Cobb SR, Buhl EH, Halasy K, Paulsen O, Somogyi P. Synchronization of neuronal activity in hippocampus by individual GABAergic interneurons. Nature. 1995;378(6552):75–8.
69. Avoli M, de Curtis M, Gnatkovsky V, Gotman J, Kohling R, Levesque M, et al. Specific imbalance of excitatory/inhibitory signaling establishes seizure onset pattern in temporal lobe epilepsy. J Neurophysiol. 2016;115(6):3229–37.
70. de Curtis M, Avoli M. GABAergic networks jump-start focal seizures. Epilepsia. 2016;57(5):679–87.
71. Lason W, Chlebicka M, Rejdak K. Research advances in basic mechanisms of seizures and antiepileptic drug action. Pharmacol Rep. 2013;65(4):787–801.
72. Sayyah M, Javad-Pour M, Ghazi-Khansari M. The bacterial endotoxin lipopolysaccharide enhances seizure susceptibility in mice: involvement of proinflammatory factors: nitric oxide and prostaglandins. Neuroscience. 2003;122(4):1073–80.
73. Dhote F, Peinnequin A, Carpentier P, Baille V, Delacour C, Foquin A, et al. Prolonged inflammatory gene response following soman-induced seizures in mice. Toxicology. 2007;238(2-3):166–76.
74. Levesque M, Avoli M, Bernard C. Animal models of temporal lobe epilepsy following systemic chemoconvulsant administration. J Neurosci Methods. 2016;260:45–52.
75. Gorter JA, van Vliet EA, da Silva FH L. Which insights have we gained from the kindling and post-status epilepticus models? J Neurosci Methods. 2016;260:96–108.
76. De Simoni MG, Perego C, Ravizza T, Moneta D, Conti M, Marchesi F, et al. Inflammatory cytokines and related genes are induced in the rat hippocampus by limbic status epilepticus. Eur J Neurosci. 2000;12(7):2623–33.
77. Turrin NP, Rivest S. Innate immune reaction in response to seizures: implications for the neuropathology associated with epilepsy. Neurobiol Dis. 2004;16(2):321–34.
78. Gorter JA, van Vliet EA, Aronica E, Breit T, Rauwerda H, da Silva FHL, et al. Potential new antiepileptogenic targets indicated by microarray analysis in a rat model for temporal lobe epilepsy. J Neurosci. 2006;26(43):11083–110.
79. Oprica M, Eriksson C, Schultzberg M. Inflammatory mechanisms associated with brain damage induced by kainic acid with special reference to the interleukin-1 system. J Cell Mol Med. 2003;7(2):127–40.
80. Vezzani A, Conti N, De Luigi A, Ravizza T, Moneta D, Marchesi F, et al. Interleukin-l beta immunoreactivity and microglia are enhanced in the rat hippocampus by focal kainate application: functional evidence for enhancement of electrographic seizures. J Neurosci. 1999;19(12):5054–65.
81. Peltola J, Laaksonen J, Haapala AM, Hurme M, Rainesalo S, Keranen T. Indicators of inflammation after recent tonic-clonic epileptic seizures correlate with plasma interleukin-6 levels. Seizure Eur J Epilepsy. 2002;11(1):44–6.
82. Peltola J, Palmio J, Korhonen L, Suhonen J, Miettinen A, Hurme M, et al. Interleukin-6 and Interleukin-1 receptor antagonist in cerebrospinal fluid from patients with recent tonic-clonic seizures. Epilepsy Res. 2000;41(3):205–11.
83. Crespel A, Coubes P, Rousset M-C, Brana C, Rougier A, Rondouin G, et al. Inflammatory reactions in human medial temporal lobe epilepsy with hippocampal sclerosis. Brain Res. 2002;952(2):159–69.
84. Kharatishvili I, Pitkanen A. Association of the severity of cortical damage with the occurrence of spontaneous seizures and hyperexcitability in an animal model of posttraumatic epilepsy. Epilepsy Res. 2010;90(1-2):47–59.
85. Kirkman NJ, Libbey JE, Wilcox KS, White HS, Fujinami RS. Innate but not adaptive immune responses contribute to behavioral seizures following viral infection. Epilepsia. 2010;51(3):454–64.
86. Vezzani A, Balosso S, Ravizza T. The role of cytokines in the pathophysiology of epilepsy. Brain Behav Immun. 2008;22(6):797–803.
87. Lloyd E, Somera-Molina K, Van Eldik LJ, Watterson DM, Wainwright MS. Suppression of acute proinflammatory cytokine and chemokine upregulation by post-injury administration of a novel small molecule improves long-term neurologic outcome in a mouse model of traumatic brain injury. J Neuroinflammation. 2008;5:28.
88. Somera-Molina KC, Robin B, Somera CA, Anderson C, Stine C, Koh S, et al. Glial activation links early-life seizures and long-term neurologic dysfunction: evidence using a small molecule inhibitor of proinflammatory cytokine upregulation. Epilepsia. 2007;48(9):1785–800.
89. Viviani B, Gardoni F, Marinovich M. Cytokines and neuronal ion channels in health and disease. Int Rev Neurobiol. 2007;82:247–63.
90. Cunningham AJ, Murray CA, O'Neill LA, Lynch MA, O'Connor JJ. Interleukin-1 beta (IL-1 beta) and tumour necrosis factor (TNF) inhibit long-term potentiation in the rat dentate gyrus in vitro. Neurosci Lett. 1996;203(1):17–20.
91. Probert L, Akassoglou K, Pasparakis M, Kontogeorgos G, Kollias G. Spontaneous inflammatory demyelinating disease in transgenic mice showing central nervous system-specific expression of tumor necrosis factor alpha. Proc Natl Acad Sci U S A. 1995;92(24):11294–8.
92. Samland H, Huitron-Resendiz S, Masliah E, Criado J, Henriksen SJ, Campbell IL. Profound increase in sensitivity to glutamatergic- but not cholinergic agonist-induced seizures in transgenic mice with astrocyte production of IL-6. J Neurosci Res. 2003;73(2):176–87.
93. Bradford HF. Glutamate, GABA and epilepsy. Prog Neurobiol. 1995;47(6):477–511.
94. Hu S, Sheng WS, Ehrlich LC, Peterson PK, Chao CC. Cytokine effects on glutamate uptake by human astrocytes. Neuroimmunomodulation. 2000;7(3):153–9.

95. Balosso S, Ravizza T, Pierucci M, Calcagno E, Invernizzi R, Di Giovanni G, et al. Molecular and functional interactions between tumor necrosis factor-alpha receptors and the glutamatergic system in the mouse hippocampus: implications for seizure susceptibility. Neuroscience. 2009;161(1):293–300.
96. Pickering M, Cumiskey D, O'Connor JJ. Actions of TNF-alpha on glutamatergic synaptic transmission in the central nervous system. Exp Physiol. 2005;90(5):663–70.
97. Godukhin OV, Levin SG, Parnyshkova EY. The effects of interleukin-10 on the development of epileptiform activity in the hippocampus induced by transient hypoxia, bicuculline, and electrical kindling. Neurosci Behav Physiol. 2009;39(7):625–31.
98. Shandra AA, Godlevsky LS, Vastyanov RS, Oleinik AA, Konovalenko VL, Rapoport EN, et al. The role of TNF-alpha in amygdala kindled rats. Neurosci Res. 2002;42(2):147–53.
99. Bilbo SD, Rudy JW, Watkins LR, Maier SF. A behavioural characterization of neonatal infection-facilitated memory impairment in adult rats. Behav Brain Res. 2006;169(1):39–47.
100. Boisse L, Mouihate A, Ellis S, Pittman QJ. Long-term alterations in neuroimmune responses after neonatal exposure to lipopolysaccharide. J Neurosci. 2004;24(21):4928–34.
101. Ellis S, Mouihate A, Pittman QJ. Neonatal programming of the rat neuroimmune response: stimulus specific changes elicited by bacterial and viral mimetics. J Physiol. 2006;571(Pt 3):695–701.
102. Galic MA, Riazi K, Henderson AK, Tsutsui S, Pittman QJ. Viral-like brain inflammation during development causes increased seizure susceptibility in adult rats. Neurobiol Dis. 2009;36(2):343–51.
103. Hesdorffer DC, Shinnar S, Lax DN, Pellock JM, Nordli Jr DR, Seinfeld S, et al. Risk factors for subsequent febrile seizures in the FEBSTAT study. Epilepsia. 2016;57(7):1042–7.
104. Baulac S, Gourfinkel-An I, Nabbout R, Huberfeld G, Serratosa J, Leguern E, et al. Fever, genes, and epilepsy. Lancet Neurol. 2004;3(7):421–30.
105. Virta M, Hurme M, Helminen M. Increased frequency of interleukin-1beta (-511) allele 2 in febrile seizures. Pediatr Neurol. 2002;26(3):192–5.
106. Hulkkonen J, Laippala P, Hurme M. A rare allele combination of the interleukin-1 gene complex is associated with high interleukin-1 beta plasma levels in healthy individuals. Eur Cytokine Netw. 2000;11(2):251–5.
107. Kanemoto K, Kawasaki J, Miyamoto T, Obayashi H, Nishimura M. Interleukin (IL)1beta, IL-1alpha, and IL-1 receptor antagonist gene polymorphisms in patients with temporal lobe epilepsy. Ann Neurol. 2000;47(5):571–4.
108. Binder DK, Steinhauser C. Functional changes in astroglial cells in epilepsy. Glia. 2006;54(5):358–68.
109. Heinemann U, Kaufer D, Friedman A. Blood-brain barrier dysfunction, TGFbeta signaling, and astrocyte dysfunction in epilepsy. Glia. 2012;60(8):1251–7.
110. Garlanda C, Dinarello CA, Mantovani A. The interleukin-1 family: back to the future. Immunity. 2013;39(6):1003–18.
111. Kim Y-J, Hwang S-Y, Oh E-S, Oh S, Han I-O. IL-1beta, an immediate early protein secreted by activated microglia, induces iNOS/NO in C6 astrocytoma cells through p38 MAPK and NF-kappaB pathways. J Neurosci Res. 2006;84(5):1037–46.
112. Lau LT, Yu AC. Astrocytes produce and release interleukin-1, interleukin-6, tumor necrosis factor alpha and interferon-gamma following traumatic and metabolic injury. J Neurotrauma. 2001;18(3):351–9.
113. Miossec P, Cavender D, Ziff M. Production of interleukin 1 by human endothelial cells. J Immunol. 1986;136(7):2486–91.
114. John GR, Lee SC, Song X, Rivieccio M, Brosnan CF. IL-1-regulated responses in astrocytes: relevance to injury and recovery. Glia. 2005;49(2):161–76.
115. Konsman JP, Vigues S, Mackerlova L, Bristow A, Blomqvist A. Rat brain vascular distribution of interleukin-1 type-1 receptor immunoreactivity: relationship to patterns of inducible cyclooxygenase expression by peripheral inflammatory stimuli. J Comp Neurol. 2004;472(1):113–29.
116. Pinteaux E, Parker LC, Rothwell NJ, Luheshi GN. Expression of interleukin-1 receptors and their role in interleukin-1 actions in murine microglial cells. J Neurochem. 2002;83(4):754–63.
117. Sato A, Ohtaki H, Tsumuraya T, Song D, Ohara K, Asano M, et al. Interleukin-1 participates in the classical and alternative activation of microglia/macrophages after spinal cord injury. J Neuroinflammation. 2012;9:65.
118. Srinivasan D, Yen J-H, Joseph DJ, Friedman W. Cell type-specific interleukin-1beta signaling in the CNS. J Neurosci. 2004;24(29):6482–8.
119. Vela JM, Molina-Holgado E, Arevalo-Martin A, Almazan G, Guaza C. Interleukin-1 regulates proliferation and differentiation of oligodendrocyte progenitor cells. Mol Cell Neurosci. 2002;20(3):489–502.
120. Moynagh PN. The interleukin-1 signalling pathway in astrocytes: a key contributor to inflammation in the brain. J Anat. 2005;207(3):265–9.
121. Fan L, Young PR, Barone FC, Feuerstein GZ, Smith DH, McIntosh TK. Experimental brain injury induces expression of interleukin-1 beta mRNA in the rat brain. Brain Res Mol Brain Res. 1995;30(1):125–30.
122. Kinoshita K, Chatzipanteli IK, Vitarbo E, Truettner JS, Alonso OF, Dietrich WD. Interleukin-1beta messenger ribonucleic acid and protein levels after fluid-percussion brain injury in rats: importance of injury severity and brain temperature. Neurosurgery. 2002;51(1):195–203. discussion.
123. Ciallella JR, Ikonomovic MD, Paljug WR, Wilbur YI, Dixon CE, Kochanek PM, et al. Changes in expression of amyloid precursor protein and interleukin-1beta after experimental traumatic brain injury in rats. J Neurotrauma. 2002;19(12):1555–67.
124. Kamm K, Vanderkolk W, Lawrence C, Jonker M, Davis AT. The effect of traumatic brain injury upon the concentration and expression of interleukin-1beta and interleukin-10 in the rat. J Trauma. 2006;60(1):152–7.
125. Acosta SA, Tajiri N, Shinozuka K, Ishikawa H, Grimmig B, Diamond DM, et al. Long-term upregulation of inflammation and suppression of cell proliferation in the brain of adult rats exposed to traumatic brain injury using the controlled cortical impact model. PLoS One. 2013;8(1):e53376.
126. Frugier T, Morganti-Kossmann MC, O'Reilly D, McLean CA. In situ detection of inflammatory mediators in post mortem human brain tissue after traumatic injury. J Neurotrauma. 2010;27(3):497–507.
127. Holmin S, Soderlund J, Biberfeld P, Mathiesen T. Intracerebral inflammation after human brain contusion. Neurosurgery. 1998;42(2):291–8.
128. Winter CD, Iannotti F, Pringle AK, Trikkas C, Clough GF, Church MK. A microdialysis method for the recovery of IL-1 beta, IL-6 and nerve growth factor from human brain in vivo. J Neurosci Methods. 2002;119(1):45–50.
129. Shiozaki T, Hayakata T, Tasaki O, Hosotubo H, Fuijita K, Mouri T, et al. Cerebrospinal fluid concentrations of anti-inflammatory mediators in early-phase severe traumatic brain injury. Shock. 2005;23(5):406–10.
130. Hunt RF, Boychuk JA, Smith BN. Neural circuit mechanisms of post-traumatic epilepsy. Front Cell Neurosci. 2013;7:89. doi:10.3389/fncel.2013.00089.
131. Clausen F, Hanell A, Bjork M, Hillered L, Mir AK, Gram H, et al. Neutralization of interleukin-1beta modifies the inflammatory response and improves histological and cognitive outcome following traumatic brain injury in mice. Eur J Neurosci. 2009;30(3):385–96.
132. Clausen F, Hanell A, Israelsson C, Hedin J, Ebendal T, Mir AK, et al. Neutralization of interleukin-1beta reduces cerebral edema and tissue loss and improves late cognitive outcome following traumatic brain injury in mice. Eur J Neurosci. 2011;34(1):110–23.
133. Lazovic J, Basu A, Lin H-W, Rothstein RP, Krady JK, Smith MB, et al. Neuroinflammation and both cytotoxic and vasogenic edema are reduced in interleukin-1 type 1 receptor-deficient mice conferring neuroprotection. Stroke. 2005;36(10):2226–31.
134. Sanderson KL, Raghupathi R, Saatman KE, Martin D, Miller G, McIntosh TK. Interleukin-1 receptor antagonist attenuates regional neuronal cell death and cognitive dysfunction after experimental brain injury. J Cereb Blood Flow Metab. 1999;19(10):1118–25.
135. Helmy A, Guilfoyle MR, Carpenter KLH, Pickard JD, Menon DK, Hutchinson PJ. Recombinant human interleukin-1 receptor antagonist in severe traumatic brain injury: a phase II randomized control trial. J Cereb Blood Flow Metab. 2014;34(5):845–51.
136. Diamond ML, Ritter AC, Failla MD, Boles JA, Conley YP, Kochanek PM, et al. IL-1beta associations with posttraumatic epilepsy development: a genetics and biomarker cohort study. Epilepsia. 2015;56(7):991–1001.
137. Dube CM, Ravizza T, Hamamura M, Zha Q, Keebaugh A, Fok K, et al. Epileptogenesis provoked by prolonged experimental febrile seizures: mechanisms and biomarkers. J Neurosci. 2010;30(22):7484–94.
138. Dube C, Vezzani A, Behrens M, Bartfai T, Baram TZ. Interleukin-1beta contributes to the generation of experimental febrile seizures. Ann Neurol. 2005;57(1):152–5.
139. Zhu G, Okada M, Yoshida S, Mori F, Ueno S, Wakabayashi K, et al. Effects of interleukin-1beta on hippocampal glutamate and GABA releases associated with Ca2+-induced Ca2+ releasing systems. Epilepsy Res. 2006;71(2-3):107–16.
140. Wetherington J, Serrano G, Dingledine R. Astrocytes in the epileptic brain. Neuron. 2008;58(2):168–78.
141. Ferrari CC, Depino AM, Prada F, Muraro N, Campbell S, Podhajcer O, et al. Reversible demyelination, blood-brain barrier breakdown, and pronounced neutrophil recruitment induced by chronic IL-1 expression in the brain. Am J Pathol. 2004;165(5):1827–37.

142. Proescholdt MG, Chakravarty S, Foster JA, Foti SB, Briley EM, Herkenham M. Intracerebroventricular but not intravenous interleukin-1beta induces widespread vascular-mediated leukocyte infiltration and immune signal mRNA expression followed by brain-wide glial activation. Neuroscience. 2002;112(3):731–49.
143. Quagliarello VJ, Wispelwey B, Long Jr WJ, Scheld WM. Recombinant human interleukin-1 induces meningitis and blood-brain barrier injury in the rat. Characterization and comparison with tumor necrosis factor. J Clin Invest. 1991;87(4):1360–6.
144. Shaftel SS, Carlson TJ, Olschowka JA, Kyrkanides S, Matousek SB, O'Banion MK. Chronic interleukin-1beta expression in mouse brain leads to leukocyte infiltration and neutrophil-independent blood brain barrier permeability without overt neurodegeneration. J Neurosci. 2007;27(35):9301–9.
145. Harting MT, Jimenez F, Adams SD, Mercer DW, Cox Jr CS. Acute, regional inflammatory response after traumatic brain injury: implications for cellular therapy. Surgery. 2008;144(5):803–13.
146. Lu K-T, Wang Y-W, Yang J-T, Yang Y-L, Chen H-I. Effect of interleukin-1 on traumatic brain injury-induced damage to hippocampal neurons. J Neurotrauma. 2005;22(8):885–95.
147. Pacifici R, Paris L, Di Carlo S, Bacosi A, Pichini S, Zuccaro P. Cytokine production in blood mononuclear cells from epileptic patients. Epilepsia. 1995;36(4):384–7.
148. Tanriverdi T, Uzan M, Sanus GZ, Baykara O, Is M, Ozkara C, et al. Lack of association between the IL1A gene (-889) polymorphism and outcome after head injury. Surg Neurol. 2006;65(1):7–10. discussion.
149. Haspolat S, Baysal Y, Duman O, Coskun M, Tosun O, Yegin O. Interleukin-1alpha, interleukin-1beta, and interleukin-1Ra polymorphisms in febrile seizures. J Child Neurol. 2005;20(7):565–8.
150. Bianchi ME, Manfredi AA. High-mobility group box 1 (HMGB1) protein at the crossroads between innate and adaptive immunity. Immunol Rev. 2007;220:35–46.
151. Stros M. HMGB proteins: interactions with DNA and chromatin. Biochim Biophys Acta. 2010;1799(1-2):101–13.
152. Yanai H, Ban T, Taniguchi T. Essential role of high-mobility group box proteins in nucleic acid-mediated innate immune responses. J Intern Med. 2011;270(4):301–8.
153. Goodwin GH, Sanders C, Johns EW. A new group of chromatin-associated proteins with a high content of acidic and basic amino acids. Eur J Biochem. 1973;38(1):14–9.
154. Gerlitz G, Hock R, Ueda T, Bustin M. The dynamics of HMG protein-chromatin interactions in living cells. Biochem Cell Biol. 2009;87(1):127–37.
155. Venters BJ, Pugh BF. How eukaryotic genes are transcribed. Crit Rev Biochem Mol Biol. 2009;44(2-3):117–41.
156. Calogero S, Grassi F, Aguzzi A, Voigtlander T, Ferrier P, Ferrari S, et al. The lack of chromosomal protein Hmg1 does not disrupt cell growth but causes lethal hypoglycaemia in newborn mice. Nat Genet. 1999;22(3):276–80.
157. Yang H, Antoine DJ, Andersson U, Tracey KJ. The many faces of HMGB1: molecular structure-functional activity in inflammation, apoptosis, and chemotaxis. J Leukoc Biol. 2013;93(6):865–73.
158. Scaffidi P, Misteli T, Bianchi ME. Release of chromatin protein HMGB1 by necrotic cells triggers inflammation. Nature. 2002;418(6894):191–5.
159. Bonaldi T, Talamo F, Scaffidi P, Ferrera D, Porto A, Bachi A, et al. Monocytic cells hyperacetylate chromatin protein HMGB1 to redirect it towards secretion. EMBO J. 2003;22(20):5551–60.
160. Lu B, Nakamura T, Inouye K, Li J, Tang Y, Lundback P, et al. Novel role of PKR in inflammasome activation and HMGB1 release. Nature. 2012;488(7413):670–4.
161. Wang H, Bloom O, Zhang M, Vishnubhakat JM, Ombrellino M, Che J, et al. HMG-1 as a late mediator of endotoxin lethality in mice. Science (New York, NY). 1999;285(5425):248–51.
162. Harris HE, Andersson U, Pisetsky DS. HMGB1: a multifunctional alarmin driving autoimmune and inflammatory disease. Nat Rev Rheumatol. 2012; 8(4):195–202.
163. Aronica E, Crino PB. Inflammation in epilepsy: clinical observations. Epilepsia. 2011;52 Suppl 3:26–32.
164. Chiavegato A, Zurolo E, Losi G, Aronica E, Carmignoto G. The inflammatory molecules IL-1 beta and HMGB1 can rapidly enhance focal seizure generation in a brain slice model of temporal lobe epilepsy. Front Cell Neurosci. 2014;8;155.
165. Maroso M, Balosso S, Ravizza T, Liu J, Aronica E, Iyer AM, et al. Toll-like receptor 4 and high-mobility group box-1 are involved in ictogenesis and can be targeted to reduce seizures. Nat Med. 2010;16(4):413–U91.
166. Iori V, Maroso M, Rizzi M, Iyer AM, Vertemara R, Carli M, et al. Receptor for advanced glycation endproducts is upregulated in temporal lobe epilepsy and contributes to experimental seizures. Neurobiol Dis. 2013;58:102–14.
167. Balosso S, Liu J, Bianchi ME, Vezzani A. Disulfide-containing high mobility group box-1 promotes n-methyl-d-aspartate receptor function and excitotoxicity by activating toll-like receptor 4-dependent signaling in hippocampal neurons. Antioxid Redox Signal. 2014;21(12):1726–40.
168. Tang D, Kang R, Zeh 3rd HJ, Lotze MT. High-mobility group box 1, oxidative stress, and disease. Antioxid Redox Signal. 2011;14(7):1315–35.
169. Waldbaum S, Patel M. Mitochondria, oxidative stress, and temporal lobe epilepsy. Epilepsy Res. 2010;88(1):23–45.
170. Chen G, Shi J, Jin W, Wang L, Xie W, Sun J, et al. Progesterone administration modulates TLRs/NF-kappa B signaling pathway in rat brain after cortical contusion. Ann Clin Lab Sci. 2008;38(1):65–74.
171. Okun E, Griffioen KJ, Lathia JD, Tang S-C, Mattson MP, Arumugam TV. Toll-like receptors in neurodegeneration. Brain Res Rev. 2009;59(2):278–92.
172. Chang ZL. Important aspects of toll-like receptors, ligands and their signaling pathways. Inflamm Res. 2010;59(10):791–808.
173. Lu Y-C, Yeh W-C, Ohashi PS. LPS/TLR4 signal transduction pathway. Cytokine. 2008;42(2):145–51.
174. Sha YG, Zmijewski J, Xu ZW, Abraham E. HMGB1 develops enhanced binding to cytokines. J Immunol. 2008;180(4):2531–7.
175. Garcia-Arnandis I, Guillen MI, Gomar F, Pelletier JP, Martel-Pelletier J, Alcaraz MJ. High mobility group box 1 potentiates the pro-inflammatory effects of interleukin-1 beta in osteoarthritic synoviocytes. Arthr Res Ther. 2010;12(4):R165.
176. Annegers JF, Grabow JD, Groover RV, Laws Jr ER, Elveback LR, Kurland LT. Seizures after head trauma: a population study. Neurology. 1980;30(7 Pt 1):683–9.
177. Shlosberg D, Benifla M, Kaufer D, Friedman A. Blood-brain barrier breakdown as a therapeutic target in traumatic brain injury. Nat Rev Neurol. 2010;6(7):393–403.
178. Kelley BJ, Lifshitz J, Povlishock JT. Neuroinflammatory responses after experimental diffuse traumatic brain injury. J Neuropathol Exp Neurol. 2007;66(11):989–1001.
179. Friedman A, Kaufer D, Heinemann U. Blood-brain barrier breakdown-inducing astrocytic transformation: novel targets for the prevention of epilepsy. Epilepsy Res. 2009;85(2-3):142–9.
180. Tomkins O, Feintuch A, Benifla M, Cohen A, Friedman A, Shelef I. Blood-brain barrier breakdown following traumatic brain injury: a possible role in posttraumatic epilepsy. Cardiovasc Psychiatr Neurol. 2011;2011:765923.
181. Tomkins O, Shelef I, Kaizerman I, Eliushin A, Afawi Z, Misk A, et al. Blood-brain barrier disruption in post-traumatic epilepsy. J Neurol Neurosurg Psychiatry. 2008;79(7):774–7.
182. Cacheaux LP, Ivens S, David Y, Lakhter AJ, Bar-Klein G, Shapira M, et al. Transcriptome profiling reveals TGF-beta signaling involvement in epileptogenesis. J Neurosci. 2009;29(28):8927–35.
183. Weissberg I, Wood L, Kamintsky L, Vazquez O, Milikovsky DZ, Alexander A, et al. Albumin induces excitatory synaptogenesis through astrocytic TGF-beta/ ALK5 signaling in a model of acquired epilepsy following blood-brain barrier dysfunction. Neurobiol Dis. 2015;78:115–25.
184. Ivens S, Kaufer D, Flores LP, Bechmann I, Zumsteg D, Tomkins O, et al. TGF-beta receptor-mediated albumin uptake into astrocytes is involved in neocortical epileptogenesis. Brain. 2007;130(Pt 2):535–47.
185. Barkai E, Grossman Y, Gutnick MJ. Long-term changes in neocortical activity after chemical kindling with systemic pentylenetetrazole: an in vitro study. J Neurophysiol. 1994;72(1):72–83.
186. Sanabria ERG, Silva AV, Spreafico R, Cavalheiro EA. Damage, reorganization, and abnormal neocortical hyperexcitability in the pilocarpine model of temporal lobe epilepsy. Epilepsia. 2002;43 Suppl 5:96–106.
187. Tigyi G, Hong L, Yakubu M, Parfenova H, Shibata M, Leffler CW. Lysophosphatidic acid alters cerebrovascular reactivity in piglets. Am J Phys. 1995;268(5 Pt 2):H2048–55.
188. Blobe GC, Schiemann WP, Lodish HF. Role of transforming growth factor beta in human disease. N Engl J Med. 2000;342(18):1350–8.
189. Gold LI, Parekh TV. Loss of growth regulation by transforming growth factor-beta (TGF-beta) in human cancers: studies on endometrial carcinoma. Semin Reprod Endocrinol. 1999;17(1):73–92.
190. Shi Y, Massague J. Mechanisms of TGF-beta signaling from cell membrane to the nucleus. Cell. 2003;113(6):685–700.
191. Szelenyi J. Cytokines and the central nervous system. Brain Res Bull. 2001;54(4):329–38.

192. Phillips DJ, Nguyen P, Adamides AA, Bye N, Rosenfeld JV, Kossmann T, et al. Activin a release into cerebrospinal fluid in a subset of patients with severe traumatic brain injury. J Neurotrauma. 2006;23(9):1283–94.
193. Brionne TC, Tesseur I, Masliah E, Wyss-Coray T. Loss of TGF-beta 1 leads to increased neuronal cell death and microgliosis in mouse brain. Neuron. 2003;40(6):1133–45.
194. Prehn JH, Bindokas VP, Marcuccilli CJ, Krajewski S, Reed JC, Miller RJ. Regulation of neuronal Bcl2 protein expression and calcium homeostasis by transforming growth factor type beta confers wide-ranging protection on rat hippocampal neurons. Proc Natl Acad Sci U S A. 1994;91(26):12599–603.
195. Plata-Salaman CR, Ilyin SE, Turrin NP, Gayle D, Flynn MC, Romanovitch AE, et al. Kindling modulates the IL-1beta system, TNF-alpha, TGF-beta1, and neuropeptide mRNAs in specific brain regions. Brain Res Mol Brain Res. 2000;75(2):248–58.
196. Aronica E, van Vliet EA, Mayboroda OA, Troost D, da Silva FH, Gorter JA. Upregulation of metabotropic glutamate receptor subtype mGluR3 and mGluR5 in reactive astrocytes in a rat model of mesial temporal lobe epilepsy. Eur J Neurosci. 2000;12(7):2333–44.
197. Frigerio F, Frasca A, Weissberg I, Parrella S, Friedman A, Vezzani A, et al. Long-lasting pro-ictogenic effects induced in vivo by rat brain exposure to serum albumin in the absence of concomitant pathology. Epilepsia. 2012;53(11):1887–97.
198. Jin X, Prince DA, Huguenard JR. Enhanced excitatory synaptic connectivity in layer v pyramidal neurons of chronically injured epileptogenic neocortex in rats. J Neurosci. 2006;26(18):4891–900.
199. Scheff SW, Price DA, Hicks RR, Baldwin SA, Robinson S, Brackney C. Synaptogenesis in the hippocampal CA1 field following traumatic brain injury. J Neurotrauma. 2005;22(7):719–32.
200. Schoderboeck L, Adzemovic M, Nicolussi E-M, Crupinschi C, Hochmeister S, Fischer M-T, et al. The "window of susceptibility" for inflammation in the immature central nervous system is characterized by a leaky blood-brain barrier and the local expression of inflammatory chemokines. Neurobiol Dis. 2009;35(3):368–75.
201. Galea I, Bechmann I, Perry VH. What is immune privilege (not)? Trends Immunol. 2007;28(1):12–8.
202. Umehara F, Qin YF, Goto M, Wekerle H, Meyermann R. Experimental autoimmune encephalomyelitis in the maturing central-nervous-system-transfer of myelin basic protein-specific T-line lymphocytes to neonatal lewis rats. Lab Investig. 1990;62(2):147–55.
203. Anthony D, Dempster R, Fearn S, Clements J, Wells G, Perry VH, et al. CXC chemokines generate age-related increases in neutrophil-mediated brain inflammation and blood-brain barrier breakdown. Curr Biol. 1998;8(16):923–6.
204. Anthony DC, Bolton SJ, Fearn S, Perry VH. Age-related effects of interleukin-1 beta on polymorphonuclear neutrophil-dependent increases in blood-brain barrier permeability in rats. Brain. 1997;120:435–44.
205. Mollgard K, Saunders NR. The development of the human blood-brain and blood-CSF barriers. Neuropathol Appl Neurobiol. 1986;12(4):337–58.
206. Elhofy A, Wang J, Tani M, Fife BT, Kennedy KJ, Bennett J, et al. Transgenic expression of CCL2 in the central nervous system prevents experimental autoimmune encephalomyelitis. J Leukoc Biol. 2005;77(2):229–37.
207. Karpus WJ, Lukacs NW, McRae BL, Strieter RM, Kunkel SL, Miller SD. An important role for the chemokine macrophage inflammatory protein-1 alpha in the pathogenesis of the T cell-mediated autoimmune disease, experimental autoimmune encephalomyelitis. J Immunol. 1995;155(10):5003–10.
208. Luo Y, Fischer FR, Hancock WW, Dorf ME. Macrophage inflammatory protein-2 and KC induce chemokine production by mouse astrocytes. J Immunol. 2000;165(7):4015–23.
209. Levy O. Innate immunity of the newborn: basic mechanisms and clinical correlates. Nat Rev Immunol. 2007;7(5):379–90.
210. Berger RP, Ta'asan S, Rand A, Lokshin A, Kochanek P. Multiplex assessment of serum biomarker concentrations in well-appearing children with inflicted traumatic brain injury. Pediatr Res. 2009;65(1):97–102.
211. Buttram SDW, Wisniewski SR, Jackson EK, Adelson PD, Feldman K, Bayir H, et al. Multiplex assessment of cytokine and chemokine levels in cerebrospinal fluid following severe pediatric traumatic brain injury: effects of moderate hypothermia. J Neurotrauma. 2007;24(11):1707–17.
212. Whalen MJ, Carlos TM, Kochanek PM, Wisniewski SR, Bell MJ, Clark RS, et al. Interleukin-8 is increased in cerebrospinal fluid of children with severe head injury. Crit Care Med. 2000;28(4):929–34.
213. Perry VH, Hume DA, Gordon S. Immunohistochemical localization of macrophages and microglia in the adult and developing mouse brain. Neuroscience. 1985;15(2):313–26.
214. Lawson LJ, Perry VH. The unique characteristics of inflammatory responses in mouse brain are acquired during postnatal development. Eur J Neurosci. 1995;7(7):1584–95.
215. Oppenheim R. Neuronal cell death and some related regressive phenomena during neurogenesis: a selective historical review and progress report. Oxford: Oxford University Press; 1981.
216. Unkeless JC. Characterization of a monoclonal antibody directed against mouse macrophage and lymphocyte Fc receptors. J Exp Med. 1979;150(3):580–96.
217. Johnston MV, Trescher WH, Ishida A, Nakajima W. Neurobiology of hypoxic-ischemic injury in the developing brain. Pediatr Res. 2001;49(6):735–41.
218. Brooks-Kayal AR. Rearranging receptors. Epilepsia. 2005;46 Suppl 7:29–38.
219. Ben-Ari Y. Excitatory actions of gaba during development: the nature of the nurture. Nat Rev Neurosci. 2002;3(9):728–39.
220. Dzhala VI, Staley KJ. Excitatory actions of endogenously released GABA contribute to initiation of ictal epileptiform activity in the developing hippocampus. J Neurosci. 2003;23(5):1840–6.
221. Khazipov R, Khalilov I, Tyzio R, Morozova E, Ben-Ari Y, Holmes GL. Developmental changes in GABAergic actions and seizure susceptibility in the rat hippocampus. Eur J Neurosci. 2004;19(3):590–600.
222. Ruffolo G, Iyer A, Cifelli P, Roseti C, Muhlebner A, van Scheppingen J, et al. Functional aspects of early brain development are preserved in tuberous sclerosis complex (TSC) epileptogenic lesions. Neurobiol Dis. 2016;95:93–101.
223. Hernan AE, Holmes GL. Antiepileptic drug treatment strategies in neonatal epilepsy. Prog Brain Res. 2016;226:179–93.
224. Stamboulian-Platel S, Legendre A, Chabrol T, Platel J-C, Pernot F, Duveau V, et al. Activation of GABA(A) receptors controls mesiotemporal lobe epilepsy despite changes in chloride transporters expression: in vivo and in silico approach. Exp Neurol. 2016;284:11–28.
225. Erecinska M, Cherian S, Silver IA. Energy metabolism in mammalian brain during development. Prog Neurobiol. 2004;73(6):397–445.
226. Holmes GL. Effects of seizures on brain development: lessons from the laboratory. Pediatr Neurol. 2005;33(1):1–11.
227. Szot P, White SS, McCarthy EB, Turella A, Rejniak SX, Schwartzkroin PA. Behavioral and metabolic features of repetitive seizures in immature and mature rats. Epilepsy Res. 2001;46(3):191–203.
228. Liu Z, Stafstrom CE, Sarkisian M, Tandon P, Yang Y, Hori A, et al. Age-dependent effects of glutamate toxicity in the hippocampus. Brain Research. Dev Brain Res. 1996;97(2):178–84.
229. Galic MA, Riazi K, Heida JG, Mouihate A, Fournier NM, Spencer SJ, et al. Postnatal inflammation increases seizure susceptibility in adult rats. J Neurosci. 2008;28(27):6904–13.
230. Harre EM, Galic MA, Mouihate A, Noorbakhsh F, Pittman QJ. Neonatal inflammation produces selective behavioural deficits and alters N-methyl-D-aspartate receptor subunit mRNA in the adult rat brain. Eur J Neurosci. 2008;27(3):644–53.
231. Insel TR, Miller LP, Gelhard RE. The ontogeny of excitatory amino-acid receptors in rat forebrain.1. N-methyl-D-aspartate and quisqualate receptors. Neuroscience. 1990;35(1):31–43.
232. Flint AC, Maisch US, Weishaupt JH, Kriegstein AR, Monyer H. NR2A subunit expression shortens NMDA receptor synaptic currents in developing neocortex. J Neurosci. 1997;17(7):2469–76.
233. Monyer H, Burnashev N, Laurie DJ, Sakmann B, Seeburg PH. Developmental and regional expression in the rat brain and functional-properties of 4 NMDA receptors. Neuron. 1994;12(3):529–40.
234. Hestrin S. Developmental regulation of NMDA receptor-mediated synaptic currents at a central synapse. Nature. 1992;357(6380):686–9.
235. Pitkanen A, McIntosh TK. Animal. models of post-traumatic epilepsy. J Neurotrauma. 2006;23(2):241–61.
236. Golarai G, Greenwood AC, Feeney DM, Connor JA. Physiological and structural evidence for hippocampal involvement in persistent seizure susceptibility after traumatic brain injury. J Neurosci. 2001;21(21):8523–37.
237. Cernak I, Vink R, Zapple DN, Cruz MI, Ahmed F, Chang T, et al. The pathobiology of moderate diffuse traumatic brain injury as identified using a new experimental model of injury in rats. Neurobiol Dis. 2004;17(1):29–43.
238. Pitkanen A, Bolkvadze T, Immonen R. Anti-epileptogenesis in rodent post-traumatic epilepsy models. Neurosci Lett. 2011;497(3):163–71.

239. Hunt RF, Scheff SW, Smith BN. Posttraumatic epilepsy after controlled cortical impact injury in mice. Exp Neurol. 2009;215(2):243–52.
240. Annegers JF, Hauser WA, Coan SP, Rocca WA. A population-based study of seizures after traumatic brain injuries. N Engl J Med. 1998;338(1):20–4.
241. Bolkvadze T, Pitkanen A. Development of post-traumatic epilepsy after controlled cortical impact and lateral fluid-percussion-induced brain injury in the mouse. J Neurotrauma. 2012;29(5):789–812.
242. D'Ambrosio R, Eastman CL, Fattore C, Perucca E. Novel frontiers in epilepsy treatments: preventing epileptogenesis by targeting inflammation. Expert Rev Neurother. 2013;13(6):615–25.
243. Polderman KH. Mechanisms of action, physiological effects, and complications of hypothermia. Crit Care Med. 2009;37(7):S186–202.
244. Atkins CM, Truettner JS, Lotocki G, Sanchez-Molano J, Kang Y, Alonso OF, et al. Post-traumatic seizure susceptibility is attenuated by hypothermia therapy. Eur J Neurosci. 2010;32(11):1912–20.
245. D'Ambrosio R, Eastman CL, Darvas F, Fender JS, Verley DR, Farin FM, et al. Mild passive focal cooling prevents epileptic seizures after head injury in rats. Ann Neurol. 2013;73(2):199–209.
246. Beattie EC, Stellwagen D, Morishita W, Bresnahan JC, Ha BK, Von Zastrow M, et al. Control of synaptic strength by glial TNF alpha. Science. 2002;295(5563):2282–5.
247. Jiang JX, Yang MS, Quan Y, Gueorguieva P, Ganesh T, Dingledine R. Therapeutic window for cyclooxygenase-2 related anti-inflammatory therapy after status epilepticus. Neurobiol Dis. 2015;76:126–36.
248. Song Y, Pimentel C, Walters K, Boller L, Ghiasvand S, Liu J, et al. Neuroprotective levels of IGF-1 exacerbate epileptogenesis after brain injury. Sci Rep. 2016;6:32095.
249. Alyu F, Dikmen M. Inflammatory aspects of epileptogenesis: contribution of molecular inflammatory mechanisms. Acta Neuropsychiatr. 2016:3:1-16. doi: 10.1017/neu.2016.47.
250. Kaltschmidt B, Widera D, Kaltschmidt C. Signaling via NF-kappa B in the nervous system. Biochim Biophys Acta Mol Cell Res. 2005;1745(3):287–99.

9

Moderate hypothermia inhibits microglial activation after traumatic brain injury by modulating autophagy/apoptosis and the MyD88-dependent TLR4 signaling pathway

Fengchen Zhang[1†], Haiping Dong[2†], Tao Lv[1], Ke Jin[1], Yichao Jin[1*], Xiaohua Zhang[1*] and Jiyao Jiang[1]

Abstract

Background: Complex mechanisms participate in microglial activation after a traumatic brain injury (TBI). TBI can induce autophagy and apoptosis in neurons and glial cells, and moderate hypothermia plays a protective role in the acute phase of TBI. In the present study, we evaluated the effect of TBI and moderate hypothermia on microglial activation and investigated the possible roles of autophagy/apoptosis and toll-like receptor 4 (TLR4).

Methods: The TBI model was induced with a fluid percussion TBI device. Moderate hypothermia was achieved under general anesthesia by partial immersion in a water bath for 4 h. All rats were killed 24 h after the TBI.

Results: Our results showed downregulation of the microglial activation and autophagy, but upregulation of microglial apoptosis, upon post-TBI hypothermia treatment. The expression of TLR4 and downstream myeloid differentiation primary response 88 (MyD88) was attenuated. Moderate hypothermia reduced neural cell death post-TBI.

Conclusions: Moderate hypothermia can reduce the number of activated microglia by inhibiting autophagy and promoting apoptosis, probably through a negative modulation between autophagy and apoptosis. Moderate hypothermia may attenuate the pro-inflammatory function of microglia by inhibiting the MyD88-dependent TLR4 signaling pathway.

Keywords: Apoptosis, Autophagy, Microglial activation, Toll-like receptor, Traumatic brain injury

Background

In developing countries, traumatic brain injury (TBI) is a major cause of morbidity and mortality. The pathological process of TBI is quite complicated and is commonly divided into two phases, primary and secondary injury. The activation of resident microglia plays a key pro-inflammatory role in the acute secondary phase post-TBI [1–3].

Autophagy is a highly conserved intracellular process, which includes the degradation of abnormal accumulations of toxic substances, proteins, and damaged organelles, so that the proteins and other substances can be recycled efficiently. After TBI, autophagy can both protect cells and damage them [4–6]. In our previous study, we found that TBI could induce autophagy and apoptosis in neurons and glial cells. However, in the acute phase of TBI, hypothermia plays a cytoprotective role. Furthermore, we demonstrated that post-TBI hypothermia could upregulate the autophagy pathway, modulate apoptosis, and reduce cell death in neurons and glial cells; a possible mechanism for this is the negative regulatory effect of autophagy on apoptosis [7, 8]. We also found autophagy induction in microglia after TBI [9], but the regulatory effect of moderate hypothermia on microglial activation remains unknown.

Among the variety of receptors involved in microglial activation, toll-like receptors are significant for microglial activation and functioning. Toll-like receptor 4 (TLR4) is mainly expressed in microglia. TLR4 activates

* Correspondence: honam612@163.com; zxh1969@aliyun.com
[†]Fengchen Zhang and Haiping Dong contributed equally to this work.
[1]Department of Neurosurgery, Ren-Ji Hospital, School of Medicine, Shanghai Jiao Tong University, No. 160 Pujian Road, Shanghai 200127, People's Republic of China

interleukin-1 receptor-associated kinase (IRAK) through the myeloid differentiation primary response 88 (MyD88)-dependent pathway; this further activates tumor necrosis factor receptor-associated factor 6 (TRAF6), which is followed by the activation of the downstream transcription factors nuclear factor kappa light chain enhancer of activated B cells (NF-κB), activator protein 1, and interferon regulatory factor-5. These transcription factors induce the expression of pro-inflammatory cytokines, such as interleukin-6 (IL-6), tumor necrosis factor alpha (TNF-α), and interleukin-12 (IL-12) [10–13].

In this study, we evaluated the effect of hypothermia on the microglial activation post-TBI and preliminarily explored the possible mechanisms, with regard to the relationship between autophagy, apoptosis, and the MyD88-dependent TLR4 pathway.

Methods

Animals and experimental design

All animal procedures in this study were approved by the Animal Care and Experimental Committee of the School of Medicine of Shanghai Jiao Tong University. Adult male Sprague–Dawley rats (280–300 g) were used. Rats were randomly divided into four groups: sham injury with normothermia group (SNG; 37 °C; $n = 60$), sham injury with hypothermia (SHG; 32 °C; $n = 60$), TBI with normothermia group (TNG; 37 °C; $n = 60$), and TBI with hypothermia group (THG; 32 °C; $n = 60$). Rats were housed in individual cages in a temperature- and humidity-controlled animal facility with a 12-h light/dark cycle. Rats were housed in the animal facility for at least 7 days before surgery, and they were given free access to food and water during this period.

Surgical preparation

Rats were anesthetized through intraperitoneal injection (i.p.) of 10% chloral hydrate (3.3 mL/kg) and were then mounted in a stereotaxic frame. An incision was made along the midline of the scalp, and a 4.8-mm diameter craniectomy was performed on the left parietal bone (midway between the bregma and the lambda). A rigid plastic injury tube (a modified Leur-loc needle hub, with an inside diameter of 2.6 mm) was secured over the exposed, intact dura by using cyanoacrylate adhesive. Two skull screws (2.1 mm in diameter, 6.0 mm in length) were placed in the burr holes, 1 mm rostral to the bregma and 1 mm caudal to the lambda. The injury tube was secured to the skull with dental cement. Bone wax was used to cover the open needle hub connector after the dental cement had hardened (5 min). The scalp was closed with sutures. The animals were returned to their cages for recovery.

Lateral fluid percussion brain injury

A fluid percussion device (VCU Biomedical Engineering, Richmond, VA) was used to cause TBI, as described in detail previously [10, 14]. The rats were subjected to TBI 24 h after the surgical procedure to minimize possible confounding factors of the surgery. In brief, the device consisted of a Plexiglas cylindrical reservoir filled with 37 °C isotonic saline. One end of the reservoir had a rubber-covered Plexiglas piston mounted on O-rings, and the opposite end had a pressure transducer housing with a 2.6-mm inside diameter male needle hub opening. On the day of the TBI, rats were anesthetized with 10% chloral hydrate (3.3 mL/kg, i.p.) and endotracheally intubated for mechanical ventilation. The suture was opened, and the bone wax was removed. The rats were disconnected from the ventilator, and the injury tube was connected to the fluid percussion cylinder. A fluid pressure pulse was then applied for 10 ms directly onto the exposed dura to produce a moderate TBI (2.1–2.2 atm). The injury was delivered within 10 s after disconnection from the ventilator. The resulting pressure pulse was measured in atmosphere by using an extracranial transducer (Statham PA 85-100; Gloud, Oxnard, CA) and recorded on a storage oscilloscope (Tektronix 5111; Tektronix, Beaverton, OR). After the initial observation, the rats were ventilated with a 2:1 nitrous oxide/oxygen mixture and the rectal and temporal muscle temperatures were recorded. The needle hub, screws, and dental cement were then removed from the skull, and the scalp was sutured closed. The rats were extubated as soon as spontaneous breathing was observed. The SNG and SHG rats were subjected to the same anesthetic and surgical procedures as the rats in the other groups but without being subjected to injury.

Manipulation of temperature

The frontal cortex brain temperature was monitored with a digital electronic thermometer (model DP 80; Omega Engineering, Stamford, CT) and a 0.15-mm diameter temperature probe (model HYP-033-1-T-G-60-SMP-M; Omega Engineering) inserted 4.0 mm ventral to the surface of the skull. The probe was removed before the fluid percussion injury and replaced immediately after the injury. Rectal temperatures were measured with an electronic thermometer with an analog display (model 43 TE; YSI, Yellow Springs, OH) and a temperature probe (series 400; YSI). A brain temperature of 32 °C was achieved by immersing the body of the anesthetized rat in ice-cold water. The skin and fur of the animals were protected from direct contact with the water by placing each animal in a plastic bag (head exposed) before immersion. Animals were removed from the water bath when the brain temperature had dropped to within 2 °C of the target temperature. It took approximately 30 min to reach the target brain temperatures, which were maintained for 4 h under general anesthesia at room temperature by intermittent application of ice packs as needed. Gradual warming of the animals to normothermia levels (37 °C) was done over a 90-min period to avoid rapid warming that may have affected the secondary injury processes.

Hematoxylin and eosin (HE) staining

Rats were subjected to deep anesthesia with 10% chloral hydrate. At 24 h after TBI, rats were perfused transcardially with 4% paraformaldehyde. The brains were removed, further fixed at 4 °C overnight, and then immersed in 30% sucrose/phosphate-buffered saline (PBS) at 4 °C overnight. Specimens were mounted in optimal cutting temperature compound (OCT). Serial sections were obtained by using a cryostat and were stained with toluidine blue for 30 min; two to three drops of glacial acetic acid were then added. Once the nucleus and granulation were clearly visible, the sections were mounted in Permount or Histoclad. Sections were cut in a microtome and adhered to glass slides with polylysine. Images of injured cortex and ipsilateral hippocampus were captured at × 100 by using a microscope (Nikon Labophot; Nikon USA, Melville, NY). There were six rats in each of the four groups.

Immunohistochemical staining

The 4-mm-thick, formalin-fixed OCT-embedded sections were subjected to immunofluorescence analysis to determine the immunoreactivity of ionized calcium-binding adapter molecule 1 (Iba-1) and cleaved caspase 3. Endogenous peroxidase was blocked by treatment with 3% hydrogen peroxide for 5 min, followed by a brief rinse in distilled water and a 15-min wash in PBS. Sections were cooled at room temperature for 20 min and rinsed in PBS. Nonspecific protein binding was blocked by incubation in 5% horse serum for 40 min. Sections were incubated with primary antibodies (goat anti-rat Iba-1, diluted 1:100, Abcam; rabbit anti-rat cleaved caspase 3, diluted 1:100, CST) for 1 h at room temperature and then subjected to a 15-min wash in PBS. Sections were incubated with Alexa Fluor 488 donkey anti-goat secondary antibodies for Iba-1 and Alexa Fluor 555 donkey anti-rabbit secondary antibodies for cleaved caspase 3, protein light chain 3 (LC3), and Beclin-1 (1:1000 dilution, Invitrogen) for 1 h at room temperature. For negative controls, sections were incubated in the absence of a primary antibody. At least 10 randomly selected microscopic fields (× 630 magnification; Zeiss LSM880; Zeiss, Germany) were used for counting the Iba-1-positive and cleaved caspase 3-positive cells. There were six rats in each of the four groups.

Immunofluorescence microscopy for cell localization

The primary antibodies for immunofluorescence were goat anti-rat Iba-1 (1:100 dilution, Abcam), rabbit anti-rat cleaved caspase 3 (1:100 dilution, CST), rabbit anti-rat LC3 (1:100 dilution, CST), and rabbit anti-rat Beclin-1 (1:100 dilution, Proteintech). The sections were incubated with the primary antibodies in PBS with 1% bovine serum albumin for 30–40 min at room temperature; this was followed by washing and application of the secondary antibodies. The secondary antibodies were Alexa Fluor 488 donkey anti-goat for Iba-1 (1:1000 dilution, Invitrogen) and Alexa Fluor 555 donkey anti-rabbit for cleaved caspase 3, LC3, and Beclin-1 (1:1000 dilution, Invitrogen). We performed double labeling for Iba-1/cleaved caspase 3, LC3, or Beclin-1 to detect expression of them in microglia. After a final wash, the sections were protected with cover slips with anti-fading mounting medium, sealed with clear nail polish, and stored at 4 °C for preservation. At least 10 randomly selected microscope fields were observed in each group, and the number of positive cells was statistically analyzed (× 630 magnifications; Zeiss LSM880; Zeiss, Germany). There were six rats in each of the four groups.

Western blot analysis

At 24 h after TBI, the injured cortex and ipsilateral hippocampus were harvested. The frozen brain samples were mechanically lysed in 20 mM tris(hydroxymethyl)aminomethane (Tris; pH 7.6), containing 0.2% sodium dodecylsulfate (SDS), 1% Triton X-100, 1% deoxycholate, 1 mM phenylmethylsulphonyl fluoride, and 0.11 IU/mL aprotinin (all purchased from Sigma–Aldrich, Inc.). The lysates were centrifuged at 12,000*g* for 20 min at 4 °C. The protein concentration was estimated by the Bradford method. The samples (60 μg/lane) were separated by 12% SDS polyacrylamide gel electrophoresis and electro-transferred onto a polyvinylidene difluoride membrane (Bio-Rad Lab, Hercules, CA). The membrane was blocked with 5% skim milk for 2 h at room temperature and incubated with primary antibodies against TLR4 (1:1000 dilution, Proteintech), MyD88 (1:1000 dilution, Proteintech), cleaved caspase 3 (1:100 dilution, CST), and Iba-1 (1:1000 dilution, Abcam). β-Actin (1:10,000 dilution, Sigma–Aldrich) was used as the loading control. After the membrane had been washed six times in a mixture of Tris-buffered saline and Tween-20 (TBST) for 10 min each time, it was incubated with the appropriate horseradish peroxidase-conjugated secondary antibody (1:10,000 dilution in TBST) for 2 h. The blotted protein bands were visualized by enhanced chemiluminescence Western blot detection reagents (Amersham, Arlington Heights, IL) and exposed to X-ray film. The developed films were digitized using an Epson Perfection 2480 scanner (Seiko Corp, Nagano, Japan). The results were quantified by Quantity One Software (Bio-Rad). The band density values were calculated as a ratio of TLR4, MyD88, Iba-1, and cleaved caspase 3/β-actin. There were six rats in each of the four groups.

Quantitative real-time polymerase chain reaction (qRT-PCR)

Total RNA was isolated from the injured cortex and the ipsilateral hippocampus by using Trizol (Invitrogen) according to the manufacturer's instructions. cDNA was synthesized by using a reverse transcription kit (TAKARA). PCR was performed by using SYBR Advantage Premix (TAKARA). The primers for TLR4 were (forward) 5′-TGT TCC TTT CCT GCC TGA GAC-3′ and (reverse) 5′-GGT TCT TGG TTG AAT AAG GGA TGT C-3′. The primers for MyD88 were (forward) 5′-GGT TCT GGA CCC GTC TTG C-3′ and (reverse) 5′-AGA ATC AGG CTC CAA GTC AGC-3′. Relative mRNA expression was calculated with the $2^{-\Delta\Delta Ct}$ method; SNG values were taken as 100%. β-Actin was used as the control. All experiments were done in triplicate. There were six rats in each of the four groups.

Enzyme-linked immunosorbent assay (ELISA) analysis of TNF-α and interleukin-1β (IL-1β)

At 24 h after TBI, rats were subjected to deep anesthesia by 10% chloral hydrate. The brains were quickly removed by dissection and kept over ice in physiologic salt solution. The injured cortex and ipsilateral hippocampus specimens were separated, cut into small pieces, dispersed by aspiration into a pipette, and suspended in 1 mL of physiologic salt solution in a test tube. Samples were kept over wet ice for 20 min before use. The homogenates were centrifuged at 7500 rpm for 20 min. The supernatants were used for measuring TNF-α and IL-1β concentrations with commercial ELISA kits (Shanghai Enzyme-linked Biotechnology Co., Ltd.) by following the manufacturer's instructions. There were six rats in each of the four groups.

Statistical analysis

All data are presented as the mean ± the standard deviation (SD). SPSS for Windows version 23.0 (SPSS, Inc., Chicago, IL) was used for statistical analysis of the data. All data were subjected to one-way analysis of variance. Post hoc comparisons were made with Fisher's least significant difference test. Statistical significance was inferred at $P < 0.05$.

Results

Histologic examination of the injured cortex and the ipsilateral hippocampus

The brains of SNG and SHG rats showed the normal neuronal structure. The gray/white matter interface showed visible contusions and hemorrhaging in TNG and THG rats (Fig. 1).

TBI caused cell apoptosis, microglial activation, and an inflammatory response, which moderate hypothermia inhibited

Immunohistochemical staining and Western blotting of cleaved caspase 3 were used to evaluate cell apoptosis in injured cortex and ipsilateral hippocampus samples. Few cleaved caspase 3-positive cells were found in both areas in SNG and SHG rats. At 24 h after TBI, the expression level of cleaved caspase 3-positive cells significantly increased relative to those in SNG rats (TNG: immunohistochemical staining: injured cortex, 23.2 ± 2.39, $P < 0.001$; ipsilateral hippocampus, 23.1 ± 2.47, $P < 0.001$, and Western blotting: injured cortex, 1.61 ± 0.26, $P < 0.001$; ipsilateral hippocampus, 1.04 ± 0.27, $P < 0.01$). However, moderate hypothermia inhibited cell apoptosis in comparison with that in TNG rats (THG: immunohistochemical staining: injured cortex, 13.3 ± 1.49, $P < 0.001$; ipsilateral hippocampus, 11.70 ± 1.57, $P < 0.001$, and Western blotting: injured cortex, 1.16 ± 0.18, $P < 0.05$; ipsilateral hippocampus, 0.55 ± 0.19, $P < 0.05$). There were no significant differences between the SNG and SHG rats (Fig. 2 and Additional file 1: Figure S1).

Changes in microglial activation were evaluated from differences in Iba-1 expression, as determined by immunohistochemical staining and Western blotting of Iba-1. The expression level of Iba-1 significantly increased 24 h after TBI (TNG: immunohistochemical staining: injured cortex, 22 ± 1.94, $P < 0.001$; ipsilateral hippocampus, 29.5 ± 1.51, $P < 0.001$, and Western blotting: injured cortex, 0.91 ± 0.06, $P < 0.001$; ipsilateral hippocampus, 0.98 ± 0.15, $P < 0.001$), whereas moderate hypothermia inhibited microglial activation in comparison with that in TNG rats (THG: immunohistochemical staining: injured cortex, 17 ± 1.25, $P < 0.001$; ipsilateral hippocampus, 12 ± 1.83, $P < 0.001$, and Western blotting: injured cortex, 0.65 ± 0.03, $P < 0.001$; ipsilateral hippocampus, 0.66 ± 0.04, $P < 0.01$). There were no significant differences between SNG and SHG rats (Fig. 3 and Additional file 2: Figure S2).

TNF-α and IL-1β are involved in the inflammatory response after TBI. To determine the differences in the inflammatory responses, we separately tested the expression of TNF-α and IL-1β in the injured cortex and ipsilateral hippocampus. The results showed that the expression levels of TNF-α and IL-1β in TNG rats were significantly increased relative to those in SNG rats (TNG: injured cortex: TNF-α, 28.73 ± 4.33, $P < 0.01$; IL-1β, 5.21 ± 0.34, $P < 0.005$, and ipsilateral hippocampus: TNF-α, 30.95 ± 3.09, $P < 0.001$; IL-1β, 5.90 ± 0.43, $P < 0.001$). Moderate hypothermia attenuated the expression of TNF-α and IL-1β in comparison with that in TNG rats (THG: injured cortex: TNF-α, 23.41 ± 1.58, $P < 0.05$; IL-1β, 4.23 ± 0.53, $P < 0.01$, and ipsilateral hippocampus: TNF-α, 19.64 ± 3.05, $P < 0.001$; IL-1β, 4.73 ± 0.21, $P < 0.001$). There were no significant differences between SNG and SHG rats (Fig. 4).

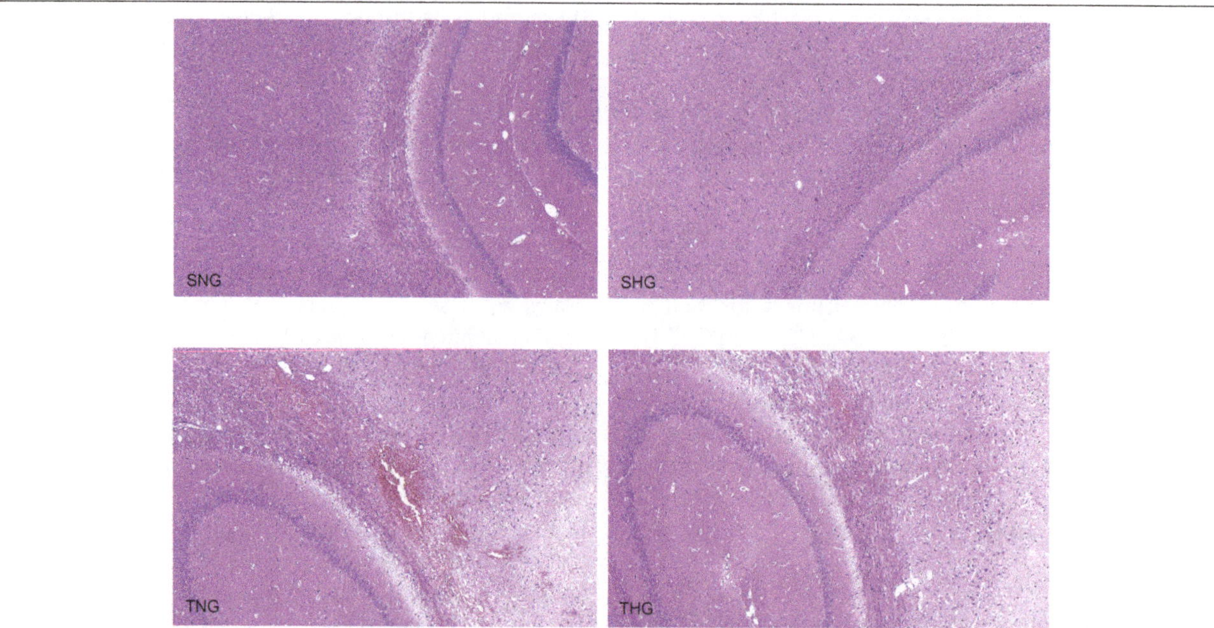

Fig. 1 HE staining of the injured cortex and ipsilateral hippocampus. HE staining of the injured cortex and ipsilateral hippocampus from SNG, SHG, TNG, and THG rats 24 h after TBI (magnification, × 100). The gray/white matter interface shows visible contusion and hemorrhaging in the TNG and THG rats

TBI caused microglial autophagy, which moderate hypothermia attenuated

A few LC3- and Beclin-1-positive microglial cells were observed in the sham groups and indicated the constitutive activity of autophagy in the normal rat brain. At 24 h after TBI, the LC3- and Beclin-1-positive microglial cells in the injured cortex and ipsilateral hippocampus were significantly increased in number compared with those in SNG rats (TNG: LC3-positive microglia: injured cortex, 18.8 ± 1.4, $P < 0.001$; ipsilateral hippocampus,

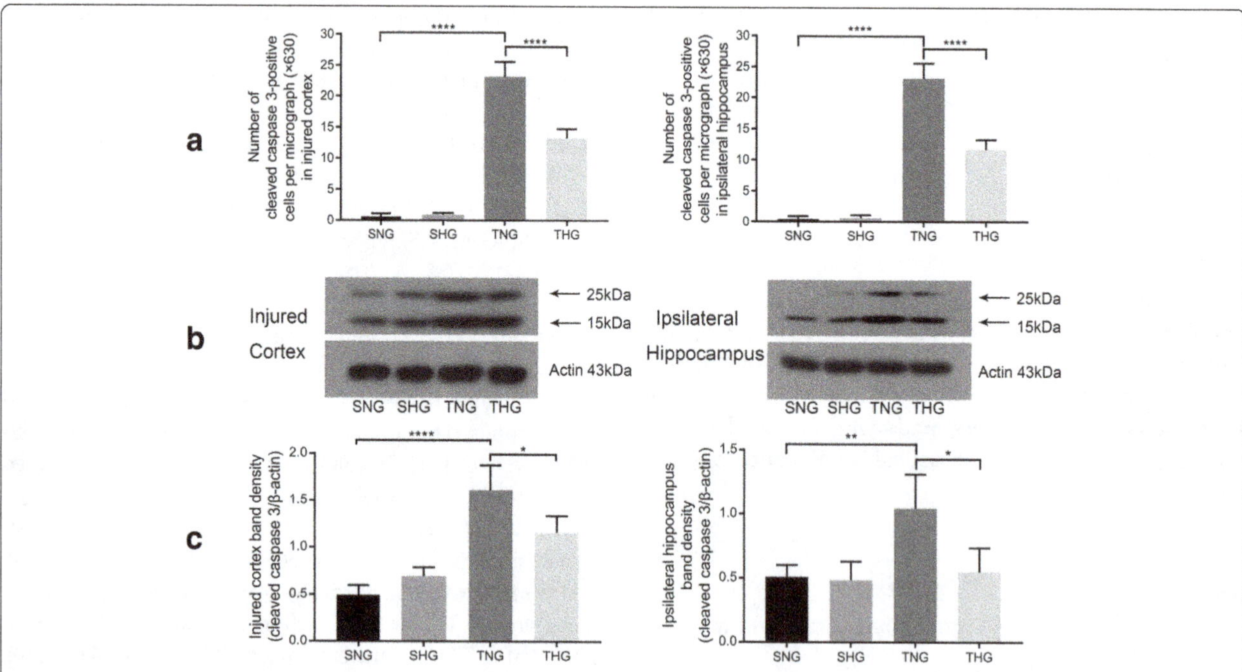

Fig. 2 Immunofluorescence analysis and Western blotting of cleaved caspase 3 expression in the injured cortex and ipsilateral hippocampus. **a** Number of cleaved caspase 3-positive cells in the injured cortex and ipsilateral hippocampus. Data in the bar graphs represent mean ± SD. ****$P < 0.001$. At least 10 randomly selected microscopic fields were used for counting (magnification, × 630). **b, c** Western blotting of cleaved caspase 3 from the injured cortex and ipsilateral hippocampus. Data in the bar graphs represent mean ± SD. β-Actin was used as the load control. *$P < 0.05$; **$P < 0.01$; ****$P < 0.001$

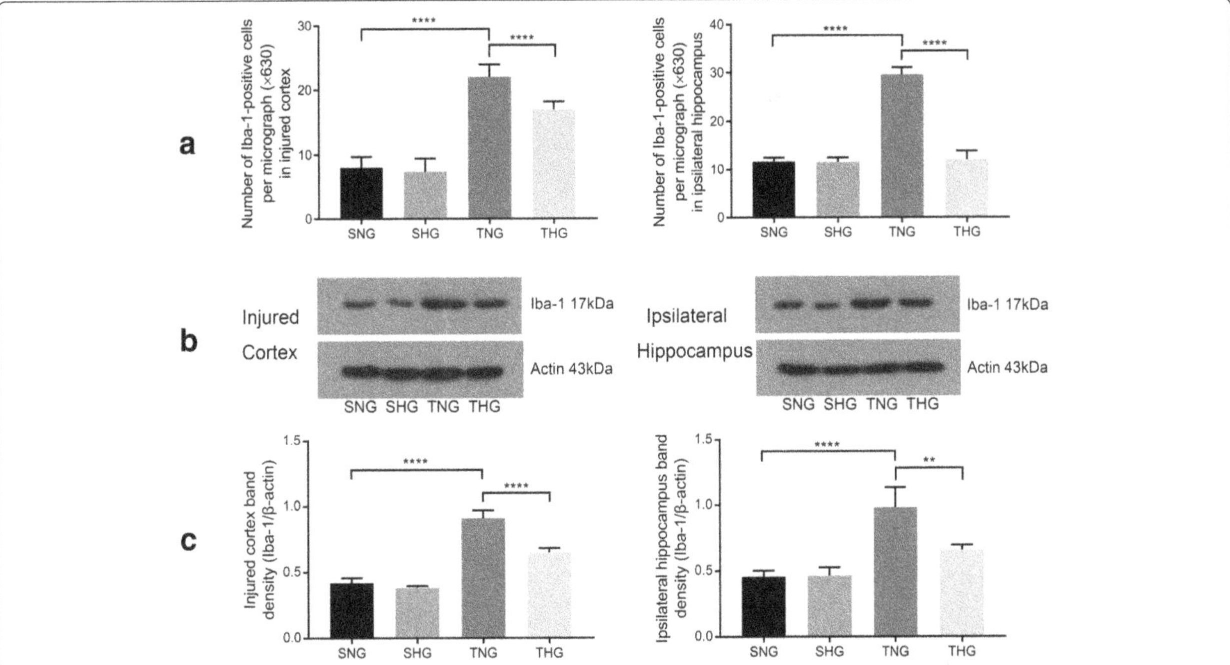

Fig. 3 Immunofluorescence analysis and Western blotting of Iba-1 expression in the injured cortex and ipsilateral hippocampus. **a** Number of Iba-1-positive cells in the injured cortex and ipsilateral hippocampus. Data in the bar graphs represent mean ± SD. ****$P < 0.001$. At least 10 randomly selected microscopic fields were used for counting (magnification, × 630). **b**, **c** Western blotting of Iba-1 from the injured cortex and ipsilateral hippocampus. Data in the bar graphs represent mean ± SD. β-Actin was used as the load control. **$P < 0.01$; ****$P < 0.001$

23.2 ± 2.74, $P < 0.001$, and Beclin-1-positive microglia: injured cortex, 16.5 ± 2.22, $P < 0.001$; ipsilateral hippocampus, 16.8 ± 2.44, $P < 0.001$). However, moderate hypothermia significantly attenuated microglial autophagy relative to that in TNG rats (THG: LC3-positive microglia: injured cortex, 5 ± 1.33, $P < 0.001$; ipsilateral hippocampus, 5.2 ± 1.55, $P < 0.001$, and Beclin-1-positive microglia: injured cortex, 4.8 ± 1.32, $P < 0.001$; ipsilateral hippocampus, 6.7 ± 1.06, $P < 0.001$). There were no significant differences between SNG and SHG rats (Figs. 5 and 6).

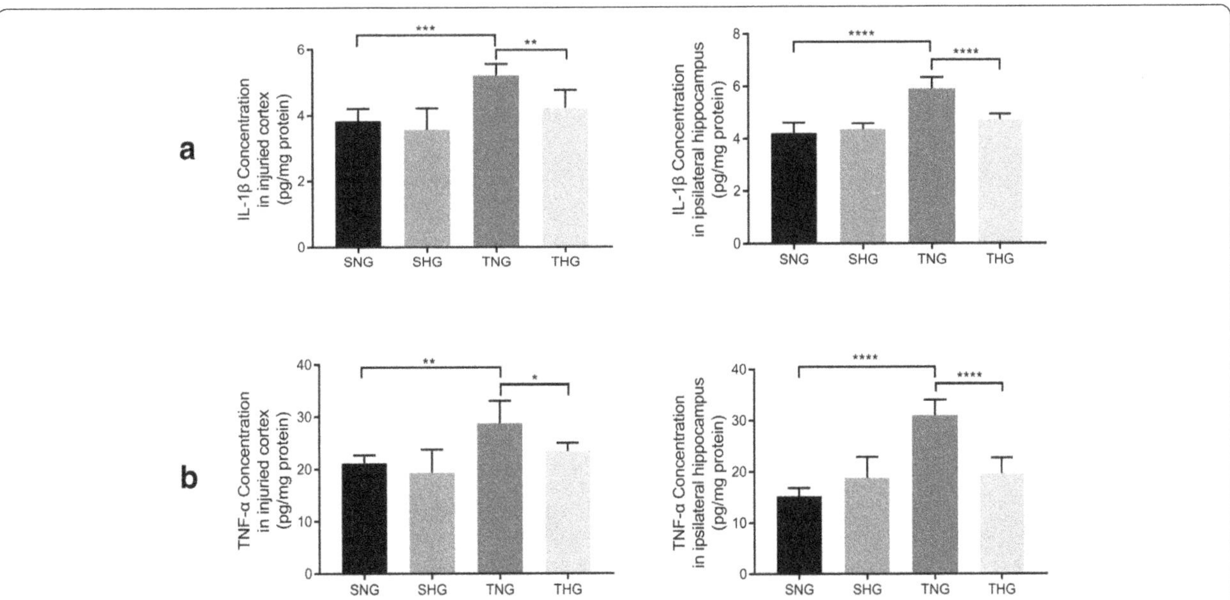

Fig. 4 ELISA of IL-1β and TNF-α from the injured cortex and ipsilateral hippocampus. The levels of IL-1β (**a**) and TNF-α (**b**) from the injured cortex and ipsilateral hippocampus with or without moderate hypothermia are shown. Data in the bar graphs represent mean ± SD. *$P < 0.05$; **$P < 0.01$; ***$P < 0.005$; ****$P < 0.001$. There were six rats in each of the four groups

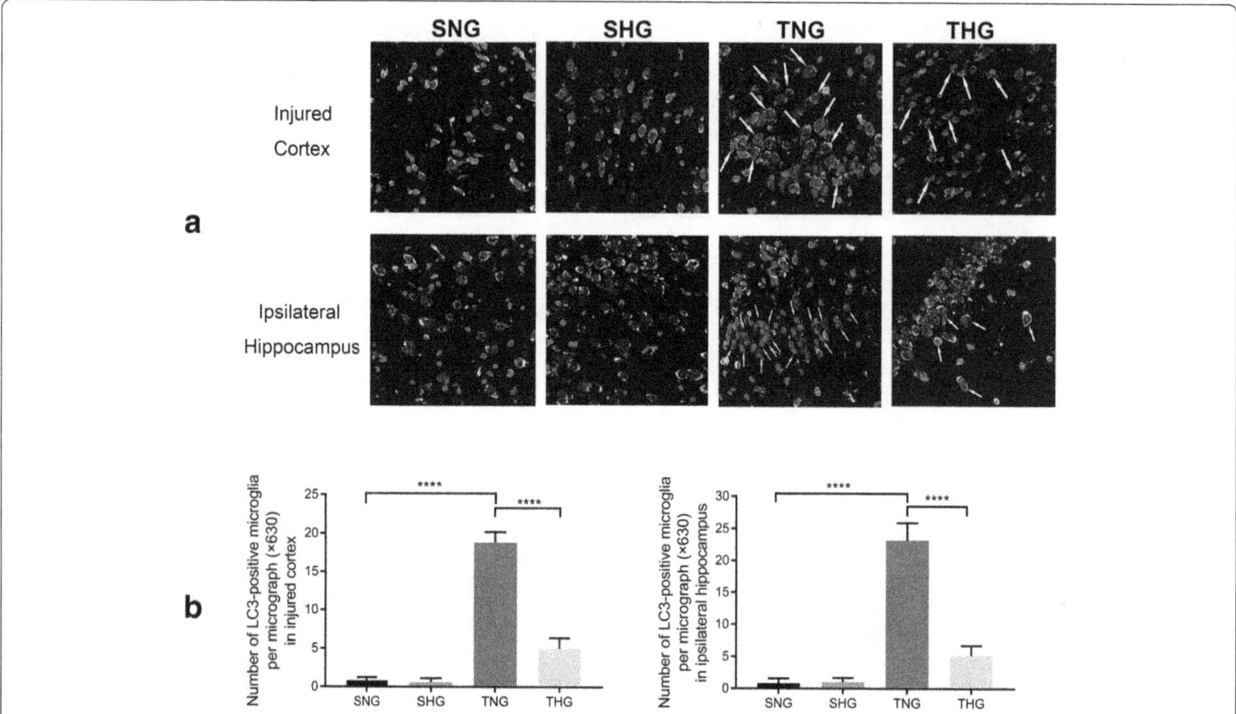

Fig. 5 Immunofluorescence analysis of LC3 (red) and Iba-1 (green) from the injured cortex and ipsilateral hippocampus. **a** Immunohistochemical staining of LC3 and Iba-1 from the injured cortex and ipsilateral hippocampus. Arrows indicate co-localization of LC3 and Iba-1 (magnification, × 630). **b** Number of LC3-positive microglia in the injured cortex and ipsilateral hippocampus. At least 10 randomly selected microscopic fields were used for counting. Data in the bar graphs represent mean ± SD. *****P* < 0.001

TBI caused microglial apoptosis, which moderate hypothermia promotion

Induction of microglial apoptosis was detected with immunohistochemical staining of Iba-1 and cleaved caspase 3. The number of cleaved caspase 3-positive microglial cells significantly increased 24 h after TBI in the injured cortex and ipsilateral hippocampus (TNG: injured cortex, 3.9 ± 0.99, $P < 0.001$; ipsilateral hippocampus, 5.3 ± 1.06, $P < 0.001$), whereas moderate hypothermia promoted microglial apoptosis, relative to that in TNG rats (THG: injured cortex, 16.9 ± 2.18, $P < 0.001$; ipsilateral hippocampus, 11.9 ± 1.20, $P < 0.001$). There were no significant differences between SNG and SHG rats (Fig. 7).

TBI activated the MyD88-dependent TLR4 pathway, which was inhibited by moderate hypothermia

Expression of TLR4 and MyD88 in microglial cells was measured with Western blotting and qRT-PCR. The protein levels of TLR4 and MyD88 significantly increased in the injured cortex and ipsilateral hippocampus 24 h after TBI (TNG: TLR4: injured cortex, 1.27 ± 0.06, $P < 0.001$; ipsilateral hippocampus, 2.03 ± 0.27, $P < 0.01$, and MyD88: injured cortex, 1.32 ± 0.002, $P < 0.005$; ipsilateral hippocampus, 1.18 ± 0.08, $P < 0.005$). Moderate hypothermia decreased the protein levels of TLR4 and MyD88 relative to those in TNG rats (THG: TLR4: injured cortex, 0.82 ± 0.08, $P < 0.001$; ipsilateral hippocampus, 1.41 ± 0.34, $P < 0.05$, and MyD88: injured cortex, 0.95 ± 0.10, $P < 0.01$; ipsilateral hippocampus, 0.86 ± 0.12, $P < 0.01$). There were no significant differences between SNG and SHG rats (Fig. 8).

Meanwhile, the mRNA levels of TLR4 and MyD88 in the injured cortex and ipsilateral hippocampus also significantly increased 24 h after TBI (TNG: TLR4: injured cortex, 4.3-fold, $P < 0.001$; ipsilateral hippocampus, 5.7-fold, $P < 0.005$, and MyD88: injured cortex, 2.3-fold, $P < 0.005$; ipsilateral hippocampus, 3.5-fold, $P < 0.001$). Moderate hypothermia also decreased the mRNA levels of TLR4 and MyD88 compared with those in TNG rats (TLR4: injured cortex, 1.4-fold, $P < 0.005$; ipsilateral hippocampus, 1.1-fold, $P < 0.005$, and MyD88: injured cortex, 1.1-fold, $P < 0.005$; ipsilateral hippocampus, 1.8-fold, $P < 0.005$). There were no significant differences between SNG and SHG rats (Fig. 9).

Discussion

Our results suggest that microglial activation post-TBI could be suppressed by moderate hypothermia and that the negative regulation of autophagy and apoptosis may play a role in this process. In addition, hypothermia may also act by inhibiting the MyD88-dependent TLR4 pathway. Thus, moderate hypothermia exerts anti-inflammatory and neuroprotective effects.

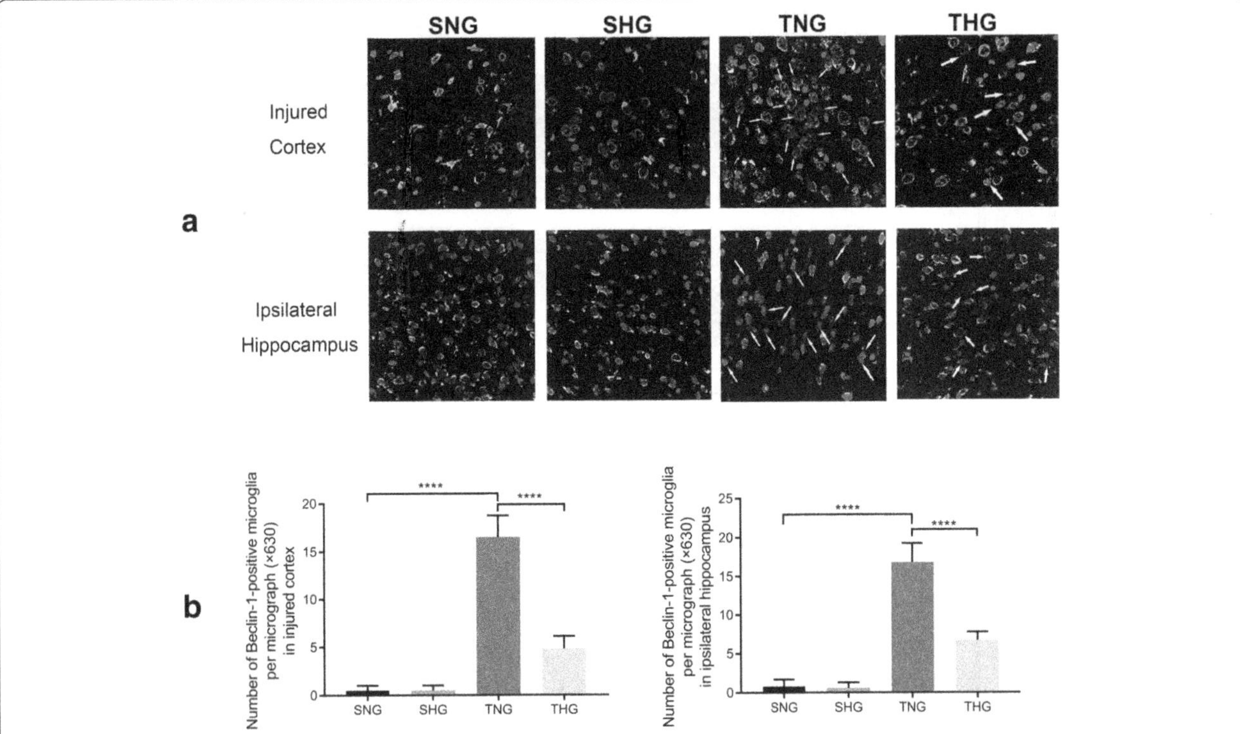

Fig. 6 Immunofluorescence analysis of Beclin-1 (red) and Iba-1 (green) from the injured cortex and ipsilateral hippocampus. **a** Immunohistochemical staining of Beclin-1 and Iba-1 from the injured cortex and ipsilateral hippocampus. Arrows indicate co-localization of Beclin-1 and Iba-1 (magnification, ×630). **b** Number of Beclin-1-positive microglia in the injured cortex and ipsilateral hippocampus. At least 10 randomly selected microscopic fields were used for counting. Data in the bar graphs represent mean ± SD. ****$P < 0.001$

In this study, we found that moderate TBI induced by fluid percussion caused cortical and ipsilateral hippocampal cell death, microglial activation, and microglial autophagy 24 h after TBI. We also found that moderate hypothermia could reduce the amount of hippocampal and cortical cell death. Furthermore, we found that microglial autophagy was suppressed, and microglial apoptosis was increased after moderate hypothermia 24 h post-TBI. In addition, the attenuation of microglial activation was observed through the downregulated expression of Iba-1, which is an important biomarker for microglial activation. These results suggest that moderate hypothermia may reduce the number of activated microglia by inhibiting autophagy and promoting apoptosis.

Apoptotic cell death is one of the most common pathologic changes after TBI [15–18]. The activation of cleaved caspase 3, which is an executioner caspase, presents an irreversible point in the complex cascade of apoptosis induction. Activated caspase-3 has been detected in neurons, astrocytes, and oligodendrocytes post-TBI in previous studies [19–23]. In this study, the number of microglia labeled by cleaved caspase-3 significantly increased after moderate hypothermia post-TBI, which indicates that hypothermia accelerated apoptosis of the microglia.

Autophagy is a highly regulated process involving the bulk degradation of cytoplasmic macromolecules and organelles in mammalian cells through the lysosomal system. Beclin-1, an autophagic biomarker, is a novel Bcl-2-homology-3 domain-only protein that participates in autophagy regulation with several co-actors [24]. LC3, a mammalian orthologue of yeast ATG8, is synthesized as pro-LC3, which is cleaved by ATG4 protease and converted into LC3-I. Once autophagy is activated, LC3-I is conjugated to phosphatidylethanolamine (lipidated) to form LC3-II. The amounts of LC3-II and p62 degraded by autophagy provide an estimate of the autophagy activity [25]. Diskin et al. first demonstrated that the Beclin-1 level increased near the site of an injury by using the closed-head injury model in mice in 2005 [26]. Viscomi et al. found that autophagy could serve as a protective mechanism for maintaining cellular homeostasis after TBI, which could be enhanced by rapamycin through inactivation of the mammalian target of rapamycin [27]. However, the role of autophagy is still controversial. In previous studies, we have demonstrated that moderate hypothermia post-TBI could activate the neuronal and glial autophagy pathway, which could negatively modulate apoptosis and reduce cell death [8, 14]. On the other hand, this negative regulatory effect of autophagy on apoptosis may play a different role in microglia and may be associated with different cell types. In this study, the use of LC3 and Beclin-1 as autophagic

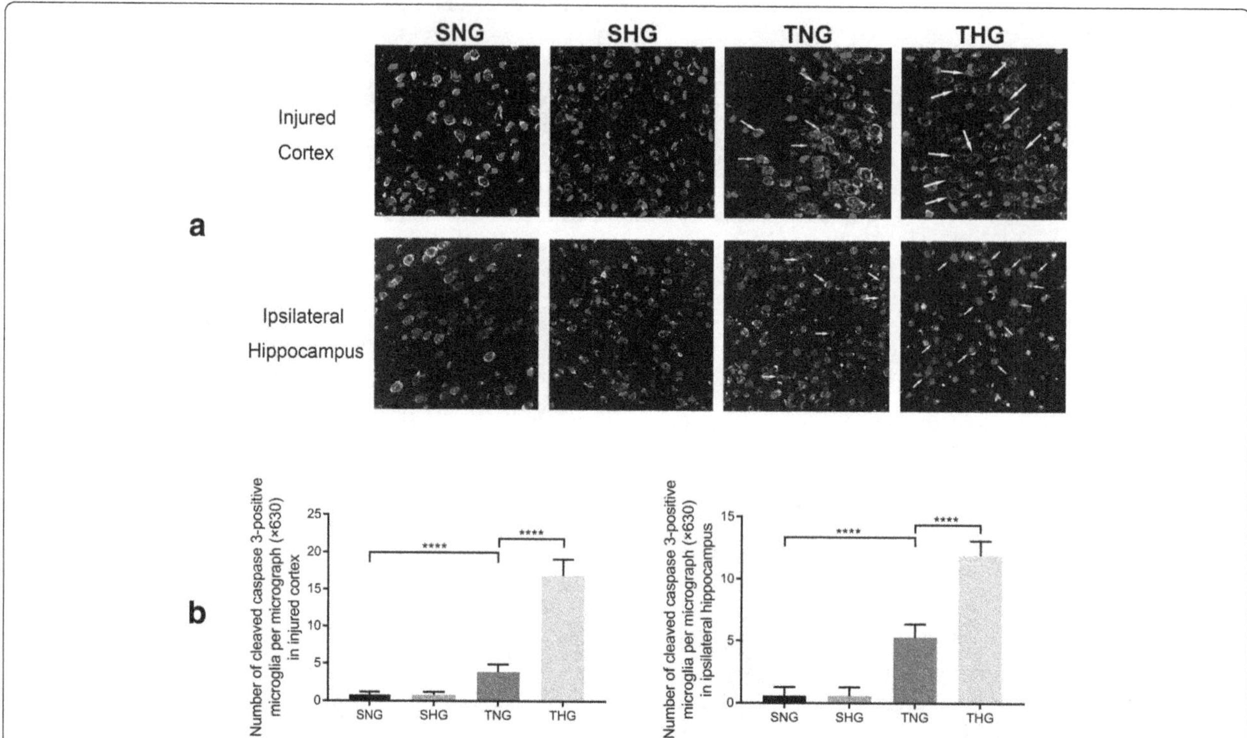

Fig. 7 Immunofluorescence analysis of cleaved caspase 3 (red) and Iba-1 (green) from the injured cortex and ipsilateral hippocampus. **a** Immunohistochemical staining of cleaved caspase 3 and Iba-1 from the injured cortex and ipsilateral hippocampus. Arrows indicate co-localization of cleaved caspase 3 and Iba-1 (magnification, ×630). **b** Number of cleaved caspase 3-positive microglia in the injured cortex and ipsilateral hippocampus. At least 10 randomly selected microscopic fields were used for counting. Data in the bar graphs represent mean ± SD. ****$P < 0.001$

biomarkers showed that microglial autophagy could be inhibited by moderate hypothermia.

From the above discussion, it can be stated that moderate hypothermia reduces the number of activated microglia. Moderate hypothermia inhibits autophagy and promotes apoptosis, which may be the possible mechanism. However, how moderate hypothermia specifically affects the autophagy and apoptosis of microglia post-TBI is not very clear. This issue needs further research.

In addition to reducing the number of activated microglia, the moderate hypothermia may also directly affect the microglial pro-inflammatory function. In the current study, we found that a moderate TBI induced by fluid percussion led to high expression of the inflammatory cytokines TNF-α and IL-1β. We also found that moderate hypothermia post-TBI could inhibit the expression of TLR4 and MyD88 and reduce the level of the inflammatory cytokines TNF-α and IL-1β after 24 h. This suggested that activated microglia might initiate neuroinflammatory responses post-TBI through the MyD88-dependent TLR4 pathway. Moderate hypothermia may reduce the release of inflammatory cytokines from activated microglia by inhibiting the MyD88-dependent TLR4 pathway.

Toll-like receptors play a role in microglial activation, and toll-like receptor-associated pathway mediates the release of pro-inflammatory cytokines [28]. TLR4 is the most abundant toll-like receptor expressed in microglia [10, 11]. TLR4 could activate IRAK and TRAF6 via the MyD88-dependent pathway. TRAF6 induces the activation of transforming growth factor-β-activated kinase 1, which leads to the activation of the mitogen-activated protein kinase and IκB kinase (IKK) cascades [29, 30]. When activated by these signals, IKK phosphorylates two serine residues located in an IκB regulatory domain, and the IκB proteins are ubiquitinated and degraded by proteasomes. After that, the NF-κB complex is freed to enter the nucleus, where it can further induce the expression of pro-inflammatory cytokines IL-6, TNF-α, IL-12, and so on [12, 13, 31, 32]. This current study demonstrated that moderate hypothermia might decrease the level of inflammatory cytokines by inhibiting the expression of relevant proteins in the MyD88-dependent TLR4 pathway.

Iba-1, also known as allograft inflammatory factor 1, is a 17-kDa EF-hand protein that is specifically expressed in macrophages/microglia and is upregulated during the activation of these cells. Ionized calcium-binding adapter molecule 1 (Iba1) expression is upregulated in microglia following nerve injury [33]. There is a constitutive expression of Iba-1 in microglial cells, but Iba-1 has also been regarded in several articles as an important biomarker to detect the activation of microglia [34–36]. After referring to these papers, we chose to detect the

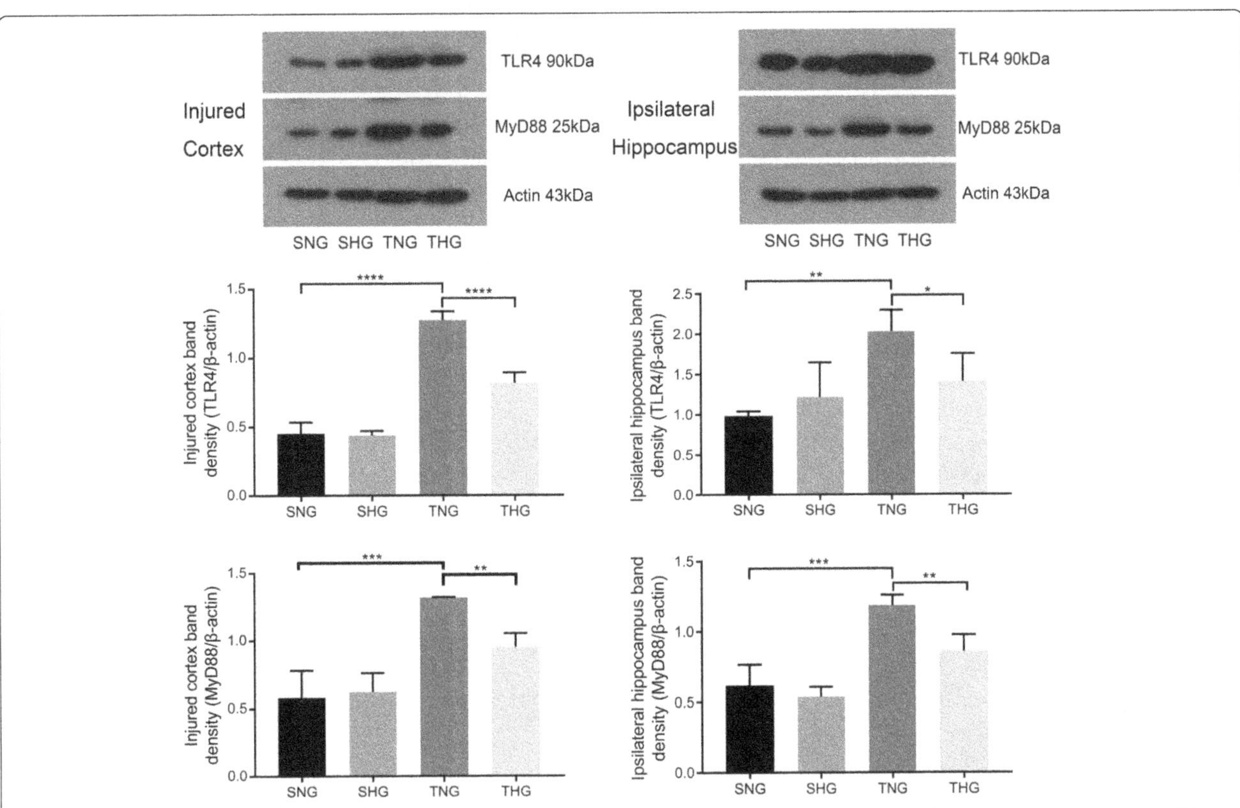

Fig. 8 Western blotting of TLR4 and MyD88 from the injured cortex and ipsilateral hippocampus. Data in the bar graphs represent mean ± SD. β-Actin was used as the load control. *$P < 0.05$; **$P < 0.01$; ***$P < 0.005$; ****$P < 0.001$

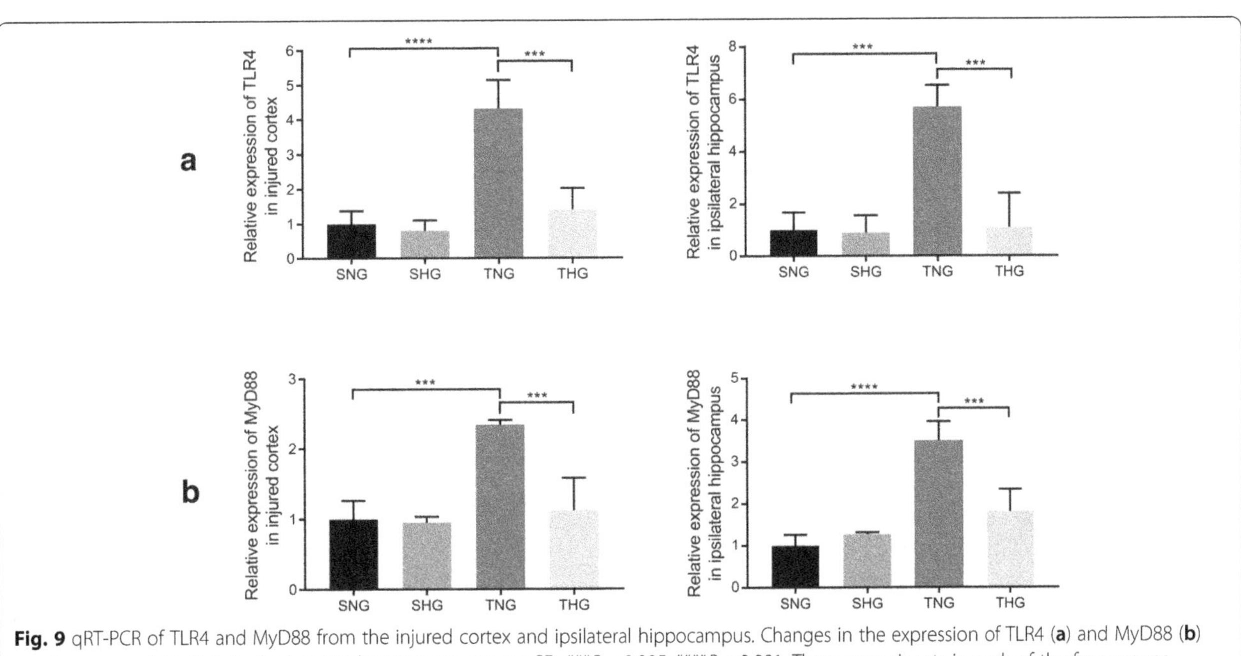

Fig. 9 qRT-PCR of TLR4 and MyD88 from the injured cortex and ipsilateral hippocampus. Changes in the expression of TLR4 (**a**) and MyD88 (**b**) are shown as *n*-fold. Data in the bar graphs represent mean ± SD. ***$P < 0.005$; ****$P < 0.001$. There were six rats in each of the four groups

expression level of Iba-1 for microglial activation by immunohistochemical staining and Western blotting. However, Iba-1 is not an ideal biomarker to distinguish microglial cells from macrophages. Other biomarkers, such as CD11b and CD68, are not of high specificity to microglia. The key to studying microglial activation after TBI is to figure out the immune subtypes of microglia. Therefore, we are planning to define the subtypes of macrophages/microglia post-TBI with a series of biomarkers in animal models in the future.

In previous studies, we estimated the role of autophagy and apoptosis in neuron and glial cells post-TBI, as well as the modulation of moderate hypothermia upon them. The term "glial cells" includes both macroglia and microglia. Macroglia, including oligodendrocytes, astrocytes, and ependymal cells, are derived from ectodermal tissues. However, microglia are derived from the earliest wave of mononuclear cells that originate in the yolk sac blood islands early in development. Microglia are resident immune cells in the central nervous system. In our opinion, microglia are distinct from macroglia, although they can be classified as glial cells. The current study is based on this opinion and extends the research that has taken place in the past. The effects of moderate hypothermia post-TBI are quite different between microglia and macroglia, which is our core concern. This study initially explored the changes in microglial autophagy and apoptosis after TBI and the regulation of hypothermia upon these processes. This study only draws preliminary conclusions.

The specific mechanism of moderate hypothermia on the TLR4 pathway of microglia post-TBI remains unclear. Logically, it would be necessary to inhibit or block the TLR4/MyD88 pathway to study the effects of hypothermia on microglial activation. But this pathway is quite important, and we are concerned that inhibition or knockout of this pathway may affect the survival rate of the experimental animals after TBI. Therefore, we are planning to establish an in vitro model of a cell stretch injury. We can then perform more efficient gene editing on microglia and study the specific mechanism of moderate hypothermia on the TLR4 pathway.

The negative correlation between autophagy and apoptosis has been widely observed in our past studies and in this study. The autophagy inhibitor 3-methyladenine (3-MA) was used after moderate hypothermia post-TBI in a previous report [9], and an increase of apoptosis was observed therewith. Therefore, we preliminarily speculated that there is a negative modulation between autophagy and apoptosis. We intend to establish in vitro or in vivo models of TBI in the future and perform moderate hypothermia on microglia with and without addition of 3-MA, to further investigate the effect of hypothermia on the pathological process of autophagy and apoptosis.

Conclusion

In the present study, microglial activation could be induced by TBI and moderate hypothermia could reduce the number of activated microglia by inhibiting autophagy and promoting apoptosis, probably through negative modulation between autophagy and apoptosis. In addition, moderate hypothermia may attenuate the pro-inflammatory function of microglia by inhibiting the MyD88-dependent TLR4 signaling pathway. This study preliminarily elucidates the possible molecular mechanism for participation of microglia in the neuroprotective effect of post-TBI moderate hypothermia and suggests new ideas for the investigation of efficacious neuroprotective methods. Further research is needed to deeply investigate the effect of moderate hypothermia on microglia after traumatic brain injury and the underlying molecular mechanism behind it.

Abbreviations

3-MA: 3-Methyladenine; ELISA: Enzyme-linked immunosorbent assay; HE: Hematoxylin and eosin; i.p.: Intraperitoneal injection; Iba1: Ionized calcium-binding adapter molecule 1; IKK: IκB kinase; IL-12: Interleukin 12; IL-1β: Interleukin 1β; IL-6: Interleukin 6; LC3: Protein light chain 3; MyD88: Myeloid differentiation primary response 88; NF-κB: Nuclear factor kappa light chain enhancer of activated B cells; OCT: Optimal cutting temperature compound; PBS: Phosphate-buffered saline; qRT-PCR: Quantitative real-time polymerase chain reaction; SD: Standard deviation; SDS: Sodium dodecylsulfate; SHG: Sham injury with hypothermia group; SNG: Sham injury with normothermia group; TBI: Traumatic brain injury; TBST: Tris-buffered saline and Tween-20; THG: TBI with hypothermia group; TLR4: Toll-like receptor 4; TNF-α: Tumor necrosis factor-α; TNG: TBI with normothermia group; TRAF6: Adaptor molecules TNF receptor-associated factor 6; Tris: Tris(hydroxymethyl)aminomethane

Acknowledgements

The authors thank Haiyang Gao and Yinyin Lin for the preparation and laboratory support, Jialin Huang for the experiment guidance, and the entire Neurosurgery Department for the critical discussions.

Funding

This work was supported by grants from the National Natural Science Foundation of China (No. 81601061 to Y. Jin and No. 81471333 to X. Zhang) and the Shanghai Youth Physician Training Assistance Scheme.

Authors' contributions

FZ and YJ designed the experiments. FZ and HD performed the majority of the experiments with the help of TL and KJ. FZ, HD, TL, and YJ performed the error analysis. XZ and JJ participated in the discussion about the results and in the manuscript preparation. YJ supervised the entire project and was responsible for finalizing and submitting the manuscript. All authors read and approved the final manuscript.

Consent for publication

Not applicable.

Competing interests

The authors declare that they have no competing interests.

Author details
[1]Department of Neurosurgery, Ren-Ji Hospital, School of Medicine, Shanghai Jiao Tong University, No. 160 Pujian Road, Shanghai 200127, People's Republic of China. [2]Department of Anesthesiology, Ren-Ji Hospital, School of Medicine, Shanghai Jiao Tong University, No. 160 Pujian Road, Shanghai 200127, People's Republic of China.

References

1. Lozano D, Gonzales-Portillo GS, Acosta S, de la Pena I, Tajiri N, Kaneko Y, Borlongan CV. Neuroinflammatory responses to traumatic brain injury: etiology, clinical consequences, and therapeutic opportunities. Neuropsychiatr Dis Treat. 2015;11:97–106.
2. Quintard H, Patet C, Suys T, Marques-Vidal P, Oddo M. Normobaric hyperoxia is associated with increased cerebral excitotoxicity after severe traumatic brain injury. Neurocrit Care. 2015;22(2):243–50.
3. Karve IP, Taylor JM, Crack PJ. The contribution of astrocytes and microglia to traumatic brain injury. Br J Pharmacol. 2016;173(4):692–702.
4. Liu CL, Chen S, Dietrich D, Hu BR. Changes in autophagy after traumatic brain injury. J Cereb Blood Flow Metab. 2008;28(4):674–83.
5. Luo CL, Li BX, Li QQ, Chen XP, Sun YX, Bao HJ, Dai DK, Shen YW, Xu HF, Ni H, et al. Autophagy is involved in traumatic brain injury-induced cell death and contributes to functional outcome deficits in mice. Neuroscience. 2011; 184:54–63.
6. Lipinski MM, Wu J, Faden AI, Sarkar C. Function and mechanisms of autophagy in brain and spinal cord trauma. Antioxid Redox Signal. 2015; 23(6):565–77.
7. Jin Y, Lin Y, Feng JF, Jia F, Gao GY, Jiang JY. Moderate hypothermia significantly decreases hippocampal cell death involving autophagy pathway after moderate traumatic brain injury. J Neurotrauma. 2015;32(14): 1090–100.
8. Jin Y, Lin Y, Feng JF, Jia F, Gao G, Jiang JY. Attenuation of cell death in injured cortex after post-traumatic brain injury moderate hypothermia: possible involvement of autophagy pathway. World Neurosurg. 2015;84(2):420–30.
9. Jin Y, Lei J, Lin Y, Gao GY, Jiang JY. Autophagy inhibitor 3-MA weakens neuroprotective effects of posttraumatic brain injury moderate hypothermia. World Neurosurg. 2016;88:433–46.
10. Bsibsi M, Ravid R, Gveric D, van Noort JM. Broad expression of Toll-like receptors in the human central nervous system. J Neuropathol Exp Neurol. 2002;61(11):1013–21.
11. Lehnardt S, Lachance C, Patrizi S, Lefebvre S, Follett PL, Jensen FE, Rosenberg PA, Volpe JJ, Vartanian T. The toll-like receptor TLR4 is necessary for lipopolysaccharide-induced oligodendrocyte injury in the CNS. J Neurosci. 2002;22(7):2478–86.
12. Kawai T, Akira S. Signaling to NF-kappaB by Toll-like receptors. Trends Mol Med. 2007;13(11):460–9.
13. Okun E, Griffioen KJ, Lathia JD, Tang SC, Mattson MP, Arumugam TV. Toll-like receptors in neurodegeneration. Brain Res Rev. 2009;59(2):278–92.
14. Jin Y, Wang R, Yang S, Zhang X, Dai J. Role of microglia autophagy in microglia activation after traumatic brain injury. World Neurosurg. 2017; 100:351–60.
15. Luo CL, Chen XP, Yang R, Sun YX, Li QQ, Bao HJ, Cao QQ, Ni H, Qin ZH, Tao LY. Cathepsin B contributes to traumatic brain injury-induced cell death through a mitochondria-mediated apoptotic pathway. J Neurosci Res. 2010; 88(13):2847–58.
16. Cui DM, Zeng T, Ren J, Wang K, Jin Y, Zhou L, Gao L. KLF4 knockdown attenuates TBI-induced neuronal damage through p53 and JAK-STAT3 signaling. CNS Neurosci Ther. 2017;23(2):106–18.
17. Xue Z, Song Z, Wan Y, Wang K, Mo L, Wang Y. Calcium-sensing receptor antagonist NPS2390 attenuates neuronal apoptosis though intrinsic pathway following traumatic brain injury in rats. Biochem Biophys Res Commun. 2017;486(2):589–94.
18. Zhang HB, Cheng SX, Tu Y, Zhang S, Hou SK, Yang Z. Protective effect of mild-induced hypothermia against moderate traumatic brain injury in rats involved in necroptotic and apoptotic pathways. Brain Inj. 2017; 31(3):406 15.
19. Slemmer JE, Zhu C, Landshamer S, Trabold R, Grohm J, Ardeshiri A, Wagner E, Sweeney MI, Blomgren K, Culmsee C, et al. Causal role of apoptosis-inducing factor for neuronal cell death following traumatic brain injury. Am J Pathol. 2008;173(6):1795–805.
20. Nakajima Y, Horiuchi Y, Kamata H, Yukawa M, Kuwabara M, Tsubokawa T. Distinct time courses of secondary brain damage in the hippocampus following brain concussion and contusion in rats. Tohoku J Exp Med. 2010; 221(3):229–35.
21. Flygt J, Gumucio A, Ingelsson M, Skoglund K, Holm J, Alafuzoff I, Marklund N. Human traumatic brain injury results in oligodendrocyte death and increases the number of oligodendrocyte progenitor cells. J Neuropathol Exp Neurol. 2016;75(6):503–15.
22. Yang H, Gu ZT, Li L, Maegele M, Zhou BY, Li F, Zhao M, Zhao KS. SIRT1 plays a neuroprotective role in traumatic brain injury in rats via inhibiting the p38 MAPK pathway. Acta Pharmacol Sin. 2017;38(2):168–81.
23. Huang CY, Lee YC, Li PC, Liliang PC, Lu K, Wang KW, Chang LC, Shiu LY, Chen MF, Sun YT, et al. TDP-43 proteolysis is associated with astrocyte reactivity after traumatic brain injury in rodents. J Neuroimmunol. 2017;313:61–8.
24. Clark RSB, Bayir H, Chu CT, Alber SM, Kochanek PM, Watkins SC. Autophagy is increased in mice after traumatic brain injury and is detectable in human brain after trauma and critical illness. Autophagy. 2008;4(1):88–90.
25. Yoshii SR, Mizushima N. Monitoring and measuring autophagy. Int J Mol Sci. 2017;18(9):1865.
26. Diskin T, Tal-Or P, Erlich S, Mizrachy L, Alexandrovich A, Shohami E, Pinkas-Kramarski R. Closed head injury induces upregulation of Beclin 1 at the cortical site of injury. J Neurotrauma. 2005;22(7):750–62.
27. Viscomi MT, D'Amelio M, Cavallucci V, Latini L, Bisicchia E, Nazio F, Fanelli F, Maccarrone M, Moreno S, Cecconi F, et al. Stimulation of autophagy by rapamycin protects neurons from remote degeneration after acute focal brain damage. Autophagy. 2012;8(2):222–35.
28. Olson JK, Miller SD. Microglia initiate central nervous system innate and adaptive immune responses through multiple TLRs. J Immunol. 2004;173(6):3916–24.
29. Palsson-McDermott EM, O'Neill LAJ. Signal transduction by the lipopolysaccharide receptor, Toll-like receptor-4. Immunology. 2004;113(2): 153–62.
30. Lu YC, Yeh WC, Ohashi PS. LPS/TLR4 signal transduction pathway. Cytokine. 2008;42(2):145–51.
31. Deptala A, Bedner E, Gorczyca W, Darzynkiewicz Z. Activation of nuclear factor kappa B (NF-kappaB) assayed by laser scanning cytometry (LSC). Cytometry. 1998;33(3):376–82.
32. Basak S, Shih VFS, Hoffmann A. Generation and activation of multiple dimeric transcription factors within the NF-kappa B signaling system. Mol Cell Biol. 2008;28(10):3139–50.
33. Ito D, Imai Y, Ohsawa K, Nakajima K, Fukuuchi Y, Kohsaka S. Microglia-specific localisation of a novel calcium binding protein, Iba1. Mol Brain Res. 1998;57(1):1–9.
34. Beschorner R, Engel S, Mittelbronn M, Adjodah D, Dietz K, Schluesener HJ, Meyermann R. Differential regulation of the monocytic calcium-binding peptides macrophage-inhibiting factor related protein-8 (MRP8/S100A8) and allograft inflammatory factor-1 (AIF-1) following human traumatic brain injury. Acta Neuropathol. 2000;100(6):627–34.
35. Schwab JM, Frei E, Klusman I, Schnell L, Schwab ME, Schluesener HJ. AIF-1 expression defines a proliferating and alert microglial/macrophage phenotype following spinal cord injury in rats. J Neuroimmunol. 2001;119(2):214–22.
36. Schluesener HJ, Seid K, Kretzschmar J, Meyermann R. Allograft-inflammatory factor-1 in rat experimental autoimmune encephalomyelitis, neuritis, and uveitis: expression by activated macrophages and microglial cells. Glia. 1998;24(2):244–51.

10

Cortisol-induced immune suppression by a blockade of lymphocyte egress in traumatic brain injury

Tingting Dong, Liang Zhi, Brijesh Bhayana and Mei X. Wu*

Abstract

Background: Acute traumatic brain injury (TBI) represents one of major causes of mortality and disability in the USA. Neuroinflammation has been regarded both beneficial and detrimental, probably in a time-dependent fashion.

Methods: To address a role for neuroinflammation in brain injury, C57BL/6 mice were subjected to a closed head mild TBI (mTBI) by a standard controlled cortical impact, along with or without treatment of sphingosine 1-phosphate (S1P) or rolipram, after which the brain tissue of the impact site was evaluated for cell morphology via histology, inflammation by qRT-PCR and T cell staining, and cell death with Caspase-3 and TUNEL staining. Circulating lymphocytes were quantified by flow cytometry, and plasma hydrocortisone was analyzed by LC-MS/MS. To investigate the mechanism whereby cortisol lowered the number of peripheral T cells, T cell egress was tracked in lymph nodes by intravital confocal microscopy after hydrocortisone administration.

Results: We detected a decreased number of circulating lymphocytes, in particular, T cells soon after mTBI, which was inversely correlated with a transient and robust increase of plasma cortisol. The transient lymphocytopenia might be caused by cortisol in part via a blockade of lymphocyte egress as demonstrated by the ability of cortisol to inhibit T cell egress from the secondary lymphoid tissues. Moreover, exogenous hydrocortisone severely suppressed periphery lymphocytes in uninjured mice, whereas administering an egress-promoting agent S1P normalized circulating T cells in mTBI mice and increased T cells in the injured brain. Likewise, rolipram, a cAMP phosphodiesterase inhibitor, was also able to elevate cAMP levels in T cells in the presence of hydrocortisone in vitro and abrogate the action of cortisol in mTBI mice. The investigation demonstrated that the number of circulating T cells in the early phase of TBI was positively correlated with T cell infiltration and inflammatory responses as well as cell death at the cerebral cortex and hippocampus beneath the impact site.

Conclusions: Decreases in intracellular cAMP might be part of the mechanism behind cortisol-mediated blockade of T cell egress. The study argues strongly for a protective role of cortisol-induced immune suppression in the early stage of TBI.

Keywords: TBI, T lymphocytes, Cortisol, Inflammation, cAMP

Abbreviations: TBI, Traumatic brain injury; mTBI, Mild traumatic brain injury; S1P, Sphingosine 1-phosphate; LC-MS/MS, Liquid chromatography-tandem mass spectrometry; cAMP, Cyclic adenosine monophosphate; IL-1α, Interleukin-1-alpha; IL6, Interleukin-6; TNF-α, Tumor necrosis factor-alpha; BBB, Blood-brain barrier; NSS, Neurological severity score; ACK, Ammonium-chloride-potassium; HCl, Hydrochloric acid; BSA, Bovine serum albumin; H&E, Hematoxylin and eosin; DAPI, 4′, 6′-diamidino-2 phenylindole; PBS, Phosphate-buffered saline; qRT-PCR, Quantitative reverse-transcription

(Continued on next page)

* Correspondence: mwu5@mgh.harvard.edu
Wellman Center for Photomedicine, Massachusetts General Hospital, Department of Dermatology, Harvard Medical School, 50 Blossom Street, Boston, MA 02114, USA

(Continued from previous page)
polymerase chain reaction; TUNEL, Terminal deoxynucleotidyl transferase dUTP nick end labeling; CMTMR, 5-(and-6)-(((4-chloromethyl) benzoyl) amino) tetramethylrhodamine; PMT, Photomultiplier tubes; SEM, Standard errors of measurement; HC, Hydrocortisone; PI, Propidium iodide; IL-1β, Interleukin-1-beta; CCL2, Chemokine (C-C motif) ligand 2; CXCL10, C-X-C motif chemokine 10; ICAM-1, Intercellular adhesion molecule 1; PDE4, Phosphodiesterase

Background

Acute traumatic brain injury (TBI) is a major cause of mortality and disability in the early decades of life in many developed countries. At least 5.3 million people in the USA currently require long-term or life-long assistance with the activities of daily living after TBI [1]. TBI results in cerebral structural damage and functional deficits due to both primary and secondary injury. The primary injury is caused directly by the external mechanical force at the moment of trauma leading to skull fractures, brain contusions, lacerations, diffused axonal injuries, vascular tearing, intracranial hemorrhages, etc. The primary injury is followed by development of secondary neuronal damage that evolves over a period of months [2], thereby providing a golden opportunity for prevention and intervention. Tremendous efforts have been made in the past decades toward exploring the cellular and molecular mechanisms underlying secondary brain damage as well as identification of specific targets for prevention and/or therapeutics against this disorder [2]. It is now believed that a cascade of molecular, neurochemical, neuronal cell apoptosis, cellular, and immune processes contribute to secondary brain damage as a consequence of mitochondrial dysfunction, cerebral hypoxia, and disruption of calcium homeostasis in cells at the impact site [2, 3].

A growing body of evidence indicates that inflammation induced by primary brain injury plays dual and opposite roles in the outcome of TBI [4]. On one hand, it contributes to reparation and regeneration processes of the primary brain injury, for instance, clearance of necrotic and apoptotic cells by phagocytic cells and promoting neuron growth at the injured site [5, 6]. On the other hand, it facilitates secondary brain injury via the production of various inflammatory cytokines such as interleukin-1-alpha (IL-1α) and interleukin-1-β (IL-1β), tumor necrosis factor alpha (TNF-α), and interleukin-6 (IL-6) [7, 8]. The brain is well known to be an immune privilege site, and infiltration of inflammatory cells to it is largely restricted by the blood-brain barrier (BBB) under a physiological condition [9]. However, TBI often results in an invasion of neutrophils, monocytes, and lymphocytes from the periphery and activation of microglia due to disruption of the BBB. This initiates a cascade of inflammatory responses [10]. Likewise, T lymphocytes have been shown to infiltrate the brain parenchyma post-injury, but their role in the secondary brain injury development following TBI remains poorly understood [11].

Both pre-clinical and clinical studies have shown significant, acute increases of cortisol levels in serum and cerebrospinal fluid in response to TBI [12, 13]. The increased cortisol might suppress inflammation in the brain in order to protect the injured brain tissues from inflammation insult, in light of the well-documented anti-inflammatory function of cortisol, a steroid hormone. The current investigation revealed that an elevated level of serum cortisol was inversely correlated with the number of peripheral lymphocytes, in particular, T cells following brain trauma. Cortisol appeared to sequester lymphocytes in the secondary lymphoid tissues by blocking their egress, contributing to reduced inflammation and cell death at injured brain tissues. The study sheds novel insight into the mechanism underlying cortisol-mediated suppression of inflammation and protective roles of cortisol in TBI at the early stage.

Methods

Animals

Eight-week-old female C57BL/6 mice were purchased from Charles River Laboratories and maintained in a 12-h light/dark cycle. All animal experiments were approved by the Institutional Animal Care and Use Committee (IACUC) of the Massachusetts General Hospital and performed according to the National Institutes of Health guidelines for the Care and Use of Laboratory Animals.

TBI induction

Mice were subjected to a closed head TBI by a standard controlled cortical impact on the left lateral with intact skull and scalp as previously described [7, 14]. In brief, the mice were anesthetized with isoflurane and placed on a mobile plate with their hair removed from the head. A flat face 2-mm diameter tip of the pneumatic impact device (AMS 201, AmScien Instruments, Richmond, VA) was positioned on the left hemisphere center, lowered gradually down to touch the scalp, and recorded as zero depth (sham control). The punch depth was then set 2 mm using a screw-mounted adjustment. A 4.9 ± 0.2 m/s velocity and 80 ms contact time were specified by setting 150 pounds per square inch (psi) for a high pressure and 30 psi for a low pressure impact. These parameters were selected to yield a trauma giving rise to a neurological severity score (NSS) of 3–5 at 1 h post-TBI also called mild TBI (mTBI). After recovery from anesthesia, the mice were returned to cages with post-operative care.

Quantification of circulating lymphocytes

Blood samples were collected from tail vein in 1 and 4 h after TBI to assess plasma cortisol and circulating lymphocytes or 4 h after hydrocortisone injection (Sigma, 10 mg/kg) to confirm suppressive effects of cortisol on peripheral leukocytes. In separate groups of mice, TBI was induced as above, immediately followed with i.p. injection of either sphingosine 1-phosphate (S1P) (Enzo Life Sciences, 5 μM/kg) or rolipram (Sigma, 30 μM/kg), and blood samples were collected 1 h later. Cells were pelleted, suspended, and treated with ammonium-chloride-potassium (ACK) buffer to lyse erythrocytes. The cells were then counted and stained with PE-anti-CD3 antibody for T cells, APC-anti-CD19 antibody for B cells, FITC-anti-Ly6G antibody for neutrophils, or PE-Cy7-anti-F4/80 antibody for monocytes, followed by flow cytometry analysis on BD FACSAria.

Quantification of plasma cortisol by liquid chromatography-tandem mass spectrometry (LC-MS/MS)

Quantitative analysis of hydrocortisone in serum samples was performed on an LC-MS/MS instrument. Fludrocortisone acetate was used as a reference standard; known amounts of this compound were added to the serum extract prior to the LC injections. The following working parameters were used for the LC-MS/MS analysis: scan type, MRM (363 → 121 transition for hydrocortisone and 423 → 239 transition for fludrocortisone acetate); polarity, positive; ionization, ESI; column, C18, 2.1 × 50 mm, 1.8 μm; gradient, solution A = acetonitrile, solution B = 10 mM ammonium acetate in water, 20 → 100 % of A over 5 min with a flow rate of 0.4 ml/min.

Intravital imaging of T cell egress in lymph nodes

T cells were isolated from lymph nodes and spleens of normal C57BL/6 mice and treated with a mixture of rat anti-mouse monoclonal antibodies against CD19, CD32, and CD16 followed by depletion of antibody-bound cells with BioMag goat anti-rat IgG (Polysciences Inc., Warrington, PA) as previously described [15]. The purified T cells were stained with 20 μM 5-(and-6)-(((4-chloromethyl) benzoyl) amino) tetramethylrhodamine (CMTMR, Invitrogen) for 20 min at 37 °C. The labeled cells were adoptively transferred to cognate C57BL/6 mice by tail intravenous injection of 1×10^7 cells per mouse. The recipient mice were then subcutaneously injected with 15 μg anti-LYVE-1 Ab (R&D Systems) conjugated with Alexa Fluor-647 (monoclonal antibody labeling kit, Invitrogen) in a hind footpad, followed by i.p. injection with 10 mg/kg of hydrocortisone or saline 16 h later. After 2 h of hydrocortisone injection, the mouse was anesthetized and placed on an electrically heated plate to maintain the temperature at 36 °C and had their popliteal lymph nodes exposed by a small skin incision. The lymph node to be imaged was bathed with a continuous flow of warm saline in order to maintain a local temperature at 36 °C during imaging. Intravital imaging of the lymph node was performed using a home-built microscope and the images were acquired using an in-house developed software [16]. The in vivo confocal microscope was equipped with three photomultiplier tubes (PMT, Hamamatsu, R9110) which were optimized to provide bright images with a high contrast. Each x-y plane spanned 250 × 250 μm at a resolution of 2 pixels per μm. Stacks of images were acquired with a z-axis resolution of 3 μm per section, and time-series images were obtained in a 20-s interval. To determine whether a cell was inside, outside, or on the border of a cortical sinus, its location relative to the sinusoid wall was assessed in the x-y and/or the z plane. The moving distances and velocities of the tacking cells were tracked for each video segment and calculated using ImageJ software.

Transwell assay for cell migration

T cell migration was analyzed in 48-well micro chemotaxis chamber (Neuro Probe) as previously described [17]. T cells isolated from normal C57BL/6 mice as above were suspended at 1×10^5 cells in 100 μl in RPMI medium supplemented with 3 % fetal bovine serum (charcoal stripped), 2 mM L-glutamine, 100 U/ml penicillin, 100 μg/ml streptomycin, and 20 μM of either hydrocortisone or vehicle followed by adding the cells to the upper chamber of the transwell. S1P at 20 nM or vehicle was prepared in the same medium and added to the lower chamber of the transwell. Migration was performed for 4 h at 37 °C in a humidified 5 % CO_2 incubator. The number of migrated cells was determined by counting the cells in the lower chamber.

S1P administration

S1P (Enzo Life Sciences) was prepared according to the manufacturer's instructions. Briefly, S1P was dissolved in methanol (0.5 mg/ml) and aliquoted, followed by evaporation of the solvent under a stream of nitrogen to deposit a thin film on the inside of the tube. Prior to use, the aliquots were resuspended in PBS with 4 mg/ml bovine serum albumin (BSA) to a final concentration of S1P at 500 μM. The S1P or the vehicle was i.p. injected into the mice at a dosage of 200 μl per mouse immediately after TBI.

Measurement of intracellular cAMP

T cells (2×10^6/ml) freshly isolated from normal C57BL/6 mice were incubated at 37 °C in serum free Aim V medium (Invitrogen) and pretreated with 10 μM rolipram (Sigma) or saline for 15 min, followed by a treatment with 100 μM hydrocortisone or vehicle at 37 °C for 5 min. Intracellular cAMP was extracted with hydrochloric acid (HCl) and measured using a cAMP EIA kit following the manufacturer's instruction (Assay Designs).

Real-time quantitative reverse transcription polymerase chain reaction (qRT-PCR)

Total RNA was extracted from mouse cortex beneath the impact site 3 days after indicated treatments. The RNA was reverse transcribed with a high capacity RNA-to-cDNA kit (Applied Biosystems, Foster City, CA, USA) and amplified by qRT-PCR) in Roche Lightcycler 480 with a SYBR Green I Master kit (Roche Diagnostics, Indianapolis, IN, USA). The PCR program was preincubation at 95 °C, 5 min, followed by 45 cycles of 95 °C, 10 s, 60 °C, 10 s, and 72 °C, 10 s. The relative levels of each target gene were normalized to endogenous β-actin and calculated using comparative Ct method (ΔΔCt method) [18]. The primer sequences used were 5′-GAA GAGCCCATCCTCTGTGA-3′ (forward) and 5′-TTCA TCTCGGAGCCTGTAGTG-3′ (reverse) for IL-1β; 5′-G GCTCAGCCAGATGCAGTTAA-3′ (forward) and 5′-C CTACTCATTGGGATCATCTTGT-3′ (reverse) for CCL 2; 5′- GCCGTCATTTTCTGCCTCA-3′ (forward) and 5′-CGTCCTTGCGAGAGGGATC-3′ (reverse) for CXCL 10; 5′- GGGCTGGCATTGTTCTCTAATGTC-3′ (forward) and 5′-GGATGGTAGCTGGAAGATCGAAAG-3′ (reverse) for ICAM-1; 5′-GTCTACTGAACTTCGGGGT GAT-3′ (forward) and 5′-ATGATCTGAGTGTGAGGGT CTG-3′ (reverse) for TNF-α; and 5′-CGAGGCCCAGAG CAAGAGAG-3′ (forward) and 5′-CGGTTGGCCTTAG GGTTCAG-3′ (reverse) for β-actin.

Histological examination

Mice were anesthetized and fixed by cardiac perfusion with cold PBS followed by 10 % formalin. Brains were carefully removed, fixed overnight in 10 % formalin, and subjected to histopathological processing and analysis. Hematoxylin and eosin (H&E)-stained sections of 5-μm-thickness were scanned by Nanozoomer Slide Scanner (Olympus America, Center Valley, PA).

Immunofluorescence assays

Acetone-fixed tissue sections were incubated with a blocking buffer (3 % BSA, 10 % goat serum and 0.4 % Triton X-100 in PBS) for 1 h at room temperature, followed with primary antibody diluted in the blocking buffer at 4 °C overnight. After reaction with a secondary antibody for 2 h at room temperature and washing, the slides were mounted with DAPI (4′, 6′-diamidino-2 phenylindole)-containing mounting medium (Invitrogen, USA). The primary antibody was rabbit anti-Caspase-3 (active) antibody at a 1:100 dilution (Millipore, USA) and rat anti-CD3 antibody at a 1:100 dilution (BioLegend, USA). TUNEL staining was carried out by an ApopTag® Fluorescein In Situ Apoptosis Detection Kit (Millipore, USA). Images were captured using a confocal microscope (Olympus FV1000, Olympus, Japan). Percentages of Caspase-3+ cells were determined by the number of Caspase-3^+ cells relatively to DAPI$^+$ cells in each field of the 20 randomly selected views of hippocampus area, which represented a total of ten sections from five injured brains in each group. Optical density of TUNEL staining was also calculated in 20 randomly selected views from a total of ten sections from five injured brains in each group by ImageJ software.

Statistical analysis

The data are presented as mean ± standard errors of measurement (SEM). The statistical analysis was performed using the non-parametric Mann-Whitney *t* test for comparison between two groups and one-way ANOVA or two-way ANOVA for comparison among multiple groups by the Graphpad Prism 6.0 software (GraphPad Software, CA, USA). A value of $P < 0.05$ was considered statistically significant.

Results

Elevation of cortisol but reduction of circulating lymphocytes following TBI

Our previous study showed that introduction of inflammation worsened secondary brain damage following mTBI [7]. The mTBI was created by a gentle hit of the brain with an intact skull and scalp by a standard controlled impact, which resulted in extensive cell death at the impact site and significant neurologic severity score (NSS) ranging from 3 to 5 [7]. However, the abnormality was fully recovered functionally and histologically in 4 weeks [7], resembling the majority of mTBI in humans [7]. To determine contributing factors to the full recovery of mTBI, we measured plasma cortisol and found that this steroid hormone rose sharply 1 h post-TBI and declined thereafter (Fig. 1a), similar to what has been reported in patients suffering from traumatic injury or after surgery [12, 13]. In parallel to the elevated level of plasma cortisol was a transient but significantly diminished number of peripheral lymphocytes, with a 42 % decrease in 1 h after injury and a 20 % decrease in 4 h as compared to control mice (Fig. 1b). The decrease appeared to be more predominant in T cells than in B cells, with a 53 % decrease of T cells (Fig. 1c) compared to only a 28 % decrease of B cells (Fig. 1d) at 1 h post-injury. There were no significant differences in the

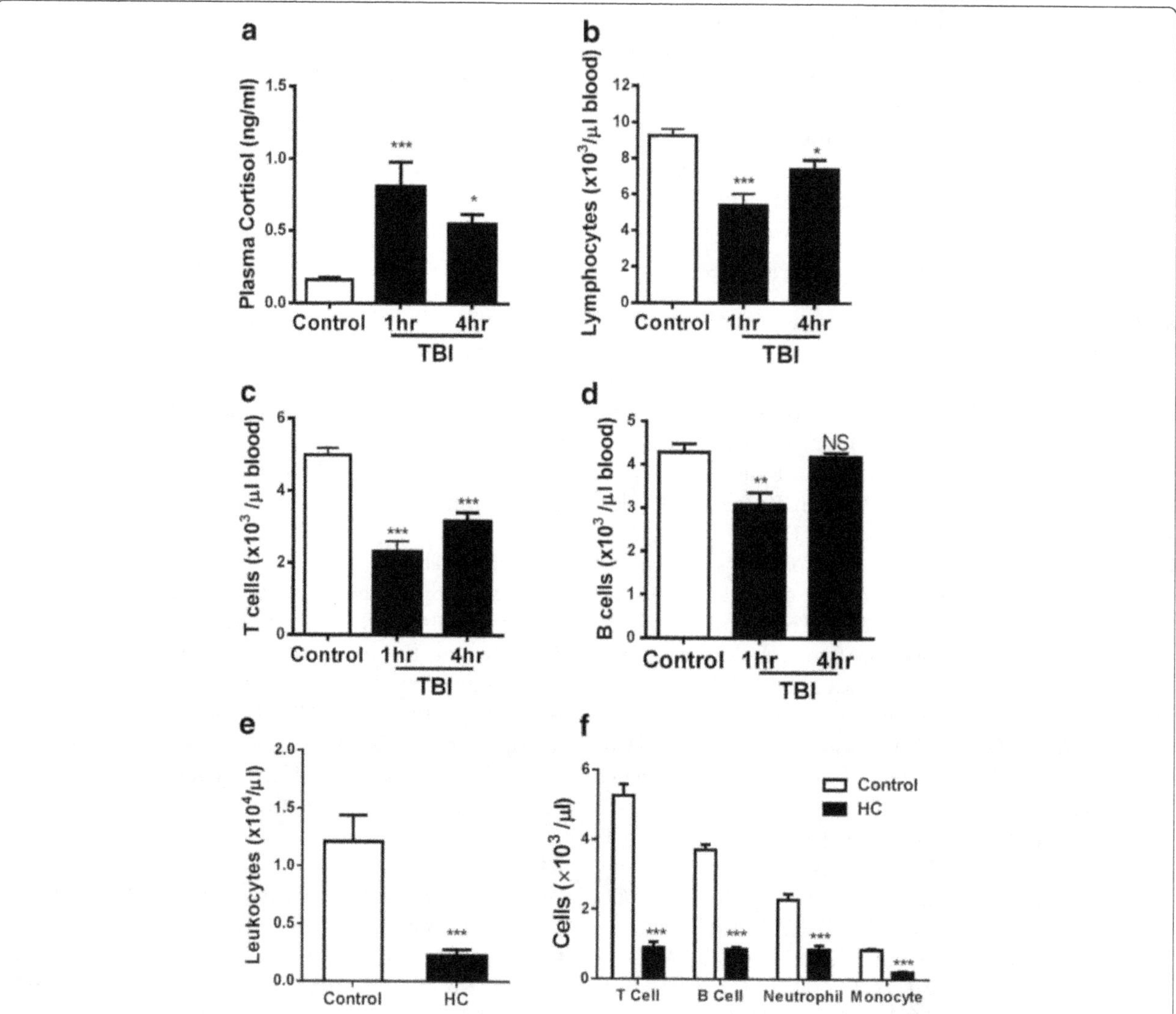

Fig. 1 Inverse relationship between cortisol and lymphocytes in blood following TBI. **a** Plasma cortisol was quantified before and 1 and 4 h after TBI. In parallel, the numbers of peripheral lymphocytes (**b**), T cells (**c**), and B cells (**d**) were analyzed at the same time points. A total number of leukocytes (**e**) or indicated cells (**f**) were measured in blood by flow cytometry 4 h after i.p. injection of 10 mg/kg hydrocortisone. Data are expressed as means ± SEM. $n = 5$ in (**a**) or 6 in (**b**, **c**, **d**, **e**, **f**). Significance was determined using one-way ANOVA (**a**, **b**, **c**, **d**) or non-parametric Mann-Whitney *t* test (**e**, **f**). $^{*}P < 0.05$, $^{**}P < 0.01$, $^{***}P < 0.001$, and NS, no significance compared before and after TBI or HC treatment. The experiment was repeated three times with similar results

number of circulating monocytes and neutrophils compared to controls at these time points examined. The finding that transient lymphocytopenia is inversely correlated with the amount of plasma cortisol in the animals is consistent with the well-documented immune suppression of cortisol [19].

Exogenous hydrocortisone depresses the number of leukocytes in the periphery

The inverse correlation between plasma cortisol and the number of circulating lymphocytes following mTBI raised an intriguing possibility that plasma cortisol might be directly responsible for TBI-induced lymphocytopenia. To determine this, mice were intraperitoneally administered hydrocortisone at a dose of 10 mg/kg followed by enumeration of circulating leukocytes. As shown in Fig. 1e, exogenous hydrocortisone reduced the number of leukocytes by 81 % in the periphery over the control mice in 4 h after administration. The reduction was most profound in T cells followed by B cells, neutrophils, and monocytes, all of which are key cellular components in the inflammatory cascade (Fig. 1f). These results corroborate that the reduced number of peripheral lymphocytes is ascribed directly to an elevated level of endogenous cortisol triggered by TBI.

Hydrocortisone blocks T cell egress from the cortical sinus in lymph nodes

Although cortisol is well known as a suppressant of inflammation, the underlying mechanism is not fully understood. Previous studies with ^{51}Cr-labeled lymphocytes suggested that a decrease in egress of lymphocytes, rather than increased homing or cell death, was the mechanism for the lymphopenia induced by traumatic stress [20]. In support of this, flow cytometric analysis of peripheral T and B cells after propidium iodide (PI) staining did not reveal any significant difference in cell death in the mice (data not shown). We questioned whether cortisol blocked lymphocyte egress, lowering the number of peripheral lymphocytes as did immune suppression drug FTY720, an analog of S1P [15, 21, 22]. We thus tracked T cell egress in part because T cells were key contributors to the acute phase of brain injury [23] and the cells appeared to be more affected by cortisol. To this end, purified naive T cells were labeled with a red vital fluorescent dye CMTMR and infused into cognate mice followed by subcutaneous injection of LYVE-1 antibody to mark lymphatic vessels. The cortical sinusoid region in and adjacent to T cell zones of the popliteal lymph node was imaged 2 h later after hydrocortisone injection by intravital confocal microscopy as we previously described [15]. As can be seen in Fig. 3a, the number of T cells was severely reduced within the cortical sinusoid in the presence compared to the absence of hydrocortisone (Fig. 2a). Consistent with this, when tracking 200 cells in 10~15 randomly selected imaging stacks, we found that the frequency of T cells entering cortical sinusoids diminished to 15 from 45 % in the presence compared to the absence of hydrocortisone (Fig. 2b). On the contrary, T cells moving away from the sinusoids increased from 40 to 75 % in the mice (Fig. 2c). It can be envisioned that as a majority of T cells are moving away from the sinusoids, their egress could be largely prevented, explaining only few T cells within the sinusoids (Fig. 2a) and a reduced number of T cells in the periphery (Fig. 1f). Cortisol also reduced the ability of T cells to adhere on the sinusoids (Fig. 2e), in a good agreement with a low entry frequency (Fig. 2b), because T cell sticking to the sinusoid facilitated entry of the cell into a sinusoid [15]. During T cell egress, T cells continuously move toward and crawl along the sinusoid to search for a "hot entry port" and upon finding the "port," the cell enters the sinusoid via it [24, 25], but many of them move away from the sinusoid prior to reaching it or after several attempts to associate with or adhere on the sinusoids [15, 26]. Hydrocortisone appeared not to affect the number of T cells that crawled on the sinusoids (Fig. 2d) but greatly increased the number of T cells moving away the sinusoids (Fig. 2c).

S1P or rolipram increases the number of peripheral T cells after TBI

We went on to determine whether a high level of S1P, an egress-promoting agent, could override cortisol-mediated blockade of T cell egress. We first assessed T cell migration toward S1P in the presence or absence of hydrocortisone in vitro, an assay that is commonly used for assessing S1P function [27]. T cells, along with hydrocortisone or vehicle, were added to the upper chamber and S1P or vehicle was included in the lower chamber of the transwell. As can be seen in Fig. 3a, S1P significantly increased migration of T cells into the lower chamber in the presence or absence of hydrocortisone, suggesting that a high level of S1P may overcome the inhibitory effect of hydrocortisone and restore the number of circulating T cells in mice with mTBI. Indeed, when mice were i.p. administered S1P immediately after TBI, the number of T cells was completely normalized in the blood 1 h post-S1P injection in TBI mice (Fig. 3c). In light of a well-established role for S1P in egress of lymphocytes, the result corroborates the ability of cortisol to block T cell egress, leading to a diminished number of lymphocytes in circulation immediately after mTBI. Moreover, the result also confirmed the ability of hydrocortisone to vigorously blunt T cell migration in the presence or absence of S1P (Fig. 3a), implicating that cortisol hampered T cell egress via an intrinsic signaling pathway of T cells, probably via regulation of cAMP degradation, a key secondary messenger molecule signaling downstream of the $S1P_1$ receptor as depicted in Fig. 6. Our previous investigation showed that FTY720 blocked T cell egress by persistent activation of heterotrimeric Gαi proteins leading to prolonged inhibition of cAMP production, apart from induction of $S1P_1$ receptor internalization [15]. We therefore measured cAMP after hydrocortisone treatment and found that hydrocortisone lowered cAMP levels significantly (Fig. 3b). The low level of cAMP induced by hydrocortisone was reversed by rolipram (Fig. 3b), a cAMP phosphodiesterase inhibitor that prevents cAMP degradation, corroborating an antagonistic effect of rolipram on cortisol-mediated reduction of cAMP, probably via the same target or the same signaling pathway as illustrated in Fig. 6. In support, i.p. injection of rolipram immediately after mTBI also significantly increased the number of T cells in the periphery, albeit to a much lesser degree in comparison with S1P (Fig. 3c). The results clearly suggest that hydrocortisone blocks T cell egress via a downstream target of the $S1P_1$ receptor.

A protective role for cortisol in TBI pathogenesis

We next verified positive correlations of circulating lymphocytes with inflammation occurring at the impact site of the brain and directly associated the low inflammation at the injured site with cortisol-mediated blockade of lymphocyte egress in mTBI mice. To this end, several inflammatory mediators, including IL-1β, CCL2, CXCL10, ICAM-1, and TNF-α, were assayed by qRT-

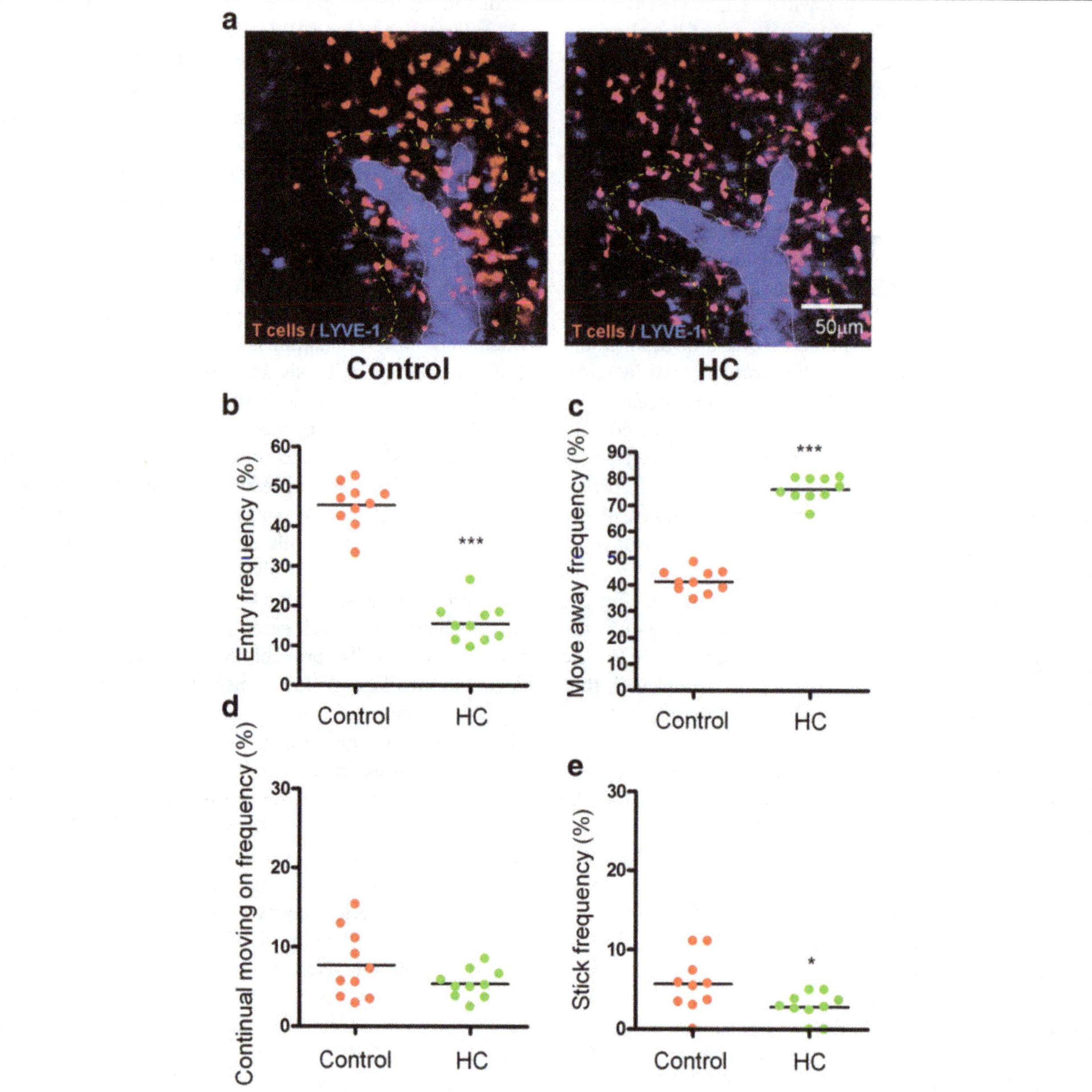

Fig. 2 T cell egress is blocked by hydrocortisone. The representative images taken from control or hydrocortisone (HC)-treated mice are shown in (**a**). LYVE-1$^+$ cortical sinuses are shown in *blue* pseudocolor in order to distinguish them with CMTMR labeled T cells (*red*) and the representative sinus area is delineated by a *dotted white line*. The *dotted yellow line* outlines the area within 30 μm of distance from the outer boundaries of cortical sinuses. Note: few T cells within cortical sinus in the presence of HC. *Scale bar*, 50 μm. Frequencies at which T cells entered (**b**), moved away (**c**), crawled on (**d**), or stuck to (**e**) (kept adhering to one point on the sinus wall and never displaced during the imaging period after they engaged the sinus) the cortical sinuses in control and HC-treated mice were calculated by manually tracking individual cells in each time-lapse image, with a total of 200 cells randomly selected in 10~15 imaging stacks. Each *dot* represents data from a single time-lapse image, and *bars* represent the means. Significance was measured using non-parametric Mann-Whitney *t* test. $*P < 0.05$, $***P < 0.001$ in the presence or absence of hydrocortisone. Data are combined from two independent experiments each with two lymph nodes imaged in each treatment. The experiment was repeated two times with similar results

PCR at the impact site 3 days after mTBI in the presence or absence of SIP or rolipram [7]. Our previous study showed that mTBI up regulated proinflammatory mediators at 6 h and dwindled down gradually [7]. Consistent with this, transcription levels of these proinflammatory mediators in the mice were not significantly different from controls (Fig. 4). In contrast, S1P robustly bolstered all five inflammatory mediators at the impact sites, confirming a positive relationship between the number of circulating lymphocytes and inflammatory responses occurring at the impact brain tissues (Fig. 4 vs Fig. 3c). Moreover, out of the five inflammatory

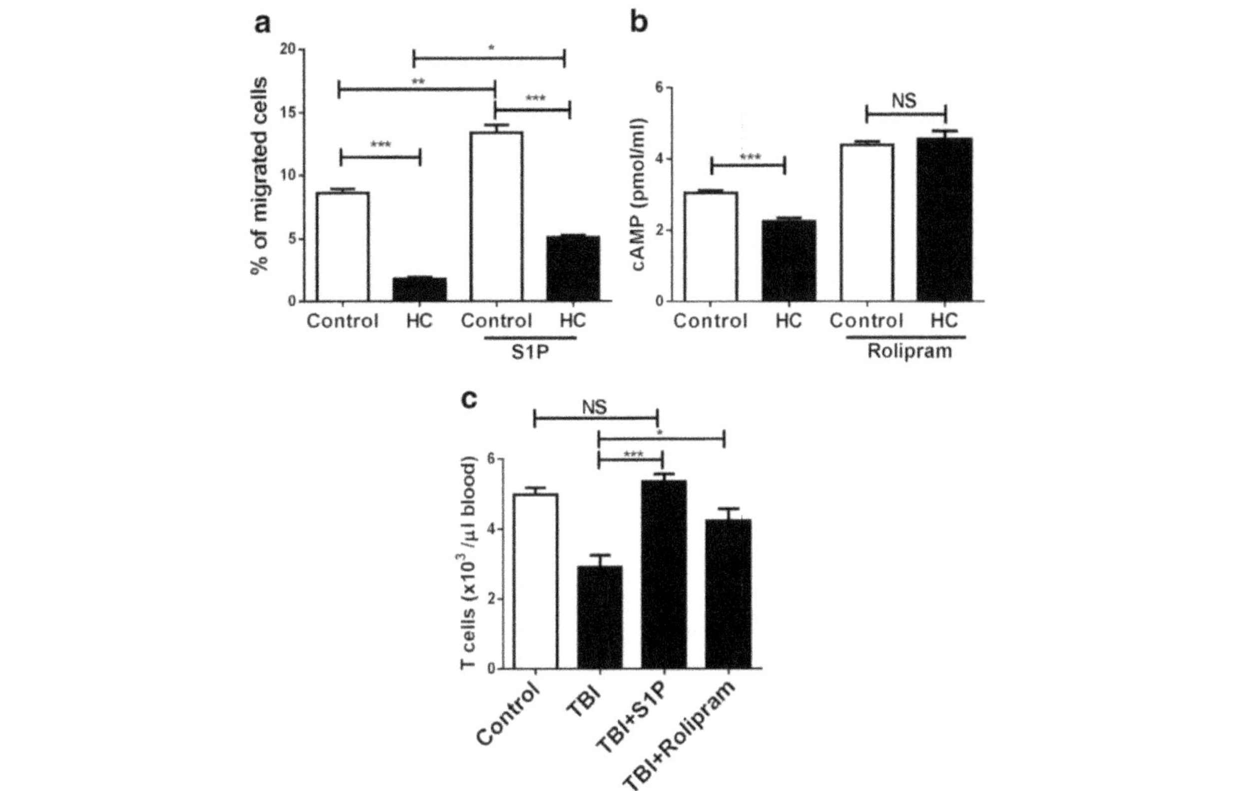

Fig. 3 S1P or rolipram increases peripheral T cells in TBI mice. **a** T cell migration was analyzed in 48-well micro chemotaxis chamber, with 20 μM hydrocortisone or vehicle in the upper chamber and 20 nM S1P or vehicle in the lower chamber. The number of migrated cells was assessed 4 h later in the lower chambers. **b** T cells were pretreated with 10 μM rolipram or saline for 15 min and then with 100 μM hydrocortisone or vehicle treatment for 5 min, after which intracellular cAMP level was measured. **c** Peripheral T cells were measured before and 1 h after TBI. S1P or rolipram was i.p. injected immediately after TBI. Results are expressed as means ± SEM. $n = 9$ for (**a**), 6 for (**c**), or 4 for (**b**). Significance was determined using two- (**a**, **b**) or one-way (**c**) ANOVA. $^*P < 0.05$, $^{**}P < 0.01$, $^{***}P < 0.001$, and NS, no significance compared between indicated groups. The experiment was repeated three times with similar results

mediators tested, CCL2 and CXCL10 were also produced at levels significantly higher in TBI mice given rolipram than those mice given vehicle control or uninjured mice (Fig. 4a–c). Histologically, we observed no overt alterations in the gross morphology or at a low magnification on day 7 after injury either in presence or in absence of S1P or rolipram (Fig. 5a). But a robust increase in the number of morphologically abnormal cells was evidenced in the cerebral cortex (B) and hippocampus (C) beneath the injured site in TBI mice receiving S1P compared to TBI controls under a high magnification (Fig. 5b, c). Notably, healthy cell nuclei were relatively large consisting of several discernible nucleoli in the nucleoplasm in the cerebral neocortex and hippocampus in the absence of S1P or normal control mice (Fig. 5b, c). In contrast, morphologically abnormal cells were characterized by dark red staining of the nucleoplasm with eosin and presented only at the injured site (Fig. 5b, c, the third pannel). Although the types of these abnormal cells were unknown, probably both neurons and glias, the cells appeared undergoing apoptosis as revealed by two apoptotic markers, Caspase-3 and TUNEL staining. S1P significantly elevated Caspase-3 activation in the hippocampus (Fig. 5f, i) and TUNEL staining in the cerebral cortex (Fig 5g, j) in comparison with TBI only or controls. When rolipram was given, morphologically abnormal cells were also increased, but largely limited to the cerebral neocortex (Fig. 5b, c bottom). The apoptosis cells were also found both in the cortex (Fig 5g, j) and hippocampus (Fig. 5f, i) in TBI mice receiving rolipram albeit to a much lesser extent in comparison with S1P, consistent with less effect of rolipram on T cell egress in vivo (Fig. 3c). The increase of cell death at the injured site of the brain was proportionally correlated with T cell infiltration in the tissue as revealed by anti-CD3 antibody staining (Fig. 5d, e, h). T cells were hardly presented in the uninjured control mice or mice with mTBI, in agreement with a complete recovery of the injury in mTBI mice. However, the number of T cells increased robustly in the injured brain after i.p. injection of S1P and to a much lesser degree rolipram, as a consequence of elevating levels of T cells

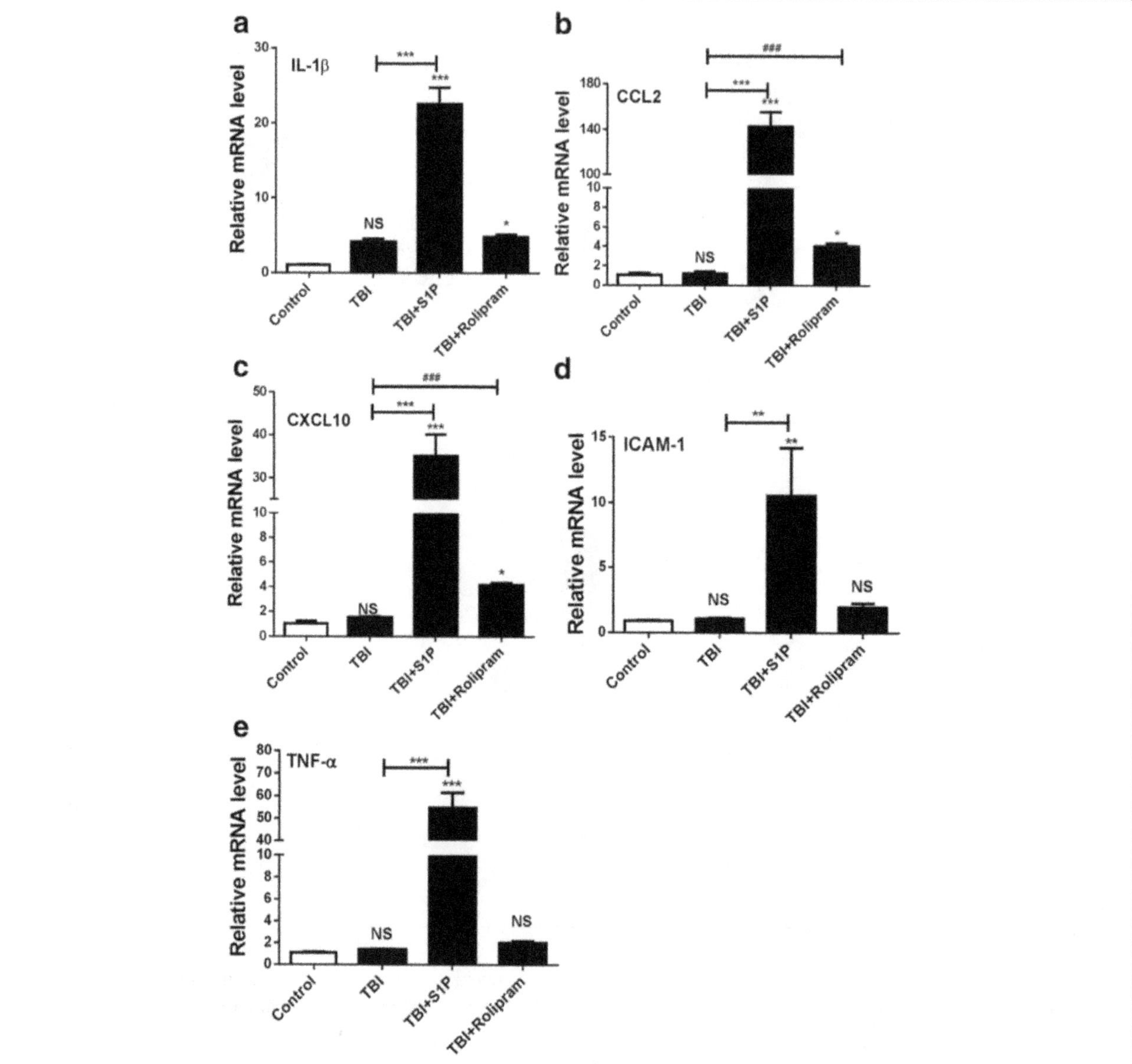

Fig. 4 S1P or rolipram exaggerates inflammatory responses in injured brain. IL-1β (**a**), CCL2 (**b**), CXCL10 (**c**), ICAM-1 (**d**), and TNF-α (**e**) were analyzed at the impact site of the cerebral cortex in 3 days after TBI by qRT-PCR. The data are expressed as means ± SEM and normalized to β-actin. $n = 5$, significance was measured using one-way ANOVA. $^{*}P < 0.05$, $^{**}P < 0.01$, $^{***}P < 0.001$ and NS, no significance compared between indicated groups. $^{\#\#\#}P < 0.001$ compared between TBI and TBI + rolipram in CCL2 and CXCL10 expression level by non-parametric Mann-Whitney *t* test. The experiment was repeated three times with similar results

in circulation. The results conclude that a high level of peripheral lymphocytes can directly contribute to the heightened inflammation at the injured site of the brain in the early phase of TBI.

Discussion

Brain has been viewed as an immune-privileged organ with little immunological and inflammatory activity under a physiological condition. This is primarily attributed to the relative impermeability of the blood-brain barrier (BBB) to cellular and molecular components of the immune and inflammatory reactions. However, upon brain injury, both immediate and secondary dysfunctions of the BBB occur as a consequence of disrupting the tight junction complexes and the integrity of the capillary basement membranes [9]. Neutrophils can be found aggregated in the microvasculature as early as 2 h post trauma [28]. Their infiltration in damaged neural tissue commences within 24 h [29], followed by macrophages within 36–48 h after trauma [30]. T lymphocytes have been shown to infiltrate the brain within 2–3 days post injury in a rat TBI model [31]. In those studies, severe or moderate TBI was induced via opening scalp and skull and infiltration of inflammatory cells was apparent

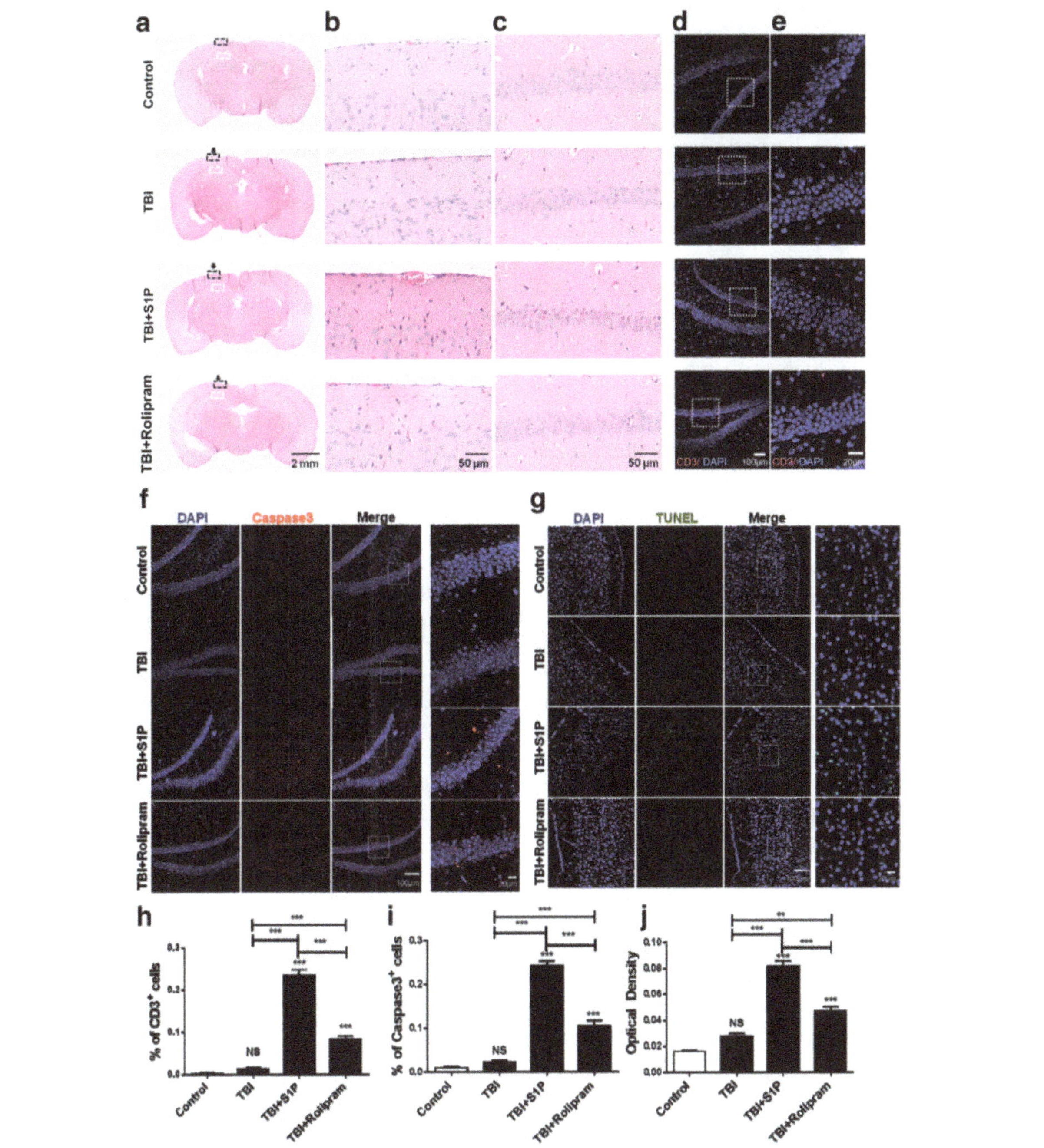

Fig. 5 A protective role for cortisol in TBI pathogenesis. **a** Histologic examination of normal control and injured brain at 7 days after TBI with or without administration of S1P or rolipram. The impact site was pointed by an *arrow*. The region of the cerebral cortex was highlighted in a *dashed black line square* and enlarged in panel (**b**); and the hippocampus was outlined by a *dashed white line square* and magnified in panel (**c**). Representative results of six mice in each group. **d** Representative immunofluorescence results of anti-CD3 antibody staining at hippocampus beneath the injured site and enlarged in panel (**e**). **f** Representative immunofluorescence staining for Caspase-3 expression at hippocampus beneath the injured site. **g** Representative TUNEL staining for apoptosis cells at the injury site. Percentages of CD3-positive cells in panel (**e**), Caspase-3-positive cells in panel (**f**), and optical density of TUNEL staining in panel (**g**) were determined by ImageJ and expressed as means ± SEM in (**h**), (**i**), or (**j**), respectively. $n = 6$, significance was measured using one-way ANOVA. $^{*}P < 0.05$, $^{**}P < 0.01$, $^{***}P < 0.001$ and NS, no significance compared between indicated groups. The experiment was repeated three times with similar results

[28–31], which is likely to be detrimental and associated with a severe loss of brain tissue and permanent impairment of cognitive neuron function [32]. Cortisol-mediated suppression of inflammation alone may be too weak to be effective in severe TBI. In contrast, mTBI was generated in our study with an intact scalp and skull and overt infiltration of inflammatory cells was not observed, which might be ascribed primarily to cortisol-mediated blockade of lymphocyte egress. In support of limiting inflammation at the injured site by cortisol-mediated blockade on lymphocyte egress at the initial phase of TBI, when the blockade was abolished by administering S1P, the number of circulating T cells was elevated significantly and positively correlated with increasing inflammatory responses (Fig. 4), T cell infiltration, and cell death (Fig. 5) at the impact site. The cortisol-mediated immune suppression observed in this TBI model is highly relevant to what happens in humans as a majority of mTBI recovers fully in humans in a few weeks. The observation hints that immediate immune suppression following TBI can prevent secondary brain damage and thus is beneficial to mTBI patients.

Pre-clinical and clinical studies have supported the use of methylprednisolone, a glucocorticoid drug, as an acute neuroprotectant after acute spinal cord injury [33, 34]. Supplement with hydrocortisone post trauma also improves neurological recovery and leads to beneficial outcomes [35]. Moreover, progesterone, an indirect precursor of cortisol, has shown promise to be a neuroprotective agent, and it is currently under clinical trials for the treatment of TBI [36, 37]. The benefit of inhibiting T cell egress by cortisol is also consistent with a better outcome of cerebral ischemia in T cell-deficient mice than in wild-type controls [38]. Moreover, lymphocyte-deficient $Rag1^{-/-}$ mice are profoundly protected from stab wound injury of the cortex [39]. Apparently, the linkage between lymphocyte infiltration and adverse outcome post-TBI contradicts the key role of T cells in the reparative process. Several studies have shown that T cells are required for neurogenesis and depletion of T cells impairs neuronal cell proliferation [5, 40]. Perhaps, dynamic regulation of the timing and degree of lymphocyte infiltration is pivotal for its neuroprotection. Yet, despite the beneficial role, excess cortisol has adverse effects on mood, cognition, and neurodegeneration [41, 42]. It is thus necessary to monitor cortisol levels post injury and give it preferably to patients with corticosteroid insufficiency [41]. Alternatively, suboptimal FTY720 or anti-S1P antibody may be used to suppress lymphocyte egress at the early phase of TBI to prevent secondary brain damage [43, 44].

Cortisol is widely recognized for its role in the stress response and for its physiologic anti-inflammatory effects. The mechanism underlying its anti-inflammatory effects may be multifaceted including transcriptional suppression of proinflammatory genes [45, 46] and inhibition of the functions of macrophages and neutrophils [47], and the like. Exogenous glucocorticosteroid administration, especially in supraphysiological doses, also induces cell death of immature T and B cells, but mature T cells and activated B cells are resistant to cell death induced by cortisol at this low dose [48]. Because the number of circulating T cells could be restored in traumatic mice by S1P or rolipram (Fig. 3c), cortisol-induced T lymphocytopenia following TBI was unlikely ascribed to cell death. Our study demonstrating a blockade of T cell egress by cortisol adds a novel mechanism to our current understanding of the anti-inflammatory activity of this steroid hormone. Substantial evidence has shown that T cell egress is initiated by binding of S1P to the $S1P_1$ receptor [21, 49]. The $S1P_1$ receptor is a G protein-coupled receptor and activates exclusively heterotrimeric Gαi proteins that inhibit adenylate cyclase, leading to brief reduction of cAMP production followed by normalization and increases of cAMP in the cells (Fig. 6) [50]. On the contrary, FTY720 binds to the $S1P_1$ receptor and causes the receptor internalization and prolonged reduction of cAMP, which promotes a sinus-moving away signal and blunts T cell egress [15]. The level of cAMP was lower in the presence than in the absence of hydrocortisone (Fig. 3b) but it was elevated by rolipram. Because rolipram can partially overcome the inhibitory effect of cortisol and increase cAMP levels in the presence of cortisol (Fig. 3b), cortisol may activate cAMP phosphodiesterase (PDE4) either directly or indirectly (Fig. 6). The secondary messenger cAMP is a signaling target downstream the $S1P_1$ receptor, and thus, hydrocortisone inhibits T cell migration (Fig. 3c) or egress (Fig. 3c), at least in part, by lowering cAMP level in the cells independent of the $S1P_1$ receptor.

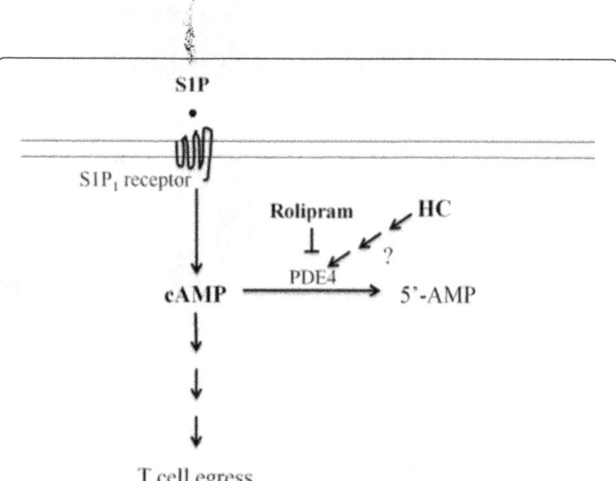

Fig. 6 Schematic illustration of a possible mechanism underlying cortisol-mediated blockade of T cell egress. cAMP is one of the important second messengers downstream the $S1P_1$ receptor and its production takes central part in the control of T cell egress. One of the cortisol (HC) activities may activate cAMP phosphodiesterase (PDE4) either directly or indirectly and enhance degradation of cAMP to 5'-AMP. Cortisol-facilitated degradation of cAMP may be one of the mechanisms where cortisol compromises T cell egress in the presence of S1P. On the contrary, rolipram inhibits PDE4, leading to increased levels of cAMP and promoting T cell egress

Conclusions

We report here that following mTBI, plasma cortisol levels are significantly and transiently elevated, which appears to be directly responsible for the brief lymphocytopenia in the periphery by its ability to block lymphocyte egress from secondary lymphoid tissues. Abrogation of cortisol action on lymphocyte egress by injection of S1P or rolipram was associated with prolonged and increased inflammatory responses and elevated cell death and T cell infiltration at the injured site of the brain cortex, concluding that lymphocyte infiltration of brain in the early phase of brain injury is detrimental. The current work highlights a protective role of cortisol-induced immune suppression in the early phase of TBI and offers valuable information with respect to prevention of TBI soon after injury by a blockade of lymphocyte egress.

Acknowledgements

The authors would like to thank members of the Photopathology Core at Wellman Center for the experimental assistance with the histopathology, flow cytometry, and microscopy services.

Funding

This work is supported by FA9550-11-1-0415 and FA9550-13-1-0068, Department of Defense/Air Force Office of Scientific Research Military Photomedicine Program, W81XWH-13-2-0067, Department of Defense, CDMRP/BAA, and the fund of Wellman Center for Photomedicine to MXW.

Authors' contributions

TD and LZ designed and performed the research and analyzed the data. BB and TD wrote the manuscript. MXW designed and supervised the research and wrote the manuscript. All authors read and approved the final manuscript.

Competing interests

The authors declare that they have no competing interests.

Consent for publication

Not applicable.

References

1. Selassie AW, Zaloshnja E, Langlois JA, Miller T, Jones P, Steiner C. Incidence of long-term disability following traumatic brain injury hospitalization, United States, 2003. J Head Trauma Rehabil. 2008;23(2):123–31.
2. Bramlett HM, Dietrich WD. Progressive damage after brain and spinal cord injury: pathomechanisms and treatment strategies. Prog Brain Res. 2007;161:125–41.
3. Marklund N, Bakshi A, Castelbuono DJ, Conte V, McIntosh TK. Evaluation of pharmacological treatment strategies in traumatic brain injury. Curr Pharm Des. 2006;12(13):1645–80.
4. Finnie JW. Neuroinflammation: beneficial and detrimental effects after traumatic brain injury. Inflammopharmacology. 2013;21(4):309–20.
5. Ziv Y, Ron N, Butovsky O, Landa G, Sudai E, Greenberg N, et al. Immune cells contribute to the maintenance of neurogenesis and spatial learning abilities in adulthood. Nat Neurosci. 2006;9(2):268–75.
6. Wieloch T, Nikolich K. Mechanisms of neural plasticity following brain injury. Curr Opin Neurobiol. 2006;16(3):258–64.
7. Zhang Q, Zhou C, Hamblin MR, Wu MX. Low-level laser therapy effectively prevents secondary brain injury induced by immediate early responsive gene X-1 deficiency. J Cereb Blood Flow Metab. 2014;34(8):1391–401.
8. Morganti-Kossman MC, Lenzlinger PM, Hans V, Stahel P, Csuka E, Ammann E, et al. Production of cytokines following brain injury: beneficial and deleterious for the damaged tissue. Mol Psychiatry. 1997;2(2):133–6.
9. Bradbury MW. The blood-brain barrier. Exp Physiol. 1993;78(4):453–72.
10. Cederberg D, Siesjo P. What has inflammation to do with traumatic brain injury? Childs Nerv Syst. 2010;26(2):221–6.
11. Clausen F, Lorant T, Lewen A, Hillered L. T lymphocyte trafficking: a novel target for neuroprotection in traumatic brain injury. J Neurotrauma. 2007;24(8):1295–307.
12. Santarsieri M, Niyonkuru C, McCullough EH, Dobos JA, Dixon CE, et al. Cerebrospinal fluid cortisol and progesterone profiles and outcomes prognostication after severe traumatic brain injury. J Neurotrauma. 2014; 31(8):699–712.
13. Wagner AK, McCullough EH, Niyonkuru C, Ozawa H, Loucks TL, et al. Acute serum hormone levels: characterization and prognosis after severe traumatic brain injury. J Neurotrauma. 2011;28(6):871–88.
14. Dong T, Zhang Q, Hamblin MR, Wu MX. Low-level light in combination with metabolic modulators for effective therapy of injured brain. J Cereb Blood Flow Metab. 2015;35(9):1435–44.
15. Zhi L, Kim P, Thompson BD, Pitsillides C, Bankovich AJ, Yun SH, et al. FTY720 blocks egress of T cells in part by abrogation of their adhesion on the lymph node sinus. J Immunol. 2011;187(5):2244–51.
16. Kim P, Puoris'haag M, Cote D, Lin CP, Yun SH. In vivo confocal and multiphoton microendoscopy. J Biomed Opt. 2008;13(1):010501.
17. Thompson BD, Jin Y, Wu KH, Colvin RA, Luster AD, Birnbaumer L, et al. Inhibition of G alpha i2 activation by G alpha i3 in CXCR3-mediated signaling. J Biol Chem. 2007;282(13):9547–55.
18. Schmittgen TD, Livak KJ. Analyzing real-time PCR data by the comparative C(T) method. Nat Protoc. 2008;3(6):1101–8.
19. Coutinho AE, Chapman KE. The anti-inflammatory and immunosuppressive effects of glucocorticoids, recent developments and mechanistic insights. Mol Cell Endocrinol. 2011;335(1):2–13.
20. Bolton PM, Kirov SM, Donald KJ. The effects of major and minor trauma on lymphocyte kinetics in mice. Aust J Exp Biol Med Sci. 1979;57:479–92.
21. Matloubian M, Lo CG, Cinamon G, Lesneski MJ, Xu Y, Brinkmann V, et al. Lymphocyte egress from thymus and peripheral lymphoid organs is dependent on S1P receptor 1. Nature. 2004;427(6972):355–60.
22. Graler MH, Goetzl EJ. The immunosuppressant FTY720 down-regulates sphingosine 1-phosphate G-protein-coupled receptors. FASEB J. 2004;18(3):551–3.
23. Kelso ML, Gendelman HE. Bridge between neuroimmunity and traumatic brain injury. Curr Pharm Des. 2014;20(26):4284–98.
24. Grigorova IL, Schwab SR, Phan TG, Pham TH, Okada T, Cyster JG. Cortical sinus probing, S1P1-dependent entry and flow-based capture of egressing T cells. Nat Immunol. 2009;10(1):58–65.
25. Wei SH, Rosen H, Matheu MP, Sanna MG, Wang SK, Jo E, et al. Sphingosine 1-phosphate type 1 receptor agonism inhibits transendothelial migration of medullary T cells to lymphatic sinuses. Nat Immunol. 2005;6(12):1228–35.
26. Sinha RK, Park C, Hwang IY, Davis MD, Kehrl JH. B lymphocytes exit lymph nodes through cortical lymphatic sinusoids by a mechanism independent of sphingosine-1-phosphate-mediated chemotaxis. Immunity. 2009;30(3):434–46.
27. Sensken SC, Nagarajan M, Bode C, Graler MH. Local inactivation of sphingosine 1-phosphate in lymph nodes induces lymphopenia. J Immunol. 2011;186(6):3432–40.
28. Schoettle RJ, Kochanek PM, Magargee MJ, Uhl MW, Nemoto EM. Early polymorphonuclear leukocyte accumulation correlates with the development of posttraumatic cerebral edema in rats. J Neurotrauma. 1990;7(4):207–17.
29. Soares HD, Hicks RR, Smith D, McIntosh TK. Inflammatory leukocytic recruitment and diffuse neuronal degeneration are separate pathological processes resulting from traumatic brain injury. J Neurosci. 1995;15(12):8223–33.
30. Giulian D, Chen J, Ingeman JE, George JK, Noponen M. The role of mononuclear phagocytes in wound healing after traumatic injury to adult mammalian brain. J Neurosci. 1989;9(12):4416–29.
31. Holmin S, Mathiesen T, Shetye J, Biberfeld P. Intracerebral inflammatory response to experimental brain contusion. Acta Neurochir (Wien). 1995;132(1-3):110–9.
32. Marklund N, Hillered L. Animal modelling of traumatic brain injury in preclinical drug development: where do we go from here? Br J Pharmacol. 2011;164(4):1207–29.
33. Bracken MB, Shepard MJ, Collins WF, Holford TR, Young W, Baskin DS, et al. A randomized, controlled trial of methylprednisolone or naloxone in the treatment of acute spinal-cord injury. Results of the Second National Acute Spinal Cord Injury Study. N Engl J Med. 1990;322(20):1405–11.

34. Bracken MB, Shepard MJ, Collins Jr WF, Holford TR, Baskin DS, Eisenberg HM, et al. Methylprednisolone or naloxone treatment after acute spinal cord injury: 1-year follow-up data. Results of the second National Acute Spinal Cord Injury Study. J Neurosurg. 1992;76(1):23–31.
35. Chen X, Zhao Z, Chai Y, Luo L, Jiang R, Dong J, et al. Stress-dose hydrocortisone reduces critical illness-related corticosteroid insufficiency associated with severe traumatic brain injury in rats. Crit Care. 2013;17(5):R241.
36. Wright DW, Kellermann AL, Hertzberg VS, Clark PL, Frankel M, Goldstein FC, et al. ProTECT: a randomized clinical trial of progesterone for acute traumatic brain injury. Ann Emerg Med. 2007;49(4):391–402. 402.
37. Xiao G, Wei J, Yan W, Wang W, Lu Z. Improved outcomes from the administration of progesterone for patients with acute severe traumatic brain injury: a randomized controlled trial. Crit Care. 2008;12(2):R61.
38. Hurn PD, Subramanian S, Parker SM, Afentoulis ME, Kaler LJ, Vandenbark AA, et al. T- and B-cell-deficient mice with experimental stroke have reduced lesion size and inflammation. J Cereb Blood Flow Metab. 2007;27(11):1798–805.
39. Fee D, Crumbaugh A, Jacques T, Herdrich B, Sewell D, Auerbach D, et al. Activated/effector CD4+ T cells exacerbate acute damage in the central nervous system following traumatic injury. J Neuroimmunol. 2003;136(1-2):54–66.
40. Wolf SA, Steiner B, Akpinarli A, Kammertoens T, Nassenstein C, Braun A, et al. CD4-positive T lymphocytes provide a neuroimmunological link in the control of adult hippocampal neurogenesis. J Immunol. 2009;182(7):3979–84.
41. De Kloet ER. Hormones and the stressed brain. Ann N Y Acad Sci. 2004;1018:1–15.
42. Lupien SJ, Maheu F, Tu M, Fiocco A, Schramek TE. The effects of stress and stress hormones on human cognition: implications for the field of brain and cognition. Brain Cogn. 2007;65(3):209–37.
43. O'Brien N, Jones ST, Williams DG, Cunningham HB, Moreno K, et al. Production and characterization of monoclonal anti-sphingosine-1-phosphate antibodies. J Lipid Res. 2009;50(11):2245–57.
44. Brinkmann V. FTY720 (fingolimod) in multiple sclerosis: therapeutic effects in the immune and the central nervous system. Br J Pharmacol. 2009;158(5):1173–82.
45. Clark AR. Anti-inflammatory functions of glucocorticoid-induced genes. Mol Cell Endocrinol. 2007;275(1-2):79–97.
46. Reichardt HM, Schutz G. Glucocorticoid signalling—multiple variations of a common theme. Mol Cell Endocrinol. 1998;146(1-2):1–6.
47. Tuckermann JP, Kleiman A, Moriggl R, Spanbroek R, Neumann A, Illing A, et al. Macrophages and neutrophils are the targets for immune suppression by glucocorticoids in contact allergy. J Clin Invest. 2007;117(5):1381–90.
48. Cox JH, Ford WL. The migration of lymphocytes across specialized vascular endothelium. IV. Prednisolone acts at several points on the recirculation pathways of lymphocytes. Cell Immunol. 1982;66(2):407–22.
49. Pappu R, Schwab SR, Cornelissen I, Pereira JP, Regard JB, Xu Y, et al. Promotion of lymphocyte egress into blood and lymph by distinct sources of sphingosine-1-phosphate. Science. 2007;316(5822):295–8.
50. Rosen H, Goetzl EJ. Sphingosine 1-phosphate and its receptors: an autocrine and paracrine network. Nat Rev Immunol. 2005;5(7):560–70.

11

Activation of the kynurenine pathway and increased production of the excitotoxin quinolinic acid following traumatic brain injury in humans

Edwin B. Yan[1*†], Tony Frugier[2†], Chai K. Lim[3†], Benjamin Heng[3†], Gayathri Sundaram[4†], May Tan[5†], Jeffrey V. Rosenfeld[6,7], David W. Walker[8], Gilles J. Guillemin[3] and Maria Cristina Morganti-Kossmann[9,10]

Abstract: During inflammation, the kynurenine pathway (KP) metabolises the essential amino acid tryptophan (TRP) potentially contributing to excitotoxicity via the release of quinolinic acid (QUIN) and 3-hydroxykynurenine (3HK). Despite the importance of excitotoxicity in the development of secondary brain damage, investigations on the KP in TBI are scarce. In this study, we comprehensively characterised changes in KP activation by measuring numerous metabolites in cerebrospinal fluid (CSF) from TBI patients and assessing the expression of key KP enzymes in brain tissue from TBI victims. Acute QUIN levels were further correlated with outcome scores to explore its prognostic value in TBI recovery.

Methods: Twenty-eight patients with severe TBI (GCS ≤ 8, three patients had initial GCS = 9–10, but rapidly deteriorated to ≤8) were recruited. CSF was collected from admission to day 5 post-injury. TRP, kynurenine (KYN), kynurenic acid (KYNA), QUIN, anthranilic acid (AA) and 3-hydroxyanthranilic acid (3HAA) were measured in CSF. The Glasgow Outcome Scale Extended (GOSE) score was assessed at 6 months post-TBI. Post-mortem brains were obtained from the Australian Neurotrauma Tissue and Fluid Bank and used in qPCR for quantitating expression of KP enzymes (indoleamine 2,3-dioxygenase-1 (IDO1), kynurenase (KYNase), kynurenine amino transferase-II (KAT-II), kynurenine 3-monooxygenase (KMO), 3-hydroxyanthranilic acid oxygenase (3HAO) and quinolinic acid phosphoribosyl transferase (QPRTase) and IDO1 immunohistochemistry.

Results: In CSF, KYN, KYNA and QUIN were elevated whereas TRP, AA and 3HAA remained unchanged. The ratios of QUIN:KYN, QUIN:KYNA, KYNA:KYN and 3HAA:AA revealed that QUIN levels were significantly higher than KYN and KYNA, supporting increased neurotoxicity. Amplified IDO1 and KYNase mRNA expression was demonstrated on post-mortem brains, and enhanced IDO1 protein coincided with overt tissue damage. QUIN levels in CSF were significantly higher in patients with unfavourable outcome and inversely correlated with GOSE scores.

Conclusion: TBI induced a striking activation of the KP pathway with sustained increase of QUIN. The exceeding production of QUIN together with increased IDO1 activation and mRNA expression in brain-injured areas suggests that TBI selectively induces a robust stimulation of the neurotoxic branch of the KP pathway. QUIN's detrimental roles are supported by its association to adverse outcome potentially becoming an early prognostic factor post-TBI.

Keywords: Patients, Traumatic brain injury, Kynurenine pathway, Tryptophan metabolism, Quinolinic acid

* Correspondence: edwin.yan@monash.edu
†Equal contributors
[1]Department of Physiology, Monash University, Clayton, VIC 3800, Australia
Full list of author information is available at the end of the article

Introduction

Traumatic brain injury (TBI) is one of the leading causes of morbidity and mortality in healthy individuals. Epidemiologic studies reported that TBI occurs more frequently in young adults due to motor vehicle accidents, sport activities and assaults as major causes of injury. Although advanced progress in pre-hospital intervention, neuroimaging, emergency management and intensive care as well as neurosurgical techniques have reduced mortality after severe TBI, the overall outcome remains poor with patients suffering from long-term disability and mental illness.

TBI is distinguished in two phases, namely primary and secondary injury. Primary injury occurs at the time of trauma resulting from either direct physical impact (focal trauma) or inertial force induced by rapid acceleration-deceleration (diffuse trauma) or a combination of both [1]. Subsequently, long-lasting secondary injury processes commence lasting for minutes, hours and days following a TBI. The combination of such pathological changes in the brain's intrinsic physiology and biochemistry aggravates brain damage and possibly underlies the causes of death. Over the past decades, compelling evidence has shown that such delayed processes represent the most destructive phase of TBI; however, the complexity and the mechanisms of secondary brain injury require further elucidation. There are few well-defined secondary pathways including inflammation, oxidative stress and excitotoxicity that terminate with the release of neurotoxins, leading to delayed cell death.

The study presented in this paper aimed to investigate changes in cerebral activation of the kynurenine pathway (KP) induced by severe TBI, with a specific focus on the potential roles of the terminal end product of the KP, the neurotoxin quinolinic acid (QUIN) [2] in predicting patients' long-term outcome.

The KP is the major cascade for metabolism of the essential amino acid tryptophan (TRP). TRP is the only amino acid bound to albumin to form a TRP-albumin complex in the blood stream [3]. This complex serves as a buffering system for maintaining a relative constant level of free TRP in blood. Free circulating TRP can be transported across the blood-brain barrier into the brain by the sodium-independent amino acid transporter system [4]. TRP is required for the synthesis of all proteins to ensure cell survival in both the periphery and central nervous system. It also strongly influences the function of the immune system in that reduction in TRP concentration suppresses the proliferation of peripheral mononuclear cells [5], decreases the activation of allogenic immune cells [6] and enhances the inhibition of T-cell responses [7]. In this regard, *in vivo* studies have shown that blocking the activity of the TRP-metabolising enzyme, indoleamine 2,3-dioxygenase-1 (IDO1), in the brain results in maintenance of the TRP pool and consequently the proliferation of T cells [8]. In the brain, TRP is metabolised to kynurenine (KYN) by IDO1 in neurons, astrocytes, microglia and infiltrated macrophages. KYN is then further metabolised into other neuroactive products of the KP such as kynurenic acid (KYNA), anthranilic acid (AA), 3-hydroxykynurenine (3HK), 3-hydroxyanthranilic acid (3HAA), QUIN, picolinic acid (PA) and nicotinic acid (NA) [9].

Numerous metabolites of the KP have received considerable attention since they display neuroactive, neurotoxic or immunomodulatory properties [10]. In fact, while QUIN acts as an excitotoxic agonist to the N-methyl-D-aspartate (NMDA) receptor, KYNA is rather considered a neuroprotectant through its antagonising action to the NMDA receptor, thus having an opposite functional role to its counterparts [11].

Therefore, understanding the changes in this complex pathway that are triggered in pathological conditions is critical for the future development of therapies to reduce secondary brain tissue damage. These KP metabolites are implicated in a variety of neuroinflammatory disorders including Alzheimer's disease, amyotrophic lateral sclerosis (ALS) and the AIDS-dementia complex [9, 12–16]. With the pathogenesis of neurological diseases, QUIN is likely one of the most important end products of the KP (review by [17]). In the primate and human brain, QUIN levels are strongly induced by interferon gamma (IFN-γ), a cytokine that is upregulated during infection and inflammation [12, 18] and following hypoxia-ischemia [19]. QUIN displays the ability to bind and activate the NMDA receptor causing prolonged Ca^{2+} influx, with loss of intra- and extra-cellular ionic balance in neurons; it increases cell membrane permeability, contributes to vasogenic oedema and ultimately leads to cell death [17].

Animal experiments employing intrastriatal injection of QUIN resulted in substantial neuronal cell loss [20, 21], whereas peripheral QUIN administration increased cerebral astrogliosis and oxidative stress [22]. Delivery of QUIN into the brain produced a progressive mitochondrial dysfunction, impaired cellular energy homeostasis [23, 24], increased oxidative stress [25] and enhanced nitric oxide (NO) synthase activities [26]. Even a modest (~200 nM) but prolonged elevation of QUIN in the adult brain is sufficient to reduce dendritic varicosities and microtubular assemblies of human neurons *in vitro* [27].

Despite the relevance of QUIN production in the pathogenesis of many neurological conditions, there are only limited studies that reported changes in the levels of QUIN and no reports at all in the TBI setting demonstrating changes of other metabolites of the KP. Published data showed that increased concentration of QUIN in cerebrospinal fluid (CSF) is strongly associated with mortality in children and adults after TBI [28, 29]. However, these early reports have not assessed how elevated QUIN production relates to other metabolites of the KP, which presents intrinsic branches potentially leading to opposite, neuroprotective or neurotoxic sequel. Therefore, further understanding of the activation of the KP consequent to TBI is pivotal to pinpoint its roles in the progress of secondary brain damage and develop a pharmacological intervention targeting the specific step of this complex pathway responsible for excessive QUIN synthesis [30].

In this study, we embarked on a comprehensive characterisation of the KP by measuring six metabolites in CSF collected from patients with severe TBI. In order to elucidate the relationship between these metabolites and the activation state of the KP, the level of expression of six enzymes of the KP was examined using post-mortem brain tissue obtained from individuals who died of TBI. This study design hinges on the hypothesis that TBI activates cerebral KP, enhances the production of neurotoxin QUIN and increases mRNA expression of enzymes regulating QUIN production in the brain. We further hypothesised that QUIN concentrations in CSF are correlative with Glasgow Outcome Scale Extended (GOSE) scores assessed at 6 months following TBI. Therefore, measuring QUIN in the clinic may aid in assessing long-term outcomes in severe TBI patients.

Materials and methods

Patient recruitment and CSF and serum sample collection

The study was conducted in accordance with the National Statement on Ethical Conduct in Research Involving Humans of the National Health and Medical Research Council of Australia and was approved by the Human Ethics Committee of the Alfred Hospital, Melbourne, Australia. Twenty-eight severe TBI patients were recruited from the Trauma Service of the Alfred Hospital (Table 1). Formal consent was obtained from the next of kin before the commencement of the study. The patient's inclusion criteria included severe TBI, established by a post-resuscitation, pre-intubation Glasgow Coma Scale (GCS) ≤ 8 (three patients had initial GCS = 9–10 but rapidly deteriorated requiring intubation at the scene) and implantation of an extraventricular drain (EVD) for monitoring and decreasing intracranial pressure via drainage of CSF. Exclusion criteria included age below 18 years, pregnancy, history of neurodegenerative disease, infectious disease, previous TBI and cancer.

Management of TBI patients included preliminary CT scans within 4 h of admission to assess the extent of injury and surgical implantation of an *in situ* intracranial pressure (ICP) probe coupled with an EVD. CSF was drained when the ICP was greater than 20 mmHg and accumulated in a drainage bag over 24 h. The CSF was collected daily by ICU research staff for six consecutive days from admission to the hospital (day 0) until day 5 post-TBI. CSF was centrifuged at 2000×*g* for 15 min at 4 °C, and the supernatant was stored at −80 °C until analysis. Blood samples were also collected daily and centrifuged, and serum was stored at −80 °C.

Table 1 Demographic information of TBI patients

Variables	Values
Age, years, median (range)	35 (21–69)
Gender, *n* (%)	
Males	22 (62.9)
Females	6 (17.1)
Type of accident, *n* (%)	
Motor vehicle	14 (50.0)
Motorbicycle	5 (17.9)
Pedestrian	4 (14.3)
Fall	3 (10.7)
Other	2 (7.1)
GCS, median (range)	5.5 (3–10)
GCS ≤ 8, n (%)	25 (89.3)
ISS, median (range)	36.5 (13–57)
GOSE, median (range)	4 (1–8)
Unfavourable outcome (1–4), *n* (%)	18 (64.3)
GOSE 1	6
GOSE 2	3
GOSE 3	4
GOSE 4	5
Favourable outcome (5–8), *n* (%)	10 (35.7)
GOSE 5	4
GOSE 6	3
GOSE 7	1
GOSE 8	2

A total of 28 patients with severe TBI were recruited in the study for longitudinal collection of CSF and serum. The following clinical parameters were recorded: Glasgow Coma Scale (GCS): severe ≤8. Injury Severity Score (ISS): 0 = no injury, 75 = maximal untreatable injury. Glasgow Outcome Scale Extended (GOSE): 1 = dead, 2 = vegetative state, 3 = lower severe disability, 4 = upper severe disability, 5 = lower moderate disability, 6 = upper moderate disability, 7 = lower good recovery, 8 = upper good recovery

Assessment of outcomes

The outcome was assessed using the Glasgow Outcome Scale Extended (GOSE) at 6 months post-injury. Phone interviews with individual patients, their family members or other informants were conducted by experienced research nurses using the questionnaire of Wilson et al. [31]. The GOSE is an examiner-dependent assessment; therefore, research staffs conducting the interviews are extensively trained to produce high-level consistency among patients. GOSE aims to gauge the patient's social, occupational, behavioural and neurological recovery after TBI, where GOSE 1 = death, 2 = vegetative state, 3 = severe disability (lower band), 4 = severe disability (upper band), 5 = moderate disability (lower band), 6 = moderate disability (upper band), 7 = good recovery (lower band) and 8 = good recovery (upper band).

Control patients and sample collection

Control CSF was obtained from patients undergoing elective neurosurgery for implantation of ventriculo-peritoneal shunts following a diagnosis of hydrocephalus (n = 11, 6 males and 5 females, between the ages of 30 and 74 years). Ethics approval was granted by the Alfred Human Ethics Board and informed consent was obtained prior surgery. Exclusion criteria included involvement of neurodegenerative diseases, cancer, infectious disease, intracerebral haemorrhages or previous TBI. Control serum samples (n = 20) were obtained from 12 female and 8 male healthy volunteers between the ages of 21 and 55 years. Both serum and CSF samples were processed using the same methods as described for TBI patients.

Measurement of tryptophan metabolites in CSF and serum

CSF samples were analysed by high-performance liquid chromatography (HPLC) and gas chromatography-mass spectrometry (GC-MS) methods to quantify the concentration of the metabolites of the KP, namely TRP, KYN, KYNA, AA, 3HAA and QUIN. TRP was only measured in serum. Proteins in CSF and serum were first precipitated by adding equal amount of 5 % trichloroacetic acid (*w/v*, Sigma-Aldrich, St. Louis, MO, USA) to the sample and then centrifuged for 10 min at 2000×*g* at 4 °C. The supernatants were filtered through 0.2-μm filters (Waters, Rydalmer, NSW, Australia) before use in HPLC.

The HPLC methods for quantification of TRP, KYN, KYNA, AA and 3HAA were based on Darlington et al. [32] with slight modification. The mobile phase of the TRP, KYN and KYNA assay consisted of 50 mM sodium acetate (Merck, Whitehouse Station, NJ, USA), 250 mM zinc acetate (Sigma-Aldrich, St. Louis, MO, USA) and 5 % acetonitrile (Merck, Whitehouse Station, NJ, USA). The mobile phase was buffered to pH 5.5 by glacial acetate acid (Merck, Whitehouse Station, NJ, USA), filtered through a 0.45-μm filter and pumped at a flow rate of 1 ml/min. The mobile phase of AA and 3HAA consisted of 25 mM sodium acetate and 2.5 % acetonitrile, buffered at pH 5.5, filtered and pumped at a flow rate of 1 ml/min. Stock standards of TRP, KYN, KYNA, AA and 3HAA were made in concentration of 250 mM using high-purity chemical from Sigma-Aldrich (St. Louis, MO, USA). The stock standard solution was kept at 4 °C for 1 month. Working standards were made by further dilution of the stock solution to establish standard curves of 1.25, 2.5, 6.25 and 12.5 μM for TRP and KYN; 10, 20, 60, 120 and 200 nM for KYNA; and 5, 15, 30 and 50 pM for AA and 3HAA. Quality control samples were prepared for each metabolite, aliquoted in multiple vials and stored at −80 °C. Deproteinised human CSF and serum samples (100 μl), standards and quality controls were injected into HPLC. The retention time and peak height of each metabolite from each sample were quantified using either WinChrom Chromatography Data System (GBC, Melbourne, Australia) or Waters Millennium Chromatography Manager (Waters, Rydalmer, NSW, Australia). TRP, KYN and KYNA were separated using a polymeric column (20 × 3.2 mm; 5-μm particle size; Agilent Technologies, Forest Hill, VIC, Australia) and detected by an absorbance detector for TRP and KYN (Photodiode Array Detector, Shimadzu SPD-M10A (Kyoto, Japan); absorbance wavelength TRP = 278 nm; KYN = 363 nm) or a fluorescent detector for KYNA (Waters 474 Scanning Fluorescence Detector, excitation = 344 nm, emission = 388 nm) connected in series. AA and 3HAA were measured by a Synergi Hydro column (250 × 4.60 mm; 4 μm particle size; Phenomenex (Torrance, CA, USA)) connected to a fluorescent detector (Waters 474 Scanning Fluorescence Detector, Ex = 320 nm, Em = 420 nm). For each set of sample measurement, fresh working standards were prepared and measured together with unknown samples and quality controls. A standard curve was plotted using linear regression of the area under the chromatograph of the corresponding concentration of the standards. The concentrations of TRP, KYN, KYNA, AA and 3HAA were calculated against the standard curves from the corresponding run of the assay. Quality controls were used to calculate inter- and intra-assay coefficient.

QUIN in CSF was measured by GC-MS as described by Smythe et al. [33]. Briefly, a standard curve of QUIN (10, 20, 50, 100, 200 and 500 nM) was prepared from a stock solution (2 μM). An internal standard containing 50–200 fmol of [$^2H_3$]-QUIN in 50 μl was added into 100-μl deproteinised samples. These samples were then dried by N_2 stream. The residues were mixed with trifluoroacetic anhydride (100 μl, Sigma-Aldrich, St. Louis, MO, USA) and hexafluoroisopropanol (100 μl; Sigma-Aldrich, St. Louis, MO, USA) and left at room temperature overnight to produce the dihexafluoroisopropyl ester from QUIN. The dihexafluoroisopropyl ester product was dissolved in toluene (1 ml, Sigma-Aldrich, St. Louis, MO, USA), washed with 5 % $NaHCO_3$ (1 ml; Sigma-Aldrich, St. Louis, MO, USA) and ddH_2O (1 ml) and dried over anhydrous sodium sulphate (~500 mg; Sigma-Aldrich, St. Louis, MO, USA). The samples were then transferred into an auto-sampler (7683, Agilent Technologies, Forest Hill, VIC, Australia), and 1 μl was injected into a HP-5MS capillary column (30 m × 0.25 mm; Agilent Technologies, Forest Hill, VIC, Australia) connected to an Agilent 6890 gas chromatograph and an Agilent mass selective detector (Agilent Technologies, Forest Hill, VIC, Australia).

Post-mortem brain tissue collection

All procedures were conducted in accordance with the Australian National Health & Medical Research Council's National Statement on Ethical Conduct in Human Research (2007), the Victorian Human Tissue Act 1982, the National Code of Ethical Autopsy Practice and the Victorian Government Policies and Practices in Relation to Post-Mortem.

Trauma brain samples from 16 individuals who died after closed head injury were obtained from the Australian Neurotrauma Tissue and Fluid Bank. Cases were aged between 18 and 78 years (mean 49.9 years), and the causes of injury include motor vehicle accident, motorbike accident, nursing home accident, household accident, stair accident and falls (see Table 2 for clinical information and epidemiological details). The post-mortem intervals varied between 40 and 129 h (mean 80.6 h).

Tissues were divided into four groups—Control, Acute Death, Delayed Death Injured Tissue and Delayed Death Normal Tissue. The Acute Death group includes nine patients (seven males and two females) who were pronounced dead upon the arrival of paramedics at the scene of accident (survival time <17 min). In those victims with an absence of visible tissue damage at post-mortem, cortical tissue was collected directly under the area having marked injury to the skull and skin. The group of delayed death includes seven patients (five males and two females) who survived more than 6 h post-TBI (range of 6–122 h, mean survival time of 40 h). At autopsy, two full coronal brain slices were taken by a forensic pathologist at 1 cm posterior to the mammillary bodies at the level of the basal ganglia. One slice was fresh frozen for PCR experiments, and the other was fixed in formalin for immunohistochemistry. The tissue used in these experiments was taken

Table 2 Details of the 16 trauma and 10 control cases

Case	Age (years)	Sex	Cause of injury	PMI (h)	Cause of death	Survival time
1	51.1	M	Motor vehicle accident	60	Brain + multiple injuries	<17 min
2	78.7	M	Nursing home accident	45	Brain injury	<17 min
3	27	M	Suicide	84	Brain + multiple injuries	<17 min
4	18.3	M	Motor vehicle accident	79	Brain + multiple injuries	<17 min
5	57.9	F	Motor vehicle accident	87	Brain + multiple injuries	<17 min
6	49	M	Motor vehicle accident	107	Brain + multiple injuries	<17 min
7	34.7	M	Motorbike accident	66	Brain + multiple injuries	<17 min
8	21.5	M	Motor vehicle accident	100	Brain injury	<17 min
9	57.6	F	Motor vehicle accident	97	Brain injury	<17 min
10	46.0	M	Fall	129	Brain injury	6 h
11	56.3	M	Motor vehicle accident	65	Brain injury	8 h
12	64.6	M	Fall	61	Brain injury	8 h
13	75.9	M	Staircase fall	89	Brain injury	10 h
14	59.6	F	Motor vehicle accident	80	Brain injury	35 h
15	61.7	M	Fall	40	Brain injury	93 h
16	38.9	F	Staircase fall	101	Brain injury	122 h
17	16	M	-	-	Suicide by hanging	-
18	48.7	M	-	50	Cardiac failure	-
19	51.6	M	-	64	Asthma	-
20	52.3	M	-	52	Cardiomyopathy	-
21	59.6	M	-	43	Pulmonary embolism	-
22	64.1	M	-	24	Ischaemic heart disease	-
23	66.9	M	-	10	Pneumonia	-
24	64.4	M	-	24	Pulmonary embolism	-
25	77.5	M	-	53	Myocardial infarction	-
26	60	F	-	48	Myocardial infarction	-

Cases 1–9: cases with a survival time between 0 and 17 min; cases 10–16: cases with a survival time between 6 and 261 h; cases 17–26: control cases. All brains were obtained at autopsy

PMI post-mortem interval (time between death and brain retrieval), *M* male, *F* female

from the cortical region of these coronal slices in areas showing visible tissue damage (Delayed Death Injured Tissue) and from a corresponding region on the contralateral side of the brain without macroscopic injury (Delayed Death Normal Tissue). These groupings were consistent with our previous reports [34–36].

For comparison, the same regions analysed in TBI tissues were obtained from control brain samples. These were provided by the National Neural Tissue Resource Centre of Australia (n = 13). These brains originated from individuals with no history of TBI or neuropathology; the age range matched that of TBI population and was between 16 and 78 years old (mean 58 years old). A neuropathologist, Prof. C. McLean, Head of the Department of Anatomical Pathology at the Alfred Hospital, performed brain tissue pathology and injury identification.

Gene expression of enzymes regulating the kynurenine pathway

The RNA isolation and cDNA preparation was performed using a well-characterised methodology as described previously in these brains by our group [36]. Briefly, TRIzol Plus RNA purification kit was used for RNA extraction from fresh frozen cortex tissue. A Nanodrop1000 spectrophotometer (Thermo Fisher Scientific, Wilmington, DE, USA) was used to determine the concentration and purity of the RNA samples. A minimum ratio of absorbance at 260 and 280 nm of 2 was considered as pure RNA. Agilent 2100 bioanalyzer (Agilent Technologies, Waldbronn, Germany) was used to assess the integrity of extracted RNA. RNA quality is considered good if the sample has a minimum RNA integrity number (RIN) value of 6. Oligo d(T)20 was then used as primers to reverse transcribed RNA fraction into cDNA using SuperScript III reverse transcriptase according to the manufacturer's protocol (Invitrogen, Carlsbad, CA, USA). Quantitative PCR was performed using TaqMan primer for kynurenase (KYNase, Hs00187 560_m1), kynurenine amino transferase-II (KAT-II, Hs0021 2039_m1), kynurenine 3-monooxygenase (KMO, Hs00175 738_m1), 3-hydroxyanthranilic acid oxygenase (3HAO, Hs 00201915_m1) and quinolinic acid phosphoribosyl transferase (QPRTase, Hs00204757_m1) (Applied Biosystems, Foster City, CA, USA). Hydroxymethylbilane synthase (HMBS, Hs00609297_m1), peptidylpropyl isomerase A (cyclophilin A) (PPIA, Hs99999904_m1), ubiquitin C (UBC, Hs00824723_m1) and glyceraldehyde-3-phosphate dehydrogenase (GAPDH, Hs99999905_m1) (Applied Biosystems, Foster City, CA, USA) have the most stable mRNA levels in post-mortem brain tissue and were used as endogenous control.

Quantitative PCR (qPCR) reaction mixture for each sample contains 1 μl of cDNA, 12.5 μl Taq-Man Universal PCR Master Mix (Applied Biosystems, Foster City, CA, USA), 1.25 μl of primer and 10.25 μl nuclease-free H_2O. Seven microlitres of the reaction mixture was added into a 384 well plate, and qPCRs were performed using the 7900HT Fast Real-Time PCR system (Applied Biosystems, Foster City, CA, USA). All experiments were performed in triplicate. The level of mRNA expression of KP enzymes was quantified using the comparative Ct method (ΔΔCt). This method used an arithmetic formula ($2^{-\Delta\Delta Ct}$) instead of a standard curve for the calculation of the relative KP enzyme expression level. This method can be used in place of the standard curve as long as both target and housekeeping genes have been validated to have approximate equal efficiencies. The mRNA levels of KP enzymes were normalised using the averaged level of endogenous control gene (HMBS, PPIA, UBC and GAPDH).

For IDO1, the primer forward (GCCAGCTTCGAGAA AGAGTTG) and reverse (TGACTTGTGGTCTGTGAG ATGA) were made based on Harvard primer bank (http://pga.mgh.harvard.edu/primerbank/, assessed on April 2012). qPCR reactions were performed in a final volume of 10 μl. Each reaction mixture contains 5 μl Fast SYBR® green master mix, 5 μM forward and reverse primers and 125 ng of cDNA template. The reaction was incubated at 95 °C for 20 s and amplified for 40 cycles of 95 °C for 1 s and 55 °C for 20 s.

IDO1 immunohistochemistry

Localisation and distribution of cells expressing IDO1 were identified using immunohistochemical staining. Cortical tissues were immersion fixed in 4 % paraformaldehyde for 72 h before paraffin-embedding process. Immunohistochemistry was performed on 7-μm sections using a Dako Autostainer XL (DakoCytomation, Carpinteria, CA, USA). In brief, sections were deparaffinised and rehydrated and then subjected to antigen retrieval in a citrate buffer (Dako (Cambridge, UK), S2367, pH 9) within a pressurised heating chamber (Dako (Cambridge, UK), S2800, 125 °C, 20 psi) for 2 min. Quenching of endogenous peroxidase activity was achieved using 3 % H_2O_2. Sections were then treated with serum-free protein blocker (Dako (Cambridge, UK), X0909) before 120-min incubation with antibody against IDO1 (IDO-MCA, 1:100, Oriental Yeast Co., Ltd., Tokyo, Japan). Envision HRP-linked polymer (Dako (Cambridge, UK), K4001) and 3,3-diaminobenzidine (Dako (Cambridge, UK), K3468) were applied to visualise positive staining. Tissue sections were counterstained with haematoxylin on a Leica Autostainer XL (North Ryde, NSW, Australia) and coverslipped using a Leica CV5030 device (North Ryde, NSW, Australia). Isotype-matched monoclonal antibody was used as a negative control. All sections were examined under a light microscope (Leica DM2500, North Ryde, NSW, Australia) and positive-stained cells were counted semi-quantitatively by ImageJ software as number of positive cell × 100/total number of cells in ten random microscopic (×200) fields in each section. Statistical analyses were performed using GraphPad Prism Version 6 software (mean ± SE). All tests were two-tailed with 95 % confidence interval values ($p < 0.05$).

Statistical analysis

Tryptophan metabolites

Statistical analyses were undertaken using GraphPad Prism 5. Generally, for all data sets, we first tested the data for homogeneity of variance using Bartlett's test prior to applying further analysis. Due to non-normally distributed metabolite data, logarithmic transformation was applied before analysis using one-way ANOVA and Dunnett *post hoc* for multiple comparisons between control group and each day after TBI. Differences in QUIN levels in CSF between favourable (GOSE 5–8) and unfavourable outcome (GOSE 1–4) was determined by Student's *t*-test following logarithmic transformation. To reflect logarithmic transformation of data, results were presented as geometric means with 95 % confidence intervals throughout. Correlation between QUIN and GOSE was conducted using Spearman's correlation coefficient. A *p* value of less than 0.05 was considered as statistically significant.

qPCR

Statistical analyses were undertaken using GraphPad Prism 5. Due to non-normally distributed data; logarithmic transformation was applied before analysed using 1-way ANOVA and Dunnett *post hoc* for multiple comparisons between each group. A *p* value of less than 0.05 was considered as statistically significant.

Results

Patient demographics and outcome

A total of 28 TBI patients were recruited immediately after resuscitation at the accident scene and admitted to the ICU. TBI patients' age ranged between 21 and 69 years (median age of 35 years) with a majority of males ($n = 22$, 62.9 %) (Table 1). Most patients ($n = 23$) were victims of road traffic accidents (82.2 %), and the remaining patients sustained a fall ($n = 3$) or other injurious mechanisms ($n = 2$). The GCS at the scene was ≤8 for all patients with the exception of three patients who had an initial GCS of 9–10 and rapidly deteriorated requiring intubation prior to admission to the hospital. The Injury Severity Scores (ISS) were recorded to assess the combined injuries sustained including brain and peripheral trauma. Median ISS for this cohort was 36.5 ranging between 13 and 57, which is indicative of a high incidence of additional injuries to TBI. Outcome assessed at 6 months post-TBI was generally poor with a median GOSE of 4. Following dichotomisation, 18 patients had an unfavourable outcome with GOSE 1–4 (64.3 %), whereas 10 patients had a favourable outcome with GOSE 5–8 (35.7 %); 6 patients died (GOSE 1) during the first 6 months from injury.

Changes in tryptophan metabolites and increases QUIN in CSF after TBI

The levels of TRP in CSF showed an apparent increase between day 0 and 5 after TBI; however, the median concentrations (average median 4255 nM, 25–75 percentile: 2088–7358 nM) were not significantly different from controls (median: 3000 nM, 25–75 %: 2260–4690 nM) (Fig. 1a). In the TBI cohort, KYN displayed median levels ranging between 115.1 and 163.6 nM over the days 0 to 3 and were similar to control with a median of 78.48 nM (25–75 %: 56.21–98.62 nM; Fig. 1b). However, later in the study at days 4 and 5 post-injury, KYN concentrations became significantly elevated of at least twofold over controls with median values of 188.0 nM (25–75 %: 105.5–249.3 nM) and 228.0 nM (25–75 %: 173.1–444.1 nM; $p < 0.05$) on each day, respectively. In CSF, TBI induced an early and gradual elevation of the NMDA antagonist KYNA, which became significantly higher than controls from day 2 onwards (control median: 73.08 nM, 25–75 %: 37.86–105.8 nM; day 2 median: 127.3 nM, 25–75 %: 80.13–237.1 nM, 1.7-fold increase; $p < 0.05$; Fig. 1c). After day 2, KYNA reached a plateau that lasted until day 5 with median concentrations between 127.3 and 143.5 nM.

In contrast to KYNA, the other potent NMDA receptor agonist, QUIN, increased over control as early as day 1 to further augment from day 2 to day 4 before showing a mild decrease on day 5, which was still significantly higher than control ($p < 0.05$; Fig. 1d). In more detail, the concentration of QUIN was unchanged at day 0 (median: 21.4 nM, 25–75 %: 12.9–43.5 nM) and began to increase from day 1 (median: 79.6 nM, 25–75 %: 47.32–127.6 nM) (Fig. 1d), reaching a peak at day 4 (median: 229.4 nM, 25–75 %: 146.4–438.2 nM), which represented a tenfold increase from control levels ($p < 0.005$). Of note, the concentrations of QUIN in control CSF (median: 3 nM, 25–75 %: 3–34.5 nM) matched the normal CSF levels reported by others in the literature (<50 nM) (see review [17]).

The median concentration of AA steadily increased after TBI with an apparent peak of 12.5 nM (25–75 %: 7.4–22.2 nM) detected at day 4, which consisted of an ~2-fold increase from the control level (Fig. 1e). In comparison, the downstream product of AA and precursor of QUIN, 3HAA, displayed a 2- to 5-fold increase between days 1 and 4, despite the large variations observed throughout the study (Fig. 1f). For both AA and 3HAA, there were no statistically significant differences to control at any time point examined.

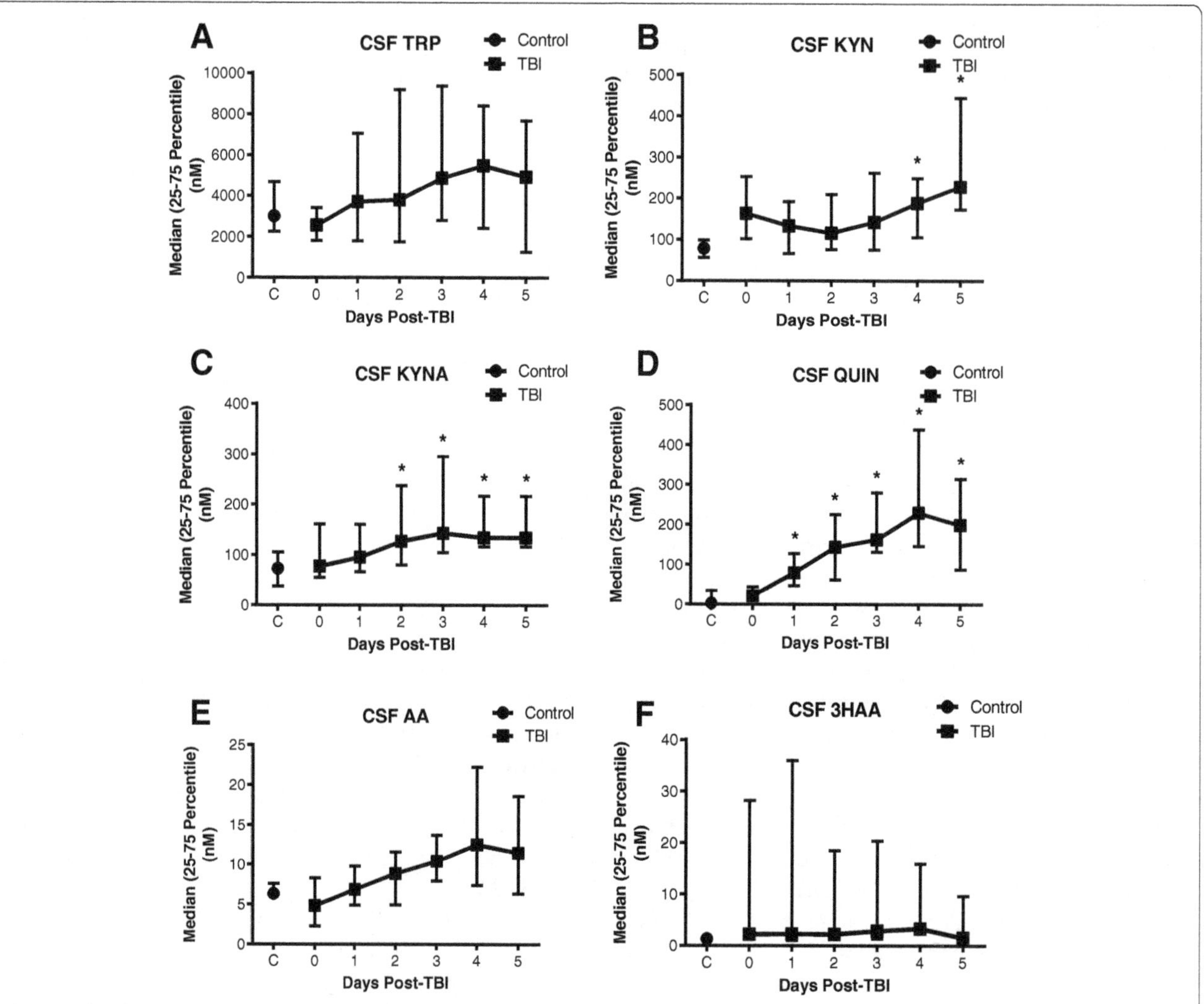

Fig. 1 Profile of the kynurenine pathway metabolites in the CSF of patients with TBI. The concentration of six tryptophan metabolites was measured in the CSF of TBI patients consecutively from the day of hospital admission (day 0) to day 5 after injury and compared to the CSF of control individuals. **a** Tryptophan (TRP), **b** kynurenine (KYN), **c** kynurenic acid (KYNA), **d** quinolinic acid (QUIN), **e** anthranilic acid (AA) and **f** 3-hydroxyanthranilic acid (3HAA). Data is presented as daily median with 25–75 percentile. *Asterisks* indicate significant differences ($p < 0.05$) to control using one-way ANOVA followed by Dunnett's multiple comparison as *post hoc*. TBI patients: $n = 25–28$ per time point; control group: $n = 9–11$. Significant increase of KYNA concentration in CSF were observed between days 2 and 5 when compared to the control level, while QUIN concentration was significantly increased between days 1 and 5 as to the controls

KP activity shifts towards the production of the excitotoxic metabolite QUIN

KYNA and QUIN are end products of two distinct branches of the KP and are released at different concentrations in both normal and disease conditions [37]. We then further explored the impact of TBI to drive the KP towards excitotoxicity and QUIN production, manifested through disproportional amounts of KYNA and QUIN; we calculated the ratios of each one of these metabolites with their common precursor KYN.

Interestingly, we found a significant and protracted increase in the ratio of QUIN and KYN from day 1 to day 5 post-TBI (Fig. 2a). This striking elevation reached a maximum of 28.8-fold over control levels on day 4 ($p < 0.05$). In contrast, the ratios of KYNA and KYN (range of median values from 0.51 to 1.1) as well as the ratios of 3HAA and AA (range of median values from 0.24 to 1.46) remained unchanged throughout the study and were not different from controls (median: 0.65) (Fig. 2b–d). The overproduction of QUIN was also supported by the ratio of QUIN and its neuroprotectant counterpart, KYNA, which presented significantly higher values from day 2 to day 5 after TBI (median: day 2 = 1.3, day 3 = 0.76, day 4 = 1.97 and day 5 = 1.3) when compared with controls (median: 0.3) (Fig. 2c).

These results demonstrate substantial changes in KP activity induced by TBI, whereby metabolism of TRP was shifted towards an enhanced release of neurotoxic

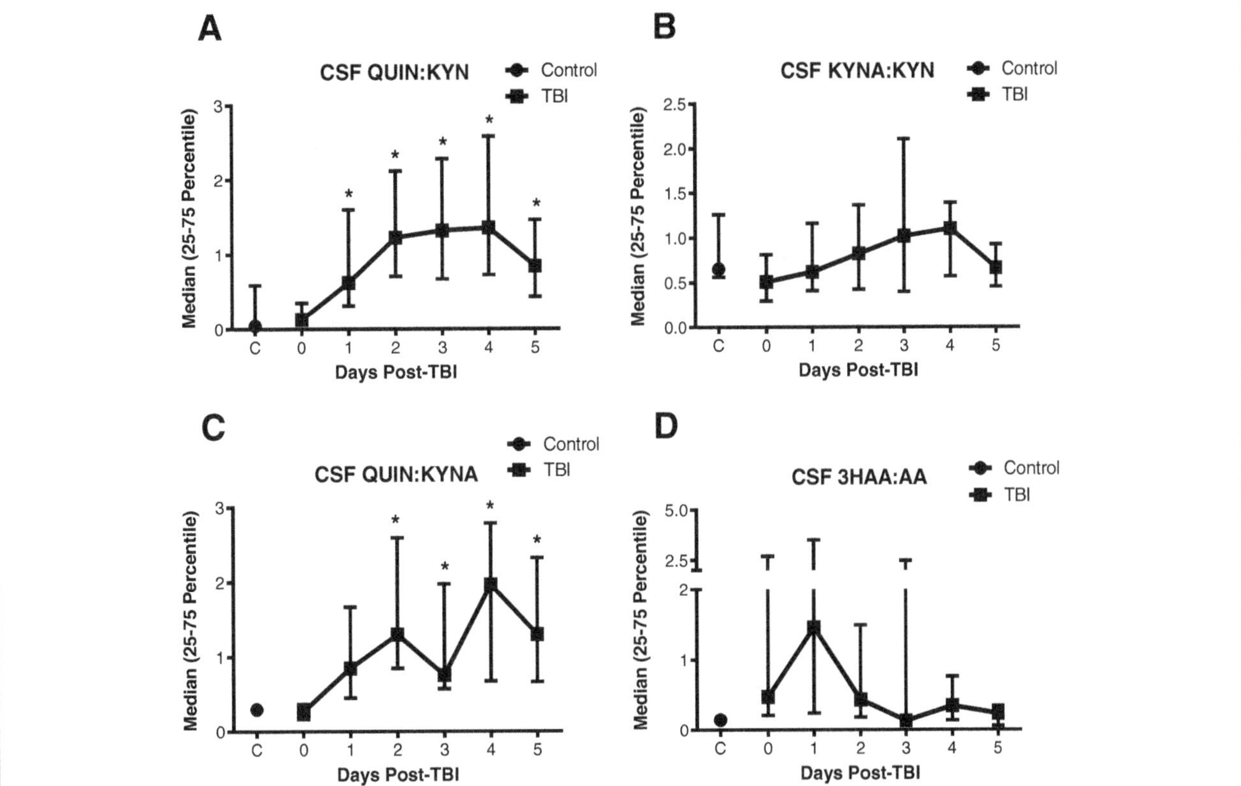

Fig. 2 Ratios of metabolites of the kynurenine pathway indicate a higher production of quinolinic acid. The daily CSF concentrations of each metabolite were used to calculate the individual ratios depicted as follows: **a** kynurenic acid (KYNA) versus kynurenine (KYN), **b** quinolinic acid (QUIN) versus KYN, **c** QUIN versus KYNA and **d** 3-hydroxyanthranilic acid (3HAA) versus anthranilic acid (AA). Data is shown as median with 25–75 percentile. *Asterisks* indicate significant differences ($p < 0.05$) to control group using one-way ANOVA followed by Dunnett's multiple comparison as *post hoc*. TBI patients: $n = 25$ per time point; control group: $n = 9$. Significant increase in the ratio of QUIN to KYN and QUIN to KYNA when compared to the control level indicating QUIN production increased after TBI

QUIN, rather than the alternative branches terminating with the end products KYNA or AA.

Serum concentrations of tryptophan decrease after TBI

We were also interested to determine how changes in the production of TRP observed in CSF relate with TRP levels in the blood. Interestingly, the concentration of serum TRP was significantly decreased from day 0 to day 4 following TBI with a reduction ranging between 25 and 50 %, $p < 0.05$ (Fig. 3). Although the medians of TRP on day 5 (36.29 μM, 25–75 %: 29.34–44.37 μM) and day 4 (35.6 μM, 25–75 %: 30.63–43.93 μM) were similar, the apparent increase of TRP on day 5 was not found to be statistically different to control levels ($p = 0.274$), possibly due to a larger data variance at this time point.

Up regulation of IDO1 mRNA in the injured brain supports the increase of QUIN in CSF

This section of the study aimed at elucidating the mechanisms leading to the alterations in KP metabolite detected in the CSF of TBI patients and substantiating the evidence of KP activation directly on the injured brain. Using post-mortem brain tissue from TBI victims, we examined changes in the expression level of six enzymes of the KP, namely IDO1, KYNase, KAT-II, KMO, 3HAO and QPRTase, which were normalised to a set of three constitutive genes to generate reliable PCR data (see the 'Materials and methods' section).

IDO1 is the first enzyme required in the initial step of the KP to metabolise TRP into KYN. KYNase is needed for metabolising 3HK into 3HAA prior to the final conversion of the latter into QUIN. IDO1 mRNA levels were significantly increased at least fivefold in the Delayed Death Injured Tissue as compared to the controls ($p < 0.05$; Fig. 4a). There were no significant differences observed on the IDO1 levels between the other groups (i.e. Acute Death vs control and Delayed Death Normal Tissue vs control). A similar pattern was also observed in the KYNase mRNA levels whereby over a sevenfold increase was detected in the Delayed Death Injured Tissue over the controls (Fig. 4b, $p < 0.05$) and no differences between the other groups. In contrast, mRNA expression of KAT-II, KMO, 3HAO and QPRTase remained unchanged in both the acute and delayed death groups (Fig. 4c–f).

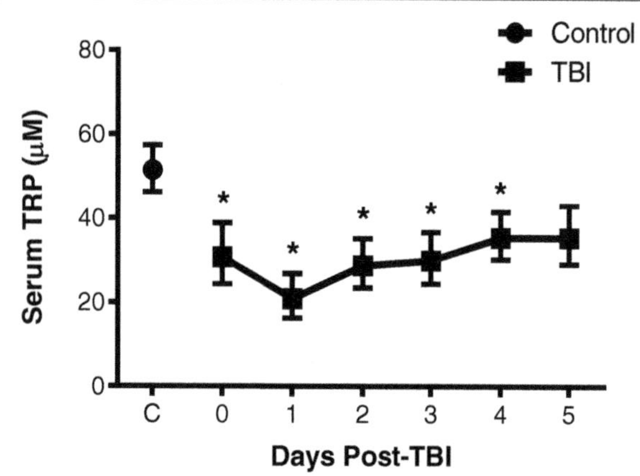

Fig. 3 The concentration of tryptophan in serum is reduced after TBI. The concentration of tryptophan in serum samples of TBI patients was measured from the day of hospital admission (day 0) to day 5 after injury and compared to the control serum. Significant decrease in serum TRP levels were observed between days 0 and 4; there was no statistical difference at day 5 to control levels, but median concentration at day 5 (36.29 μM) was similar to day 4 (35.6 μM). Data is shown as daily median with 25–75 percentile. *Asterisks* indicate significant differences ($p < 0.05$) between TBI and control using one-way ANOVA followed by Dunnett's multiple comparison as *post hoc*. TBI patients: n = 25–28 per time point; control group: n = 9–11

Thus, the marked increase in QUIN production observed in CSF following TBI is supported by the upregulation of mRNA expression of those enzymes of the KP involved in the synthesis of QUIN, IDO1 and KYNase.

Expression of active IDO1 protein is increased in the injured brain

We next seek to determine the localisation of active IDO1 enzyme on post-mortem brain tissue to be related to the findings of upregulated IDO1 mRNA shown above. Using an antibody that specifically recognises activated IDO1, immunohistochemistry revealed a significant increase in the number of IDO1-positive cells after TBI, which peaked in acute TBI and gradually declined in the injured and normal tissue of delayed death patients.

The highest amounts of cells expressing IDO1 were detected in the brains of patients with acute death after TBI (19.1 ± 3.1 % of total cells; Fig. 5a(III,IV), Fig. 5b) compared to control tissues (6.2 ± 0.8 %; p = 0.0286; Fig. 5a(I,II)). Although the number of IDO1-positive cells was lower in the Delayed Death Injured Tissue, they were still significantly elevated (12.1 ± 2.3 %) compared to control (Fig. 5a(V,VI), Fig. 5b). For comparison, analysis of the brain region of the delayed death that did not present evident tissue pathology showed no increase in IDO1 protein expression, having similar numbers of IDO1-positive cells to control brains (Fig. 5a(VII,VIII), Fig. 5b). Based on the microscopic evaluation, cells expressing IDO1 have morphology typical of pyramidal cortical neurons, thus suggesting their potential contribution to the activation of the KP. Together, this immunohistochemical data supports the hypothesis that IDO1 is indeed activated in the injured brain.

QUIN concentrations in CSF correlate with outcomes scores

Previous studies reported that higher concentrations of QUIN in CSF correlated with mortality in adult and paediatric TBI patients [28, 29]. We, therefore, investigated the relationship of QUIN with outcome scores at 6 months post-TBI. We performed a Pearson correlation of coefficient between the GOSE scores and maximal CSF concentration of QUIN between days 1 and 5 after TBI. A significant inverse correlation was observed between QUIN and GOSE with $r = -0.46$ and $p < 0.02$ (Fig. 6a). This correlation indicates a potential prognostic value for QUIN, whereby patients with higher QUIN production in the acute phase after injury have poor recovery at 6 months post-injury. Furthermore, we dichotomised TBI patients according to favourable (GOSE 5–8) and unfavourable outcome (GOSE 1–4) scores. Patients with unfavourable outcome had a close to significant higher concentration of QUIN (median: 0.28 μM, 25–75 %: 0.20–0.48 μM) than patients with favourable outcome (median: 0.17 μM, 25–75 %: 0.08–0.26 μM) (p = 0.056; Fig. 6b).

Discussion

Clinical studies have shown that secondary injury processes induced by TBI generate ongoing disease-like characteristics that cause progressive brain damage, delay physical recovery and contribute to the onset of mental illness. Therefore, early treatment aimed to reduce acute pathological sequel is the major focus in the development of therapeutic strategies in TBI patients. It is well established that excitotoxicity, neuroinflammation and oxidative stress are pivotal pathways of secondary brain damage following TBI [38]. Studies of neurodegenerative diseases and infection of the nervous system have shown that TRP metabolism participates in the regulation of immune activation, generation of oxidative radicals and production of excitotoxic substances [17]. Despite robust evidence showing that the KP plays an important role in neuropathology, this pathway has only been sporadically examined in the context of TBI. This gap spurred the current investigation aimed at measuring a number of metabolites of the KP in live, severely injured TBI patients' CSF and understanding how these metabolites relate to the expression of critical enzymes of the KP in post-mortem brain tissues of TBI victims. Our data demonstrates that the KP is profoundly activated after brain trauma by showing increased concentration of a number of TRP metabolites in CSF, including KYN, KYNA and QUIN. Enhanced production of the excitotoxic

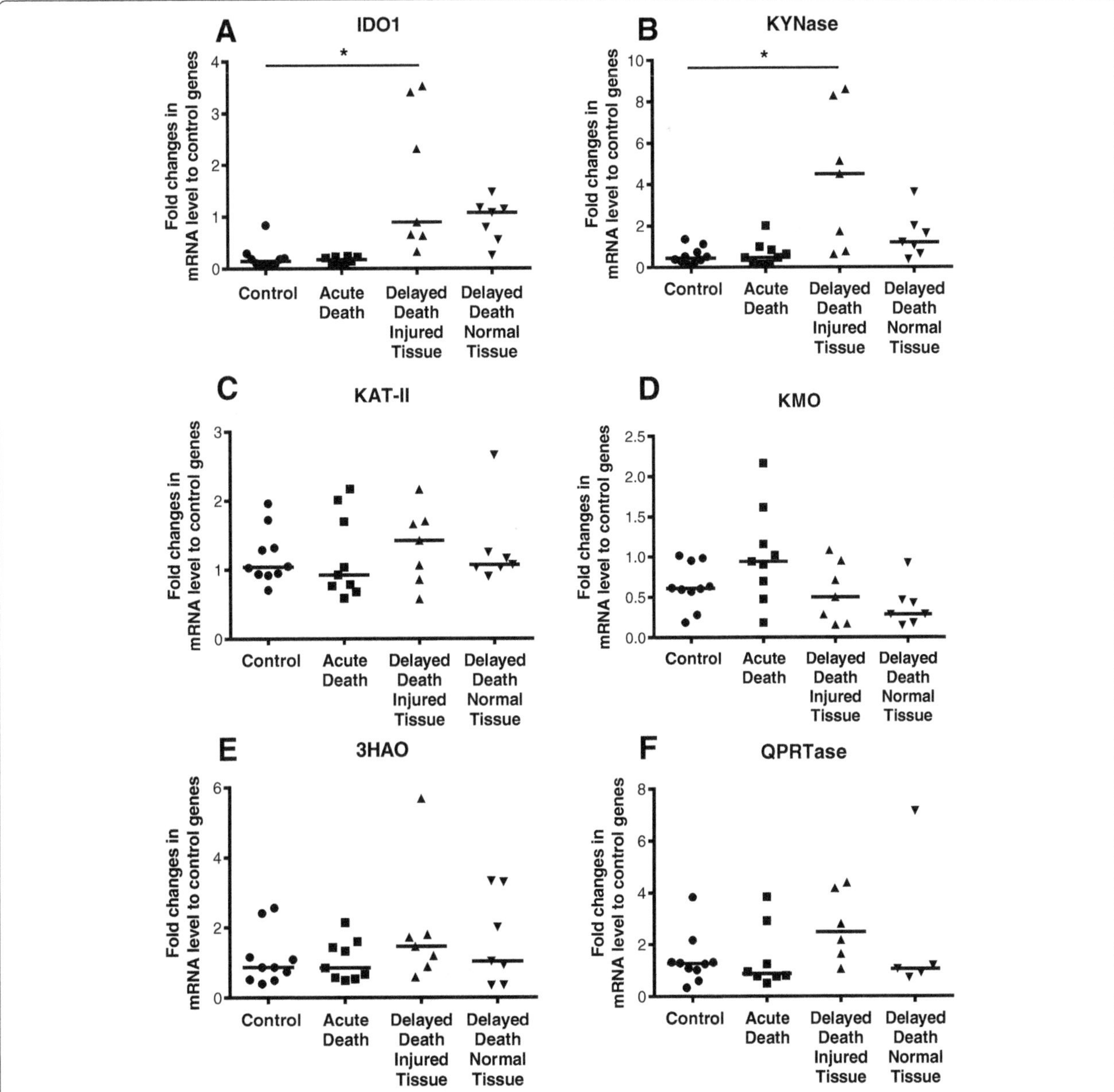

Fig. 4 qPCR analysis of enzymes of the kynurenine pathway in brains of TBI victims demonstrates enhanced IDO1 and KYNase expression. Gene expression of six enzymes of the kynurenine pathway was determined by qPCR in four groups of post-mortem brains obtained from the temporal cortex after TBI and uninjured control individuals ($n = 10$). Groups comprise the following: TBI patients with acute death (survived <17 min after injury, $n = 9$), TBI patients with delayed death (survival between 6 and 122 h, $n = 7$) with tissue collected from brain regions having evident tissue pathology (Delay Death Injured Tissue) and brain regions without macroscopic damage obtained from the contralateral uninjured side (Delay Death Normal Tissue) ($n = 7$). **a** Indoleamine-pyrrole 2,3-dioxygenase (IDO1), **b**. kynurenase (KYNase), **c** kynurenine amino transferase-II (KAT-II), **d** kynurenine 3-monooxygenase (KMO), **e** 3-hydroxyanthranilic acid oxygenase (3HAO) and **f** quinolinic acid phosphoribosyl transferase (QPRTase). *Asterisks* indicate significant differences ($p < 0.05$) between TBI and control groups using one-way ANOVA followed by Dunnett's multiple comparison as *post hoc*. Data shown as median with 25–75 percentile. IDO1 and KYNase were significantly increased in the Delay Death Injured Tissue group as to the control samples

metabolite QUIN likely arises from the activation and overexpression of the enzyme IDO1 subsequently driving the pathway into the production of intermediate metabolites 3HK (passive intermediate) and 3HAA via the activation of KYNase.

We need to distinguish between IDO1 enzyme activation detected by immunohistochemistry and upregulation of IDO1 mRNA measured by PCR to explain the different timing of the changes observed. IDO1 is stored in a dephosphorylated form (inactive) with its activation by

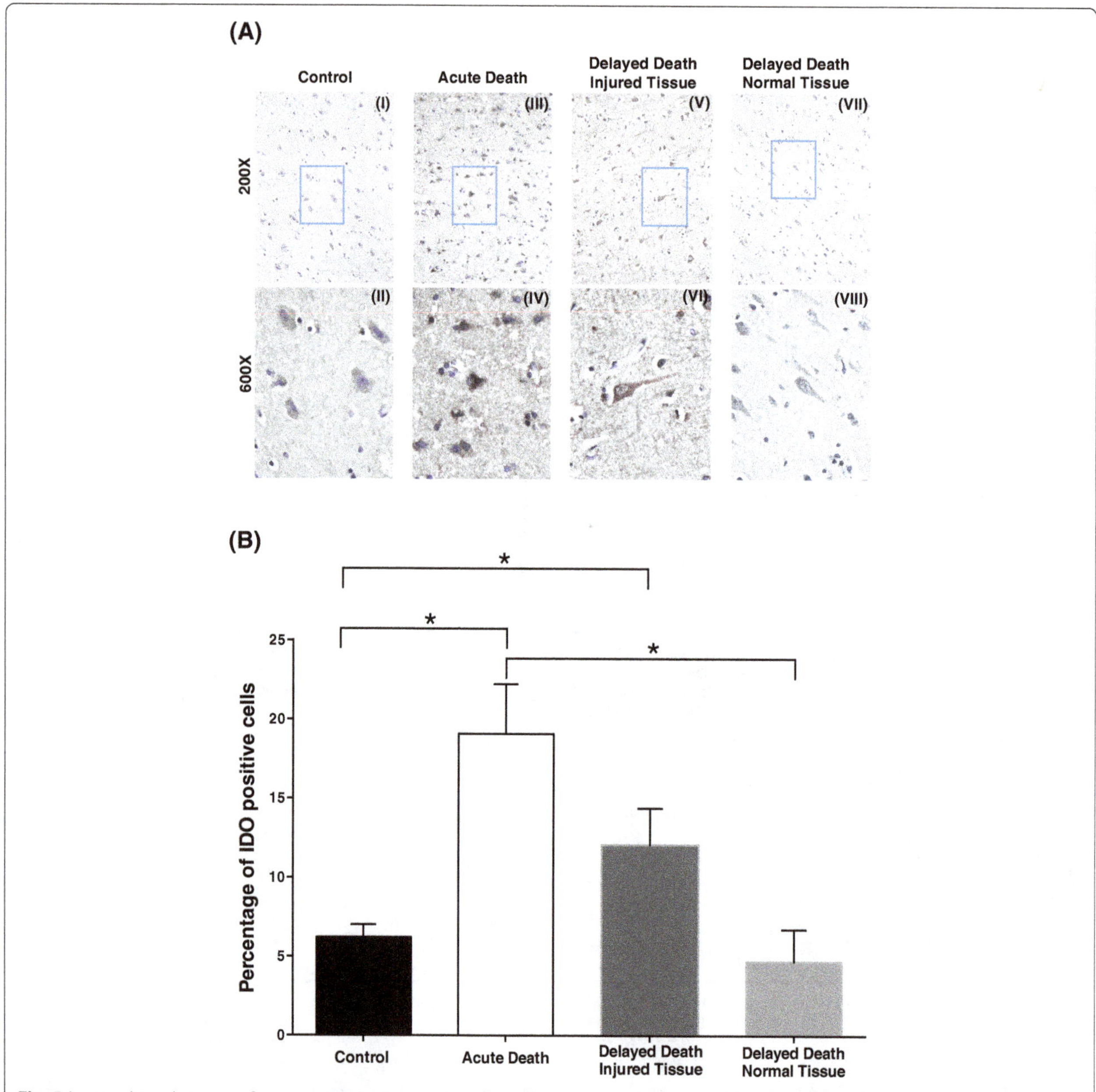

Fig. 5 Immunohistochemistry of post-mortem brains reveals increased IDO1 acutely after TBI. **a** IDO1 immunohistochemistry was performed on post-mortem brains as described in the 'Materials and methods' section. IDO1 is found increasingly expressed in Acute Death and Delayed Death Injured Tissue samples compared to the control. Top panels (i, iii, v, vii) indicate ×200 magnification; bottom panels (ii, iv, vi, viii) indicate ×600 magnification. Figures represent IDO1 immunohistochemistry of the cortex of the uninjured control group (i and ii), acute death (<17 min after injury; Acute Death) (iii and iv), tissue obtained from injured cortex of TBI patients with delayed death (survival between 6 and 122 h; Delay Death Injured Tissue) (v and vi) and tissue collected from regions without macroscopic damage of the contralateral uninjured side (Delay Death Normal Tissue) (vii and viii). *Rectangular boxes* in the ×200 panels indicate the magnified regions of ×600. Brain sections were counterstained with haematoxylin. **b** IDO immunohistochemistry staining was semi-quantitatively assessed in post-mortem brain samples and presented as the percentage of positively stained cells relative to the total number of cells per field. Statistical differences were calculated as described in the Materials and methods section, $*p \leq 0.05$. Data are mean ± SEM. Significant increase in the number of IDO1-positive cells was observed in Acute Death and Delayed Death Injured Tissue as compared to the controls; similar levels of IDO1-positive cells were between Control and Delayed Death Normal Tissue groups

phosphorylation occurring within a few minutes from stimulation [39, 40]. This activation process makes IDO1 recognisable to the mAb used in immunohistochemistry of post-mortem early-injured brains presented in Fig. 5. Unfortunately, there is no commercially available antibody for the dephosphorylated/inactive form of IDO1 to allow for its detection *in situ*. Moreover, activated IDO1 has the capacity of auto-amplification, a fact that may explain the

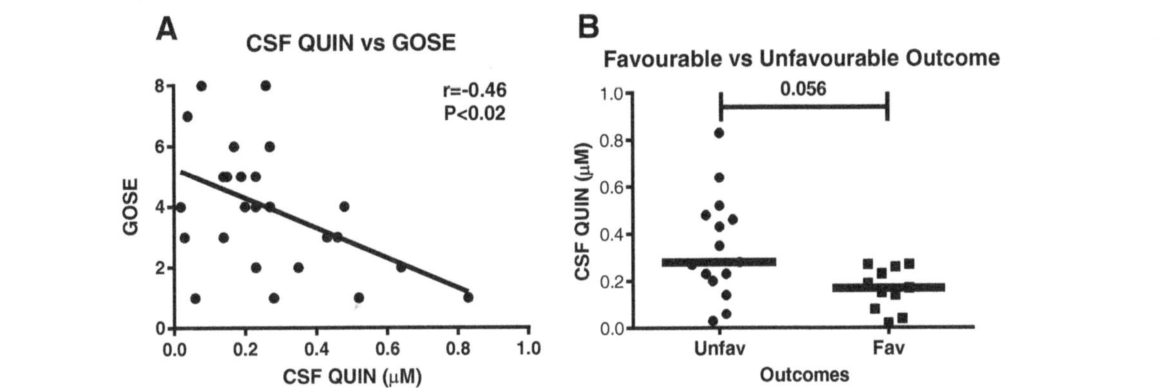

Fig. 6 The concentration of QUIN in CSF is inversely correlated with GOSE scores and is significantly more elevated in patients with unfavourable outcome. **a** Correlative analysis was undertaken using maximal concentration of QUIN in CSF of each patient between day 0 (admission to hospital) and day 5 post-TBI and the GOSE scores assessed at 6 months after TBI. A significant negative correlation ($p < 0.05$) was observed between QUIN and GOSE scores with $r = -0.46$ ($n = 28$). **b** TBI patients were grouped into favourable (GOSE 5–8, $n = 11$) and unfavourable outcome (GOSE 1–4, $n = 15$) and their maximal QUIN concentration compared between the groups. Patients with unfavourable outcome showed a close to significant ($p = 0.056$) higher concentration of QUIN in CSF compared to patients with favourable outcome

later upregulation of IDO1 mRNA in post-mortem brains of delayed survival times between 6 and 122 h post-TBI [39] (Fig. 4a).

In regard to the immunohistochemistry experiments, our data has to be taken with caution given the limited number of tissues stained and the variety of brain regions analysed. Importantly, however, these experiments confirm that active IDO1 protein is indeed present in the brain early after trauma, corroborating the hypothesis that IDO1 activation is actually increased within a few minutes after TBI (Fig. 5a,b). We are aware that these results warrant further investigations to explore the mechanisms and profiles of IDO1 activation after TBI to allow for a comprehensive quantification and understanding of its role in the ultimate activation of the KP.

Collectively, the analysis of the KP metabolite in CSF and the expression of the KP enzymes in post-mortem brain tissue suggests that the QUIN production is increased via the activation of the minor branch of the KP, beginning from the metabolism of KYN to AA, the production of 3HAA and finally the accumulation of QUIN. This hypothesis is also supported by the gradual increase in the concentration of AA in CSF (Fig. 1e), which, although not significant, displays a pattern strikingly similar to the pattern observed for QUIN production (Fig. 1d).

In addition, we report of an inverse correlation between elevated QUIN in CSF and the adverse long-term outcome, corroborating both a detrimental role of QUIN in the pathophysiology of secondary brain damage as well as the potential therapeutic implications of targeting QUIN production to reduce morbidity in this patient population.

The KP represents the major metabolic cascade of TRP metabolism, which degrades up to 90 % of available amino acid. The KP is dramatically enhanced in disease conditions that particularly involve the activation of the immune system. We and others have focused much of our research efforts in characterising the inflammatory response resulting from TBI, via clinical and experimental investigations (reviews [41, 42]).

During an inflammatory response, the release of cytokines, in particular IFN-γ, by activated monocytes and leukocytes increases the degradation of TRP via the KP [43]. This likely occurs through the ability of IFN-γ to activate the upstream enzyme IDO1 of the KP, which may become highly processed to release bioproducts such as QUIN, known to promoting excitotoxicity. We have previously shown that IFN-γ is rapidly upregulated in the CSF of severe TBI patients. In addition, using the same brain homogenates analysed in this study, we demonstrated that IFN-γ was already found enhanced in early death brains with even greater concentrations in the delayed death brains by a sixfold increase from controls [36, 44]. In fact, among the eight cytokines analysed, IFN-γ was the third highest cytokine following IL-6 and IL-8 [36].

We cannot exclude, however, the contribution of other factors in the activation/upregulation of IDO1. In fact, *in vitro* studies on cultured microglia have demonstrated IFN-γ-independent activation of IDO1 by TNF-α and IL-1β [45]. This point is pertinent to our study as we have previously shown a fourfold elevation of TNF-α at protein/mRNA levels in the same post-mortem brains harvested within 17 min post-injury while a nonsignificant increase of IL-1β mRNA was observed early (17 min) which was followed by a substantial and significant upregulation of over fivefold in the delayed group dying beyond 6 h from TBI [36]. It is conceivable that combined increase of these cytokines early after TBI results in subsequent and significant induction of IDO1 mRNA that was observed in the injured brain of delayed death patients (Fig. 4a).

In our study, the levels of TRP in CSF remained within a normal range whereas the blood concentrations were found below physiological values during almost the entire acute phase post-TBI. It is important to note that in healthy conditions the concentration of TRP in serum is tenfold higher than the CSF level. Although serum TRP decreased up to 50 % after injury, its blood levels were still higher compared to CSF. The striking difference between these two compartments may allow sufficient amounts of TRP to be transported to the brain or CSF via the brain/CSF barrier to maintaining a constant CSF concentration, which may explain the lack of changes of TRP in CSF.

Decreased concentrations of TRP in serum were reported previously in patients with infectious and neurodegenerative diseases and cancers. The authors speculated that this phenomenon is caused by an enhancement in peripheral IDO1/TDO enzyme activity [46]. Our observation of a significant decrease of TRP in serum after TBI confirms the findings reported by others in multiple trauma patients showing that blood TRP was significantly attenuated [46].

Although cytokines can strongly affect the KP, it has been demonstrated that TRP itself possesses important immune-regulatory properties. TRP depletion suppresses the proliferation of mononuclear cells [5], decreases immune cell activation [6, 47] and inhibits parasitic growth [48]. Therefore, a low concentration of serum TRP may provide some beneficial effects in the early stage after severe brain injury by reducing acute inflammatory responses. However, with the current setting, our study is unable elucidate the underlining mechanisms leading to the reduction of TRP in blood, a question which warrants further investigations.

Analysis of gene expression of the KP enzymes indicated that KP is strongly activated after TBI. The enzyme KAT has four isoforms, which are responsible for the synthesis of the neuroprotectant KYNA from its precursor KYN [49]. In this study, we have only examined KAT-II, one of the major KATs involved in both normal and disease conditions, which is considered as a promising target for pharmaceutical intervention. The expression of KAT-II in post-mortem brain did not vary between the three groups of TBI patients, Acute Death, Delayed Death Injured Tissue and Delayed Death Normal Tissue relative to control tissues. The unchanged expression levels of KAT-II observed in these brains are consistent with the unaltered concentration of its bioproduct KYNA in CSF between days 0, 1 and 2 and controls (Fig. 1c). It is important to consider that the average survival time of the delayed group is 40 h; thus, the tissue sample collected from these victims occurred well before the observed increase of KYNA in CSF, which was only found to be significant at 3 days post-injury. Here, we cannot adequately explain the mechanisms leading to enhanced KYNA and whether this is due to the increase of KAT expression/activation or as a result of an elevated concentration of the precursor KYN. However, we have to bear in mind that mRNA expression levels do not reflect changes in enzyme activation, thus posing a limitation in this study, solely based on qPCR. Previous work by Han et al. has shown that the Km of KAT-II is 1.7 ± 0.5 mM [50], a concentration that greatly exceeds the concentration of KYN in the CSF samples we found in the control and TBI cases (mean 0.08 ± 0.01 μM and 0.21 ± 0.02 μM, respectively). Therefore, we cannot state without doubt that the marked increase in the KYNA on days 3, 4 and 5 is attributed to the elevation of KYN following injury.

KMO is the key enzyme converting KYN into 3HK and subsequently into QUIN. This step of the KP has been suggested to be the main pathway for QUIN production. Inhibition of KMO was effectively ameliorating QUIN-mediated neurodegeneration in rodent [51]. However, in our study, KMO did not change significantly after TBI with median levels remaining similar among the four groups examined (Fig. 4d).

Newly emerged evidence demonstrated the important roles of 3HAA and AA in both brain and periphery in normal and disease conditions (see review by Darlington et al. 2010 [52]). Studies on osteoporosis [53], Huntington's disease [54, 55], stroke [32] and depression [56] have shown a simultaneous increase in AA and reduction in 3HAA in blood. In the brain, AA is an effective inhibitor of 3HAO [57]; therefore, the increase in AA in neurodegenerative diseases may provide some degree of inhibition of 3HAO that is required for the synthesis of the neurotoxin QUIN. Our study demonstrated that the ratios of 3HAA and AA are higher in the early days after TBI and gradually decreased, suggesting an overproduction in AA compared to 3HAA over time.

Despite the lack of changes in those metabolites upstream to QUIN synthesis (3HAA, 3HK not measured) and despite the elevation of KYNA—a metabolite generated via a separate branch from the one responsible for QUIN production—evidence for enhanced activation of the branch of the KP pathway leading to increased QUIN reported in this study is based on the following data: (1) prolonged elevation of QUIN in CSF of TBI patients, (2) increased QUIN:KYN and QUIN:KYNA ratios from CSF measurements of these metabolites, (3) increased IDO1 and KYNase mRNA expression in human brains and (4) enhanced acute expression of IDO1 protein on neurons in the injured brain region but not in tissue areas of normal appearance.

QUIN exerts its neurotoxic activity by interacting with a subgroup of NMDA receptors leading to a widespread destruction of neuronal terminals and sparing fibres [58]. In cultured cortico-striatal neurons, prolonged exposure to submicromolar concentrations of QUIN caused excitotoxic damage [59]. Further, *in vivo* studies using intrastriatal injection of QUIN showed tissue lesions similarly located in the basal nuclei as occurring in Huntington's disease patients [60]. Another recent *in vivo* study also demonstrated that brain regions, i.e. cerebellar cortex, hippocampus and cerebellum, have different susceptibility to QUIN-induced oxidative stress [61].

Our recent studies in NSC-34, a mouse motor neuron cell line, demonstrated that 2 μM QUIN is highly toxic and that uptake of QUIN by NSC-34 cells occurs as early as 30 min after exposure to QUIN [62]. QUIN neurotoxicity is mediated by both direct and indirect mechanisms. It has been reported that QUIN can directly increase free radical generations once entering the cells [63–65]. Free radical production following hypoxia-ischemia in association with inflammation plays a prominent role in the ultimate death of cells. Free radicals can cause cellular injury via several mechanisms, including membrane lipid peroxidation, oxidative damage of proteins and DNA and RNA fragmentation [66]. QUIN has been shown to chelate Fe^{2+} to form a QUIN-Fe^{2+} complex, which results in the production of the most toxic hydroxyl radical via the Fenton reaction [67]. Accumulation of QUIN in neurons has been shown in Alzheimer's disease [9], motor neurons in ALS [68] and neuronal cell line [62]. Collectively, these multiple biochemical pathways in which QUIN may be involved have been demonstrated to be contributing elements within the complex mechanisms of secondary brain damage arising from TBI.

Studies have shown significant associations between QUIN concentration and severity of the infectious diseases of the nervous system. Concentration of CSF QUIN is elevated 3.5-fold in the early stage of immunodeficiency syndrome (AIDS) patients [18], while it increased over 20-fold in patients at the late stage of the disease [18]. A higher level of CSF QUIN in individuals with HIV infection was positively correlated with more severe motor deficits [69]. In the context of outcome following TBI, these observations are consistent with the finding of our study, whereby we detected a significant negative correlation between patients' GOSE scores and QUIN concentrations in CSF, including the evidence of higher QUIN in patients with unfavourable when compared to those with favourable outcomes. This suggests a critical role of QUIN as a potential biomarker for the early prediction of long-term outcome following TBI.

Conclusion

Highly neuroactive products of TRP metabolism have received considerable attention in the last two decades. Numerous studies have demonstrated the importance of TRP and its metabolites in both normal physiology and disease conditions such as neuroinflammatory, infectious and neurodegenerative diseases. However, limited reports have examined changes and roles of TRP metabolism in TBI. This study is the first to investigate longitudinal changes in key metabolites of the KP in patients with severe TBI including investigations in brain gene expression of key regulatory enzymes of the KP in individuals who died due to TBI. We have obtained novel and convincing data of enhanced KYNase expression occurring in the acute phase following TBI. These results indicate that TBI may selectively activate the branch of the KP leading to increased QUIN production in the injured brain. This novel finding supports the concept that blocking the activity of KYNase (with existing compounds such as oestrone sulphate or nicotinylalanine) may become an effective therapeutic strategy in attenuating QUIN production and its driven excitotoxicity, thus diminishing the detrimental consequences of secondary brain damage.

Authors' contributions

EBY carried out the overall study design, tryptophan metabolite measurements, data analysis and manuscript preparation. TF carried out enzyme gene expression analysis and data analysis and assisted in manuscript preparation. CKL carried out metabolite measurements and data analysis and assisted in manuscript preparation. BH carried out enzyme gene expression analysis and data analysis and assisted in manuscript preparation. GS carried out immunohistochemistry and data analysis and assisted in manuscript preparation. MT carried out tryptophan metabolite measurements and data analysis. JVR collected human control samples and assisted in TBI sample collection. DWW advised on sample measurement and validation process. GJG and MCM-K contributed significantly in study design, oversighted the study and contributed to draft the manuscript. GJG and MCM-K are the senior authors of this study. All authors read and approved the final manuscript.

Acknowledgements

This study was funded by the Victorian Neurotrauma Initiative/Traffic Accident Commission project grant D009 and Research Fellowships to EBY and MCM.-K and National Health Medical Research Council Project Grant #436815. GJG is funded by the Australian Research Council (Future Fellowship). Post-mortem brain tissues were received from the Victorian Brain Bank Network, supported by The Florey Institute of Neuroscience and Mental Health, The Alfred and the Victorian Forensic Institute of Medicine and funded by Australia's National Health & Medical Research Council and Parkinson's Victoria.

Author details

[1]Department of Physiology, Monash University, Clayton, VIC 3800, Australia. [2]Department of Pharmacology and Therapeutics, The University of Melbourne, Melbourne, Australia. [3]Neuroinflammation group, Faculty of Medicine and Health Sciences, Macquarie University, Sydney, Australia. [4]Applied Neurosciences Program, Peter Duncan Neurosciences Research Unit, St Vincent's Centre for Applied Medical Research, Sydney, Australia. [5]Hospital Queen Elizabeth, Karung Berkunci No. 2029, 88586 Kota Kinabalu, Sabah, Malaysia. [6]Department of Neurosurgery, The Alfred Hospital, Melbourne, Australia. [7]Department of Surgery, Central Clinical School and Monash Institute of Medical Engineering, Monash University, Melbourne, Australia. [8]The Ritchie Centre, Hudson Institute of Medical Research, Monash Medical Centre, Melbourne, Australia. [9]Australian New Zealand Intensive Care Research Centre, Department of Epidemiology and Preventive Medicine, Monash University, Melbourne, Australia. [10]Department of Child Health, Barrow Neurological Institute, University of Arizona, Phoenix, AZ, USA.

Competing interests

The authors declare that they have no competing interests.

References

1. Miller JD. Head injury. J Neurol Neurosurg Psychiatry. 1993;56:440–7.
2. Guillemin GJ. Quinolinic acid: neurotoxicity. FEBS J. 2012;279:1355.
3. McMenamy RH. Binding of indole analogues to human serum albumin. Effects of fatty acids. J Biol Chem. 1965;240:4235–43.
4. Christensen HN, Albritton LM, Kakuda DK, MacLeod CL. Gene-product designations for amino acid transporters. J Exp Biol. 1994;196:51–7.
5. Sarkhosh K, Tredget EE, Li Y, Kilani RT, Uludag H, Ghahary A. Proliferation of peripheral blood mononuclear cells is suppressed by the indoleamine 2,3-dioxygenase expression of interferon-gamma-treated skin cells in a co-culture system. Wound Repair Regen. 2003;11:337–45.
6. Sarkhosh K, Tredget EE, Karami A, Uludag H, Iwashina T, Kilani RT, et al. Immune cell proliferation is suppressed by the interferon-gamma-induced indoleamine 2,3-dioxygenase expression of fibroblasts populated in collagen gel (FPCG). J Cell Biochem. 2003;90:206–17.
7. Meisel R, Zibert A, Laryea M, Gobel U, Daubener W, Dilloo D. Human bone marrow stromal cells inhibit allogeneic T-cell responses by indoleamine 2,3-dioxygenase-mediated tryptophan degradation. Blood. 2004;103:4619–21.
8. Swanson KA, Zheng Y, Heidler KM, Mizobuchi T, Wilkes DS. CDllc + cells modulate pulmonary immune responses by production of indoleamine 2,3-dioxygenase. Am J Respir Cell Mol Biol. 2004;30:311–8.
9. Guillemin GJ, Brew BJ, Noonan CE, Takikawa O, Cullen KM. Indoleamine 2,3 dioxygenase and quinolinic acid immunoreactivity in Alzheimer's disease hippocampus. Neuropathol Appl Neurobiol. 2005;31:395–404.
10. Schwarcz R, Bruno JP, Muchowski PJ, Wu HQ. Kynurenines in the mammalian brain: when physiology meets pathology. Nat Rev Neurosci. 2012;13:465–77.
11. Foster AC, Vezzani A, French ED, Schwarcz R. Kynurenic acid blocks neurotoxicity and seizures induced in rats by the related brain metabolite quinolinic acid. Neurosci Lett. 1984;48:273–8.
12. Heyes MP, Saito K, Crowley JS, Davis LE, Demitrack MA, Der M, et al. Quinolinic acid and kynurenine pathway metabolism in inflammatory and non-inflammatory neurological disease. Brain. 1992;115(Pt 5):1249–73.
13. Moroni F. Tryptophan metabolism and brain function: focus on kynurenine and other indole metabolites. Eur J Pharmacol. 1999;375:87–100.
14. Guillemin GJ, Brew BJ. Implications of the kynurenine pathway and quinolinic acid in Alzheimer's disease. Redox Rep. 2002;7:199–206.
15. Ting KK, Brew B, Guillemin G. The involvement of astrocytes and kynurenine pathway in Alzheimer's disease. Neurotox Res. 2007;12:247–62.
16. Guillemin GJ, Williams KR, Smith DG, Smythe GA, Croitoru-Lamoury J, Brew BJ. Quinolinic acid in the pathogenesis of Alzheimer's disease. Adv Exp Med Biol. 2003;527:167–76.
17. Guillemin GJ. Quinolinic acid, the inescapable neurotoxin. FEBS J. 2012;279:1356–65.
18. Heyes MP, Brew BJ, Martin A, Price RW, Salazar AM, Sidtis JJ, et al. Quinolinic acid in cerebrospinal fluid and serum in HIV-1 infection: relationship to clinical and neurological status. Ann Neurol. 1991;29:202–9.
19. Baratte S, Molinari A, Veneroni O, Speciale C, Benatti L, Salvati P. Temporal and spatial changes of quinolinic acid immunoreactivity in the gerbil hippocampus following transient cerebral ischemia. Brain Res Mol Brain Res. 1998;59:50–7.
20. Haberny KA, Pou S, Eccles CU. Potentiation of quinolinate-induced hippocampal lesions by inhibition of NO synthesis. Neurosci Lett. 1992;146:187–90.
21. Kheramin S, Body S, Mobini S, Ho MY, Velazquez-Martinez DN, Bradshaw CM, et al. Effects of quinolinic acid-induced lesions of the orbital prefrontal cortex on inter-temporal choice: a quantitative analysis. Psychopharmacology (Berl). 2002;165:9–17.
22. Yan E, Castillo-Melendez M, Smythe G, Walker D. Quinolinic acid promotes albumin deposition in Purkinje cell, astrocytic activation and lipid peroxidation in fetal brain. Neuroscience. 2005;134:867–75.
23. Stone TW. Kynurenines in the CNS: from endogenous obscurity to therapeutic importance. Prog Neurobiol. 2001;64:185–218.
24. Stone TW, Perkins MN. Quinolinic acid: a potent endogenous excitant at amino acid receptors in CNS. Eur J Pharmacol. 1981;72:411–2.
25. Kalonia H, Kumar P, Kumar A, Nehru B. Effect of caffeic acid and rofecoxib and their combination against intrastriatal quinolinic acid induced oxidative damage, mitochondrial and histological alterations in rats. Inflammopharmacology. 2009;17:211–9.
26. Braidy N, Grant R, Adams S, Brew BJ, Guillemin GJ. Mechanism for quinolinic acid cytotoxicity in human astrocytes and neurons. Neurotox Res. 2009;16:77–86.
27. Kerr SJ, Armati PJ, Guillemin GJ, Brew BJ. Chronic exposure of human neurons to quinolinic acid results in neuronal changes consistent with AIDS dementia complex. AIDS. 1998;12:355–63.
28. Bell MJ, Kochanek PM, Heyes MP, Wisniewski SR, Sinz EH, Clark RS, et al. Quinolinic acid in the cerebrospinal fluid of children after traumatic brain injury. Crit Care Med. 1999;27:493–7.
29. Sinz EH, Kochanek PM, Heyes MP, Wisniewski SR, Bell MJ, Clark RS, et al. Quinolinic acid is increased in CSF and associated with mortality after traumatic brain injury in humans. J Cereb Blood Flow Metab. 1998;18:610–5.
30. Costantino G. Inhibitors of quinolinic acid synthesis: new weapons in the study of neuroinflammatory diseases. Future Med Chem. 2014;6:841–3.
31. Wilson JT, Pettigrew LE, Teasdale GM. Structured interviews for the Glasgow Outcome Scale and the extended Glasgow Outcome Scale: guidelines for their use. J Neurotrauma. 1998;15:573–85.
32. Darlington LG, Mackay GM, Forrest CM, Stoy N, George C, Stone TW. Altered kynurenine metabolism correlates with infarct volume in stroke. Eur J Neurosci. 2007;26:2211–21.
33. Smythe GA, Braga O, Brew BJ, Grant RS, Guillemin GJ, Kerr SJ, et al. Concurrent quantification of quinolinic, picolinic, and nicotinic acids using electron-capture negative-ion gas chromatography–mass spectrometry. Anal Biochem. 2002;301:21–6.
34. Frugier T, Conquest A, McLean C, Currie P, Moses D, Goldshmit Y. Expression and activation of EphA4 in the human brain after traumatic injury. J Neuropathol Exp Neurol. 2012;71:242–50.
35. Frugier T, Crombie D, Conquest A, Tjhong F, Taylor C, Kulkarni T, et al. Modulation of LPA receptor expression in the human brain following neurotrauma. Cell Mol Neurobiol. 2011;31:569–77.
36. Frugier T, Morganti-Kossmann C, O'Reilly D, McLean C. *In situ* detection of inflammatory mediators in post-mortem human brain tissue following traumatic injury. J Neurotrauma. 2010;27:497–507.
37. Nemeth H, Toldi J, Vecsei L. Role of kynurenines in the central and peripheral nervous systems. Curr Neurovasc Res. 2005;2:249–60.
38. Werner C, Engelhard K. Pathophysiology of traumatic brain injury. Br J Anaesth. 2007;99:4–9.
39. Fallarino F, Grohmann U, Puccetti P. Indoleamine 2,3-dioxygenase: from catalyst to signaling function. Eur J Immunol. 2012;42:1932–7.
40. Salazar C, Hofer T. Multisite protein phosphorylation–from molecular mechanisms to kinetic models. FEBS J. 2009;276:3177–98.
41. Ziebell JM, Morganti-Kossmann MC. Involvement of pro- and anti-inflammatory cytokines and chemokines in the pathophysiology of traumatic brain injury. Neurotherapeutics. 2010;7:22–30.
42. Woodcock T, Morganti-Kossmann MC. The role of markers of inflammation in traumatic brain injury. Front Neurol. 2013;4:18.
43. Yamada A, Akimoto H, Kagawa S, Guillemin GJ, Takikawa O. Proinflammatory cytokine interferon-gamma increases induction of indoleamine 2,3-dioxygenase in monocytic cells primed with amyloid beta peptide 1–42: implications for the pathogenesis of Alzheimer's disease. J Neurochem. 2009;110:791–800.
44. Yan EB, Satgunaseelan L, Paul E, Bye N, Nguyen P, Agyapomaa D, et al. Post-traumatic hypoxia is associated with prolonged cerebral cytokine production, higher serum biomarker levels, and poor outcome in patients with severe traumatic brain injury. J Neurotrauma. 2014;31:618–29.
45. Wang Y, Lawson MA, Dantzer R, Kelley KW. LPS-induced indoleamine 2,3-dioxygenase is regulated in an interferon-gamma-independent manner by a JNK signaling pathway in primary murine microglia. Brain Behav Immun. 2010;24:201–9.
46. Ploder M, Spittler A, Schroecksnadel K, Neurauter G, Pelinka LE, Roth E, et al. Tryptophan degradation in multiple trauma patients: survivors compared with non-survivors. Clin Sci (Lond). 2009;116:593–8.
47. Pellegrin K, Neurauter G, Wirleitner B, Fleming AW, Peterson VM, Fuchs D. Enhanced enzymatic degradation of tryptophan by indoleamine 2,3-dioxygenase contributes to the tryptophan-deficient state seen after major trauma. Shock. 2005;23:209–15.
48. Pfefferkorn ER. Interferon gamma blocks the growth of Toxoplasma gondii in human fibroblasts by inducing the host cells to degrade tryptophan. Proc Natl Acad Sci U S A. 1984;81:908–12.
49. Han Q, Cai T, Tagle DA, Li J. Structure, expression, and function of kynurenine aminotransferases in human and rodent brains. Cell Mol Life Sci. 2010;67:353–68.
50. Han Q, Cai T, Tagle DA, Robinson H, Li J. Substrate specificity and structure of human aminoadipate aminotransferase/kynurenine aminotransferase II. Biosci Rep. 2008;28:205–15.
51. Zwilling D, Huang SY, Sathyasaikumar KV, Notarangelo FM, Guidetti P, Wu HQ, et al. Kynurenine 3-monooxygenase inhibition in blood ameliorates neurodegeneration. Cell. 2011;145:863–74.

52. Darlington LG, Forrest CM, Mackay GM, Smith RA, Smith AJ, Stoy N, et al. On the Biological Importance of the 3-hydroxyanthranilic Acid: anthranilic acid ratio. Int J Tryptophan Res. 2010;3:51–9.
53. Forrest CM, Mackay GM, Oxford L, Stoy N, Stone TW, Darlington LG. Kynurenine pathway metabolism in patients with osteoporosis after 2 years of drug treatment. Clin Exp Pharmacol Physiol. 2006;33:1078–87.
54. Stoy N, Mackay GM, Forrest CM, Christofides J, Egerton M, Stone TW, et al. Tryptophan metabolism and oxidative stress in patients with Huntington's disease. J Neurochem. 2005;93:611–23.
55. Forrest CM, Mackay GM, Stoy N, Spiden SL, Taylor R, Stone TW, et al. Blood levels of kynurenines, interleukin-23 and soluble human leucocyte antigen-G at different stages of Huntington's disease. J Neurochem. 2010;112:112–22.
56. Mackay GM, Forrest CM, Christofides J, Bridel MA, Mitchell S, Cowlard R, et al. Kynurenine metabolites and inflammation markers in depressed patients treated with fluoxetine or counselling. Clin Exp Pharmacol Physiol. 2009;36:425–35.
57. Guillemin GJ, Cullen KM, Lim CK, Smythe GA, Garner B, Kapoor V, et al. Characterization of the kynurenine pathway in human neurons. J Neurosci. 2007;27:12884–92.
58. Schwarcz R, Whetsell Jr WO, Mangano RM. Quinolinic acid: an endogenous metabolite that produces axon-sparing lesions in rat brain. Science. 1983;219:316–8.
59. Whetsell Jr WO, Schwarcz R. Prolonged exposure to submicromolar concentrations of quinolinic acid causes excitotoxic damage in organotypic cultures of rat corticostriatal system. Neurosci Lett. 1989;97:271–5.
60. Beal MF, Kowall NW, Ellison DW, Mazurek MF, Swartz KJ, Martin JB. Replication of the neurochemical characteristics of Huntington's disease by quinolinic acid. Nature. 1986;321:168–71.
61. Vandresen-Filho S, Martins WC, Bertoldo DB, Mancini G, De Bem AF, Tasca CI. Cerebral cortex, hippocampus, striatum and cerebellum show differential susceptibility to quinolinic acid-induced oxidative stress. Neurol Sci 2015.
62. Chen Y, Brew BJ, Guillemin GJ. Characterization of the kynurenine pathway in NSC-34 cell line: implications for amyotrophic lateral sclerosis. J Neurochem. 2011;118:816–25.
63. Iwahashi H, Kawamori H, Fukushima K. Quinolinic acid, alpha-picolinic acid, fusaric acid, and 2,6-pyridinedicarboxylic acid enhance the Fenton reaction in phosphate buffer. Chem Biol Interact. 1999;118:201–15.
64. Santamaria A, Galvan-Arzate S, Lisy V, Ali SF, Duhart HM, Osorio-Rico L, et al. Quinolinic acid induces oxidative stress in rat brain synaptosomes. Neuroreport. 2001;12:871–4.
65. Santamaria A, Jimenez-Capdeville ME, Camacho A, Rodriguez-Martinez E, Flores A, Galvan-Arzate S. *In vivo* hydroxyl radical formation after quinolinic acid infusion into rat corpus striatum. Neuroreport. 2001;12:2693–6.
66. von Ruecker AA, Han-Jeon BG, Wild M, Bidlingmaier F. Protein kinase C involvement in lipid peroxidation and cell membrane damage induced by oxygen-based radicals in hepatocytes. Biochem Biophys Res Commun. 1989;163:836–42.
67. Goda K, Kishimoto R, Shimizu S, Hamane Y, Ueda M. Quinolinic acid and active oxygens. Possible contribution of active oxygens during cell death in the brain. Adv Exp Med Biol. 1996;398:247–54.
68. Chen Y, Stankovic R, Cullen KM, Meininger V, Garner B, Coggan S, et al. The kynurenine pathway and inflammation in amyotrophic lateral sclerosis. Neurotox Res. 2010;18:132–42.
69. Martin A, Heyes MP, Salazar AM, Kampen DL, Williams J, Law WA, et al. Progressive slowing of reaction time and increasing cerebrospinal fluid concentrations of quinolinic acid in HIV-infected individuals. J Neuropsychiatry Clin Neurosci. 1992;4:270–9.

STING-mediated type-I interferons contribute to the neuroinflammatory process and detrimental effects following traumatic brain injury

Amar Abdullah[1], Moses Zhang[1], Tony Frugier[1], Sammy Bedoui[2], Juliet M. Taylor[1*†] and Peter J. Crack[1*†]

Abstract

Background: Traumatic brain injury (TBI) represents a major cause of disability and death worldwide with sustained neuroinflammation and autophagy dysfunction contributing to the cellular damage. Stimulator of interferon genes (STING)-induced type-I interferon (IFN) signalling is known to be essential in mounting the innate immune response against infections and cell injury in the periphery, but its role in the CNS remains unclear. We previously identified the type-I IFN pathway as a key mediator of neuroinflammation and neuronal cell death in TBI. However, the modulation of the type-I IFN and neuroinflammatory responses by STING and its contribution to autophagy and neuronal cell death after TBI has not been explored.

Methods: C57BL/6J wild-type (WT) and STING$^{-/-}$ mice (8–10-week-old males) were subjected to controlled cortical impact (CCI) surgery and brains analysed by QPCR, Western blot and immunohistochemical analyses at 2 h or 24 h. STING expression was also analysed by QPCR in post-mortem human brain samples.

Results: A significant upregulation in STING expression was identified in late trauma human brain samples that was confirmed in wild-type mice at 2 h and 24 h after CCI. This correlated with an elevated pro-inflammatory cytokine profile with increased TNF-α, IL-6, IL-1β and type-I IFN (IFN-α and IFN-β) levels. This expression was suppressed in the STING$^{-/-}$ mice with a smaller lesion volume in the knockout animals at 24 h post CCI. Wild-type mice also displayed increased levels of autophagy markers, LC3-II, p62 and LAMP2 after TBI; however, STING$^{-/-}$ mice showed reduced LAMP2 expression suggesting a role for STING in driving dysfunctional autophagy after TBI.

Conclusion: Our data implicates a detrimental role for STING in mediating the TBI-induced neuroinflammatory response and autophagy dysfunction, potentially identifying a new therapeutic target for reducing cellular damage in TBI.

Keywords: STING, Type-I interferon, Traumatic brain injury, Neuroinflammation, Autophagy

Background

Traumatic brain injury (TBI) remains the leading cause of death and permanent disability in adolescents worldwide [1]. Current treatments are inadequate, with the majority of potential therapeutics failing in clinical trials [2–4]. This can be attributed to the complexities of the secondary damage and the pathways involved in the neuronal cell death after TBI that are not fully understood. TBI is characterised by an initial, irreversible damage at the site of impact with the brain, in severe cases, suffering extensive cell loss. This is followed by secondary injury leading to progressive neuronal cell death within the surrounding area [5] that is associated with priming of resident brain cells, mainly microglia and astrocytes, infiltration of peripheral leukocytes [6] and the subsequent release of inflammatory cytokines, chemokines [7] and other secondary messengers. Mounting evidence suggests neuroinflammation contributes to the neurological deficits

* Correspondence: juliett@unimelb.edu.au; pcrack@unimelb.edu.au
†Juliet M. Taylor and Peter J. Crack contributed equally to this work.
[1]Neuropharmacology Laboratory, Department of Pharmacology & Therapeutics, University of Melbourne, Parkville, Melbourne 3010, Australia

observed after TBI [8–11]. It has been proposed that while this neuroinflammatory response contributes to a pro-survival milieu in the early stages of brain injury [12, 13], prolonged or chronic neuroinflammation is detrimental, leading to cell death in both animal studies and post mortem human brain samples [14–16]. Specifically, activation of microglia and astrocytes and the sustained release of pro-inflammatory cytokines such as TNF-α [17–19], IL-6 [20] and IL-1β [21–23] creates a toxic microenvironment detrimental to neuronal cell viability after brain injury.

The type-I interferons (IFNs) are known to be critical mediators of the inflammatory response in the periphery [24, 25]. Classically, the activation of type-I IFN signalling involves recognition of IFN-α and -β by their cognate receptors, composed of interferon receptor 1 (IFNAR1) and interferon receptor 2 (IFNAR2) subunits which are readily associated with the Janus activated kinases (JAKs) tyrosine kinase 2 (TYK2) and JAK1, respectively [26]. Upon activation, JAKs will in turn phosphorylate signal transducer and activator of transcription 2 (STAT2) or STAT1/3 at a tyrosine residue and subsequently activate the interferon regulatory factors (IRFs) (IRF3 and 7) [27, 28] leading to the production of type-I IFN and other pro-inflammatory cytokines [25]. Several recent studies have implicated the type-I IFNs in neuropathologies with increased expression linked to progression of neurological diseases including Gaucher disease [29], Aicardi-Goutieres syndrome [30] and model of prion disease [31]. In support of this, our group has identified a detrimental role for the type-I IFNs in animal models of Alzheimer's (AD) [32, 33] and Parkinson's disease (PD) [33] with elevated expression of type-I IFNs found in post-mortem human AD [33] and PD [34] brains. Furthermore, we also reported an increased expression of the type-I IFNs in human trauma brains (with greater than 6 h survival time) with attenuated type-I IFN signalling conferring a reduced neuroinflammatory response and smaller lesion volume in the controlled cortical impact (CCI) TBI animal model [35]. However, the underlying mechanisms that trigger the type-I IFN-mediated neuro-inflammatory response after TBI warrants further investigation.

The type-I IFNs can be alternatively activated through the stimulator of interferon genes (STING)-tumour necrosis factor (TNF) receptor-associated factor NF-κB activator (TANK)-binding kinase 1 (TBK1)-IRF3 signalling axis which requires the presence of cytosolic DNA in the cells. The STING-TBK1-IRF3 signalling pathway has long been appreciated as a trigger for DNA-dependent-IFN production. Aberrant IFN production signalling through a STING-dependent pathway has been implicated in autoinflammatory diseases [36] including vascular and pulmonary syndrome [37] and lupus [38]. STING has also been found to be upregulated in neurons infected by Japanese encephalitis viral RNA [39]. More recently, a study using cultured myeloid cells and mouse model of multiple sclerosis found that the antiviral drug ganciclovir (GCV) induces a type-I IFN response in microglia in a STING-dependent manner with activation of the STING pathway reducing microglial reactivity and the neuroinflammatory response [40]. Together, these studies suggest a role for STING in modulating immunological responses involving the type-I IFNs in the brain, with both neurotoxic and neuroprotective properties observed. However, the contribution of STING to the neuroinflammation occurring in acute and chronic neuropathologies is largely unknown.

Autophagy, a very well-characterised cellular degradation and/or recycling process, has also been implicated in human and animal models of TBI [41–44]. Following stimuli, autophagy is initiated by the formation of phagophore, which gradually elongates and envelops parts of cytoplasm such as damaged and old organelles. Eventually, propagating ends of the phagophore will come together to form a double-membrane vesicle termed the autophagosome, which subsequently fuse with the lysosome that degrades the materials captured by lysosomal hydrolases [45, 46]. Evidence in the literature reports increased autophagy markers after TBI, with both protective and detrimental effects observed. This double-edged sword role of autophagy reported after brain trauma may be due to the lack of understanding of its mechanisms and cell-type specificity within the CNS. Recently, a role for the STING and type-I IFN pathways in autophagy has also been proposed [47–50]. Specifically, STING and its downstream TBK1 protein are required for autophagy activation to eliminate bacterial infection in macrophages [51]. Subsequently, it was found that cyclic GMP-AMP synthase (cGAS), upstream activator of STING is required for activating type-I IFN production via the STING/TBK1/IRF3 pathway in this infection setting [52]. Intriguingly, cGAS is known to be degraded by p62-dependent selective autophagy upon sensing cytoplasmic DNA [53]. A recent report confirmed cGAS-STING degradation through this pathway is mediated by TBK1 [54] suggesting that the anti-microbial response and autophagy activation via STING is a tightly controlled event to prevent an excessive inflammatory response in the cells. However, the regulation of autophagy by STING and the type-I IFNs within the CNS is unknown. We were interested to investigate this in our CCI model and the possible role for STING and type-I IFN signalling in influencing this critical event after TBI.

In this study, we employed a similar CCI model as previously described by Karve et al. [35] to further elucidate the instigator of the type-I IFNs and its contribution to the neuroinflammatory environment after TBI. We hypothesise that type-I IFN expression is induced following TBI in part, through a DNA sensing pathway involving STING. Here, we report for the first time a critical role for STING in mediating the type-I IFN production and neuroinflammatory response after TBI. We found that STING$^{-/-}$ mice subjected to CCI surgery have a smaller lesion size as compared to their wild-type (WT) littermates. Importantly, this neuroprotection can be attributed in part to reduced pro-inflammatory cytokine levels and reduced astrocyte activation. In addition, we observed increased STING mRNA levels in post mortem human TBI brains implicating a role for STING in acute brain injury. This study also provides the first evidence for a critical role for STING in modulating autophagy activity after TBI. STING$^{-/-}$ mice had sustained and higher expression of autophagy markers including LC3 and p62 after TBI as compared to WT mice. Further, increased and impaired autophagic activity as measured by lysosomal-associated membrane protein 2 (LAMP2) expression levels was detected in WT mice at 24 h following CCI. However, reduced LAMP2 levels were identified in STING$^{-/-}$ brains at 24 h post-TBI suggesting an adaptation to normal autophagic activity in the absence of STING after TBI. This increased autophagic activity might serve as protective mechanism to remove injured cells and promote a protective environment thus partially contributing to the neuroprotection observed in STING$^{-/-}$ mice after TBI. Collectively, this study has identified a deleterious role for STING in mediating type-I IFN signalling and proposes STING as a potential target for therapeutic intervention following TBI.

Methods

Antibodies

Primary antibodies used for Western blot analysis:

Primary antibodies	Origin	Dilution	Company	Catalogue no
Anti-TMEM173/STING	Rabbit	1 in 500	Abcam	ab92605
Anti-LC3	Rabbit	1 in 1000	MBL	PM036
Anti-SQSTM1/p62	Mouse	1 in 1000	Abcam	ab56416
Anti-GFAP(GA5)	Mouse	1 in 1000	Cell Signalling	#3670
Anti-β-Actin	Mouse	1 in 1000	Sigma-Aldrich	A5441
Anti-LAMP2	Rat	1 in 1000	Abcam	ab25339

Secondary antibodies used: horseradish peroxidize conjugated goat anti-rabbit (1: 1000, Dako, P0488), goat anti-mouse (1: 1000, Dako, P0447) and rabbit anti-rat (1:1000, Abcam, ab6734).

Primary antibodies used for immunohistochemical analysis:

Primary antibodies	Origin	Dilution	Vendor	Catalogue no
Anti-TMEM173/STING	Rabbit	1 in 50	Abcam	ab92605
Anti-GFAP (GA5)	Mouse	1 in 1000	Cell Signalling	#3670
Anti-FOX3a	Mouse	1 in 250	Abcam	ab104224
Anti-IBA1	Rabbit	1 in 200	Wako	019–19741

Secondary antibodies used: Alexa fluor 488 goat anti-rabbit (1:1000, Life Technologies, A11008), Alexa fluor 594 goat anti-mouse (1:1000, Life Technologies, A11012).

Animals

Adult male mice of 8–10 week of age with average body weight 23 ± 3 g were used in all experiments. WT mice of C57BL/6J background were purchased from the Animal Resource Centre while STING$^{-/-}$ mice were a kind gift from Dr. Sammy Bedoui (Peter Doherty Institute, University of Melbourne) and Professor Ben Kile (Walter and Eliza Hall Institute, University of Melbourne).

Controlled cortical impact

The controlled cortical impact (CCI) procedures performed in this study were based on standard protocols as previously described and reported by our group [11]. Briefly, mice were anaesthetised using ketamine (100 mg/kg, Parnell)/Xylazine (10 mg/kg, Parnell) via intra-peritoneal injection. Craniotomy was then performed with hand-held electrical drill (Dremel 10.8 V) removing the bone flap to expose the right parietal cortex. Mice were restrained by stereotaxic device and were subjected to a 1.5-mm deep impact (velocity of 5 m/s) using the computer-controlled impactor device (LinMot-Talk 1100) (impactor diameter of 2 mm). Sham control mice underwent identical procedures as those for CCI without actual injury by the impactor. Following successful CCI, all mice were euthanized at 2 h and 24 h post injury and brains removed for further analysis.

Lesion size analysis

Twenty-four hours after CCI surgery, mice were transcardially perfused with 0.1% heparinised phosphate-buffered saline (Pfizer), followed by 4% paraformaldehyde (Scharlab S.L.) and their brains were isolated. Isolated brains were sectioned using a mouse brain matrix to 500 μm thickness followed by incubation in a 2% 2,3,5-triphenyltetrazolium chloride (TTC) in PBS solution at 35 °C for 15 min. Images of the stained brain sections were photomicrographed using a Zeiss Axioskop microscope and lesion area was determined using the ImageJ software (v1.47; NIH). White TTC staining of the lesion region within the brain was calculated using Cavalieri formula to find total lesion volume; [volume = $\Sigma A \times t \times ISF$] where A = sum of the corrected infarct areas, t = section thickness (500 μm) and ISF = inverse of the sampling fraction.

RNA extractions and cDNA synthesis

Cortical and striatal regions of the brain were isolated from the ipsilateral and contralateral hemispheres and were homogenised in 1 ml Trizol (Invitrogen) before incubation at room temperature for 10 min. Then, 0.2 ml Chloroform (Chem Supply) per 1 ml Trizol was added to the samples, and samples were centrifuged at 12,000 g for 15 min at 4 °C to separate samples into phases. The colourless, aqueous phase of each sample, which contained RNA, was transferred into a fresh 1.7 ml microcentrifuge tube. RNA was precipitated by adding 0.5 ml Propan-2-ol (Chem Supply) per 1 ml Trizol, and samples were again centrifuged at 12,000 g for 10 min at 4 °C. The supernatant from the tubes was discarded, and the RNA pellet was washed with 75% Ethanol (Chem Supply) in diethyl pyrocarbonate (DEPC)-treated water (Sigma), vortexed and centrifuged at 7500 g for 5 min at 4 °C. The RNA pellet was air-dried, and redissolved in RNAse-free H_20 (Invitrogen). Concentration of the RNA samples was measured using the NanoDrop 1000 Spectrophotometer (Thermo Scientific).

Quantitative real time polymerase chain reaction

cDNA was transcribed from 1 μg RNA using a high-capacity cDNA reverse transcription kit (Applied Biosystems) as previously described [33]. Genes of interest was detected using Taqman (Applied Biosciences) (Table 1) or SYBR green (GeneWorks) (Table 2) primers. Ct values were obtained for each sample, and relative transcript levels for each gene were calculated using the δδCT method [55]. For quantifying STING mRNA expression from human trauma samples, four control genes were used with the comparative C_T method (δC_T) applied as previously described [11].

QPCR analysis of human samples

Trauma brain samples from individuals who had died following closed head injury and non-head trauma controls were obtained from the Victorian Brain Bank Network (VBBN) [56] (Additional file 1: Table S1). RNA extractions and CDNA synthesis were performed as above with STING expression determined using Taqman primers (Table 1).

Western blot analysis

Protein concentration was measured using Braford assay with 50 μg of protein used for Western blot analysis. Extracted proteins were incubated in 2× Novex® Tris-glycine SDS sample buffer (Invitrogen) for 10 min at 100 °C and were resolved on 8% or 12% acrylamide SDS PAGE gels. Blots were then transferred to polyvinylidene fluoride (PVDF) membranes using a semi-dry transfer apparatus (BioRad). Membranes were blocked with 5% *w*/*v* skim milk in TBS-T for 1 h and incubated with primary antibodies in 2% *w*/*v* skim milk in TBS-T at 4 °C overnight. Membranes were washed three times for 10 min each with TBS-T prior to being incubated with HRP-conjugated secondary antibodies (diluted in 2% skim milk in TBS-T) for 60 min at room temperature. Again, membranes were washed with TBS-T and signals were detected using an ECL prime® Western blotting detection kit (Amersham) and visualised with the IQ350 imaging machine (GE Healthcare). Post-image densitometry was performed using ImageJ software (NIH), whereby signal intensity was calculated in arbitrary units. For densitometry calculations, phosphorylation intensity was measured in arbitrary units and normalised to the β-actin loading control. These values were then calculated as fold change compared to control.

Immunohistochemistry

Animals were perfused with ice-cold PBS followed by 4% PFA before hemispheres were removed and fixed in 5 ml of chilled 4% *w*/*v* paraformaldehyde, pH 7.4 (Sigma-Aldrich) overnight at 4 °C. These were then incubated at 4 °C overnight in 30% *w*/*v* sucrose before being embedded in OCT and cryosectioned into 30 μm coronal sections.

For immunohistochemistry, sections were permeabilised in 0.2% Triton X-100/PBS (PBS-T) for 20 min before being blocked for 1 h in 10% normal donkey serum/5% BSA/PBS at RT°C. The following antibodies were diluted in 1% BSA and incubated overnight at 4 °C: anti-mouse FOX3a (1:250, Abcam), anti-rabbit ionised calcium-binding adaptor molecule 1 (IBA1) (1:200, WAKO), anti-mouse glial fibrillary acidic protein (GFAP) (1:1000, Cell signalling) and anti-rabbit STING (1:50, Abcam). Sections were then washed

Table 1 Taqman primers used for QPCR analysis

Gene	Species	Refseq	Amplicon length (bp)	Catalogue no
GAPDH	Mouse	NM_008084.2	107	Mm99999915_m1
IFN-β	Mouse	NM_010510.1	69	Mm00439552_s1
IL1-β	Mouse	NM_008361.3	63	Mm01336189_m1
TNF-α	Mouse	NM_013693.3	81	Mm00443258_m1
IL6	Mouse	NM_031168.1	78	Mm00446190_m1
IRF3	Mouse	NM_016849.4	59	Mm00516779_m1
IRF7	Mouse	NM_001252600.1 NM_001252601.1 NM_016850.3	67	Mm00516788_m1
STING	Mouse	NM_028261.1	173	Mm01158117_m1
STING	Human	NM_001301738.1	89	Hs00736955_g1

Table 2 Sybr green primer sequences used QPCR analysis

Gene	Forward primer (5'-3')	Reverse primer (5'-3')
GAPDH	ATCTTCTTGTGCAGTGCCAGC	ACTCCACGACATACTCAGCACC
IFN-α	GCAATCCTCCTAGACTCACTTCTGCA	TATAGTTCCTCACAGCCAGCAG
IFNαE4	–	TATTTCTTCATAGCCAGCTG
TGF-β	TGCGCTTGCAGAGATTAAAA	CGTCAAAAGACAGCCACTCA

three times in PBS before 2-h incubation at room temperature with Alexa Fluor 594-conjugated donkey anti-mouse and Alexa Fluor 488-conjugated donkey anti-rabbit secondary antibodies. Sections were again washed in three washes of PBS before being mounted in Vectashield plus DAPI (Vectashield). Slides were viewed using a Ziess Axio 123,672,641 microscope and images captured using an Axio Cam Mrm camera and Zen 2011 software. Three fields of view were taken of three sections/animal (Additional file 2: Figure S1).

Statistical analysis

Data are expressed as mean ± SEM and were analysed using Graph Pad Prism 7.0 software. For QPCR data, a one-way analysis of variance (ANOVA) was performed followed by Bonferroni's post-hoc analysis, with a value of $p < 0.05$ considered statistically significant. Lesion volume were analysed using an unpaired student's t test, with a value of $p < 0.05$ considered statistically significant.

Results

STING expression is elevated in post-mortem human TBI brains

To investigate a possible role for STING in TBI, mRNA expression was analysed by QPCR in post mortem human brain tissue. Details of post mortem human brain tissue can be found as previously described [35]. We found that STING mRNA level was significantly upregulated in both ipsilateral (2.729 ± 0.5082; $^{***}p = 0.0003$) and contralateral (2.193 ± 0.4101; $^{*}p = 0.0139$) regions of late trauma group (patients died 6 h after TBI) as compared to control subjects (Fig. 1). This data implicates for the first time increased STING expression after TBI in human trauma brains.

Increased levels of STING are detected following TBI

To further investigate the role of STING after TBI, WT mice were subjected to CCI surgery and brains removed at 2 h and 24 h after CCI for QPCR, Western blot and immunohistochemical analysis. Mice brains were divided into ipsilateral and contralateral regions, which were further divided into cortex and striatum. This allowed a critical assessment of the severity of the CCI model and its effects on gene expression in specific regions of the brain. STING mRNA expression was increased at 2 h with significant and robust upregulation at 24 h across ipsilateral and contralateral regions of the brain with the highest upregulation seen in the ipsilateral cortex (5.632 ± 0.8245; $p = 0.0095$) (Fig. 2a). This suggests that our CCI model induces global effects on the brain with the effect of the injury spreading throughout the brain. Elevated STING expression was confirmed at the protein level at 2 h and 24 h by Western blot analysis (Fig. 2b), although densitometric analysis found this to be not significant as compared to sham control; Sham IC VS 24 h TBI IC = 2.033 ± 0.6579; p = n.s. (Fig. 2c).

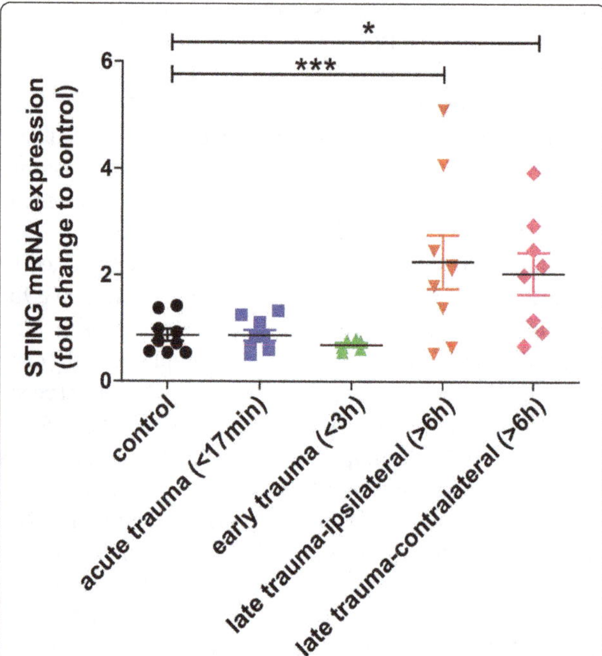

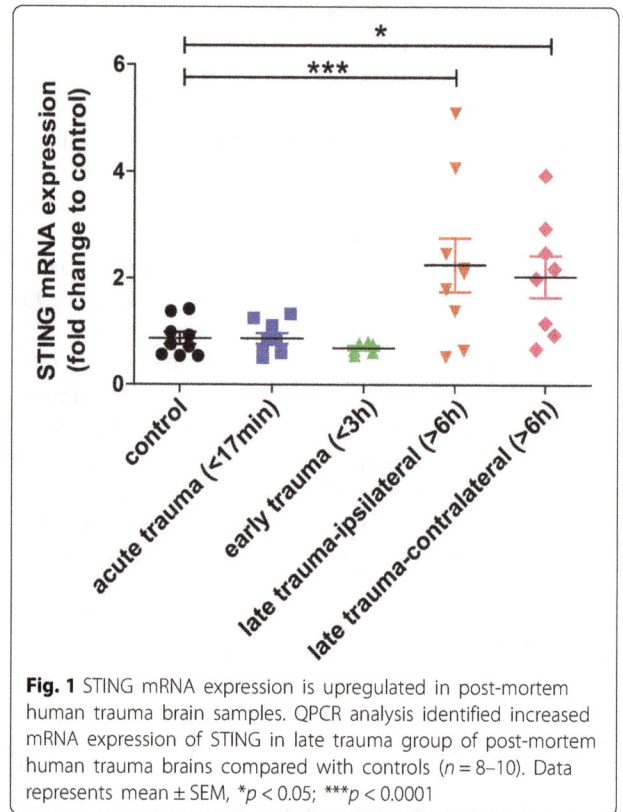

Fig. 1 STING mRNA expression is upregulated in post-mortem human trauma brain samples. QPCR analysis identified increased mRNA expression of STING in late trauma group of post-mortem human trauma brains compared with controls (n = 8–10). Data represents mean ± SEM, $^{*}p < 0.05$; $^{***}p < 0.0001$

STING colocalized with neuronal and astrocyte marker after TBI

To determine the cellular localisation of STING activation in the brain, we performed immunostaining on brain sections from WT mice after 24 h CCI. STING expression was detected near the lesion region and colocalized with FOX3a (neuronal marker) (Fig. 3f) with its expression barely detectable in the contralateral region (Fig. 3h) of the brain and sham sections (Fig. 3b). More interestingly, STING expression colocalized with GFAP (astrocyte marker) at 24 h after CCI in both the ipsilateral (Fig. 3o) and contralateral (Fig. 3r) regions. This suggests that

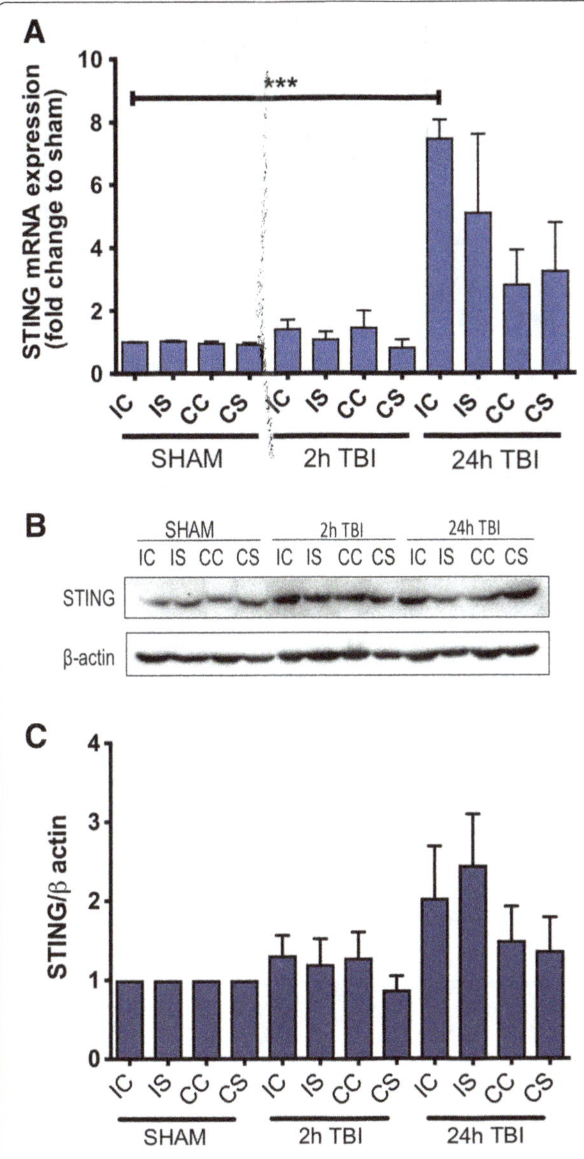

Fig. 2 TBI induces STING expression in WT mice. Increased STING mRNA was detected by QPCR as shown in **a** ($n = 6$ for each time point) and Western blot analysis **b** ($n = 3$). Quantification of STING protein expression in (**b**) shown in (**c**). All data is expressed as mean ± SEM, ***$p < 0.001$. *IC* ipsilateral cortex, *IS* ipsilateral striatum, *CC* contralateral cortex, *CS* contralateral striatum

astrocytic STING expression is widespread following TBI whilst neuronal expression of STING is restricted near the site of injury.

$STING^{-/-}$ mice exhibit a smaller lesion volume following TBI

We recently reported that mice with reduced type-I IFN signalling ($IFNAR1^{-/-}$ mice) displayed neuroprotection with reduced lesion size compared to their sham control group [35]. In this study, to further characterise the role of STING, TTC staining was performed on brain sections of WT and $STING^{-/-}$ mice to measure the lesion size after CCI (Fig. 4a). $STING^{-/-}$ mice had significantly smaller lesion size compared to their WT littermates (WT = 4.159 ± 0.2672 VS $STING^{-/-}$ = 3.21 ± 0.1729; $p = 0.0137$) (Fig. 4b).

TBI induces type-I IFN signalling in a STING-dependent manner

To further characterise the STING pathway activation after CCI, we measured downstream STING effectors including IRF3 and IRF7 mRNA levels after 2 h and 24 h CCI (Table 3). Consistent with STING activation, we detected upregulation of IRF3 transcript levels at 2 h and 24 h TBI that was reduced in $STING^{-/-}$ mice (Fig. 5a). Further, we also identified increased IRF7 mRNA levels in WT mice at 2 h and 24 h after CCI while $STING^{-/-}$ mice showed an upregulation of IR7 at 24 h after CCI (Fig. 5b). These results suggest CCI induces IRF3 activation that is STING-dependent whilst IRF7 can be activated independently of STING at later time points after CCI. Next, to determine the role of STING in mediating the type-I IFN pathway after TBI, we analysed the type-I IFN expression profile (IFN-α and IFN-β) in WT and $STING^{-/-}$ mice after CCI (Table 3). A significant and robust upregulation in IFN-β levels was detected in the ipsilateral cortex 2 h after CCI in the WT, but not $STING^{-/-}$ mice (Fig. 5d). Twenty-four hours after CCI, we found that IFN-β expression returned to control levels in WT mice with $STING^{-/-}$ mice showing reduced levels as compared to the control group. Similarly, increased expression of IFN-α was also detected in WT mice 2 h after CCI but reduced in $STING^{-/-}$ mice as compared to the control group (Fig. 5c). Taken together, our data confirms the STING pathway is activated and supports our hypothesis that STING is an instigator of the type-IFN pathway after TBI.

TBI-induced pro-inflammatory cytokines levels are reduced in $STING^{-/-}$ mice

To elucidate the underlying mechanisms that contribute to the deleterious effect of STING after TBI, we determined the expression profile of the pro-inflammatory genes, TNF-α, IL-1β and IL-6 in WT and $STING^{-/-}$ mice after CCI (Table 3). A significant and robust upregulation of TNF-α (Fig. 6a) and IL-1β (Fig. 6b) was detected in the ipsilateral side of WT mice with this diminished in $STING^{-/-}$ mice at 2 h and 24 h after CCI. IL-6 levels were elevated in the ipsilateral cortex of WT mice 2 h after CCI compared to controls, while $STING^{-/-}$ mice showed reduced expression at similar time point (Fig. 6c). However, 24 h after CCI, we observed an upregulation in IL-6 levels in the ipsilateral cortex both in WT and $STING^{-/-}$ mice suggesting an

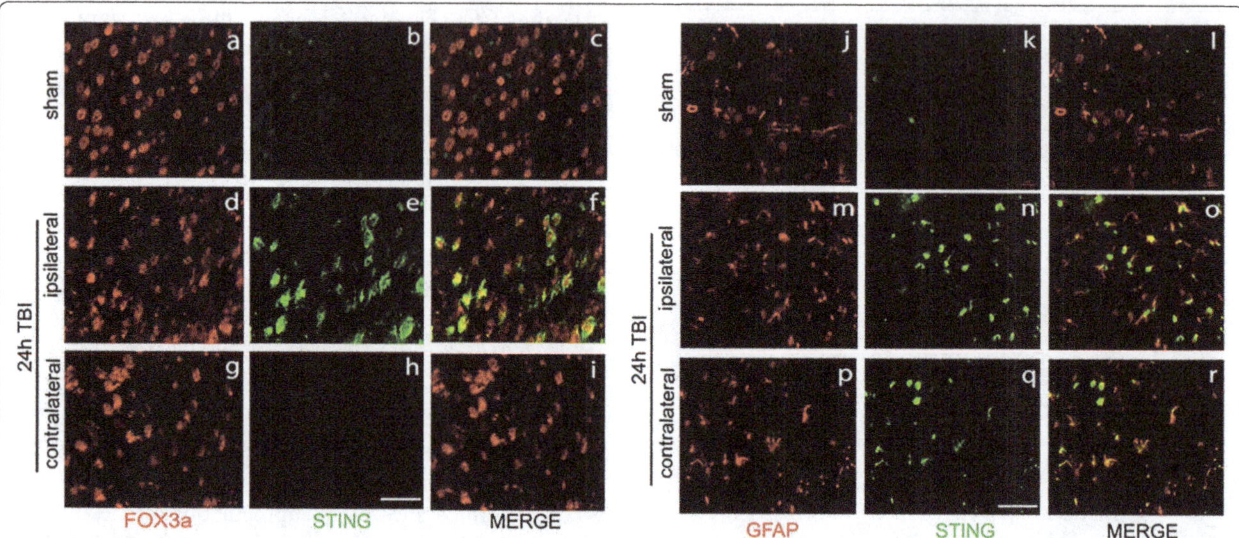

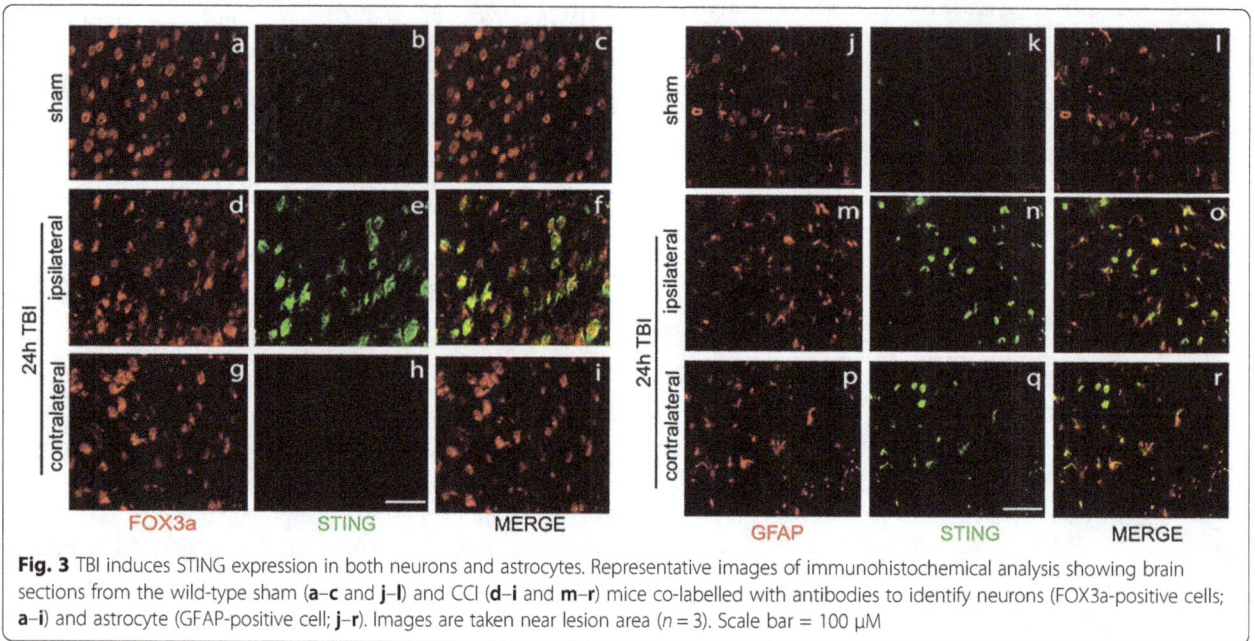

Fig. 3 TBI induces STING expression in both neurons and astrocytes. Representative images of immunohistochemical analysis showing brain sections from the wild-type sham (**a**–**c** and **j**–**l**) and CCI (**d**–**i** and **m**–**r**) mice co-labelled with antibodies to identify neurons (FOX3a-positive cells; **a**–**i**) and astrocyte (GFAP-positive cell; **j**–**r**). Images are taken near lesion area ($n = 3$). Scale bar = 100 μM

alternative pathway that induces its expression independent of STING.

STING contributes to astrocyte and microglia reactivity after TBI

To further understand the modulation of the neuroinflammatory response by STING after TBI, GFAP protein expression (an indicator of astrogliosis) was assessed in WT and STING$^{-/-}$ mice 2 h and 24 h after CCI. An increase in GFAP protein expression was observed in WT TBI mice in the ipsilateral cortex and striatum 24 h after TBI (24 h IC = 1.909 ± 0.3485, 24 h IS = 2.788 ± 0.898; $^{*}p < 0.05$ VS sham) with levels unchanged in STING$^{-/-}$ (24 h IC = 0.6724 ± 0.222, 24 h IS = 1.519 ± 0.4144) mice

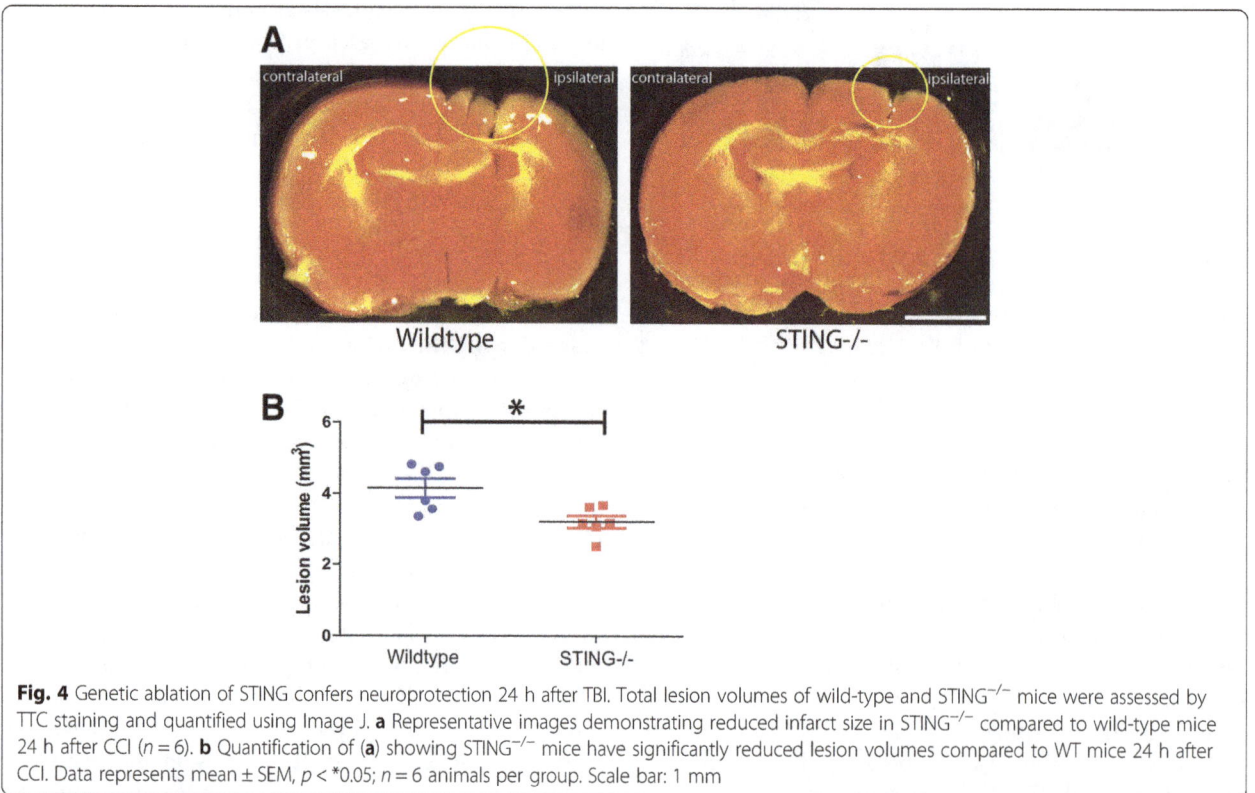

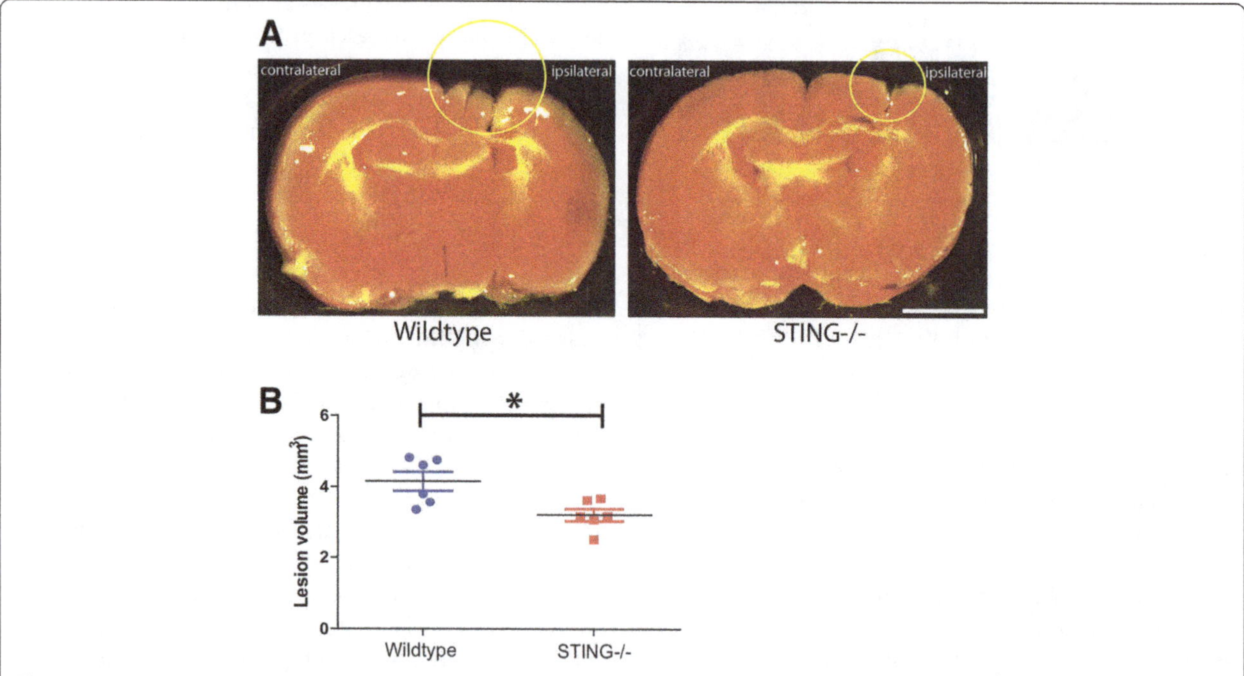

Fig. 4 Genetic ablation of STING confers neuroprotection 24 h after TBI. Total lesion volumes of wild-type and STING$^{-/-}$ mice were assessed by TTC staining and quantified using Image J. **a** Representative images demonstrating reduced infarct size in STING$^{-/-}$ compared to wild-type mice 24 h after CCI ($n = 6$). **b** Quantification of (**a**) showing STING$^{-/-}$ mice have significantly reduced lesion volumes compared to WT mice 24 h after CCI. Data represents mean ± SEM, $p < {}^{*}0.05$; $n = 6$ animals per group. Scale bar: 1 mm

Table 3 Neuroinflammatory gene expression changes in wild-type (WT) and STING$^{-/-}$ mice at 2 h and 24 h post-TBI

	WT (2 h)	STING$^{-/-}$ (2 h)	*p* value	WT (24 h)	STING$^{-/-}$ (24 h)	*p* value
Expression cortex (relative to sham)						
IRF3	1.982 ± 0.269	0.883 ± 0.179	$p = 0.7604$	2.519 ± 0.496	0.973 ± 0.173	$p = 0.0306$
IRF7	2.417 ± 0.55	0.954 ± 0.104	$p = 0.3106$	4.938 ± 0.968	4.014 ± 0.721	$p > 0.9999$
IFN-α	2.450 ± 0.903	0.024 ± 0.007	$p < 0.0001$	0.180 ± 0.065	0.174 ± 0.082	$p > 0.9999$
IFN-β	2.191 ± 0.623	0.077 ± 0.044	$p = 0.0492$	0.963 ± 0.166	0.372 ± 0.3101	$p > 0.9999$
TNF-α	173.176 ± 23.243	1.170 ± 0.280	$p < 0.0001$	30.906 ± 14.556	0.136 ± 0.020	$p = 0.6004$
IL1-β	62.860 ± 18.641	2.340 ± 0.244	$p < 0.0001$	15.237 ± 5.301	3.290 ± 2.251	$p > 0.9999$
IL-6	6.322 ± 1.037	1.679 ± 0.489	$p = 0.6419$	10.198 ± 4.661	9.126 ± 2.532	$p > 0.9999$
Expression striatum (relative to sham)						
IRF3	0.715 ± 0.106	0.112 ± 0.039	$p > 0.9999$	0.856 ± 0.118	0.320 ± 0.053	$p > 0.9999$
IRF7	0.909 ± 0.130	0.971 ± 0.160	$p > 0.9999$	1.172 ± 0.148	2.727 ± 0.384	$p = 0.1696$
IFN-α	0.972 ± 0.394	0.159 ± 0.080	$p > 0.9999$	0.205 ± 0.133	0.012 ± 0.010	$p > 0.9999$
IFN-β	0.751 ± 0.231	0.315 ± 0.619	$p > 0.9999$	1.136 ± 0.534	0.045 ± 0.0268	$p > 0.9999$
TNF-α	138.223 ± 20.547	3.354 ± 0.868	***$p < 0.0001$	12.332 ± 4.273	0.388 ± 0.029	$p > 0.9999$
IL1-β	46.589 ± 10.443	6.324 ± 1.440	***$p < 0.0001$	3.260 ± 0.536	1.648 ± 0.362	n.s $p > 0.9999$
IL-6	8.086 ± 1.463	4.342 ± 0.690	$p = 0.9244$	0.484 ± 0.103	4.722 ± 0.884	$p = 0.7951$

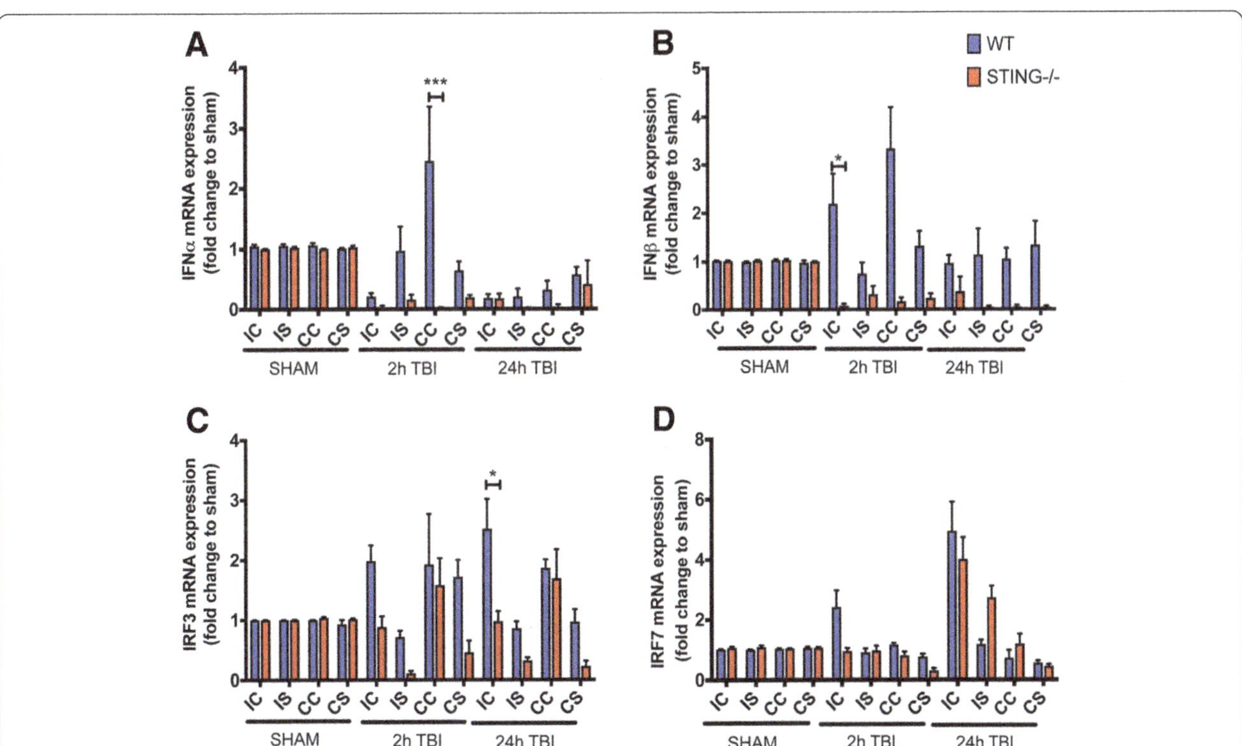

Fig. 5 STING$^{-/-}$ mice display reduced type-I IFN signalling after TBI. QPCR analysis identified increased mRNA expression of IRF3 (**a**), IRF7 (**b**), IFNα (**c**) and IFN-β (**d**) in WT brains mice as compared to STING$^{-/-}$ mice after CCI ($n = 6$). Data represents mean ± SEM, *$p < 0.05$; ***$p < 0.0001$. *IC* ipsilateral cortex, *IS* ipsilateral striatum, *CC* contralateral cortex, *CS* contralateral striatum

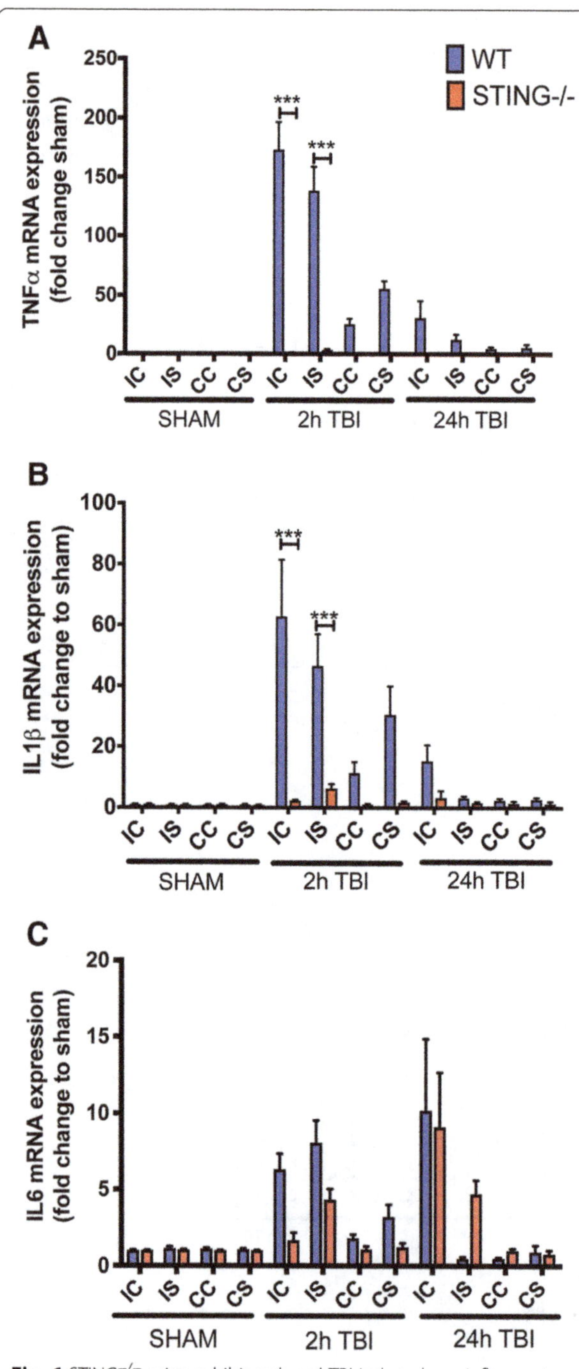

Fig. 6 STING$^{-/-}$ mice exhibit reduced TBI-induced pro-inflammatory cytokines in vivo. mRNA expression of IL-1β (**a**), IL-6 (**b**) and TNF-α (**c**) in brain tissue of wild-type and STING$^{-/-}$ mice subjected to CCI. ($n = 6$ mice for each timepoint). Data represents mean ± SEM, *$p <$ 0.05; **$p < 0.01$; ***$p < 0.001$. *IC* ipsilateral cortex, *IS* ipsilateral striatum, *CC* contralateral cortex, *CS* contralateral striatum

as compared to sham as quantified by Western blot analysis (Fig. 7a, b). This was supported by immunohistochemical analysis with GFAP staining in WT and STING$^{-/-}$ mice 24 h after CCI (WT = 726.4 ± 35.19 vs STING$^{-/-}$ = 497.7 ± 45.5; *$p = 0.0165$) (Fig. 8c. Microglial activation is a common marker for neuroinflammation after CCI. We analysed IBA-1 immunofluorescence to determine a role for STING in modulating microglia activity after CCI in WT and STING$^{-/-}$ mice. An activated form of microglia characterised by an amoeboid shape with a larger cell size was identified in the WT mice 24 h after CCI (Fig. 9b). In contrast, STING$^{-/-}$ brains at 24 h post CCI displayed ramified morphologies with branches and fine processes indicative of a less reactive microglial phenotype (Fig. 9d). Further, 24 h after TBI the quantification of IBA-1 immunofluorescence intensity in STING$^{-/-}$ mice showing significantly reduced staining as compared to wild-type brains (WT = 35.09 ± 2.637 vs STING$^{-/-}$ 19.92 ± 1.709; **$p = 0.0085$). These results strongly support a role for STING in contributing to the detrimental neuroinflammatory environment by driving glial reactivity after CCI.

STING contributes to autophagy dysfunction after TBI

STING has been implicated in influencing autophagy activity; therefore, we assessed its role in modulating autophagy after CCI. Hallmark autophagy markers, LC3, p62 and LAMP2, were measured 2 h and 24 h after CCI by Western blot analysis. An increase in LC3-II protein expression was observed in both WT and STING$^{-/-}$ mice after CCI (Fig. 10b). Interestingly, our data showed a significant increase in LC3-II levels in the ipsilateral striatum 2 h after CCI in the STING$^{-/-}$ mice as compared to the sham control but reduced in the WT mice (*LC3-II*/*LC3-I* ratio; WT 2 h IC = 1.598 ± 0.154 VS sham; n.s. $p = 0.3509$, WT 2 h IS = 1.877 ± 0.265 vs sham; *$p = 0.0296$, WT 24 h IC = 1.199 ± 0.080 vs sham; n.s. $p = 0.9983$, WT 24 h IS = 1.224 ± 0.085 vs sham; n.s. $p = 0.9960$, STING$^{-/-}$ 2 h IC = 1.774 ± 0.209 VS sham; n.s. $p = 0.0844$, STING$^{-/-}$ 2 h IS = 3.202 ± 0.372 vs sham; ***$p < 0.0001$, STING$^{-/-}$ 24 h IC = 1.494 ± 0.116 vs sham; n.s. $p = 0.6188$, STING$^{-/-}$ 24 h IS = 1.635 ± 0.095 vs sham; n.s. $p =$ 0.2722). Further, elevated expression of p62 proteins levels was also detected in both WT and STING$^{-/-}$ mice after CCI with STING$^{-/-}$ mice showing higher expression at 2 h and 24 h as compared to control genotypes (Fig. 10d) (*p62*/*β-actin*; WT 2 h IC = 3.175 ± 0.145 vs sham; ***$p <$ 0.0001, WT 2 h IS = 2.052 ± 0.209 VS sham; n.s. $p =$ 0.1292, WT 24 h IC = 0.931 ± 0.104 vs sham; n.s. $p >$ 0.9999, WT 24 h IS = 2.422 ± 0.281 vs sham; **$p = 0.0088$, STING$^{-/-}$ 2 h IC = 2.300 ± 0.206 vs sham; *$p = 0.0231$, STING$^{-/-}$ 2 h IS = 3.783 ± 0.427 VS sham; ***$p < 0.0001$, STING$^{-/-}$ 24 h IC = 1.8688 ± 0.192 vs sham; n.s. $p =$ 0.3461, STING$^{-/-}$ 24 h IS = 4.572 ± 0.486 vs sham; ***$p <$ 0.0001). To determine whether the increases in LC3-II and P62 levels were due to an increase in autophagy activity or impaired autophagy flux as a result of a block in the autophagosome-lysosomal degradation step, we examined

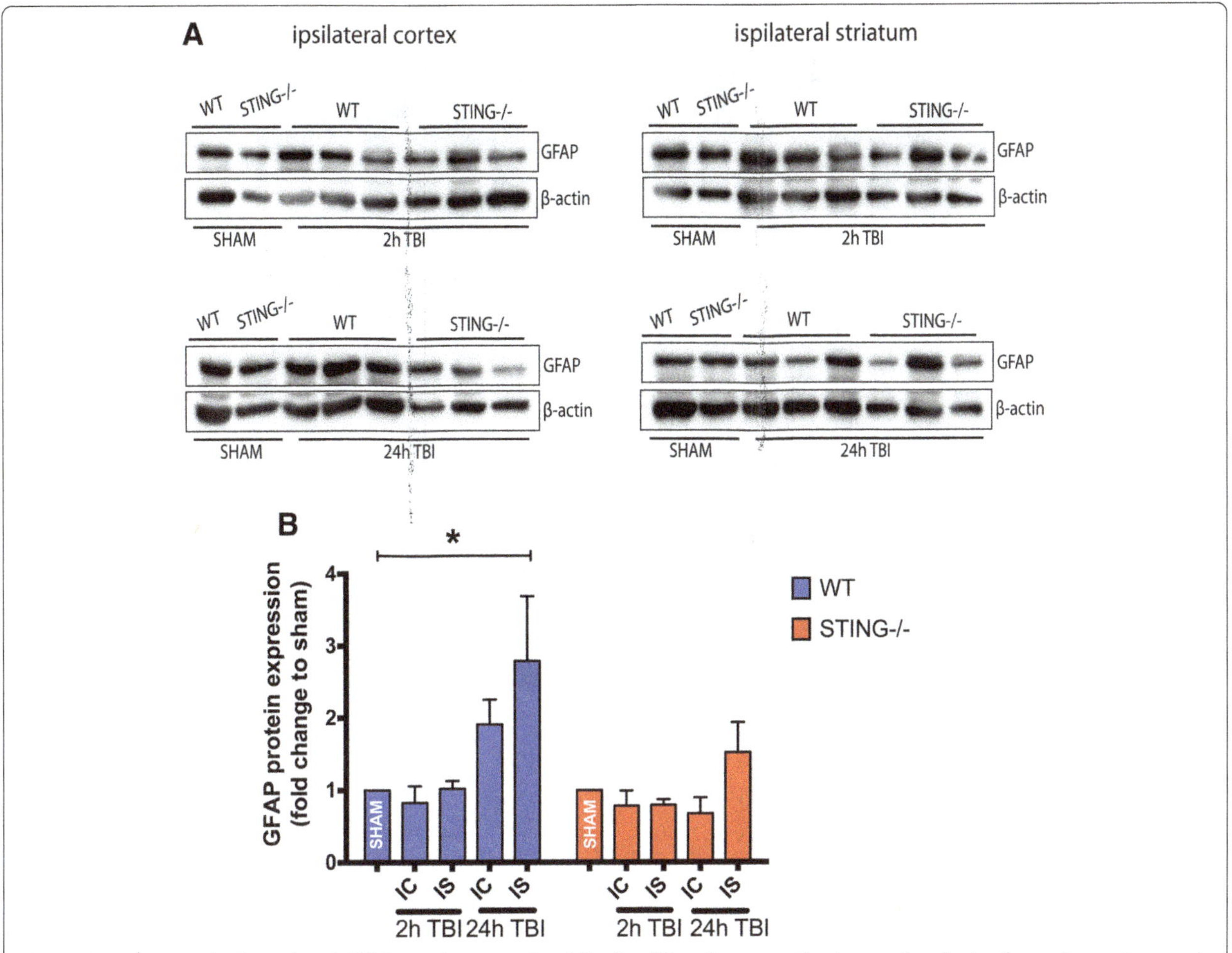

Fig. 7 $STING^{-/-}$ mice display reduced GFAP protein expression following TBI. **a** Representative images ($n = 6$ mice for each genotype and timepoint) showing GFAP protein levels in wild-type and $STING^{-/-}$ mice after TBI as assessed by western blot analysis. Significantly increased expression of GFAP was observed in the ipsilateral striatum of wild-type mice 24 h post-TBI but not in $STING^{-/-}$ mice as compared with sham group, as quantified in (**b**). Data represent mean ± SEM, $^*p < 0.05$. *IC* ipsilateral cortex, *IS* ipsilateral striatum, *CC* contralateral cortex, *CS* contralateral striatum

LAMP2 levels. As expected, WT mice showed a significant increase in LAMP2 levels in the ipsilateral cortex 24 h after CCI as compared to sham control (WT 24 h IC = 7.761 ± 2.927 vs sham; $^{***}p < 0.0001$). However, reduced LAMP2 levels were detected in the $STING^{-/-}$ mice at 24 h after CCI as compared to the control and WT genotypes ($STING^{-/-}$ 24 h IC = 1.440 ± 0.190 vs sham; n.s. $p >$ 0.9999) (Fig. 10e). It is noteworthy that LC3 and p62 levels were also higher as compared to LAMP2 levels in the $STING^{-/-}$ mice subjected to CCI, suggesting enhanced normal autophagy activity with complete autophagosome-lysosomal degradation. This increased autophagic flux could contribute to the neuroprotective effects observed in the $STING^{-/-}$ mice after CCI.

Discussion

Neuroinflammation is known to be a key driver of secondary injury progression after TBI; however, its precise mechanisms remain unclear. Identifying key molecules that regulate neuroinflammatory processes could lead to a potential therapeutic target to improve patients' outcome following TBI. This study stems from our previous finding that type-I IFNs contribute to the detrimental neuroinflammatory environment in a CCI animal model of TBI. Mice lacking the type-I IFN receptor ($IFNAR1^{-/-}$) or by targeting the IFNAR1 receptor with a blocking monoclonal antibody conferred protection after TBI [35]. Here, we sought to determine the instigator of this type-I IFN production that leads to an increased pro-inflammatory environment in this CCI model. For the first time, we report a novel role for STING in mediating neuroinflammatory processes after TBI. Genetic ablation of STING leads to decreased type-I IFN production, a reduction in pro-inflammatory cytokine expression including TNF-α, IL-6 and IL-Iβ and significantly a reduced lesion volume 24 h post CCI. In addition, this study highlights for the first time a role for STING in regulating autophagy activity with $STING^{-/-}$

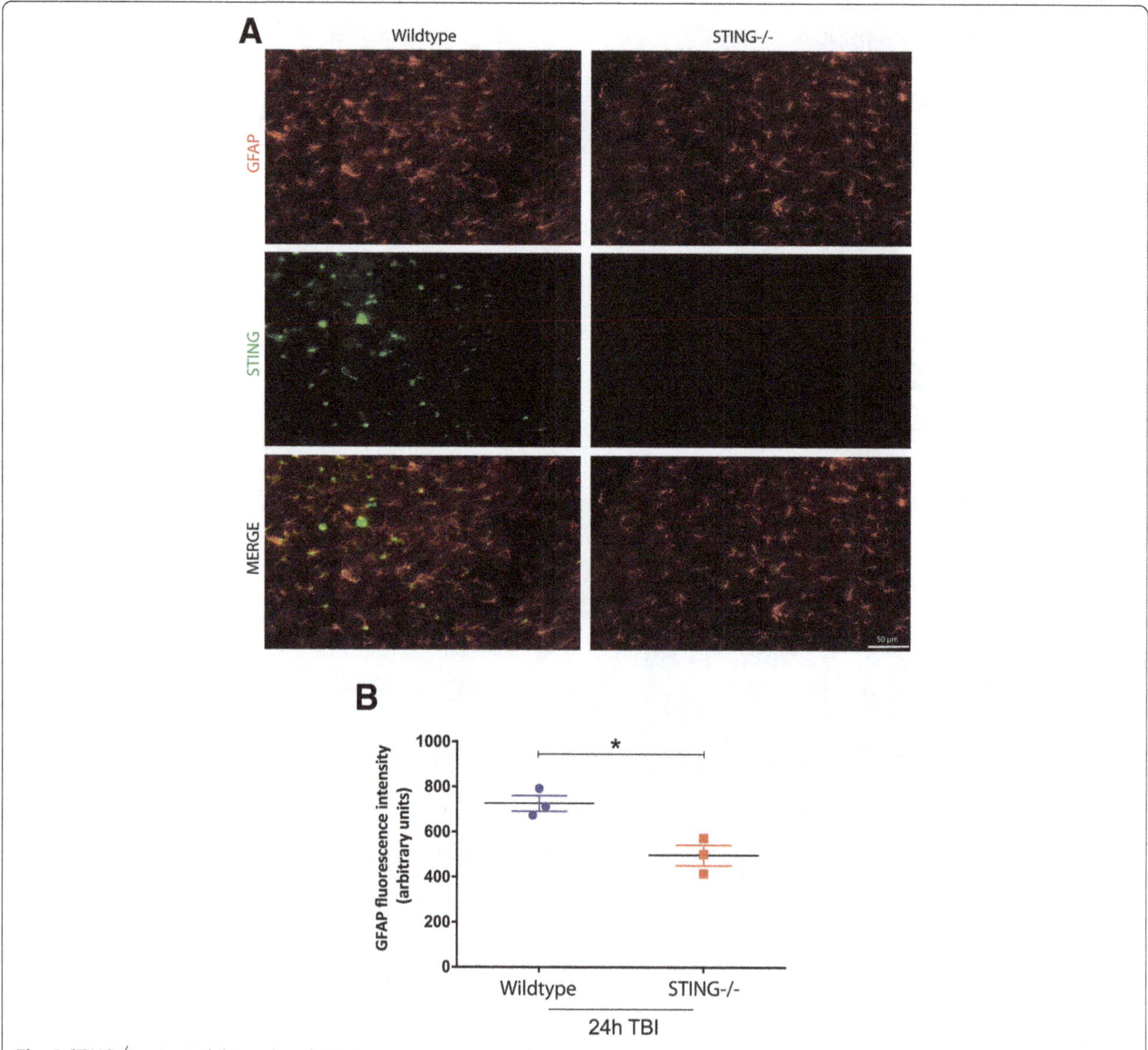

Fig. 8 STING$^{-/-}$ mice exhibit reduced GFAP immunostaining compared with WT mice after TBI. **a** High-power GFAP (red) staining co-labelled with STING (green) in the ipsilateral side of the brain. GFAP intensity is measured in (**b**) showing reduced GFAP immunoreactivity in the STING$^{-/-}$ mice 24 h after TBI ($n = 3$ mice for each genotype and timepoint). Data represent mean ± SEM, *$p < 0.05$

mice displaying increased autophagic flux in their brains after CCI.

We have previously demonstrated a detrimental role for the type-I IFNs in acute and chronic neurodegenerative diseases with increased type-I IFN expression found in both animal models and post-mortem human brains from TBI [35], AD [33] and PD [34] patients. In these animal models, reduced type-I IFN signalling was associated with an attenuated neuroinflammatory response and subsequent neuroprotection. The underlying mechanisms mediating the detrimental effects of the type-I IFNs are still not well understood. This study aimed to further characterise the signalling pathways that contributed to the increased type-I IFN production, specifically in the CCI model. Type-I IFNs can signal through the classical JAK/STAT-IRF7 pathway leading to an upregulation in pro-inflammatory cytokines and release of the type-IFN themselves [57]. The released type-I IFNs can further bind to the IFNAR1 receptor in a positive-feedback mechanism thus enhancing this signalling [58]. Alternatively, type-I IFNs can be activated through cytosolic DNA via the STING-TBK1-IRF3 pathway. The STING-dependent type-I IFNs signalling has been very well characterised in infectious disease settings; however, its role in neuroinflammation is unclear. Here, for the first time, we confirmed increased STING mRNA levels in post-mortem human TBI brains. Increased STING expression was detected in the late trauma group

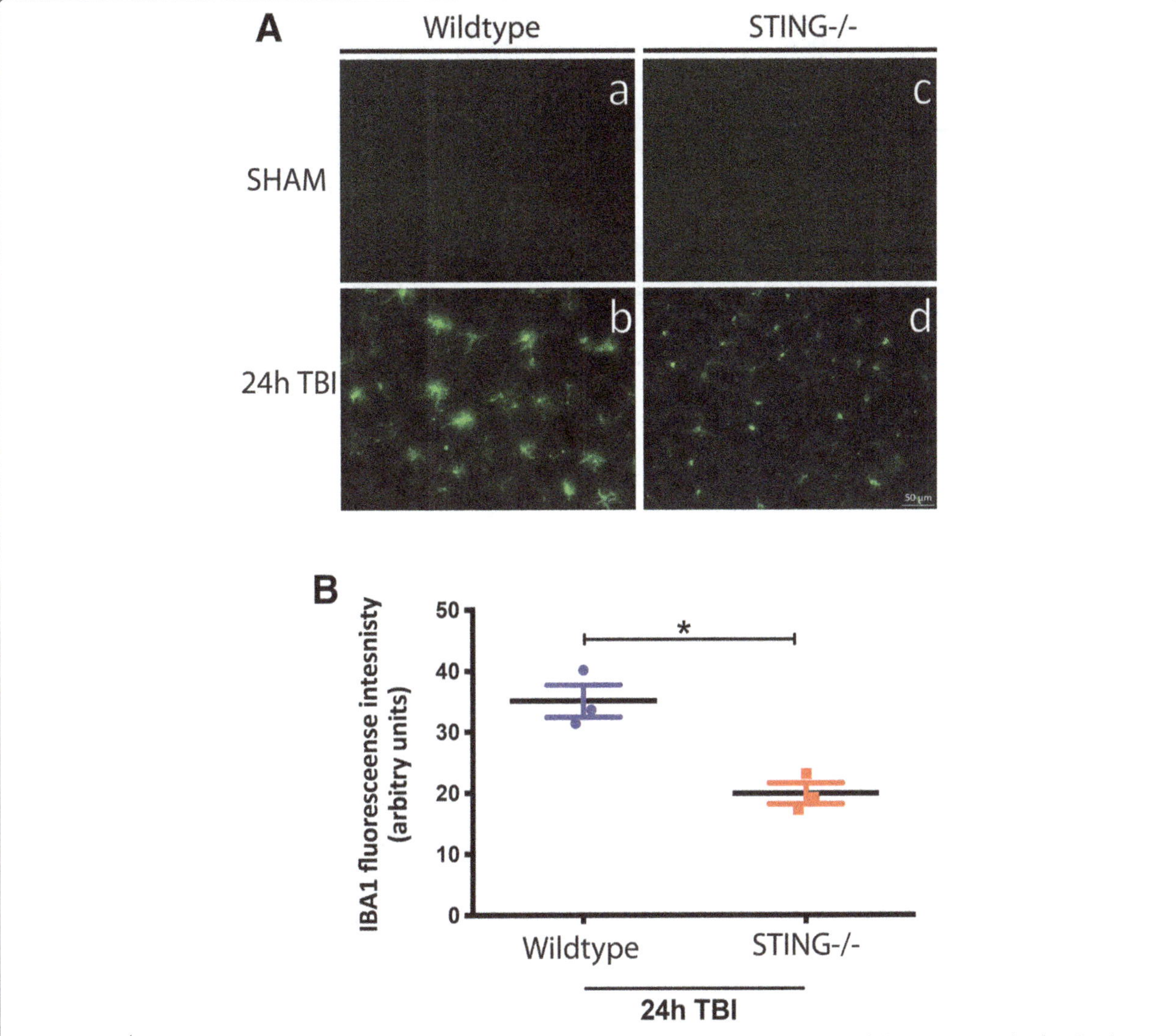

Fig. 9 STING$^{-/-}$ brains exhibit ramified microglial morphologies and reduced IBA-1 immunostaining following TBI. 24 h after TBI, brains from STING$^{-/-}$ mice displayed microglia with ramified morphologies as identified by IBA-1 staining (*d*) as compared to WT mice (*b*). IBA-1 expression was significantly reduced in the STING$^{-/-}$ mice at 24 h post-TBI as quantified in (**b**) ($n = 3$ mice for each genotype and timepoint)

(patients who died > 6 h after TBI) in both the ipsilateral and contralateral sides as compared with the control group. Interestingly, IFN-β was only increased in the ipsilateral side (not in the contralateral side) of the late trauma group while IFN-α was significantly reduced in the early trauma group (patients who died < 3 h after TBI) as previously reported [35]. This implies a co-activation of the STING and type-I IFN pathways after TBI and suggests a dominant IFN-β production after injury. The increased STING expression in both the contra- and ipsilateral sides of human TBI brains in the late trauma group implicates STING in mediating the progression of the neural injury.

Consistent with our findings in human TBI samples, we confirmed increased STING mRNA expression at 2 h after CCI with a robust and a significant upregulation at 24 h in the ipsilateral cortex as compared to the sham control. STING mRNA expression was also higher across both the ipsilateral and contralateral sides at 24 h after TBI as compared to the control group with Western blot confirming this at the protein level. In addition, we confirmed downstream STING and type-I IFN signalling activation in our CCI model with increased IRF3 and IRF7 mRNA levels detected in WT mice at 2 h and 24 h after TBI. However, STING$^{-/-}$ mice showed reduced IRF3 expression in the ipsilateral cortex at 2 h and 24 h after TBI as compared to the WT genotypes. Further, increased IRF7 mRNA was only detected at 24 h after TBI in the STING$^{-/-}$ mice as compared to the WT brains suggesting that there is alternative pathway

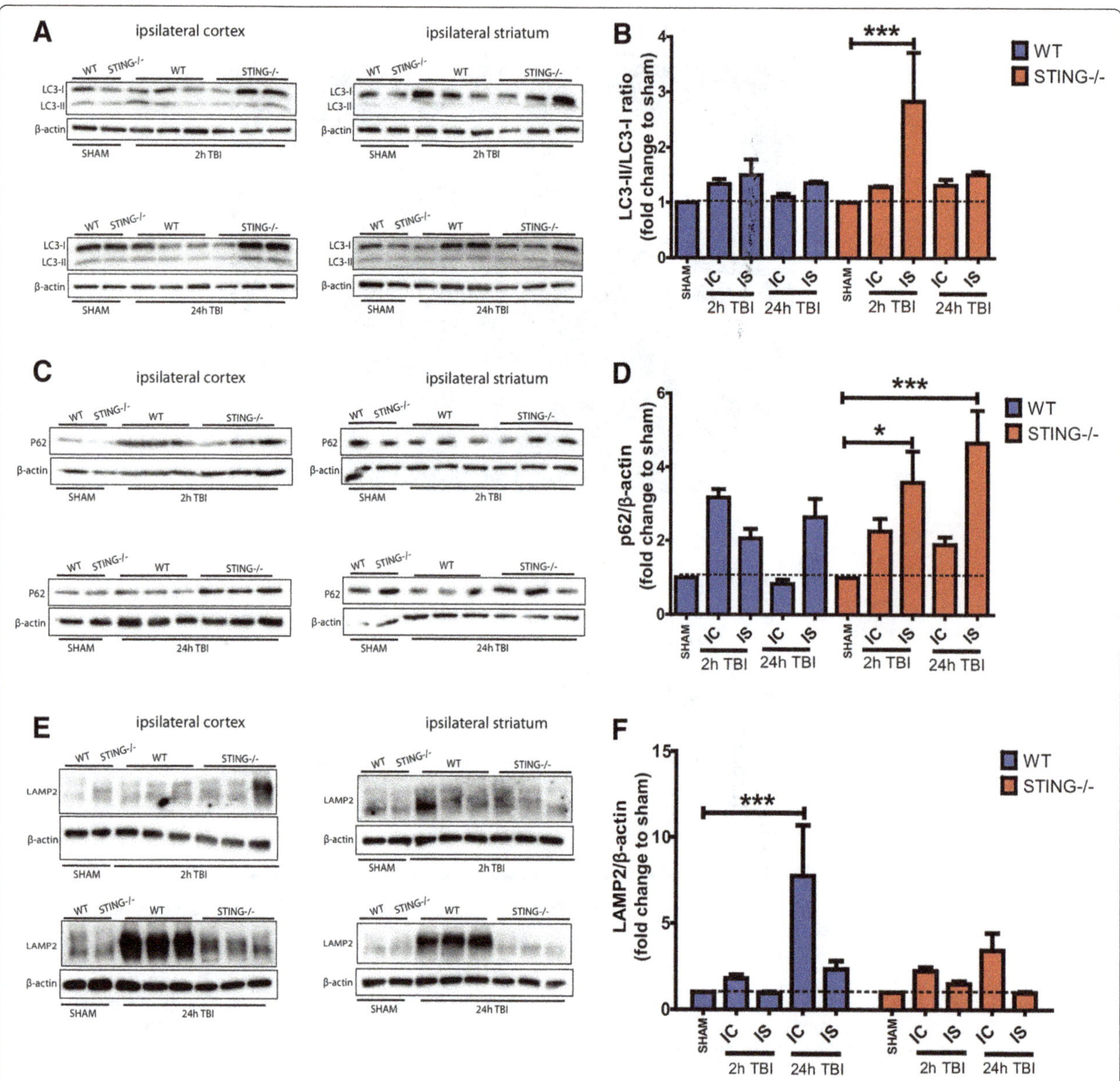

Fig. 10 STING$^{-/-}$ brains exhibit ramified microglial flux 24 h post-TBI. **a** LC3, (**c**) p62 and (**e**) LAMP2 expression was detected in wild-type and STING$^{-/-}$ brains ($n = 6$) by Western blot. LC3-I, LC3-II, p62 and LAMP2 levels were normalised to β-actin levels respectively. For densitometry calculations, **b** LC3-II/LC3-I ratio, **d** p62/β-actin ratio and **f** LAMP2/β-actin ratio was then determined from these values and was calculated as a fold change relative to genotype sham control. Data is expressed as mean ± SEM, $^{**}p < 0.01$; $^{***}p < 0.001$. *IC* ipsilateral cortex, *IS* ipsilateral striatum

mediating IRF7 activation at later timepoints in the absence of STING. These results suggest that CCI induces both IRF3 and IRF7 production and is partially STING-mediated. Numerous reports have confirmed that STING can be activated by cyclic dinucleotides and/or double-stranded (ds) DNA produced by bacteria or virally transfected cells [59–61]. STING has also been shown to be upregulated by self-DNA released during cell death in animal models of liver disease [62–64] and UV-irradiation-induced cell death [65]. More recently, activation of the STING-IRF3 axis has been implicated in driving the inflammatory response and apoptosis in fatty liver disease [66]. As CCI induces injury and tissue damage in the proximity of cortical regions of the brain, it can be implied that STING expression is induced by the release of self-DNA from the injured or dying cells after CCI. It is also possible that other type of damage-associated molecule patterns (DAMPs) might activate STING after TBI. The exact molecules or mechanism of action activating STING in our CCI model warrants further investigation. In addition, it would be of interest to further investigate the long-term contribution of STING by extending the period after injury up to 7 days or longer and/or increasing the depth and velocity of impact which correlates with severity of cortical deformation [41, 67–69].

Microglial and astrocyte reactivity are common neuroinflammatory features after TBI. We found that STING contributes to the increased IBA1 staining and altered microglial morphology after CCI. We also observed increased GFAP expression at 24 h after TBI in WT mice but significantly reduced in STING$^{-/-}$ mice at similar time points. This reduction in STING-dependent glial reactivity after TBI may contribute to the neuroprotective effects seen in STING$^{-/-}$ mice. Recently, it was reported that STING activation reduces microglial reactivity in a multiple sclerosis (MS) animal model [40]. This dual function of STING in regulating microglial reactivity observed may be attributed to the different disease models; however, it does suggest an important role for STING in contributing to the neuroinflammatory response in these CNS pathologies. We confirmed STING expression near the lesion site colocalized with GFAP (astrocyte) and FOX3a (neurons) positive cells. However, only GFAP-positive cells coexpressing STING were found in both the ipsilateral and contralateral sides 24 h after TBI suggesting that astrocytes are the major cell involved in the STING-mediated response after TBI. Utilising a bone marrow chimera approach, we have previously confirmed that type-I IFNs produced by the peripheral tissue compartment are a major contributor to the pro-inflammatory response after TBI [35]. The possibility that the TBI-induced activation of the STING pathway is systemic or brain-derived in origin warrants further investigation; however, we did confirm a critical role for STING in mediating the neuronal cell death in our CCI model. STING$^{-/-}$ mice exhibited a reduced lesion volume compared to their wild-type littermates consistent with our observation with IFNAR1$^{-/-}$ mice which display a significantly smaller lesion area compared to sham controls [35]. This implies that both STING and type-I IFN signalling are crucial players in exacerbating the outcome of TBI. TBI is known to induce a pro-inflammatory environment with a prolonged or chronic response exacerbating TBI outcome. IFN-β mRNA levels were upregulated at 2 h after TBI in WT mice but not in STING$^{-/-}$ mice, suggesting that the increased type-I IFN expression is through a STING-dependent pathway. We also found a dramatic reduction in mRNA expression of TNF-α and IL-1β in STING$^{-/-}$ mice as compared to their WT littermates at 2 h and 24 h after TBI. Whilst it is known that STING modulates pro-inflammatory cytokine production in a bacterial or viral infection setting [70, 71], its role in CNS injury is unknown. Based on our findings, we conclude that the attenuated pro-inflammatory cytokine and IFN-β levels contribute to the neuroprotective effects observed in STING$^{-/-}$ mice.

The role of autophagy has been widely implicated in TBI with increased autophagic marker expression observed in both human and animal models [41, 44, 72]. However, its precise role and the mechanisms that trigger its induction after TBI remain unclear. Both the STING and type-I IFN pathways have emerged as key players in autophagy activation in cellular and other disease models [47, 51] but their interaction and regulation following brain injury is unknown. Our results demonstrated increased expression of autophagy markers in both WT and STING$^{-/-}$ mice at 2 h and 24 h after TBI as compared to their sham controls validating our CCI model in inducing autophagy as previously reported [44, 73, 74]. Interestingly, after CCI, we observed increased and sustained expression of LC3 and p62 in STING$^{-/-}$ brains as compared to their WT counterparts. Autophagy is a dynamic and complex cellular degradation process that requires a careful analysis to accurately identify and interpret its activity to understand if dysfunction is occurring due to increased initiation or decreased flux. In this study, we assessed hallmark markers of autophagy including microtubule-associated protein 1 light chain 3 (LC3), SQSTM1/p62, and lysosomal-associated membrane protein 2 (LAMP2) in our CCI model. Conversion of LC3-I to LC3-II is representative of increased autophagy activation [75] while the degradation of p62 and LAMP2 at the late step of the autophagy process serves as a marker for normal autophagic flux. The increased expression of LC3-II and p62 levels at 2 h and 24 h time points in the WT mice after CCI in this study corresponds to other studies that detected increased expression of these autophagic markers up to 7 days after TBI [44]. Interestingly, our data showed higher and sustained expression of LC3-II and p62 levels in STING$^{-/-}$ mice at 2 h and 24 h after TBI as compared to their WT counterparts. Given that we observed a neuroprotective effect in STING$^{-/-}$ at 24 h after TBI, this suggests that the increased LC3-II and p62 levels observed are not an indication of impaired autophagy flux but rather enhanced autophagy activity that serves as a protective mechanism to reduce cellular damage following TBI. Indeed, we confirmed decreased expression of LAMP2 levels at 2 h and 24 h in the ipsilateral cortex after CCI in STING$^{-/-}$ mice as compared to their WT counterparts. This reduced LAMP2 expression in the STING$^{-/-}$ mice indicates that there is a completion of the autophagy process suggesting that STING might be a key regulator driving autophagic dysfunction seen after TBI. The dynamic process of autophagy and a clear understanding of STING function in regulating this event after TBI can be tackled by incorporating longer time points after CCI which are lacking in the current study.

Conclusions

Taken together, this study provides evidence to suggest a novel role for STING in mediating the type-I IFN pathway in the CCI model of TBI. This is also the first study to demonstrate the influence of STING in regulating the autophagy pathway following TBI. Our finding that STING is a key regulatory protein involved in TBI has identified a novel potential therapeutic strategy for the reducing the damage following brain injury.

Abbreviations

AD: Alzheimer's disease; CCI: Controlled cortical impact; GFAP: Glial fibrillary acidic protein; IBA1: Ionised calcium-binding adaptor molecule 1; IFN: Interferon; IFNAR1: Interferon alpha receptor 1; IFNAR2: Interferon alpha receptor 2; IL: Interleukin; IRF: Interferon regulatory factor; JAK: Janus activated kinase; LAMP2: Lysosomal-associated membrane protein 2; LC3: Including microtubule-associated protein 1 light chain 3; PD: Parkinson's disease; STAT: Signal transducer and activator of transcription; STING: Stimulator of interferon genes; TBI: Traumatic brain injury; TBK: Tumour necrosis factor (TNF) receptor-associated factor NF-κB activator (TANK)-binding kinase 1 (TBK1); TNF: Tumour necrosis factor; TYK2: Tyrosine kinase 2

Acknowledgments

The authors thank Professor Ben Kile for his STING expertise.

Funding

This study was supported by grants from the National Health and Medical Research Council (NHMRC) of Australia to PJC and JMT.

Authors' contributions

AA, SB, JMT and PJC conceived the study. AA, MZ and TF conducted the experiments. AA, SB, JMT and PJC analysed the data and interpreted the results. AA, JMT and PJC wrote the manuscript. All authors read and approved the final manuscript.

Consent for publication

Not applicable

Competing interests

The authors declare that they have no competing interests.

Author details

[1]Neuropharmacology Laboratory, Department of Pharmacology & Therapeutics, University of Melbourne, Parkville, Melbourne 3010, Australia. [2]Department of Microbiology & Immunology, Peter Doherty Institute, Melbourne 3010, Australia.

References

1. Lingsma HF, Roozenbeek B, Steyerberg EW, Murray GD, Maas AIR. Early prognosis in traumatic brain injury: from prophecies to predictions. Lancet Neurol. 2010;9:543–54.
2. Kim DY, O'Leary M, Nguyen A, Kaji A, Bricker S, Neville A, Bongard F, Putnam B, Plurad D. The effect of platelet and desmopressin administration on early radiographic progression of traumatic intracranial hemorrhage. J Neurotrauma. 2015;32:1815–21.
3. Skolnick BE, Maas AI, Narayan RK, van der Hoop RG, MacAllister T, Ward JD, Nelson NR, Stocchetti N. A clinical trial of progesterone for severe traumatic brain injury. N Engl J Med. 2014;371:2467–76.
4. Wright DW, Yeatts SD, Silbergleit R, Palesch YY, Hertzberg VS, Frankel M, Goldstein FC, Caveney AF, Howlett-Smith H, Bengelink EM, et al. Very early administration of progesterone for acute traumatic brain injury. N Engl J Med. 2014;371:2457–66.
5. Blennow K, Hardy J, Zetterberg H. The neuropathology and neurobiology of traumatic brain injury. Neuron. 2012;76:886–99.
6. Kigerl KA, de Rivero Vaccari JP, Dietrich WD, Popovich PG, Keane RW. Pattern recognition receptors and central nervous system repair. Exp Neurol. 2014;258:5–16.
7. Ziebell JM, Morganti-Kossmann MC. Involvement of pro- and anti-inflammatory cytokines and chemokines in the pathophysiology of traumatic brain injury. Neurotherapeutics. 2010;7:22–30.
8. Tajiri N, Acosta SA, Shahaduzzaman M, Ishikawa H, Shinozuka K, Pabon M, Hernandez-Ontiveros D, Kim DW, Metcalf C, Staples M, et al. Intravenous transplants of human adipose-derived stem cell protect the brain from traumatic brain injury-induced neurodegeneration and motor and cognitive impairments: cell graft biodistribution and soluble factors in young and aged rats. J Neurosci. 2014;34:313–26.
9. Hellewell S, Semple BD, Morganti-Kossmann MC. Therapies negating neuroinflammation after brain trauma. Brain Res. 2016;1640(Part A):36–56.
10. Witcher KG, Eiferman DS, Godbout JP. Priming the inflammatory pump of the CNS after traumatic brain injury. Trends Neurosci. 2015;38:609–20.
11. Xu X, Yin D, Ren H, Gao W, Li F, Sun D, Wu Y, Zhou S, Lyu L, Yang M, Xiong J, Han L, Jiang R, Zhang J. Selective NLRP3 inflammasome inhibitor reduces neuroinflammation and improves long-term neurological outcomes in a murine model of traumatic brain injury. Neurobiol Dis. 2018;117:15–27.
12. Woodcock T, Morganti-Kossmann MC. The role of markers of inflammation in traumatic brain injury. Front Neurol. 2013;4:18.
13. Correale J, Villa A. The neuroprotective role of inflammation in nervous system injuries. J Neurol. 2004;251:1304–16.
14. Holmin S, Mathiesen T, Shetye J, Biberfeld P. Intracerebral inflammatory response to experimental brain contusion. Acta Neurochir. 1995;132:110–9.
15. Loane DJ, Kumar A, Stoica BA, Cabatbat R, Faden AI. Progressive neurodegeneration after experimental brain trauma: association with chronic microglial activation. J Neuropathol Exp Neurol. 2014;73:14–29.
16. Block ML, Hong JS. Microglia and inflammation-mediated neurodegeneration: multiple triggers with a common mechanism. Prog Neurobiol. 2005;76:77–98.
17. Knoblach SM, Fan L, Faden AI. Early neuronal expression of tumor necrosis factor-alpha after experimental brain injury contributes to neurological impairment. J Neuroimmunol. 1999;95:115–25.
18. Trembovler V, Beit-Yannai E, Younis F, Gallily R, Horowitz M, Shohami E. Antioxidants attenuate acute toxicity of tumor necrosis factor-alpha induced by brain injury in rat. J Interf Cytokine Res. 1999;19:791–5.
19. Longhi L, Perego C, Ortolano F, Aresi S, Fumagalli S, Zanier ER, Stocchetti N, De Simoni MG. Tumor necrosis factor in traumatic brain injury: effects of genetic deletion of p55 or p75 receptor. J Cereb Blood Flow Metab. 2013; 33:1182–9.
20. Sandhir R, Puri V, Klein RM, Berman NE. Differential expression of cytokines and chemokines during secondary neuron death following brain injury in old and young mice. Neurosci Lett. 2004;369:28–32.
21. Hayakata T, Shiozaki T, Tasaki O, Ikegawa H, Inoue Y, Toshiyuki F, Hosotubo H, Kieko F, Yamashita T, Tanaka H, et al. Changes in CSF S100B and cytokine concentrations in early-phase severe traumatic brain injury. Shock. 2004;22: 102–7.
22. Shiozaki T, Hayakata T, Tasaki O, Hosotubo H, Fuijita K, Mouri T, Tajima G, Kajino K, Nakae H, Tanaka H, et al. Cerebrospinal fluid concentrations of anti-inflammatory mediators in early-phase severe traumatic brain injury. Shock. 2005;23:406–10.
23. Lu KT, Wang YW, Yang JT, Yang YL, Chen HI. Effect of interleukin-1 on traumatic brain injury-induced damage to hippocampal neurons. J Neurotrauma. 2005;22:885–95.
24. Kawai T, Akira S. Innate immune recognition of viral infection. Nat Immunol. 2006;7:131–7.
25. de Weerd NA, Samarajiwa SA, Hertzog PJ. Type I interferon receptors: biochemistry and biological functions. J Biol Chem. 2007; 282:20053–7.
26. Platanias LC. Mechanisms of type-I- and type-II-interferon-mediated signalling. Nat Rev Immunol. 2005;5:375–86.
27. Ning S, Pagano JS, Barber GN. IRF7: activation, regulation, modification and function. Genes Immun. 2011;12:399–414.
28. Takaoka A, Wang Z, Choi MK, Yanai H, Negishi H, Ban T, Lu Y, Miyagishi M,

Kodama T, Honda K, et al. DAI (DLM-1/ZBP1) is a cytosolic DNA sensor and an activator of innate immune response. Nature. 2007;448:501–5.
29. Vitner EB, Farfel-Becker T, Ferreira NS, Leshkowitz D, Sharma P, Lang KS, Futerman AH. Induction of the type I interferon response in neurological forms of Gaucher disease. J Neuroinflammation. 2016;13:104.
30. Crow YJ, Hayward BE, Parmar R, Robins P, Leitch A, Ali M, Black DN, van Bokhoven H, Brunner HG, Hamel BC, et al. Mutations in the gene encoding the 3'-5' DNA exonuclease TREX1 cause Aicardi-Goutieres syndrome at the AGS1 locus. Nat Genet. 2006;38:917–20.
31. Field R, Campion S, Warren C, Murray C, Cunningham C. Systemic challenge with the TLR3 agonist poly I:C induces amplified IFNα/β and IL-1β responses in the diseased brain and exacerbates chronic neurodegeneration. Brain Behav Immun. 2010;24:996–1007.
32. Minter MR, Moore Z, Zhang M, Brody KM, Jones NC, Shultz SR, Taylor JM, Crack PJ. Deletion of the type-1 interferon receptor in APPSWE/PS1DeltaE9 mice preserves cognitive function and alters glial phenotype. Acta Neuropathol Commun. 2016;4:016–0341.
33. Taylor JM, Minter MR, Newman AG, Zhang M, Adlard PA, Crack PJ. Type-1 interferon signaling mediates neuro-inflammatory events in models of Alzheimer's disease. Neurobiol Aging. 2014;35:1012–23.
34. Main BS, Zhang M, Brody KM, Ayton S, Frugier T, Steer D, Finkelstein D, Crack PJ, Taylor JM. Type-1 interferons contribute to the neuroinflammatory response and disease progression of the MPTP mouse model of Parkinson's disease. Glia. 2016;64:1590–604.
35. Karve IP, Zhang M, Habgood M, Frugier T, Brody KM, Sashindranath M, Ek CJ, Chappaz S, Kile BT, Wright D, et al. Ablation of Type-1 IFN signaling in hematopoietic cells confers protection following traumatic brain injury. eNeuro. 2016;3:0128–15.
36. Vogan K. STING-mediated autoinflammatory disease. Nat Genet. 2014;46:933.
37. Liu Y, Jesus AA, Marrero B, Yang D, Ramsey SE, Montealegre Sanchez GA, Tenbrock K, Wittkowski H, Jones OY, Kuehn HS, et al. Activated STING in a vascular and pulmonary syndrome. N Engl J Med. 2014;371:507–18.
38. Jeremiah N, Neven B, Gentili M, Callebaut I, Maschalidi S, Stolzenberg M-C, Goudin N, et al. Inherited STING-activating mutation underlies a familial inflammatory syndrome with lupus-like manifestations. J Clin Invest. 2014; 124:5516–20.
39. Nazmi A, Mukhopadhyay R, Dutta K, Basu A. STING mediates neuronal innate immune response following Japanese encephalitis virus infection. Sci Rep. 2012;2:347.
40. Mathur V, Burai R, Vest RT, Bonanno LN, Lehallier B, Zardeneta ME, Mistry KN, Do D, Marsh SE, Abud EM, et al. Activation of the STING-dependent type I interferon response reduces microglial reactivity and neuroinflammation. Neuron. 2017;96:1290–302. e1296
41. Clark RS, Bayir H, Chu CT, Alber SM, Kochanek PM, Watkins SC. Autophagy is increased in mice after traumatic brain injury and is detectable in human brain after trauma and critical illness. Autophagy. 2008;4:88–90.
42. Smith CM, Chen Y, Sullivan ML, Kochanek PM, Clark RS. Autophagy in acute brain injury: feast, famine, or folly? Neurobiol Dis. 2011;43:52–9.
43. Choi AM, Ryter SW, Levine B. Autophagy in human health and disease. N Engl J Med. 2013;368:651–62.
44. Sarkar C, Zhao Z, Aungst S, Sabirzhanov B, Faden AI, Lipinski MM. Impaired autophagy flux is associated with neuronal cell death after traumatic brain injury. Autophagy. 2014;10:2208–22.
45. Klionsky DJ, Emr SD. Autophagy as a regulated pathway of cellular degradation. Science. 2000;290:1717–21.
46. Mizushima N, Yoshimori T, Ohsumi Y. The role of Atg proteins in autophagosome formation. Annu Rev Cell Dev Biol. 2011;27:107–32.
47. Schmeisser H, Bekisz J, Zoon KC. New function of type I IFN: induction of autophagy. J Interf Cytokine Res. 2014;34:71–8.
48. Schmeisser H, Fey SB, Horowitz J, Fischer ER, Balinsky CA, Miyake K, Bekisz J, Snow AL, Zoon KC. Type I interferons induce autophagy in certain human cancer cell lines. Autophagy. 2013;9:683–96.
49. Liu C, Yue R, Yang Y, Cui Y, Yang L, Zhao D, Zhou X. AIM2 inhibits autophagy and IFN-beta production during M. bovis infection. Oncotarget. 2016;7:46972–87.
50. Woo S-R, Fuertes M, Furdyna M, Leung M, Duggan R, Gajewski T. Autophagy in tumor cells and the host STING pathway are critical for innate immune sensing of tumors and bridging to an adaptive immune response (P2183). J Immunol. 2013;190:170.148.
51. Watson RO, Manzanillo PS, Cox JS. Extracellular M. tuberculosis DNA targets bacteria for autophagy by activating the host DNA-sensing pathway. Cell. 2012;150:803–15.
52. Watson RO, Bell SL, MacDuff DA, Kimmey JM, Diner EJ, Olivas J, Vance RE, Stallings CL, Virgin HW, Cox JS. The cytosolic sensor cGAS detects Mycobacterium tuberculosis DNA to induce type I interferons and activate autophagy. Cell Host Microbe. 2015;17:811–9.
53. Chen M, Meng Q, Qin Y, Liang P, Tan P, He L, Zhou Y, Chen Y, Huang J, Wang RF, Cui J. TRIM14 inhibits cGAS degradation mediated by selective autophagy receptor p62 to promote innate immune responses. Mol Cell. 2016;64:105–19.
54. Prabakaran T, Bodda C, Krapp C, Zhang BC, Christensen MH, Sun C, Reinert L, Cai Y, Jensen SB, Skouboe MK, et al. Attenuation of cGAS-STING signaling is mediated by a p62/SQSTM1-dependent autophagy pathway activated by TBK1. EMBO J. 2018;37(8). https://doi.org/10.15252/embj.201797858.
55. Livak KJ, Schmittgen TD. Analysis of relative gene expression data using real-time quantitative PCR and the 2(−Delta Delta C(T)) method. Methods. 2001;25:402–8.
56. Frugier T, Conquest A, McLean C, Currie P, Moses D, Goldshmit Y. Expression and activation of EphA4 in the human brain after traumatic injury. J Neuropathol Exp Neurol. 2012;71(3):242–50.
57. de Weerd NA, Nguyen T. The interferons and their receptors—distribution and regulation. Immunol Cell Biol. 2012;90:483–91.
58. Gough DJ, Messina NL, Hii L, Gould JA, Sabapathy K, Robertson APS, Trapani JA, Levy DE, Hertzog PJ, Clarke CJP, Johnstone RW. Functional crosstalk between type I and II interferon through the regulated expression of STAT1. PLoS Biol. 2010;8:e1000361.
59. Burdette DL, Vance RE. STING and the innate immune response to nucleic acids in the cytosol. Nat Immunol. 2013;14:19–26.
60. Burdette DL, Monroe KM, Sotelo-Troha K, Iwig JS, Eckert B, Hyodo M, Hayakawa Y, Vance RE. STING is a direct innate immune sensor of cyclic di-GMP. Nature. 2011;478:515–8.
61. Cai X, Chiu YH, Chen ZJ. The cGAS-cGAMP-STING pathway of cytosolic DNA sensing and signaling. Mol Cell. 2014;54:289–96.
62. Seki E, Brenner DA. Toll-like receptors and adaptor molecules in liver disease: update. Hepatology. 2008;48:322–35.
63. Petrasek J, Iracheta-Vellve A, Csak T, Satishchandran A, Kodys K, Kurt-Jones EA, Fitzgerald KA, Szabo G. STING-IRF3 pathway links endoplasmic reticulum stress with hepatocyte apoptosis in early alcoholic liver disease. Proc Natl Acad Sci U S A. 2013;110:16544–9.
64. Gehrke N, Garcia-Bardon D, Mann A, Schad A, Alt Y, Worns MA, Sprinzl MF, Zimmermann T, Menke J, Engstler AJ, et al. Acute organ failure following the loss of anti-apoptotic cellular FLICE-inhibitory protein involves activation of innate immune receptors. Cell Death Differ. 2015;22:826–37.
65. Klarquist J, Hennies CM, Lehn MA, Reboulet RA, Feau S, Janssen EM. STING-mediated DNA sensing promotes antitumor and autoimmune responses to dying cells. J Immunol (Baltimore, Md : 1950). 2014;193:6124–34.
66. Qiao JT, Cui C, Qing L, Wang LS, He TY, Yan F, Liu FQ, Shen YH, Hou XG, Chen L. Activation of the STING-IRF3 pathway promotes hepatocyte inflammation, apoptosis and induces metabolic disorders in nonalcoholic fatty liver disease. Metabolism. 2017;81:13–24.
67. Saatman KE, Feeko KJ, Pape RL, Raghupathi R. Differential behavioral and histopathological responses to graded cortical impact injury in mice. J Neurotrauma. 2006;23(8):1241–53.
68. Goodman JC, Cherian L, Bryan RM, Robertson CS. Lateral cortical impact injury in rats: pathologic effects of varying cortical compression and impact velocity. J Neurotrauma. 1994;11:587–97.
69. Xiong Y, Mahmood A, Chopp M. Animal models of traumatic brain injury. Nat Rev Neurosci. 2013;14:128–42.
70. Blaauboer SM, Gabrielle VD, Jin L. MPYS/STING-mediated TNF-alpha, not type I IFN, is essential for the mucosal adjuvant activity of (3'-5')-cyclic-di-guanosine-monophosphate in vivo. J Immunol. 2014;192:492–502.
71. Paludan Søren R, Bowie Andrew G. Immune Sensing of DNA. Immunity. 2013;38:870–80.
72. Luo CL, Li BX, Li QQ, Chen XP, Sun YX, Bao HJ, Dai DK, Shen YW, Xu HF, Ni H, et al. Autophagy is involved in traumatic brain injury-induced cell death and contributes to functional outcome deficits in mice. Neuroscience. 2011; 184:54–63.
73. Zhang JY, Lee J, Gu X, Wei Z, Harris MJ, Yu SPP, Wei L. Intranasally delivered Wnt3a improves functional recovery after traumatic brain injury by modulating Autophagic, apoptotic and regenerative pathways in the mouse brain. J Neurotrauma. 2017;35(5):802–13.

13

Neurogenic inflammation after traumatic brain injury and its potentiation of classical inflammation

Frances Corrigan[1*], Kimberley A. Mander[1], Anna V. Leonard[1] and Robert Vink[2]

Abstract

Background: The neuroinflammatory response following traumatic brain injury (TBI) is known to be a key secondary injury factor that can drive ongoing neuronal injury. Despite this, treatments that have targeted aspects of the inflammatory pathway have not shown significant efficacy in clinical trials.

Main body: We suggest that this may be because classical inflammation only represents part of the story, with activation of neurogenic inflammation potentially one of the key initiating inflammatory events following TBI. Indeed, evidence suggests that the transient receptor potential cation channels (TRP channels), TRPV1 and TRPA1, are polymodal receptors that are activated by a variety of stimuli associated with TBI, including mechanical shear stress, leading to the release of neuropeptides such as substance P (SP). SP augments many aspects of the classical inflammatory response via activation of microglia and astrocytes, degranulation of mast cells, and promoting leukocyte migration. Furthermore, SP may initiate the earliest changes seen in blood-brain barrier (BBB) permeability, namely the increased transcellular transport of plasma proteins via activation of caveolae. This is in line with reports that alterations in transcellular transport are seen first following TBI, prior to decreases in expression of tight-junction proteins such as claudin-5 and occludin. Indeed, the receptor for SP, the tachykinin NK1 receptor, is found in caveolae and its activation following TBI may allow influx of albumin and other plasma proteins which directly augment the inflammatory response by activating astrocytes and microglia.

Conclusions: As such, the neurogenic inflammatory response can exacerbate classical inflammation via a positive feedback loop, with classical inflammatory mediators such as bradykinin and prostaglandins then further stimulating TRP receptors. Accordingly, complete inhibition of neuroinflammation following TBI may require the inhibition of both classical and neurogenic inflammatory pathways.

Keywords: Caveolae, Neuroinflammation, Neurokinin 1 receptor, Substance P, Traumatic brain injury

Background

The role of inflammation in perpetuating the secondary injury response following traumatic brain injury (TBI) has received a significant amount of attention over the last two decades and is clearly an important factor in exacerbating neuronal injury. However, while many pre-clinical studies have shown that therapeutics targeting the immune response are effective in improving outcome when administered in the immediate aftermath of the injury [1–3], reports from clinical trials have been less promising. Agents with known anti-inflammatory properties such as corticosterone, progesterone, and erythropoietin (EPO) have all shown no benefit to date [4–6]. Specifically, the CRASH trial, a prospective, randomized, placebo-controlled multicenter trial of the corticosteroid, methylprednisolone, in TBI, reported an increased mortality following TBI [4]. The ProTECT III trial utilizing progesterone was halted due to failure to demonstrate improved outcome by the Glasgow Outcome Scale-Extended Score at 6 months post-injury [6], with similar findings in another clinical trial utilizing progesterone, the SyNAPse study [5]. In addition, promising anti-inflammatory agents identified in pre-clinical studies often have narrow therapeutic windows. For

* Correspondence: frances.corrigan@adelaide.edu.au
[1]Adelaide Centre for Neuroscience Research, School of Medicine, The University of Adelaide, Adelaide, South Australia, Australia
Full list of author information is available at the end of the article

example, interleukin-1 antagonists appear most efficacious when first administered within hours following injury [1, 2], with minocycline also typically delivered within the first hour post-injury [7–9]. This may be, in part, due to the duality of the immune response following TBI, with some aspects of the inflammatory response necessary to promote repair [10]. In addition, this may also reflect that classical inflammation may be only be half the story, with neurogenic inflammation recently reported as playing a key initiating role [11–13], augmenting many aspects of the classical inflammatory response [14, 15]. This review will outline the interrelationship between classical and neurogenic inflammation, promoting a better understanding of the entire neuroinflammatory cascade and potentially facilitating the development of targeted anti-inflammatory regimes that can improve outcome following TBI.

Traumatic brain injury

TBI results from the head impacting with an object or from acceleration/deceleration forces that produce vigorous movement of the brain within the skull or varying combinations of these mechanical forces [16]. The resultant injury is caused by two mechanisms, either primary or secondary, although there is some degree of overlap [17, 18]. Primary injury is the result of mechanical forces (rotation, acceleration/deceleration, and direct force applied to the head) acting at the moment of the injury that damage the blood vessels, axons, nerve cells, and glia of the brain in a focal, multifocal, or diffuse pattern of involvement. The type and severity of the resulting injury depends upon the nature of the initiating force, as well as the site, direction, and magnitude of the force [19]. Contact forces generated when the head strikes or is struck by an object generally produce focal injuries, such as skull fractures, extradural hemorrhages, and contusions. In contrast, acceleration/deceleration forces that result from violent unrestrained head movement, such as in a motor vehicle accident, are associated with diffuse axonal injury (DAI) [20]. In contrast, secondary injury is a gradual process that occurs over minutes to days as the result of cellular, neurochemical, and metabolic alterations initiated by the primary insult [21]. Injury factors that contribute to this phenomenon include metabolic changes, edema formation, calcium influx, increased oxidative stress, excitotoxicity, inflammation, and ultimately, cell death via necrosis or apoptosis [22]. In particular, inflammation is thought to contribute to much of the secondary cell injury, directly injuring cells, and facilitating other injury factors such as oxidative stress [23] and edema formation [24, 25].

Classical inflammatory response following TBI

A robust inflammatory response develops acutely post-TBI and is characterized by the activation of resident cells, migration and recruitment of peripheral leukocytes, and the release of inflammatory mediators [26]. Cellular damage associated with the mechanical impact causes the release of a number of endogenous factors such as RNA, DNA, heat shock proteins, and HMGB1 (high mobility group box 1) which act as damage-associated molecular patterns (DAMPs) [27]. These bind to toll-like receptors (TLRs) activating the nuclear-factor-κB (NFκB) and MAPK pathways leading to the release of a variety of pro-inflammatory factors including cytokines (IL-1β, IL-6), chemokines, and immune receptors [28]. Members of the TLR family are expressed by a number of resident cells within the central nervous system (CNS), including astrocytes, microglia, and the cerebrovascular endothelium [29–31]. Apart from DAMPs, the classical inflammatory response is also initiated by the presence of extravasated blood products, complement fragments, and reactive oxygen and nitrogen species [27, 32, 33].

This inflammatory response is signaled by a rapid rise in the levels of cytokines and chemokines following TBI, with release from microglia, astrocytes, cerebrovascular endothelial cells, peripheral immune cells, and even neurons [32, 34, 35]. Following a moderate diffuse TBI in mice, for example, levels of IL-1β, tumor necrosis factor alpha (TNFα) and IL-6 within the cortex peak at 3–9 h post-injury, before gradually subsiding [36]. Similarly, within clinical studies, increased levels of IL-6, TNFα, IL-10, C-C motif chemokine ligand 2 (CCL2), and IL-8 peak within the first 2 days following moderate-severe TBI and then return to normal over a period of several weeks [37–39]. This spike in cytokine release has been correlated with astrogliosis, microglial activation, and axonal dysfunction, providing evidence of the association between the activated immune response and brain pathology [40].

Immune cells are recruited to the area of injury by the release of chemokines from the damaged neuronal tissue [41, 42]. This cellular response to injury appears to differ slightly depending on whether the initiating insult is primarily focal or diffuse in nature. A focal injury is characterized by the early infiltration of neutrophils (peaking within a few days), followed by the migration of microglia, astrocytes, macrophages, and lymphocytes to the injured site [43]. Flow cytometric analysis indicates that there is a 10- to 20-fold increase in numbers of microglia compared to peripheral macrophages, suggesting that this is predominantly a central rather than peripheral response [44]. In diffuse injury, little to no neutrophil infiltration is seen, with the early cellular response consisting of microglial accumulation and astrocytosis most prominent in the white matter tracts [45]. This response amplifies over-time with Hellewell et al. indicating that the highest numbers of microglia are present at

14 days post-injury, the latest time-point investigated in their study [45]. Even mild TBI is associated with the induction of an inflammatory response, with diffuse mTBI in pigs showing enhanced microglial activation associated with thalamic axonal injury at 6 h post-injury [46].

The function of this inflammatory response can be both detrimental and potentially beneficial. Both microglia and astrocytes can serve a neuroprotective role immediately following injury by clearing damaged cell debris by phagocytosis, releasing anti-inflammatory cytokines and neurotrophic factors, [33, 47, 48]. Indeed, numerous studies have shown that at least some inflammation is necessary following an insult to the CNS to assist in clearing damage and preparing for remodeling [10, 26]. For example, ablation of proliferating reactive astrocytes following a moderate controlled cortical impact injury significantly exacerbated cortical neuronal loss and inflammation [49]. A potential protective role for astrocytes following injury includes removal of glutamate to reduce the effects of excitotoxicity [50], with the glial scar also thought to act as a physical barrier to prevent spread of toxic molecules. [51] However, this glial scar can also have a later inhibitory effect on axonal regrowth and regeneration [52, 53]. Furthermore, even pro-inflammatory cytokines have an important role to play with Scherbel et al. showing that although knockout of TNFα was beneficial in the acute phase following injury, it had long-term deleterious consequences as demonstrated by TNFα−/− mice showing worsening of motor outcome at 1 month following a focal TBI, which was associated with enhanced cortical tissue loss [54]. This may relate to purported associated neuroprotective functions of TNFα, including the ability to reduce oxidative stress [55] and promote neurotrophic factor synthesis [56, 57], indicating that the presence of at least some TNFα is needed following injury.

In addition, activated microglia demonstrate phenotypic subpopulations, characterized by a specific molecular signature of gene expression: M1 microglia promote a classic pro-inflammatory state releasing pro-inflammatory cytokines and oxidative metabolites, while M2 microglia are important for tissue remodeling and suppress the inflammatory response [58–60]. Reports from TBI studies suggest that there is an early peak in M2-like activated microglia in the week following injury [61, 62], but this then shifts to a maladaptive M1-like activation at later time points. The importance of M2 microglia after TBI is demonstrated by a study by Kumar et al., where aged mice with an impaired M2 response had increased lesion size following a focal injury [63]. Indeed, M1 activation can exacerbate neuronal injury by triggering downstream pathways that culminate in oxidative damage, activation of apoptotic cell death, and increases in permeability of the blood-brain barrier (BBB) through modifications in its tight junctions (Tight junctions) and matrix metalloproteinase (MMP) activation [64, 65]. Furthermore, prolonged M1-like activation hampers repair and can allow tissue damage to persist for years after the initial injury; in a subset of TBI patients, there is incomplete resolution of the acute neuroinflammatory response [66]. A vicious cycle is initiated following the original insult, where the release of pro-inflammatory factors by resident glial cells promotes further glial activation, leading to a progressive chronic cycle of neuroinflammation [67], which can have neurotoxic effects on neurons through mechanisms such as oxidative stress, apoptosis, and excitotoxicity [68].

Neurogenic inflammation

Activation of sensory unmyelinated neurons by noxious stimuli causes the simultaneous release of neuropeptides such as SP, neurokinin A (NKA), neurokinin B (NKB), and calcitonin gene-related peptide (CGRP) [69]. Their release invokes neurogenic inflammation, a neurally elicited response with the typical features of an inflammatory response involving vasodilation and increased vascular permeability [70]. CGRP is chiefly responsible for promoting vasodilation, while SP primarily induces plasma extravasation, although it also produces a brief period of vasodilation [71]. Indeed, although NKA, NKB, and SP act synergistically [72], increases in capillary permeability are principally mediated by SP [73, 74].

SP is an 11-amino acid peptide that is a member of the tachykinin family which includes NKA and NKB [75]; both NKA and SP derived from the preprotachykinin-A (PPT-A) gene by alternative splicing [76]. SP is widely distributed throughout the CNS, peripheral nervous system (PNS), and enteric nervous systems. In the CNS, it is present in dorsal root ganglion (primary sensory) neurons [77] of the spinal cord and many regions of the brain including the hippocampus, cortex, basal ganglia, hypothalamus, amygdala, and caudate nucleus, being more abundant in the gray matter compared to the white matter [78]. The biological effects of SP are mediated by the tachykinin NK receptors, with SP preferentially binding to the NK1 receptor, although it has some affinity for the NK2 and NK3 receptors. NK1 receptors are expressed on endothelial cells, astrocytes, microglia, and various types of circulating and inflammation-activated immune cells [79]. Transduction of the SP signal through the NK1 receptor occurs via G protein signaling and the secondary messenger cAMP, ultimately leading to the regulation of ion channels, enzyme activity, and alterations in gene expression [80]. There are two versions of the NK1 receptor: the full-length version and a truncated form which lacks the 96 residues at the C terminus [81]. This truncated form has a diminished binding affinity for SP [79], and its activation produces a much diminished inflammatory response when compared to the full-length receptor [82]. Higher levels of expression of the shorter isoform are found in peripheral tissues, while in the brain, the longer isoform is expressed at much higher concentrations than the truncated version [83]. This suggests that for pathology within the CNS, the full-length version of the NK1 receptor is the most critical.

Role of SP following TBI

Extensive research has shown that levels of SP rise acutely following TBI in both pre-clinical animal models and in human tissue. Virtually, all blood vessels of the body are surrounded by sensory nerve fibers that contain SP [84]. Cerebral arteries, in particular, appear to receive a dense supply of these nerve fibers, and our studies in TBI have demonstrated that perivascular SP immunoreactivity increases in pre-clinical models, irrespective of injury model [13, 85, 86], and also in humans [87]. It appears that SP is released early following TBI, with increases noted in the plasma at 30 min following TBI in rodents [13]. Furthermore, this release of SP appears to depend on the magnitude of the insult, with a graded increase in SP immunoreactivity seen with increasing severity of injury [85, 88]. Indeed, SP appears to be a key injury marker, as levels in the plasma over the first 4 h following injury are significantly correlated with early mortality in clinical populations, with non-surviving TBI patients showing significantly higher levels than survivors [88].

Moreover, it has been shown that attenuating SP activity following TBI is beneficial to outcome [89]. The first demonstration of neurogenic inflammation in TBI showed that depletion of sensory neuropeptides by pretreatment with capsaicin results in the attenuation of post-traumatic BBB permeability, edema formation, and improved functional outcome [11]. Later studies, specifically targeted SP by administering an NK1 antagonist showed beneficial effects in both male [13] and female rats [90], with a significant attenuation of post-traumatic BBB permeability and a resultant significant reduction in edema formation with improvement in motor and cognitive outcome.

What promotes the release of SP following TBI?

It appears likely that the initial release of SP from sensory neurons following TBI may be mediated by mechanical activation of members of the transient receptor potential (TRP) family, predominantly TRPV1 and TRPA1 [91]. Like all TRP receptors, TRPV1 and TRPA1 are comprised of six-transmembrane proteins that assemble as tetramers to form cation-permeable pores [92, 93]. Their activation allows the influx of cations, primarily sodium and calcium, triggering the release of neuropeptides [94, 95]. TRPV1 appears to be co-expressed in most if not all of TRPA1 expressing dorsal root ganglion neurons [96, 97], with co-expression of both these receptors with neuropeptides including SP [98]. Indeed, suppression of the TRPV1 receptor, with the antagonist capsazepine, has been shown to significantly reduce SP levels in a number of inflammatory models, including a model of sepsis [99], alcohol-induced gastric injury [100], and formalin-induced asthma [101], with the latter study showing a similar reduction in SP with administration of the TRPA1 antagonist, HC-030031 [101]. Furthermore, activation of both TRPV1 and TRPA1 [102–104] has been linked to increased vascular permeability, a key downstream effect of SP release. TRPV1 immunoreactivity is prominent in astrocytes and pericytes, which are closely associated with the vasculature, as well as neurons [105], with the administration of capsazepine able to reduce BBB disruption following an ischemia-reperfusion injury [106].

TRPV1 and TRPA1 channels are considered as polymodal receptors that are activated by a wide range of stimuli. For TRPV1, this includes capsaicin (the active ingredient in chilies) [107], heat (43–52 °C) [108], protons [107], bradykinin [109], prostaglandins [110], and arachidonic acid metabolites amongst others [111]. For TRPA1, agonists include exogenous noxious agents such as components of wasabi and cinnamon [98], oxidized lipids [112], protons [113], and potentially cold (<17 °C) [113, 114]. Notably, both TRPV1 and TRPA1 are also putative mechanoreceptors. Early reports identified that the long ankyrin repeat region within the N-terminal domain of TRPA1, which assists in anchoring the receptor to the plasma membrane, could form a spring-like structure to sense mechanical forces [115, 116]. Indeed, TRPA1 knockout mice were found to be less sensitive to low-intensity mechanical stimuli compared to wild-type mice, and responses to high-intensity mechanical stimulation were notably impaired [113]. Furthermore, inhibition of TRPA1 via either gene knockout or treatment with the antagonist HC-03001 reduced mechanically induced action firing in dermal C fibers [117, 118], wide dynamic range, and nociceptive-specific neurons within the spinal cord [119] and mechanosensitive visceral afferents in the colon [120, 121]. Studies have also suggested that TRPV1 detects mechanical stimuli in a variety of tissues including the urothelium cells of the bladder [122], colonic primary afferent neurons [123], renal pelvis [124], and retinal ganglion cells [125, 126]. The threshold for the stimulation of both TRPV1 and TRPA1 appears to be lowered when there is pre-existing inflammation. Indeed, blockade of TRPA1 was only effective in reducing low-intensity mechanical stimulation of spinal neurons in animals with inflammatory arthritis [119], and application of a TRPV1 antagonist reduced Aδ-fiber unit responses only in inflamed skin [127].

In regard to TBI, a report by Zacest et al. showed that TBI mechanical stimulation of sensory nerves, presumably via TRPV1 and TRPA1, facilitates the perivascular release of SP, with SP co-localizing with amyloid precursor protein positive (injured) neurons that supply the blood vessels [87]. Apart from the initial external mechanical insult to the brain, another acute mechanical stimulus could be related to a brief but highly significant spike in blood pressure (BP) seen following injury. In a sheep model of TBI, BP was reported to rise markedly immediately after impact, peaking at a MAP of 176 mmHg before gradually returning to baseline over a 10-min period [128]. Similar findings have been shown in other models of experimental TBI [129–131]. TRPV1 receptors have indeed been shown to respond to increased intraluminal pressure [132, 133], with Scotland et al. showing that the normal myogenic response to elevation of increased transmural pressure in mesenteric small arteries in vitro was suppressed with the application of the TRPV1 antagonist capsazepine. As such release of neuropeptides including SP may be one of the earliest responses to TBI, highlighting its integral role in facilitating the inflammatory response.

How does neurogenic inflammation potentiate classical inflammation?

Direct interaction between SP and the classical inflammatory response

SP induces and augments many aspects of the classical inflammatory response (Fig 1), including leukocyte activation, endothelial cell adhesion molecule expression, and the production of inflammatory mediators such as histamine, nitric oxide, cytokines (such as IL-6), and kinins [14, 15]. SP is a potent mast cell activator [134]. Mast cells are found within the brain on the adluminal side of the BBB and in the leptomeninges [135], with their degranulation found to potentiate excitotoxicity [136] and augment and prolong numerous vasoactive, neuroactive, and immunoactive cellular and molecular responses to injury [137, 138].

SP also directly activates microglia and astrocytes. Injury induces the expression of NK1 receptors on astrocytes, and their activation is thought to contribute to the transformation to reactive astrocytes, with the resultant production of inflammatory mediators such as cytokines, prostaglandins, and thromboxane derivatives [139–141]. Similarly SP can promote microglial activation, initiating signaling via the NFκB pathway, which leads to the production of pro-inflammatory cytokines [142], with microglia producing IL-1 in response to SP [143]. Moreover, following TBI, NK1 antagonists have been shown to significantly reduce the production of the pro-inflammatory cytokine IL-6, as well as to decrease microglial proliferation [144].

Role of SP in altering BBB permeability

Apart from directly augmenting the local classical inflammatory response, SP-related BBB disruption may also play a role in perpetuating the inflammatory

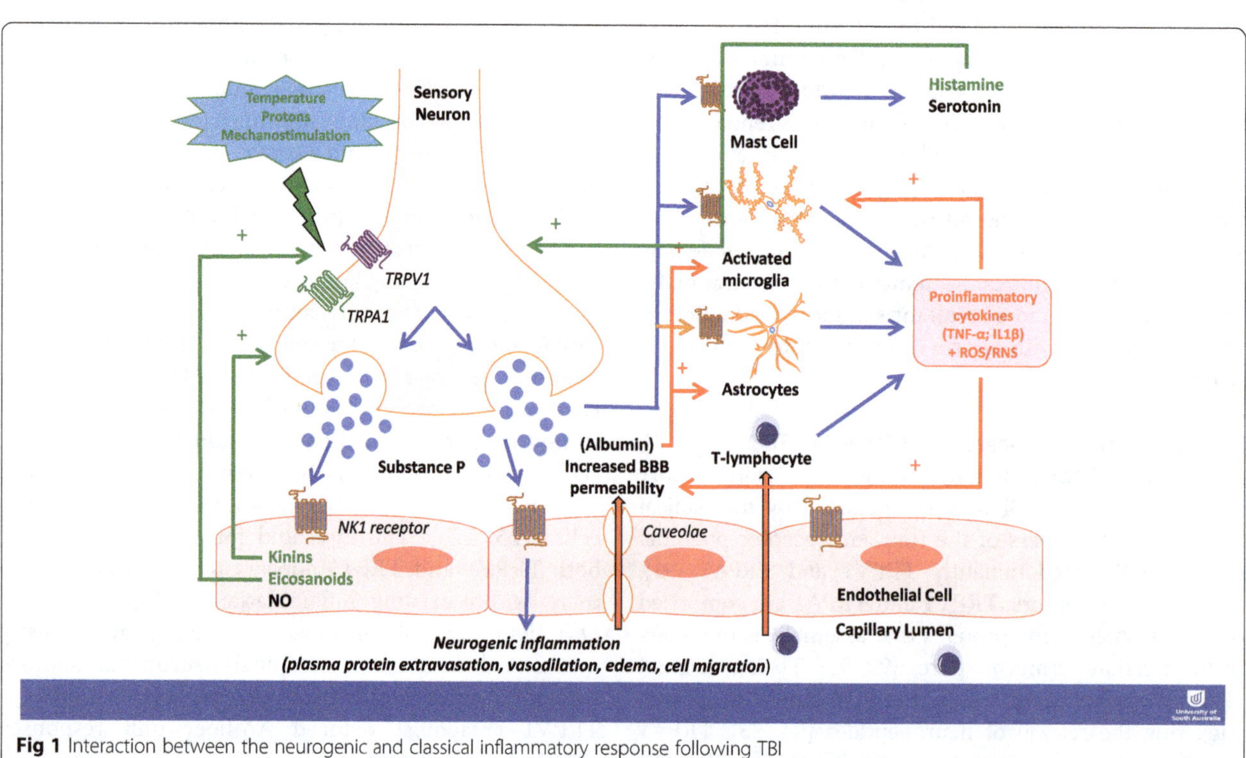

Fig 1 Interaction between the neurogenic and classical inflammatory response following TBI

response. The BBB is a highly selective barrier formed by a layer of endothelial cells joined together by tight junctions including proteins such as claudins, occludin, junctional adhesion molecules (JAMs), and zonula occluden (ZO) proteins, which are supported by the endfeet of astrocytes that act to support and enhance the tight junctions [145]. Tight junctions are present at the apical end of the interendothelial junction and closely rely on the integrity of the corresponding cadherin junction located in the basolateral region. Ultrastructural studies of cerebral endothelial cells indicate the circumferential arrangement of the TJs which provide the barrier formation required to actively restrict the movement of small hydrophilic molecules such as sodium and particular permeability tracers between cells [146]. Given the restrictions on paracellular transport, cerebral endothelial cells have tightly controlled mechanisms that enable the bidirectional transcellular passage of essential molecules and the efflux of potentially neurotoxic substances and waste products [147]. Smaller molecules can be ferried across via carrier-mediated transport or ion pumps while macromolecules employ transcytosis, which can be either receptor-mediated transport (RMT) or adsorptive-mediated transport (AMT), where positively charged macromolecules are nonspecifically transported across the cerebral endothelium [148]. Although the cerebral endothelium has relatively few pinocytotic vesicles compared to peripheral endothelial cells [149], they can still transport macromolecules via one of three vesicles: clathrin-coated pits, the most numerous and through which most of the RMT occurs, the smaller and less numerous caveolae, capable of both AMT and RMT, and large macropinocytic vesciles with nonspecific cargo [150].

Following TBI, the BBB is disrupted and this encompasses not just potential disruption to tight junctions but also increased transcytosis and altered transport properties [151–153]. This increase in the transcellular permeability of the BBB permits the extravasation of proteins and solutes from the cerebral vasculature into the extracellular space within the brain, promoting edema formation, perpetuating the inflammatory response, and causing further neuronal injury. Importantly, it appears that this transcytotic activity is the initial alteration to the BBB following TBI, which is then followed by later loss of tight junctions and movement via the paracellular pathway [151, 152]. An early study by Povlishock (1978) found an increase in BBB permeability as early as 3 min following a mild central fluid percussion injury, despite the apparent integrity of the endothelial tight junctions [154]. Notably, endothelial vesicles assume a modified appearance and initiate the formation of extensive networks for intracellular transport after injury, particularly in the setting of inflammation within the CNS [155]. Indeed, ultrastructural studies have shown that within minutes of brain injury, endothelial caveolae are significantly increased in vessel segments showing loss of BBB integrity [152, 155], with evidence for increased vesicular formation in the BBB of TBI patients [156, 157]. In a rat cortical cold injury model that produces a pure vasogenic edema, an increase in expression of caveolin-1, the key protein found in caveolae, occurred prior to the loss of tight junctions, represented by a reduction in the expression of occludin and claudin-5 [152]. Notably, caveolin-1 expression was seen in blood vessels which exhibited increased permeability to proteins, indicating that this may be the initial mechanism by which the BBB is disrupted [152]. These findings were replicated in a controlled cortical impact model of TBI, where caveolin-1 was increased at 1 day following injury, prior to a decrease in claudin-5 which occurred at day 3 following injury [151].

SP is known to promote increased permeability of the BBB leading to increased extravasation of vascular protein into the brain extracellular space. Indeed, injured animals show a strong co-localization of SP immunofluorescence with a marker of vascular permeability, Evan's blue, within the cortical vasculature at 5 h post-TBI [13]. Administration of an NK1 antagonist also leads to a dose-dependent decrease in permeability of the BBB following TBI, with an accompanying reduction in cerebral edema [13]. The exact mechanisms by which SP promotes an increase in BBB permeability are less clear. There are previous reports that application of SP can decrease the expression of ZO-1 and claudin-5 in cerebral capillary endothelial cells [158], but immediately following TBI tight junctions are intact. Alternatively, SP may initially act to increase transcytosis via activation of transport via caveolae.

Caveolae have been shown to mediate the transport of molecules such as albumin, transferrin, insulin, low-density lipoproteins, cytokines, and chemokines through the specific localization of corresponding receptors within the caveolae coats [159, 160]. Indeed, caveolin-1 knockout mice were unable to transcytose albumin as evaluated via gold-labeled immunostaining [161, 162], supporting a key role for caveolae in the early BBB changes seen following TBI, and consistent with the increases seen in expression of caveolin-1 in the immediate phase following injury [151–153]. Caveolae constitute an entire membrane system responsible for the formation of unique endo- and exocytotic compartments [163]. During transcytosis, caveolae "pinch off" from the plasma membrane to form vesicular carriers that rapidly and efficiently shuttle to the opposite membrane of the endothelial cells, fuse and release their contents via exocytosis [164]. In addition to the structural caveolin proteins, a number of signaling molecules, including specific receptors, are known to localize to the caveolae pit [160, 165]. Receptor tyrosine kinase, G-protein-coupled receptors, transforming growth factor-beta (TGF-β) type 1 and 2, certain steroid receptors and enzymes have a confirmed presence within endothelial caveolae and may play a role in facilitating macromolecular transcytosis [166–168]. Of particular note, the NK1 receptor, to which SP preferentially binds, has been reported to localize within the endothelial caveolae and can be manipulated to upregulate or relocate upon stimulation, indicating that its presence and function is dynamic and subject to the environment [169, 170]. Indeed, stimulation of the NK1 receptor within caveolae by SP causes PKCα to relocate to caveolae [170], with this process previously shown to regulate the internalization of caveolae [171], the first step in transcytosis. Although not directly studied for the NK1 receptor, in vitro studies have demonstrated increased receptor-mediated transendothelial transport of target molecules in the setting of inflammation [172]. This suggests that the activation of a caveolae-housed receptor may also internalize additional proteins in their cargo, such as albumin, facilitating their entry into the brain.

Within the CNS, albumin is able to activate microglia and astrocytes leading to the release of pro-inflammatory cytokines and chemokines (e.g., IL-1β, TNFα, MCP-1, CXC3L1), glutamate, and free radicals promoting neuronal injury and amplifying the classical inflammatory response [173–178]. Although the majority of these studies apply albumin to isolated glial cultures [174–177], Chacheaux et al. were able to demonstrate that direct application of a solution containing bovine serum albumin to the rat cortex produced similar changes in gene expression when compared to application of an agent (deoxcycholic acid) that directly opens the BBB [179]. Microarray analysis showed a comparable gene expression profile to either treatment, with an early and persistent upregulation of genes associated with immune response activation, including NF-κB pathway-related genes, cytokines, and chemokines (IL-6, CCL2, CCL7) [179]. Indeed, recent evidence suggests that following activation by albumin, microglia are neurotoxic, with media taken from microglial cultures exposed to albumin promoting the upregulation of caspase 3 and 7 in cerebellar granule neuronal cultures with an accompanying increase in cell death [174]. Furthermore, when exposure to albumin was combined with TLR4 activation via lipopolysaccharide (LPS), a synergistic increase in the release of pro-inflammatory cytokines was noted from cultured microglia [174]. As the neuronal injury associated with TBI leads to the production of DAMPs [180] that act as TLR4 agonists, influx of albumin through a disrupted BBB would lead to more potent activation of microglia. This provides another key intersection between the classical inflammatory response, in TLR4 activation by DAMPs, and the neurogenic inflammatory response, with SP release promoting albumin influx via caveolae promoting further activation of resident immune cells.

The effects of SP on the BBB relates not only to increases in permeability but also on promoting immune cell trafficking into the CNS. Activation of SP's preferred receptor, NK1, has been shown to enhance leukocyte migration by exerting a chemotactic effect on monocytes and neutrophils [181–183], increasing the expression of adhesion molecules on endothelial cells [184–187] and augmenting local chemokine production [188]. Indeed, application of SP to cerebral endothelial cultures led to a dose-dependent increase in ICAM-1 expression [184], with this associated with an increase in T lymphocyte adherence, suggesting facilitation of immune cell movement across the BBB [187]. Thus, the release of SP following TBI may facilitate the influx of peripheral immune cells like T cells, macrophages, and neutrophils into the CNS, which then further augments the local neuroinflammatory response via production of pro-inflammatory cytokines, reactive oxygen species, and metalloproteinases.

Exacerbation of neurogenic inflammation by classical inflammation

Although this discussion has focused on how neurogenic inflammation can facilitate the classical inflammatory response, this is a two-way interaction with classical inflammation further enhancing the release of neuropeptides (Fig 1). As discussed previously, TPRV1 and TRPA1 are responsive to a number of stimuli including the classical inflammatory mediators bradykinin [109] and prostaglandins [110], which are produced as part of the inflammatory response following TBI [189, 190]; their production would potentiate further SP release. For example, the kallikrein-kinin system is believed to be one of the first inflammatory pathways activated after tissue damage [191]. Bradykinin, a nonpeptide found in blood and tissue, is cleaved from its pro-form kininogen by the protease kallikrein [192], with levels found to peak within the brain at 2 h following a focal brain injury [193]. TBI is also known to increase the activity of cyclooxygenase (COX) enzymes, principally Cox-2 found in microglia and endothelial cells, increasing the synthesis of prostaglandins such as PGE_2 and $PGF_{2\alpha}$. Indeed, levels of PGE_2 have been shown to be elevated within 5 min following TBI [194]. In addition to these direct activators or TRP channels, cytokines like IL-1, IL-6, and TNFα may sensitize sensory neurons, lowering the threshold for release of neuropeptides [195, 196].

Conclusion

Following TBI activation of a classical inflammatory response only represents part of the neuroinflammatory response. The mechanical and shear stress associated with TBI also activates TRP receptors leading to the release of neuropeptides, including SP, instigating a neurogenic inflammatory response. SP both directly and indirectly, through alterations in BBB permeability with influx of plasma proteins, augments the classical inflammatory response, with both classical and neurogenic inflammation providing positive feedback to the other to amplify and propagate inflammation with the release of pro-inflammatory mediators, oxidative metabolites, and metalloproteinases amongst others, which cause further neuronal damage. As such, modulation of neuroinflammation following TBI may require addressing both inflammatory pathways with the aim to prevent the deleterious effects of the response, while facilitating repair.

Abbreviations

AMT: Absorptive-mediated transcytosis; BBB: Blood-brain barrier; CNS: Central nervous system; EPO: Erythropoietin; RMT: Receptor-mediated transcytosis; SP: Substance P; TLR: Toll-like receptor; TRP channels: Transient receptor potential cation channels; TBI: Traumatic brain injury

Acknowledgements

None to declare.

Funding

The authors received funding from the Australian National Health and Medical Research Council (NHMRC) and the Neurosurgical Research Foundation (NRF).

Authors' contributions

FC, KM, and AL performed the literature review and drafted the paper under the supervision of RV. RV graphed the illustration. All authors discussed and edited the manuscript. All authors read and approved the final manuscript.

Competing interests

The authors declare that they have no competing interests.

Consent for publication

Not applicable.

Author details

[1]Adelaide Centre for Neuroscience Research, School of Medicine, The University of Adelaide, Adelaide, South Australia, Australia. [2]Sansom Institute for Health Research, The University of South Australia, Adelaide, South Australia, Australia.

References

1. Jones NC, Prior MJ, Burden-Teh E, Marsden CA, Morris PG, Murphy S. Antagonism of the interleukin-1 receptor following traumatic brain injury in the mouse reduces the number of nitric oxide synthase-2-positive cells and improves anatomical and functional outcomes. Eur J Neurosci. 2005;22:72–8.
2. Sanderson KL, Raghupathi R, Saatman KE, Martin D, Miller G, McIntosh TK. Interleukin-1 receptor antagonist attenuates regional neuronal cell death and cognitive dysfunction after experimental brain injury. J Cereb Blood Flow Metab. 1999;19:1118–25.
3. Shohami E, Gallily R, Mechoulam R, Bass R, Ben-Hur T. Cytokine production in the brain following closed head injury: dexanabinol (HU-211) is a novel TNF-alpha inhibitor and an effective neuroprotectant. J Neuroimmunol. 1997;72:169–77.
4. Roberts I, Yates D, Sandercock P, Farrell B, Wasserberg J, Lomas G, Cottingham R, Svoboda P, Brayley N, Mazairac G, et al. Effect of intravenous corticosteroids on death within 14 days in 10008 adults with clinically significant head injury (MRC CRASH trial): randomised placebo-controlled trial. Lancet. 2004;364:1321–8.
5. Skolnick BE, Maas AI, Narayan RK, van der Hoop RG, MacAllister T, Ward JD, Nelson NR, Stocchetti N, Investigators ST. A clinical trial of progesterone for severe traumatic brain injury. N Engl J Med. 2014;371:2467–76.
6. Wright DW, Yeatts SD, Silbergleit R, Palesch YY, Hertzberg VS, Frankel M, Goldstein FC, Caveney AF, Howlett-Smith H, Bengelink EM, et al. Very early administration of progesterone for acute traumatic brain injury. N Engl J Med. 2014;371:2457–66.
7. Bye N, Habgood MD, Callaway JK, Malakooti N, Potter A, Kossmann T, Morganti-Kossmann MC. Transient neuroprotection by minocycline following traumatic brain injury is associated with attenuated microglial activation but no changes in cell apoptosis or neutrophil infiltration. Exp Neurol. 2007;204:220–33.
8. Teng YD, Choi H, Onario RC, Zhu S, Desilets FC, Lan S, Woodard EJ, Snyder EY, Eichler ME, Friedlander RM. Minocycline inhibits contusion-triggered mitochondrial cytochrome c release and mitigates functional deficits after spinal cord injury. Proc Natl Acad Sci U S A. 2004;101:3071–6.
9. Wells JE, Hurlbert RJ, Fehlings MG, Yong VW. Neuroprotection by minocycline facilitates significant recovery from spinal cord injury in mice. Brain. 2003;126:1628–37.
10. Russo MV, McGavern DB. Inflammatory neuroprotection following traumatic brain injury. Science. 2016;353:783–5.
11. Nimmo AJ, Cernak I, Heath DL, Hu X, Bennett CJ, Vink R. Neurogenic inflammation is associated with development of edema and functional deficits following traumatic brain injury in rats. Neuropeptides. 2004;38:40–7.
12. Donkin JJ, Cernak I, Blumbergs PC, Vink R. A substance P antagonist reduces axonal injury and improves neurologic outcome when administered up to 12 hours after traumatic brain injury. J Neurotrauma. 2011;28:217–24.
13. Donkin JJ, Nimmo AJ, Cernak I, Blumbergs PC, Vink R. Substance P is associated with the development of brain edema and functional deficits after traumatic brain injury. J Cereb Blood Flow Metab. 2009;29:1388–98.
14. Marriott I, Bost KL. Substance P receptor mediated macrophage responses. Adv Exp Med Biol. 2001;493:247–54.
15. Quinlan KL, Song IS, Naik SM, Letran EL, Olerud JE, Bunnett NW, Armstrong CA, Caughman SW, Ansel JC. VCAM-1 expression on human dermal microvascular endothelial cells is directly and specifically up-regulated by substance P. J Immunol. 1999;162:1656–61.
16. Finnie JW, Blumbergs PC. Traumatic brain injury. Vet Pathol. 2002;39:679–89.
17. Maas AI, Stocchetti N, Bullock R. Moderate and severe traumatic brain injury in adults. Lancet Neurol. 2008;7:728–41.
18. Gaetz M. The neurophysiology of brain injury. Clin Neurophysiol. 2004;115:4–18.
19. Smith DH, Meaney DF, Shull WH. Diffuse axonal injury in head trauma. J Head Trauma Rehabil. 2003;18:307–16.
20. Blumbergs P. Pathology. In: Reilly P, Bullock R, editors. Head injury: pathophysiology and management of severe closed injury. London: Chapman & Hall Medical; 1997. p. 39–70.
21. Hall ED, Gibson TR, Pavel KM. Lack of a gender difference in post-traumatic neurodegeneration in the mouse controlled cortical impact injury model. J Neurotrauma. 2005;22:669–79.
22. Saatman KE, Bozyczko-Coyne D, Marcy V, Siman R, McIntosh TK. Prolonged calpain-mediated spectrin breakdown occurs regionally following experimental brain injury in the rat. J Neuropathol Exp Neurol. 1996;55:850–60.
23. Liao Y, Liu P, Guo F, Zhang ZY, Zhang Z. Oxidative burst of circulating neutrophils following traumatic brain injury in human. PLoS One. 2013;8:e68963.
24. Vink R, Young A, Bennett CJ, Hu X, Connor CO, Cernak I, Nimmo AJ. Neuropeptide release influences brain edema formation after diffuse traumatic brain injury. Acta Neurochir Suppl. 2003;86:257–60.
25. Chodobski A, Zink BJ, Szmydynger-Chodobska J. Blood-brain barrier pathophysiology in traumatic brain injury. Transl Stroke Res. 2011;2:492–516.

26. Ziebell JM, Morganti-Kossmann MC. Involvement of pro- and anti-inflammatory cytokines and chemokines in the pathophysiology of traumatic brain injury. Neurotherapeutics. 2010;7:22–30.
27. Manson J, Thiemermann C, Brohi K. Trauma alarmins as activators of damage-induced inflammation. Br J Surg. 2012;99 Suppl 1:12–20.
28. Buchanan MM, Hutchinson M, Watkins LR, Yin H. Toll-like receptor 4 in CNS pathologies. J Neurochem. 2010;114:13–27.
29. Farina C, Aloisi F, Meinl E. Astrocytes are active players in cerebral innate immunity. Trends Immunol. 2007;28:138–45.
30. Gurley C, Nichols J, Liu S, Phulwani NK, Esen N, Kielian T. Microglia and astrocyte activation by toll-like receptor ligands: modulation by PPAR-gamma agonists. PPAR Res. 2008;2008:453120.
31. Nagyoszi P, Wilhelm I, Farkas AE, Fazakas C, Dung NT, Hasko J, Krizbai IA. Expression and regulation of toll-like receptors in cerebral endothelial cells. Neurochem Int. 2010;57:556–64.
32. Woodcock T, Morganti-Kossmann MC. The role of markers of inflammation in traumatic brain injury. Front Neurol. 2013;4:18.
33. Corps KN, Roth TL, McGavern DB. Inflammation and neuroprotection in traumatic brain injury. JAMA Neurol. 2015;72:355–62.
34. Bergold PJ. Treatment of traumatic brain injury with anti-inflammatory drugs. Exp Neurol. 2016;275(Pt 3):367–80.
35. Hellewell S, Semple BD, Morganti-Kossmann MC. Therapies negating neuroinflammation after brain trauma. Brain Res. 2016;1640:36–56.
36. Bachstetter AD, Rowe RK, Kaneko M, Goulding D, Lifshitz J, Van Eldik LJ. The p38alpha MAPK regulates microglial responsiveness to diffuse traumatic brain injury. J Neurosci. 2013;33:6143–53.
37. Csuka E, Morganti-Kossmann MC, Lenzlinger PM, Joller H, Trentz O, Kossmann T. IL-10 levels in cerebrospinal fluid and serum of patients with severe traumatic brain injury: relationship to IL-6, TNF-alpha, TGF-beta1 and blood-brain barrier function. J Neuroimmunol. 1999;101:211–21.
38. Semple BD, Bye N, Rancan M, Ziebell JM, Morganti-Kossmann MC. Role of CCL2 (MCP-1) in traumatic brain injury (TBI): evidence from severe TBI patients and CCL2–/– mice. J Cereb Blood Flow Metab. 2010;30:769–82.
39. Morganti-Kossman MC, Lenzlinger PM, Hans V, Stahel P, Csuka E, Ammann E, Stocker R, Trentz O, Kossmann T. Production of cytokines following brain injury: beneficial and deleterious for the damaged tissue. Mol Psychiatry. 1997;2:133–6.
40. Frugier T, Morganti-Kossmann MC, O'Reilly D, McLean CA. In situ detection of inflammatory mediators in post mortem human brain tissue after traumatic injury. J Neurotrauma. 2010;27:497–507.
41. Cardona AE, Gonzalez PA, Teale JM. CC chemokines mediate leukocyte trafficking into the central nervous system during murine neurocysticercosis: role of gamma delta T cells in amplification of the host immune response. Infect Immun. 2003;71:2634–42.
42. Wilson EH, Weninger W, Hunter CA. Trafficking of immune cells in the central nervous system. J Clin Invest. 2010;120:1368–79.
43. Gyoneva S, Ransohoff RM. Inflammatory reaction after traumatic brain injury: therapeutic potential of targeting cell-cell communication by chemokines. Trends Pharmacol Sci. 2015;36:471–80.
44. Al Nimer F, Lindblom R, Strom M, Guerreiro-Cacais AO, Parsa R, Aeinehband S, Mathiesen T, Lidman O, Piehl F. Strain influences on inflammatory pathway activation, cell infiltration and complement cascade after traumatic brain injury in the rat. Brain Behav Immun. 2013;27:109–22.
45. Hellewell SC, Yan EB, Agyapomaa DA, Bye N, Morganti-Kossmann MC. Post-traumatic hypoxia exacerbates brain tissue damage: analysis of axonal injury and glial responses. J Neurotrauma. 2010;27:1997–2010.
46. Lafrenaye AD, Todani M, Walker SA, Povlishock JT. Microglia processes associate with diffusely injured axons following mild traumatic brain injury in the micro pig. J Neuroinflammation. 2015;12:186.
47. Lull ME, Block ML. Microglial activation and chronic neurodegeneration. Neurotherapeutics. 2010;7:354–65.
48. Luo XG, Chen SD. The changing phenotype of microglia from homeostasis to disease. Transl Neurodegener. 2012;1:9.
49. Myer DJ, Gurkoff GG, Lee SM, Hovda DA, Sofroniew MV. Essential protective roles of reactive astrocytes in traumatic brain injury. Brain. 2006;129:2761–72.
50. Rothstein JD, Dykes-Hoberg M, Pardo CA, Bristol LA, Jin L, Kuncl RW, Kanai Y, Hediger MA, Wang Y, Schielke JP, Welty DF. Knockout of glutamate transporters reveals a major role for astroglial transport in excitotoxicity and clearance of glutamate. Neuron. 1996;16:675–86.
51. Fitch MT, Silver J. Glial cell extracellular matrix: boundaries for axon growth in development and regeneration. Cell Tissue Res. 1997;290:379–84.
52. Ribotta MG, Menet V, Privat A. Glial scar and axonal regeneration in the CNS: lessons from GFAP and vimentin transgenic mice. Acta Neurochir Suppl. 2004;89:87–92.
53. Silver J, Miller JH. Regeneration beyond the glial scar. Nat Rev Neurosci. 2004;5:146–56.
54. Scherbel U, Raghupathi R, Nakamura M, Saatman KE, Trojanowski JQ, Neugebauer E, Marino MW, McIntosh TK. Differential acute and chronic responses of tumor necrosis factor-deficient mice to experimental brain injury. Proc Natl Acad Sci U S A. 1999;96:8721–6.
55. Bruce-Keller AJ, Geddes JW, Knapp PE, McFall RW, Keller JN, Holtsberg FW, Parthasarathy S, Steiner SM, Mattson MP. Anti-death properties of TNF against metabolic poisoning: mitochondrial stabilization by MnSOD. J Neuroimmunol. 1999;93:53–71.
56. Saha RN, Liu X, Pahan K. Up-regulation of BDNF in astrocytes by TNF-alpha: a case for the neuroprotective role of cytokine. J Neuroimmune Pharmacol. 2006;1:212–22.
57. Hattori A, Tanaka E, Murase K, Ishida N, Chatani Y, Tsujimoto M, Hayashi K, Kohno M. Tumor necrosis factor stimulates the synthesis and secretion of biologically active nerve growth factor in non-neuronal cells. J Biol Chem. 1993;268:2577–82.
58. Loane DJ, Kumar A. Microglia in the TBI brain: the good, the bad, and the dysregulated. Exp Neurol. 2016;275(Pt 3):316–27.
59. Colton CA. Heterogeneity of microglial activation in the innate immune response in the brain. J Neuroimmune Pharmacol. 2009;4:399–418.
60. David S, Kroner A. Repertoire of microglial and macrophage responses after spinal cord injury. Nat Rev Neurosci. 2011;12:388–99.
61. Jin X, Ishii H, Bai Z, Itokazu T, Yamashita T. Temporal changes in cell marker expression and cellular infiltration in a controlled cortical impact model in adult male C57BL/6 mice. PLoS One. 2012;7:e41892.
62. Wang G, Zhang J, Hu X, Zhang L, Mao L, Jiang X, Liou AK, Leak RK, Gao Y, Chen J. Microglia/macrophage polarization dynamics in white matter after traumatic brain injury. J Cereb Blood Flow Metab. 2013;33:1864–74.
63. Kumar A, Stoica BA, Sabirzhanov B, Burns MP, Faden AI, Loane DJ. Traumatic brain injury in aged animals increases lesion size and chronically alters microglial/macrophage classical and alternative activation states. Neurobiol Aging. 2013;34:1397–411.
64. da Fonseca AC, Matias D, Garcia C, Amaral R, Geraldo LH, Freitas C, Lima FR. The impact of microglial activation on blood-brain barrier in brain diseases. Front Cell Neurosci. 2014;8:362.
65. Huang WC, Sala-Newby GB, Susana A, Johnson JL, Newby AC. Classical macrophage activation up-regulates several matrix metalloproteinases through mitogen activated protein kinases and nuclear factor-kappaB. PLoS One. 2012;7:e42507.
66. Bigler ED. Neuroinflammation and the dynamic lesion in traumatic brain injury. Brain. 2013;136:9–11.
67. Lozano D, Gonzales-Portillo GS, Acosta S, de la Pena I, Tajiri N, Kaneko Y, Borlongan CV. Neuroinflammatory responses to traumatic brain injury: etiology, clinical consequences, and therapeutic opportunities. Neuropsychiatr Dis Treat. 2015;11:97–106.
68. Faden AI, Wu J, Stoica BA, Loane DJ. Progressive inflammation-mediated neurodegeneration after traumatic brain or spinal cord injury. Br J Pharmacol. 2016;173:681–91.
69. Escott KJ, Connor HE, Brain SD, Beattie DT. The involvement of calcitonin gene-related peptide (CGRP) and substance P in feline pial artery diameter responses evoked by capsaicin. Neuropeptides. 1995;29:129–35.
70. Maggi CA, Giuliani S. Role of tachykinins as excitatory mediators of NANC contraction in the circular muscle of rat small intestine. J Auton Pharmacol. 1995;15:335–50.
71. Schlereth T, Schukraft J, Kramer-Best HH, Geber C, Ackermann T, Birklein F. Interaction of calcitonin gene related peptide (CGRP) and substance P (SP) in human skin. Neuropeptides. 2016.
72. Brain SD, Williams TJ. Interactions between the tachykinins and calcitonin gene-related peptide lead to the modulation of oedema formation and blood flow in rat skin. Br J Pharmacol. 1989;97:77–82.
73. Inoue H, Nagata N, Koshihara Y. Involvement of substance P as a mediator in capsaicin-induced mouse ear oedema. Inflamm Res. 1995;44:470–4.
74. Lembeck F, Donnerer J, Tsuchiya M, Nagahisa A. The non-peptide tachykinin antagonist, CP-96,345, is a potent inhibitor of neurogenic inflammation. Br J Pharmacol. 1992;105:527–30.
75. Schaffer M, Beiter T, Becker HD, Hunt TK. Neuropeptides: mediators of inflammation and tissue repair? Arch Surg. 1998;133:1107–16.

76. Severini C, Improta G, Falconieri-Erspamer G, Salvadori S, Erspamer V. The tachykinin peptide family. Pharmacol Rev. 2002;54:285–322.
77. Hokfelt T, Pernow B, Wahren J. Substance P: a pioneer amongst neuropeptides. J Intern Med. 2001;249:27–40.
78. Ebner K, Singewald N. The role of substance P in stress and anxiety responses. Amino Acids. 2006;31:251–72.
79. Douglas SD, Leeman SE. Neurokinin-1 receptor: functional significance in the immune system in reference to selected infections and inflammation. Ann N Y Acad Sci. 2011;1217:83–95.
80. Lundy FT, Linden GJ. Neuropeptides and neurogenic mechanisms in oral and periodontal inflammation. Crit Rev Oral Biol Med. 2004;15:82–98.
81. Fong TM, Anderson SA, Yu H, Huang RR, Strader CD. Differential activation of intracellular effector by two isoforms of human neurokinin-1 receptor. Mol Pharmacol. 1992;41:24–30.
82. Lai JP, Lai S, Tuluc F, Tansky MF, Kilpatrick LE, Leeman SE, Douglas SD. Differences in the length of the carboxyl terminus mediate functional properties of neurokinin-1 receptor. Proc Natl Acad Sci U S A. 2008;105:12605–10.
83. Caberlotto L, Hurd YL, Murdock P, Wahlin JP, Melotto S, Corsi M, Carletti R. Neurokinin 1 receptor and relative abundance of the short and long isoforms in the human brain. Eur J Neurosci. 2003;17:1736–46.
84. Donkin JJ, Turner RJ, Hassan I, Vink R. Substance P in traumatic brain injury. Prog Brain Res. 2007;161:97–109.
85. Corrigan F, Vink R, Turner RJ. Inflammation in acute CNS injury: a focus on the role of substance P. Br J Pharmacol. 2016;173:703–15.
86. Gabrielian L, Helps SC, Thornton E, Turner RJ, Leonard AV, Vink R. Substance P antagonists as a novel intervention for brain edema and raised intracranial pressure. Acta Neurochir Suppl. 2013;118:201–4.
87. Zacest AC, Vink R, Manavis J, Sarvestani GT, Blumbergs PC. Substance P immunoreactivity increases following human traumatic brain injury. Acta Neurochir Suppl. 2010;106:211–6.
88. Lorente L, Martin MM, Almeida T, Hernandez M, Ramos L, Argueso M, Caceres JJ, Sole-Violan J, Jimenez A. Serum substance P levels are associated with severity and mortality in patients with severe traumatic brain injury. Crit Care. 2015;19:192.
89. Donkin JJ, Vink R. Mechanisms of cerebral edema in traumatic brain injury: therapeutic developments. Curr Opin Neurol. 2010;23:293–9.
90. Corrigan F, Leonard A, Ghabriel M, Van Den Heuvel C, Vink R. A substance P antagonist improves outcome in female Sprague Dawley rats following diffuse traumatic brain injury. CNS Neurosci Ther. 2012;18:513–5.
91. Geppetti P, Bertrand C, Ricciardolo FL, Nadel JA. New aspects on the role of kinins in neurogenic inflammation. Can J Physiol Pharmacol. 1995;73:843–7.
92. Minke B. TRP channels and Ca2+ signaling. Cell Calcium. 2006;40:261–75.
93. Pan Z, Yang H, Reinach PS. Transient receptor potential (TRP) gene superfamily encoding cation channels. Hum Genomics. 2011;5:108–16.
94. Parenti A, De Logu F, Geppetti P, Benemei S. What is the evidence for the role of TRP channels in inflammatory and immune cells? Br J Pharmacol. 2016;173:953–69.
95. Vriens J, Appendino G, Nilius B. Pharmacology of vanilloid transient receptor potential cation channels. Mol Pharmacol. 2009;75:1262–79.
96. Anand U, Otto WR, Facer P, Zebda N, Selmer I, Gunthorpe MJ, Chessell IP, Sinisi M, Birch R, Anand P. TRPA1 receptor localisation in the human peripheral nervous system and functional studies in cultured human and rat sensory neurons. Neurosci Lett. 2008;438:221–7.
97. Bautista DM, Jordt SE, Nikai T, Tsuruda PR, Read AJ, Poblete J, Yamoah EN, Basbaum AI, Julius D. TRPA1 mediates the inflammatory actions of environmental irritants and proalgesic agents. Cell. 2006;124:1269–82.
98. Jordt SE, Bautista DM, Chuang HH, McKemy DD, Zygmunt PM, Hogestatt ED, Meng ID, Julius D. Mustard oils and cannabinoids excite sensory nerve fibres through the TRP channel ANKTM1. Nature. 2004;427:260–5.
99. Ang SF, Moochhala SM, MacAry PA, Bhatia M. Hydrogen sulfide and neurogenic inflammation in polymicrobial sepsis: involvement of substance P and ERK-NF-kappaB signaling. PLoS One. 2011;6:e24535.
100. Gazzieri D, Trevisani M, Springer J, Harrison S, Cottrell GS, Andre E, Nicoletti P, Massi D, Zecchi S, Nosi D, et al. Substance P released by TRPV1-expressing neurons produces reactive oxygen species that mediate ethanol-induced gastric injury. Free Radic Biol Med. 2007;43:581–9.
101. Wu Y, You H, Ma P, Li L, Yuan Y, Li J, Ye X, Liu X, Yao H, Chen R, et al. Role of transient receptor potential ion channels and evoked levels of neuropeptides in a formaldehyde-induced model of asthma in BALB/c mice. PLoS One. 2013;8:e62827.
102. Trevisani M, Siemens J, Materazzi S, Bautista DM, Nassini R, Campi B, Imamachi N, Andre E, Patacchini R, Cottrell GS, et al. 4-Hydroxynonenal, an endogenous aldehyde, causes pain and neurogenic inflammation through activation of the irritant receptor TRPA1. Proc Natl Acad Sci U S A. 2007;104:13519–24.
103. Andre E, Campi B, Materazzi S, Trevisani M, Amadesi S, Massi D, Creminon C, Vaksman N, Nassini R, Civelli M, et al. Cigarette smoke-induced neurogenic inflammation is mediated by alpha, beta-unsaturated aldehydes and the TRPA1 receptor in rodents. J Clin Invest. 2008;118:2574–82.
104. Nassini R, Materazzi S, Andre E, Sartiani L, Aldini G, Trevisani M, Carnini C, Massi D, Pedretti P, Carini M, et al. Acetaminophen, via its reactive metabolite N-acetyl-p-benzo-quinoneimine and transient receptor potential ankyrin-1 stimulation, causes neurogenic inflammation in the airways and other tissues in rodents. FASEB J. 2010;24:4904–16.
105. Toth A, Boczan J, Kedei N, Lizanecz E, Bagi Z, Papp Z, Edes I, Csiba L, Blumberg PM. Expression and distribution of vanilloid receptor 1 (TRPV1) in the adult rat brain. Brain Res Mol Brain Res. 2005;135:162–8.
106. Hu DE, Easton AS, Fraser PA. TRPV1 activation results in disruption of the blood-brain barrier in the rat. Br J Pharmacol. 2005;146:576–84.
107. Vellani V, Mapplebeck S, Moriondo A, Davis JB, McNaughton PA. Protein kinase C activation potentiates gating of the vanilloid receptor VR1 by capsaicin, protons, heat and anandamide. J Physiol. 2001;534:813–25.
108. Huang J, Zhang X, McNaughton PA. Inflammatory pain: the cellular basis of heat hyperalgesia. Curr Neuropharmacol. 2006;4:197–206.
109. Chuang HH, Prescott ED, Kong H, Shields S, Jordt SE, Basbaum AI, Chao MV, Julius D. Bradykinin and nerve growth factor release the capsaicin receptor from PtdIns(4,5)P2-mediated inhibition. Nature. 2001;411:957–62.
110. Shibata T, Takahashi K, Matsubara Y, Inuzuka E, Nakashima F, Takahashi N, Kozai D, Mori Y, Uchida K. Identification of a prostaglandin D2 metabolite as a neuritogenesis enhancer targeting the TRPV1 ion channel. Sci Rep. 2016;6:21261.
111. Szallasi A, Di Marzo V. New perspectives on enigmatic vanilloid receptors. Trends Neurosci. 2000;23:491–7.
112. Choi SI, Yoo S, Lim JY, Hwang SW. Are sensory TRP channels biological alarms for lipid peroxidation? Int J Mol Sci. 2014;15:16430–57.
113. Kwan KY, Allchorne AJ, Vollrath MA, Christensen AP, Zhang DS, Woolf CJ, Corey DP. TRPA1 contributes to cold, mechanical, and chemical nociception but is not essential for hair-cell transduction. Neuron. 2006;50:277–89.
114. Caspani O, Heppenstall PA. TRPA1 and cold transduction: an unresolved issue? J Gen Physiol. 2009;133:245–9.
115. Howard J, Bechstedt S. Hypothesis: a helix of ankyrin repeats of the NOMPC-TRP ion channel is the gating spring of mechanoreceptors. Curr Biol. 2004;14:R224–226.
116. Sotomayor M, Corey DP, Schulten K. In search of the hair-cell gating spring elastic properties of ankyrin and cadherin repeats. Structure. 2005;13:669–82.
117. Kerstein PC, del Camino D, Moran MM, Stucky CL. Pharmacological blockade of TRPA1 inhibits mechanical firing in nociceptors. Mol Pain. 2009;5:19.
118. Kwan KY, Glazer JM, Corey DP, Rice FL, Stucky CL. TRPA1 modulates mechanotransduction in cutaneous sensory neurons. J Neurosci. 2009;29:4808–19.
119. McGaraughty S, Chu KL, Perner RJ, Didomenico S, Kort ME, Kym PR. TRPA1 modulation of spontaneous and mechanically evoked firing of spinal neurons in uninjured, osteoarthritic, and inflamed rats. Mol Pain. 2010;6:14.
120. Brierley SM, Castro J, Harrington AM, Hughes PA, Page AJ, Rychkov GY, Blackshaw LA. TRPA1 contributes to specific mechanically activated currents and sensory neuron mechanical hypersensitivity. J Physiol. 2011;589:3575–93.
121. Brierley SM, Hughes PA, Page AJ, Kwan KY, Martin CM, O'Donnell TA, Cooper NJ, Harrington AM, Adam B, Liebregts T, et al. The ion channel TRPA1 is required for normal mechanosensation and is modulated by algesic stimuli. Gastroenterology. 2009;137:2084–95. e2083.
122. Birder LA, Nakamura Y, Kiss S, Nealen ML, Barrick S, Kanai AJ, Wang E, Ruiz G, De Groat WC, Apodaca G, et al. Altered urinary bladder function in mice lacking the vanilloid receptor TRPV1. Nat Neurosci. 2002;5:856–60.
123. Jones 3rd RC, Xu L, Gebhart GF. The mechanosensitivity of mouse colon afferent fibers and their sensitization by inflammatory mediators require transient receptor potential vanilloid 1 and acid-sensing ion channel 3. J Neurosci. 2005;25:10981–9.
124. Feng NH, Lee HH, Shiang JC, Ma MC. Transient receptor potential vanilloid type 1 channels act as mechanoreceptors and cause substance P release and sensory activation in rat kidneys. Am J Physiol Renal Physiol. 2008;294:F316–325.

125. Sappington RM, Sidorova T, Long DJ, Calkins DJ. TRPV1: contribution to retinal ganglion cell apoptosis and increased intracellular Ca2+ with exposure to hydrostatic pressure. Invest Ophthalmol Vis Sci. 2009;50:717–28.
126. Sappington RM, Sidorova T, Ward NJ, Chakravarthy R, Ho KW, Calkins DJ. Activation of transient receptor potential vanilloid-1 (TRPV1) influences how retinal ganglion cell neurons respond to pressure-related stress. Channels (Austin). 2015;9:102–13.
127. Brederson JD, Chu KL, Reilly RM, Brown BS, Kym PR, Jarvis MF, McGaraughty S. TRPV1 antagonist, A-889425, inhibits mechanotransmission in a subclass of rat primary afferent neurons following peripheral inflammation. Synapse. 2012;66:187–95.
128. Byard RW, Gabrielian L, Helps SC, Thornton E, Vink R. Further investigations into the speed of cerebral swelling following blunt cranial trauma. J Forensic Sci. 2012;57:973–5.
129. Lewis SB, Finnie JW, Blumbergs PC, Scott G, Manavis J, Brown C, Reilly PL, Jones NR, McLean AJ. A head impact model of early axonal injury in the sheep. J Neurotrauma. 1996;13:505–14.
130. Marmarou A, Foda MA, van den Brink W, Campbell J, Kita H, Demetriadou K. A new model of diffuse brain injury in rats. Part I: pathophysiology and biomechanics. J Neurosurg. 1994;80:291–300.
131. McIntosh TK, Vink R, Noble L, Yamakami I, Fernyak S, Soares H, Faden AL. Traumatic brain injury in the rat: characterization of a lateral fluid-percussion model. Neuroscience. 1989;28:233–44.
132. Sun H, Li DP, Chen SR, Hittelman WN, Pan HL. Sensing of blood pressure increase by transient receptor potential vanilloid 1 receptors on baroreceptors. J Pharmacol Exp Ther. 2009;331:851–9.
133. Scotland RS, Chauhan S, Davis C, De Felipe C, Hunt S, Kabir J, Kotsonis P, Oh U, Ahluwalia A. Vanilloid receptor TRPV1, sensory C-fibers, and vascular autoregulation: a novel mechanism involved in myogenic constriction. Circ Res. 2004;95:1027–34.
134. Okabe T, Hide M, Koro O, Nimi N, Yamamoto S. The release of leukotriene B4 from human skin in response to substance P: evidence for the functional heterogeneity of human skin mast cells among individuals. Clin Exp Immunol. 2001;124:150–6.
135. Florenzano F, Bentivoglio M. Degranulation, density, and distribution of mast cells in the rat thalamus: a light and electron microscopic study in basal conditions and after intracerebroventricular administration of nerve growth factor. J Comp Neurol. 2000;424:651–69.
136. Patkai J, Mesples B, Dommergues MA, Fromont G, Thornton EM, Renauld JC, Evrard P, Gressens P. Deleterious effects of IL-9-activated mast cells and neuroprotection by antihistamine drugs in the developing mouse brain. Pediatr Res. 2001;50:222–30.
137. Hendrix S, Warnke K, Siebenhaar F, Peters EM, Nitsch R, Maurer M. The majority of brain mast cells in B10.PL mice is present in the hippocampal formation. Neurosci Lett. 2006;392:174–7.
138. Taiwo OB, Kovacs KJ, Larson AA. Chronic daily intrathecal injections of a large volume of fluid increase mast cells in the thalamus of mice. Brain Res. 2005;1056:76–84.
139. Fiebich BL, Schleicher S, Butcher RD, Craig A, Lieb K. The neuropeptide substance P activates p38 mitogen-activated protein kinase resulting in IL-6 expression independently from NF-kappa B. J Immunol. 2000;165:5606–11.
140. Lieb K, Schaller H, Bauer J, Berger M, Schulze-Osthoff K, Fiebich BL. Substance P and histamine induce interleukin-6 expression in human astrocytoma cells by a mechanism involving protein kinase C and nuclear factor-IL-6. J Neurochem. 1998;70:1577–83.
141. Lin RC. Reactive astrocytes express substance-P immunoreactivity in the adult forebrain after injury. Neuroreport. 1995;7:310–2.
142. Rasley A, Bost KL, Olson JK, Miller SD, Marriott I. Expression of functional NK-1 receptors in murine microglia. Glia. 2002;37:258–67.
143. Martin FC, Anton PA, Gornbein JA, Shanahan F, Merrill JE. Production of interleukin-1 by microglia in response to substance P: role for a non-classical NK-1 receptor. J Neuroimmunol. 1993;42:53–60.
144. Carthew HL, Ziebell JM, Vink R. Substance P-induced changes in cell genesis following diffuse traumatic brain injury. Neuroscience. 2012;214:78–83.
145. Huber JD, Egleton RD, Davis TP. Molecular physiology and pathophysiology of tight junctions in the blood-brain barrier. Trends Neurosci. 2001;24:719–25.
146. Ballabh P, Braun A, Nedergaard M. The blood-brain barrier: an overview: structure, regulation, and clinical implications. Neurobiol Dis. 2004;16:1–13.
147. Cecchelli R, Berezowski V, Lundquist S, Culot M, Renftel M, Dehouck MP, Fenart L. Modelling of the blood-brain barrier in drug discovery and development. Nat Rev Drug Discov. 2007;6:650–61.
148. Luissint AC, Artus C, Glacial F, Ganeshamoorthy K, Couraud PO. Tight junctions at the blood brain barrier: physiological architecture and disease-associated dysregulation. Fluids Barriers CNS. 2012;9:23.
149. Villegas JC, Broadwell RD. Transcytosis of protein through the mammalian cerebral epithelium and endothelium. II. Adsorptive transcytosis of WGA-HRP and the blood-brain and brain-blood barriers. J Neurocytol. 1993;22:67–80.
150. Preston JE, Joan Abbott N, Begley DJ. Transcytosis of macromolecules at the blood-brain barrier. Adv Pharmacol. 2014;71:147–63.
151. Badaut J, Ajao DO, Sorensen DW, Fukuda AM, Pellerin L. Caveolin expression changes in the neurovascular unit after juvenile traumatic brain injury: signs of blood-brain barrier healing? Neuroscience. 2015;285:215–26.
152. Nag S, Manias JL, Stewart DJ. Expression of endothelial phosphorylated caveolin-1 is increased in brain injury. Neuropathol Appl Neurobiol. 2009;35:417–26.
153. Nag S, Venugopalan R, Stewart DJ. Increased caveolin-1 expression precedes decreased expression of occludin and claudin-5 during blood-brain barrier breakdown. Acta Neuropathol. 2007;114:459–69.
154. Povlishock JT, Becker DP, Sullivan HG, Miller JD. Vascular permeability alterations to horseradish peroxidase in experimental brain injury. Brain Res. 1978;153:223–39.
155. Lossinsky AS, Shivers RR. Structural pathways for macromolecular and cellular transport across the blood-brain barrier during inflammatory conditions. Review. Histol Histopathol. 2004;19:535–64.
156. Castejon OJ. Formation of transendothelial channels in traumatic human brain edema. Pathol Res Pract. 1984;179:7–12.
157. Vaz R, Sarmento A, Borges N, Cruz C, Azevedo I. Ultrastructural study of brain microvessels in patients with traumatic cerebral contusions. Acta Neurochir (Wien). 1997;139:215–20.
158. Lu TS, Avraham HK, Seng S, Tachado SD, Koziel H, Makriyannis A, Avraham S. Cannabinoids inhibit HIV-1 Gp120-mediated insults in brain microvascular endothelial cells. J Immunol. 2008;181:6406–16.
159. Ge S, Song L, Serwanski DR, Kuziel WA, Pachter JS. Transcellular transport of CCL2 across brain microvascular endothelial cells. J Neurochem. 2008;104:1219–32.
160. Sowa G. Caveolae, caveolins, cavins, and endothelial cell function: new insights. Front Physiol. 2012;2:120.
161. Razani B, Engelman JA, Wang XB, Schubert W, Zhang XL, Marks CB, Macaluso F, Russell RG, Li M, Pestell RG, et al. Caveolin-1 null mice are viable but show evidence of hyperproliferative and vascular abnormalities. J Biol Chem. 2001;276:38121–38.
162. Schubert W, Frank PG, Razani B, Park DS, Chow CW, Lisanti MP. Caveolae-deficient endothelial cells show defects in the uptake and transport of albumin in vivo. J Biol Chem. 2001;276:48619–22.
163. Anderson RG. The caveolae membrane system. Annu Rev Biochem. 1998;67:199–225.
164. Predescu SA, Predescu DN, Malik AB. Molecular determinants of endothelial transcytosis and their role in endothelial permeability. Am J Physiol Lung Cell Mol Physiol. 2007;293:L823–842.
165. Cameron PL, Ruffin JW, Bollag R, Rasmussen H, Cameron RS. Identification of caveolin and caveolin-related proteins in the brain. J Neurosci. 1997;17:9520–35.
166. Chen YG. Endocytic regulation of TGF-beta signaling. Cell Res. 2009;19:58–70.
167. Mitchell H, Choudhury A, Pagano RE, Leof EB. Ligand-dependent and -independent transforming growth factor-beta receptor recycling regulated by clathrin-mediated endocytosis and Rab11. Mol Biol Cell. 2004;15:4166–78.
168. Zschocke J, Manthey D, Bayatti N, Behl C. Functional interaction of estrogen receptor alpha and caveolin isoforms in neuronal SK-N-MC cells. J Steroid Biochem Mol Biol. 2003;84:167–70.
169. Kubale V, Abramovic Z, Pogacnik A, Heding A, Sentjurc M, Vrecl M. Evidence for a role of caveolin-1 in neurokinin-1 receptor plasma-membrane localization, efficient signaling, and interaction with beta-arrestin 2. Cell Tissue Res. 2007;330:231–45.
170. Monastyrskaya K, Hostettler A, Buergi S, Draeger A. The NK1 receptor localizes to the plasma membrane microdomains, and its activation is dependent on lipid raft integrity. J Biol Chem. 2005;280:7135–46.
171. Mineo C, Ying YS, Chapline C, Jaken S, Anderson RG. Targeting of protein kinase Calpha to caveolae. J Cell Biol. 1998;141:601–10.
172. Fillebeen C, Dehouck B, Benaissa M, Dhennin-Duthille I, Cecchelli R, Pierce A. Tumor necrosis factor-alpha increases lactoferrin transcytosis through the blood-brain barrier. J Neurochem. 1999;73:2491–500.

173. Calvo CF, Amigou E, Tence M, Yoshimura T, Glowinski J. Albumin stimulates monocyte chemotactic protein-1 expression in rat embryonic mixed brain cells. J Neurosci Res. 2005;80:707–14.
174. Hooper C, Pinteaux-Jones F, Fry VA, Sevastou IG, Baker D, Heales SJ, Pocock JM. Differential effects of albumin on microglia and macrophages; implications for neurodegeneration following blood-brain barrier damage. J Neurochem. 2009;109:694–705.
175. Hooper C, Taylor DL, Pocock JM. Pure albumin is a potent trigger of calcium signalling and proliferation in microglia but not macrophages or astrocytes. J Neurochem. 2005;92:1363–76.
176. Ralay Ranaivo H, Hodge JN, Choi N, Wainwright MS. Albumin induces upregulation of matrix metalloproteinase-9 in astrocytes via MAPK and reactive oxygen species-dependent pathways. J Neuroinflammation. 2012;9:68.
177. Ralay Ranaivo H, Wainwright MS. Albumin activates astrocytes and microglia through mitogen-activated protein kinase pathways. Brain Res. 2010;1313:222–31.
178. Tabernero A, Velasco A, Granda B, Lavado EM, Medina JM. Transcytosis of albumin in astrocytes activates the sterol regulatory element-binding protein-1, which promotes the synthesis of the neurotrophic factor oleic acid. J Biol Chem. 2002;277:4240–6.
179. Cacheaux LP, Ivens S, David Y, Lakhter AJ, Bar-Klein G, Shapira M, Heinemann U, Friedman A, Kaufer D. Transcriptome profiling reveals TGF-beta signaling involvement in epileptogenesis. J Neurosci. 2009;29:8927–35.
180. Hinson HE, Rowell S, Schreiber M. Clinical evidence of inflammation driving secondary brain injury: a systematic review. J Trauma Acute Care Surg. 2015;78:184–91.
181. Cao T, Pinter E, Al-Rashed S, Gerard N, Hoult JR, Brain SD. Neurokinin-1 receptor agonists are involved in mediating neutrophil accumulation in the inflamed, but not normal, cutaneous microvasculature: an in vivo study using neurokinin-1 receptor knockout mice. J Immunol. 2000;164:5424–9.
182. Schratzberger P, Reinisch N, Prodinger WM, Kahler CM, Sitte BA, Bellmann R, Fischer-Colbrie R, Winkler H, Wiedermann CJ. Differential chemotactic activities of sensory neuropeptides for human peripheral blood mononuclear cells. J Immunol. 1997;158:3895–901.
183. Souza DG, Mendonca VA, De A Castro MS, Poole S, Teixeira MM. Role of tachykinin NK receptors on the local and remote injuries following ischaemia and reperfusion of the superior mesenteric artery in the rat. Br J Pharmacol. 2002;135:303–12.
184. Annunziata P, Cioni C, Santonini R, Paccagnini E. Substance P antagonist blocks leakage and reduces activation of cytokine-stimulated rat brain endothelium. J Neuroimmunol. 2002;131:41–9.
185. Li PC, Chen WC, Chang LC, Lin SC. Substance P acts via the neurokinin receptor 1 to elicit bronchoconstriction, oxidative stress, and upregulated ICAM-1 expression after oil smoke exposure. Am J Physiol Lung Cell Mol Physiol. 2008;294:L912–920.
186. Toneatto S, Finco O, van der Putten H, Abrignani S, Annunziata P. Evidence of blood-brain barrier alteration and activation in HIV-1 gp120 transgenic mice. AIDS. 1999;13:2343–8.
187. Vishwanath R, Mukherjee R. Substance P promotes lymphocyte-endothelial cell adhesion preferentially via LFA-1/ICAM-1 interactions. J Neuroimmunol. 1996;71:163–71.
188. Ramnath RD, Bhatia M. Substance P treatment stimulates chemokine synthesis in pancreatic acinar cells via the activation of NF-kappaB. Am J Physiol Gastrointest Liver Physiol. 2006;291:G1113–1119.
189. Homayoun P, de Rodriguez Turco EB, Parkins NE, Lane DC, Soblosky J, Carey ME, Bazan NG. Delayed phospholipid degradation in rat brain after traumatic brain injury. J Neurochem. 1997;69:199–205.
190. Hellal F, Pruneau D, Palmier B, Faye P, Croci N, Plotkine M, Marchand-Verrecchia C. Detrimental role of bradykinin B2 receptor in a murine model of diffuse brain injury. J Neurotrauma. 2003;20:841–51.
191. Golias C, Charalabopoulos A, Stagikas D, Charalabopoulos K, Batistatou A. The kinin system—bradykinin: biological effects and clinical implications. Multiple role of the kinin system—bradykinin. Hippokratia. 2007;11:124–8.
192. Dobo J, Major B, Kekesi KA, Szabo I, Megyeri M, Hajela K, Juhasz G, Zavodszky P, Gal P. Cleavage of kininogen and subsequent bradykinin release by the complement component: mannose-binding lectin-associated serine protease (MASP)-1. PLoS One. 2011;6:e20036.
193. Trabold R, Eros C, Zweckberger K, Relton J, Beck H, Nussberger J, Muller-Esterl W, Bader M, Whalley E, Plesnila N. The role of bradykinin B(1) and B(2) receptors for secondary brain damage after traumatic brain injury in mice. J Cereb Blood Flow Metab. 2010;30:130–9.
194. Dewitt DS, Kong DL, Lyeth BG, Jenkins LW, Hayes RL, Wooten ED, Prough DS. Experimental traumatic brain injury elevates brain prostaglandin E2 and thromboxane B2 levels in rats. J Neurotrauma. 1988;5:303–13.
195. Liu B, Li H, Brull SJ, Zhang JM. Increased sensitivity of sensory neurons to tumor necrosis factor alpha in rats with chronic compression of the lumbar ganglia. J Neurophysiol. 2002;88:1393–9.
196. Richardson JD, Vasko MR. Cellular mechanisms of neurogenic inflammation. J Pharmacol Exp Ther. 2002;302:839–45.

14

Ccr2 deletion dissociates cavity size and tau pathology after mild traumatic brain injury

Stefka Gyoneva[1,3,4*], Daniel Kim[2,3], Atsuko Katsumoto[1,3], O. Nicole Kokiko-Cochran[1,3], Bruce T. Lamb[1,3] and Richard M. Ransohoff[1,3,4*]

Abstract

Background: Millions of people experience traumatic brain injury (TBI) as a result of falls, car accidents, sports injury, and blast. TBI has been associated with the development of neurodegenerative conditions such as Alzheimer's disease (AD) and chronic traumatic encephalopathy (CTE). In the initial hours and days, the pathology of TBI comprises neuronal injury, breakdown of the blood–brain barrier, and inflammation. At the cellular level, the inflammatory reaction consists of responses by brain-resident microglia, astrocytes, and vascular elements as well as infiltration of peripheral cells. After TBI, signaling by chemokine (C-C motif) ligand 2 (CCL2) to the chemokine (C-C motif) receptor 2 (CCR2) is a key regulator of brain infiltration by monocytes.

Methods: We utilized mice with one or both copies of *Ccr2* disrupted by red fluorescent protein (RFP, $Ccr2^{RFP/+}$ and $Ccr2^{RFP/RFP}$). We subjected these mice to the mild lateral fluid percussion model of TBI and examined several pathological outcomes 3 days later in order to determine the effects of altered monocyte entry into the brain.

Results: *Ccr2* deletion reduced monocyte infiltration, diminished lesion cavity volume, and lessened axonal damage after mild TBI, but the microglial reaction to the lesion was not affected. We further examined phosphorylation of the microtubule-associated protein tau, which aggregates in brains of people with TBI, AD, and CTE. Surprisingly, *Ccr2* deletion was associated with increased tau mislocalization to the cell body in the cortex and hippocampus by tissue staining and increased levels of phosphorylated tau in the hippocampus by Western blot.

Conclusions: Disruption of CCR2 enhanced tau pathology and reduced cavity volume in the context of TBI. The data reveal a complex role for $CCR2^+$ monocytes in TBI, as monitored by cavity volume, axonal damage, and tau phosphorylation.

Keywords: Traumatic brain injury, CCR2, Tau, MAPT, Monocyte

Background

Traumatic brain injury (TBI) is a common condition in today's society. It is variable in extent and circumstance and imposes enormous suffering and expense. The injury can be sustained in a single event or in a repetitive fashion, can be either closed head or penetrating, and ranges in severity from mild to severe. About 75 % of TBI is closed head in nature and mild in intensity [1]. Further contributing to patient suffering and impact on society, TBI is linked to the development of neurodegenerative conditions. For example, TBI of varying intensity is associated with increased risk or earlier onset of Alzheimer's disease (AD), and repetitive mild TBI is associated with chronic traumatic encephalopathy (CTE) [2–8].

One common pathological feature of TBI, AD, and CTE is the hyperphosphorylation and mislocalization of the microtubule-associated protein tau (MAPT, here termed tau) [9]. Tau contains numerous potential phosphorylation sites and is a target of multiple kinases. In physiological conditions, tau is phosphorylated at a few sites and is located in axons where it binds to microtubules to stabilize the axonal cytoskeleton. However, in pathological conditions, tau can be phosphorylated at multiple additional sites. The (hyper)phosphorylated tau (pTau) dissociates from microtubules in the axon, translocates to the cell body and proximal dendrites, and

* Correspondence: stefka.gyoneva@biogen.com; richard.ransohoff@biogen.com
[1]Department of Neurosciences, Lerner Research Institute, Cleveland Clinic Foundation, Cleveland, OH, USA

aggregates in structures termed neurofibrillary tangles, leading to impaired axonal function [9]. While the mechanisms driving tau phosphorylation and tangle formation are not well established, there is substantial evidence suggesting that inflammation can promote this process [10–12].

A prominent feature of TBI is the development of an inflammatory reaction within minutes of the injury event [13–17]. Cells at the site of injury secrete cytokines and chemokines that lead to the recruitment of peripheral immune cells—initially neutrophils, which are quickly replaced by monocytes. Concurrently, there is activation of brain-resident astrocytes and microglia. The inflammatory reaction could contribute to the progression of axonal pathology and tissue damage and is thus a potential target to ameliorate TBI pathology [13, 17, 18].

Although inflammation increases tau phosphorylation and pTau is detected in central nervous system (CNS) tissues of TBI patients and in animal models, whether post-injury inflammation affects pTau levels in the context of TBI has not been addressed. Here, we used the lateral fluid percussion injury (LFPI) model of TBI [19, 20] to study how modulation of the monocytic reaction after TBI influences tau phosphorylation. In the context of TBI, the monocytic population is primarily represented by $CD45^{lo}CX3CR1^{hi}CCR2^{-}$ microglia, $CD45^{hi}CX3CR1^{lo}CCR2^{hi}$ inflammatory monocytes, and $CD45^{hi}CX3CR1^{hi}CCr2^{lo}$ patrolling monocytes [21–24], but perivascular and meningeal macrophages may also play a role. We employed mice deficient for either chemokine (C-X3-C motif) receptor 1 ($Cx3cr1^{GFP/GFP}$ mice) or chemokine (C-C motif) receptor 2 ($Ccr2^{RFP/RFP}$ mice). $Ccr2^{RFP/RFP}$ mice display reduced infiltration of $Ly6C^{hi}$ inflammatory monocytes into the brain after TBI [25]. Here, $Cx3cr1^{GFP/GFP}$ mice showed no difference in TBI pathology compared to wild type (WT) mice, but $Ccr2^{RFP/RFP}$ mice had reduced lesion volume and axonal pathology. Surprisingly, $Ccr2^{RFP/RFP}$ mice also exhibited increased levels and mislocalization of pTau in the cortex and hippocampus, suggesting that monocyte-dependent inflammation exerts distinct effects on tissue loss as compared to tau phosphorylation after TBI.

Methods

Animals and TBI induction

All procedures performed on animals were reviewed and approved by the Institutional Animal Care and Use Committee of the Cleveland Clinic. We employed two mouse strains ($Cx3cr1^{GFP/GFP}$ and $Ccr2^{RFP/RFP}$) that allowed us to manipulate the cellular reaction after TBI and at the same time visualize the inflammatory cells of interest [26]. $Cx3cr1^{GFP/GFP}$ mice (green fluorescent protein (GFP) expression in microglia and patrolling $CCR2^{lo}$ monocytes) were maintained on the $Ccr2^{RFP/+}$ background in which only one copy of *Ccr2* is disrupted (red fluorescent protein (RFP) expression in inflammatory $CCR2^{hi}$ monocytes, some T cells). Similarly, for some experiments $Ccr2^{RFP/RFP}$ mice were maintained on the $Cx3cr1^{GFP/+}$ background. There were no statistical differences in the responses to TBI by $Ccr2^{RFP/RFP}$; $Cx3cr1^{+/+}$ and $Ccr2^{RFP/RFP}$; $Cx3cr1^{GFP/+}$ mice (data not shown) and the two genotypes were pooled together for analysis. Microglia were identified by Iba1 staining in $Ccr2^{RFP/RFP}$ mice at 3 days post injury (dpi), before other cell types have upregulated Iba1 expression [27].

To induce TBI, we performed lateral fluid percussion injury as described before [19]. Briefly, 8–10-week-old male and female mice were anesthetized with 100 mg/kg ketamine/10 mg/kg xylazine; the fur on top of the head was shaved, and the skin was cut and moved to the side. A craniotomy with ~3 mm diameter was opened on the right side of the central suture, halfway between Bregma and Lambda, without disturbing the underlying dura mater. A modified Leur-Lok hub was placed around the craniotomy and sealed in place with dental acrylic. The mice were allowed to recover from anesthesia and returned to their home cages. On the next day, the mice were anesthetized again and attached to a fluid percussion device (AmScien Instruments FP-302) by the Leur-Lok hub. The device was calibrated to deliver mild injury with pressure intensities between 0.4 and 0.6 atm. After injury, the hub was removed, the skin was sutured, and mice were returned to their home cages to recover. For all experiments, the mice were euthanized 3 dpi.

Tissue staining

Tissue staining was used to evaluate the extent of the inflammatory reaction after TBI, lesion volume, axonal pathology, and tau phosphorylation and localization. At 3 dpi, mice were deeply anesthetized with ketamine/xylazine and perfused with ice-cold phosphate-buffered saline (PBS) followed by 4 % paraformaldehyde (PFA) in PBS. The brains were isolated and postfixed in 4 % PFA overnight and sectioned on a sliding microtome at 30 μm thickness. During staining, all washes were performed three times for 5 min each in 0.1 % triton X-100 in PBS. Antibody solutions were prepared in PBS unless otherwise noted.

To visualize the inflammatory reaction after TBI, serial sections spaced 150 μm apart and spanning ~4 mm thickness around the injury cavity were blocked in 10 % normal goat serum (NGS) and stained overnight at 4 °C with mouse anti-GFP (UCDavis/NIH NeuroMab Facility #75-132, 1:8000 dilution), or rabbit anti-Iba1 (Wako #019-19741, 1:1000) antibodies to identify microglia, and rabbit or rat anti-RFP (Abcam #ab62341, 1:1000 and Chromotek #5 F8 α-Red, 1:1000, respectively) antibodies to identify infiltrating monocytes. The secondary antibodies (Goat anti-mouse-Alexa 488, Invitrogen

#A11029; anti-Rabbit IgG-Alexa Fluor 488, Invitrogen #A11008; anti-rabbit-Alexa 594, Invitrogen #A11037; anti-Rat IgG-Alexa Fluor 594, Invitrogen #A11007, all at 1:1000 dilution) were applied for 1 h at room temperature (RT). The sections were mounted on large glass slides, coverslipped and imaged.

Axonal pathology was assessed with amyloid precursor protein (APP) staining which accumulates in axonal swellings of damaged neurons [28]. The sections were incubated in 0.3 % H_2O_2 for 30 min at RT to inactivate endogenous peroxidases. Antigen retrieval was performed in 1× Target retrieval solution (Dako Cytomation #S1699) containing 0.5 % Tween in PBS at 95 °C for 10–15 min. After blocking in 10 % NGS, primary rabbit anti-APP antibody (Invitrogen #51-2700) was applied overnight at 4 °C and secondary biotinylated goat anti-rabbit antibody (Vector BA-1000) was applied for 1 h at RT. The signal was detected using the ABC Elite Kit (Vector PK-6100) and DAB substrate kit (Vector SK-4100) according to the manufacturer's instructions. Sections were allowed to dry and coverslipped with hardset mounting medium (Fisher Scientific #SP15).

For phosphorylated tau, after antigen retrieval and blocking in 5 % NGS and 0.3 % Triton X-100 in PBS for 2 h at RT, the localization of pTau was detected with the mouse anti-AT8 antibody (ThermoSci mn1020, 1:500 dilution in 5 % NGS, 0.3 % Triton X-100 in PBS) overnight at 4 °C. The secondary antibody used, goat anti-mouse-Alexa 647 (Invitrogen #A21235, 1:1000 dilution), was chosen not to interfere with the signal of genetically encoded GFP and RFP and was applied for 1 h at RT. The sections were mounted on glass slides and coverslipped with VectaShield with DAPI medium (Vector H-1200).

Imaging and image quantification

Sections stained with GFP (or Iba1) and RFP were imaged on a Leica CTR5500 microscope equipped with a QImaging Retiga EXi FAST 13941 MONO camera at 10× magnification. Tiling of consecutive fields of view was employed to capture the whole section and all sections from a mouse using ImagePro Plus software to drive the microscope. Both GFP/Iba1 (microglia) and RFP (monocyte) channels were recorded. The resulting images were then analyzed with ImageJ software (National Institutes of Health) to calculate (1) lesion cavity volume, (2) the volume of brain tissue (in 4 mm slab) occupied by microglial immunoreactivity, and (3) volume of brain tissue occupied by monocyte immunoreactivity. Initially, each slice was manually outlined; for slices with a TBI-induced cavity, the "whole slice" outline was generated based on where the tissue would be if it were not missing. Then, the cavity, the region around the cavity with increased GFP/Iba1 immunoreactivity, and the region around the cavity with increased RFP immunoreactivity were manually outlined for each brain section. Finally, all sections (~22) for an animal were multiplied by the distance between sections (150 μm) and summed up to obtain the corresponding volumes (cavity, microglia, and monocyte immunoreactivity) as a percentage of the brain volume analyzed (4 mm thickness).

APP-stained sections were also imaged with tiling but in brightfield mode. To quantify axonal damage, the corpus callosum in the ipsilateral side to the injury was manually outlined in ImageJ and the percentage of the corpus callosum with APP immunoreactivity above threshold was calculated. Two sections were stained for each animal and averaged after quantification.

AT8-stained sections were imaged on a fluorescent Leica DM4000 microscope equipped with a QImaging Retiga EXi FAST 1394 MONO camera. Images were acquired at 10–20× magnification with a Cy5 filter cube (band-pass excitation 620/60 nm, band-pass emission 700/75 nm filters, 660 nm dichroic mirror). The same fields were also acquired through a DAPI filter cube (band-pass 360/40 nm excitation, band-pass 470/40 emission, 400 nm dichroic mirror) to localize cell nuclei. Images were taken of the ipsilateral cortex (close to the injury cavity), the underlying ipsilateral hippocampus and the contralateral cortex and hippocampus.

Western blot and pTau quantification

pTau levels after TBI were quantified by Western blot. TBI and sham mice were anesthetized with ketamine/xylazine at 3 dpi and perfused with ice-cold PBS. Naïve mice that did not undergo any surgery were used as a control for the effect of surgery itself; naïve mice were simply anesthetized and perfused. The brains were isolated, the ipsilateral and contralateral hemispheres were separated (right and left for naïve mice), and the cortices and hippocampi were microdissected from each hemisphere. Tissues were homogenized in Tissue Protein Extraction Reagent (Pierce #78150) containing 1 % each of protease and phosphatase inhibitors (Sigma #P8340 and #P5726, respectively).

Fifty nanograms of total protein were separated on 4–12 % bis-tris gels (Invitrogen #NP0322) and transferred to 0.45 μm PVDF membranes (Millipore #IPFL10100). Separate membranes were run for the detection of phosphorylated tau (with mouse anti-AT8 antibody, 1:5000 dilution) and total tau (mouse anti-Tau5 antibody, Invitrogen #ahb0042. 1:5000). After running, the membranes were activated in methanol, blocked, and incubated in primary antibodies overnight at 4 °C. GAPDH (Trevigen #2275-PC-100, 1:10,000) was used as loading control on all membranes. Proteins were detected with goat anti-mouse IRDye 800CW (for AT8 or Tau5, Li-Cor #926-68171) and goat anti-rabbit IRDye 680RD (for GAPDH, Li-Cor #827-08364) fluorescent antibodies.

Images of the developed membranes were acquired on a Li-Cor Odyssey CLx imager.

To quantify the relative levels of pTau across samples, the channels for tau and GAPDH were split and analyzed separately with the ImageJ Gel tool. Both AT8 and Tau5 signals were first normalized to GAPDH to ensure equal sample loading. Then, the relative AT8 signal was normalized to total tau. There were no significant differences in total tau between samples after TBI (data not shown).

Statistical analysis

Data points on the graphs represent individual mice. The average and standard error of the mean are also shown. The effects of genotype and injury intensity were examined by two-way analysis of variance (ANOVA); statistical differences between groups were determined with Tukey's *post hoc* tests. All significant values in *post hoc* tests were adjusted for multiple comparisons. Groups were considered to be statistically different if $p < 0.05$ for both factor effect (in ANOVA) and *post hoc* tests.

Results

Preventing CCR2$^+$ monocyte infiltration after TBI reduces lesion pathology

The inflammatory reaction is a common feature of TBI. Here, we addressed how modulating monocytic inflammation might affect pathological features of neurodegeneration. We altered the inflammatory reaction in two different ways: by inactivation of *Cx3cr1* (in *Cx3cr1*$^{GFP/GFP}$ mice), which affects the activation of brain-resident microglia [29] and Ly6C^{lo} patrolling monocytes, or by inactivation of *Ccr2* (in *Ccr2*$^{RFP/RFP}$ mice), which reduces the infiltration of Ly6C^{hi} inflammatory monocytes and a subset of T cells into the brain after TBI [25]. Intercrossing these two mouse strains allowed us to not only inactivate the genes of interest, but also directly visualize chemokine (C-X3-C motif) receptor 1 (CX3CR1)- and CCR2-positive cells in tissue sections [26]. CX3CR1$^+$ patrolling monocytes and CCR2$^+$ T cells represent only a small proportion of infiltrating cells after TBI compared to CX3CR1$^+$ microglia and CCR2$^+$ inflammatory monocytes, respectively (data not shown). Hence, we herein refer to GFP-positive cells as microglia and RFP-positive cells as infiltrating inflammatory monocytes.

Ccr2$^{RFP/RFP}$, *Cx3cr1*$^{GFP/GFP}$, and control double-heterozygous mice were subjected to mild LFPI, and the inflammatory reaction and cavity pathology were analyzed 3 dpi from brain sections spanning a 4-mm portion of the brain that encompassed the whole lesion area (Fig. 1). As expected, the injury induced microglial morphological transformation (seen as increased GFP/Iba1 signal) and infiltration of hematogenous monocytes (presence of RFP$^+$ cells) at the site of damage in control double-heterozygous *Cx3cr1*$^{GFP/+}$; *Ccr2*$^{RFP/+}$ mice (Fig. 1a). The increased GFP signal and presence of RFP$^+$ cells were mostly restricted to the site of tissue damage and brain cavitation. Moreover, the GFP$^+$ cells had mainly ramified, bushy, morphology, suggesting that at this early time point, these cells were likely activated microglia rather than infiltrating CX3CR1$^+$ monocytes. Interestingly, although care was taken not to disturb the dura mater and underlying brain during craniotomy, the "sham" surgery itself induced a low level of microglial activation and monocyte infiltration (Fig. 1a). Consistent with previous studies [23, 30], deletion of *Ccr2* prevented the infiltration of peripheral CCR2-positive cells into the brain after TBI as evident by the absence of RFP$^+$ cell staining at the injury site (Fig. 1b). However, there was still prominent microglial reaction as monitored by GFP or Iba1 staining (Fig. 1b). In contrast, neither microglial activation nor monocyte infiltration in response to TBI appeared altered in *Cx3cr1*$^{GFP/GFP}$ mice at 3 dpi (Fig. 1c).

We quantified the inflammatory reaction and the cavity pathology by calculating the percentage of the brain parenchyma (in a 4-mm brain portion around the injury) that was occupied by reactive microglia, infiltrating monocytes or size of tissue cavity (Fig. 2). Both injury and genotype had a significant effect on the cavity volume (Fig. 2a; two-way ANOVA, $p < 0.001$ for Injury and $p < 0.05$ for Genotype) and monocytic reaction (Fig. 2b; two-way ANOVA, $p = 0.0010$ for Injury and $p < 0.01$ for Genotype), but there was no significant change in the microglial reaction under any conditions examined (Fig. 2c; two-way ANOVA, $p = 0.0501$ for Injury and $p = 0.1116$ for Genotype). Consistent with the tissue staining (Fig. 1), *Ccr2* deletion resulted in a significant decrease in cavity volume (Fig. 2a; two-way ANOVA and Tukey's *post hoc* test, $p < 0.05$ compared to heterozygous control) and portion of the brain parenchyma containing monocytes (Fig. 2b; two-way ANOVA and Tukey's *post hoc* test, $p < 0.05$ compared to heterozygous control). Despite this, there was no change in the microglial reaction in *Ccr2*$^{RFP/RFP}$ mice (Fig. 2c; two-way ANOVA and Tukey's *post hoc* test, $p = 0.9606$).

Deletion of *Cx3cr1* did not affect the inflammatory reaction or cavity volume when comparing knockout to heterozygous mice (Fig. 2a-c; two-way ANOVA and Tukey's *post hoc* test, $p = 0.2205$ for cavity volume, $p = 0.0781$ for monocytic reaction, and $p = 0.1463$ for microglial reaction). Because *Cx3cr1* deletion did not affect either the inflammatory reaction or cavity volume after mild injury here, we continued all subsequent studies only with *Ccr2*$^{RFP/RFP}$ mice and appropriate controls.

Ccr2 deletion reduces TBI-induced axonal pathology

After TBI, axonal pathology is characterized by APP-positive axonal swellings and axonal retraction bulbs

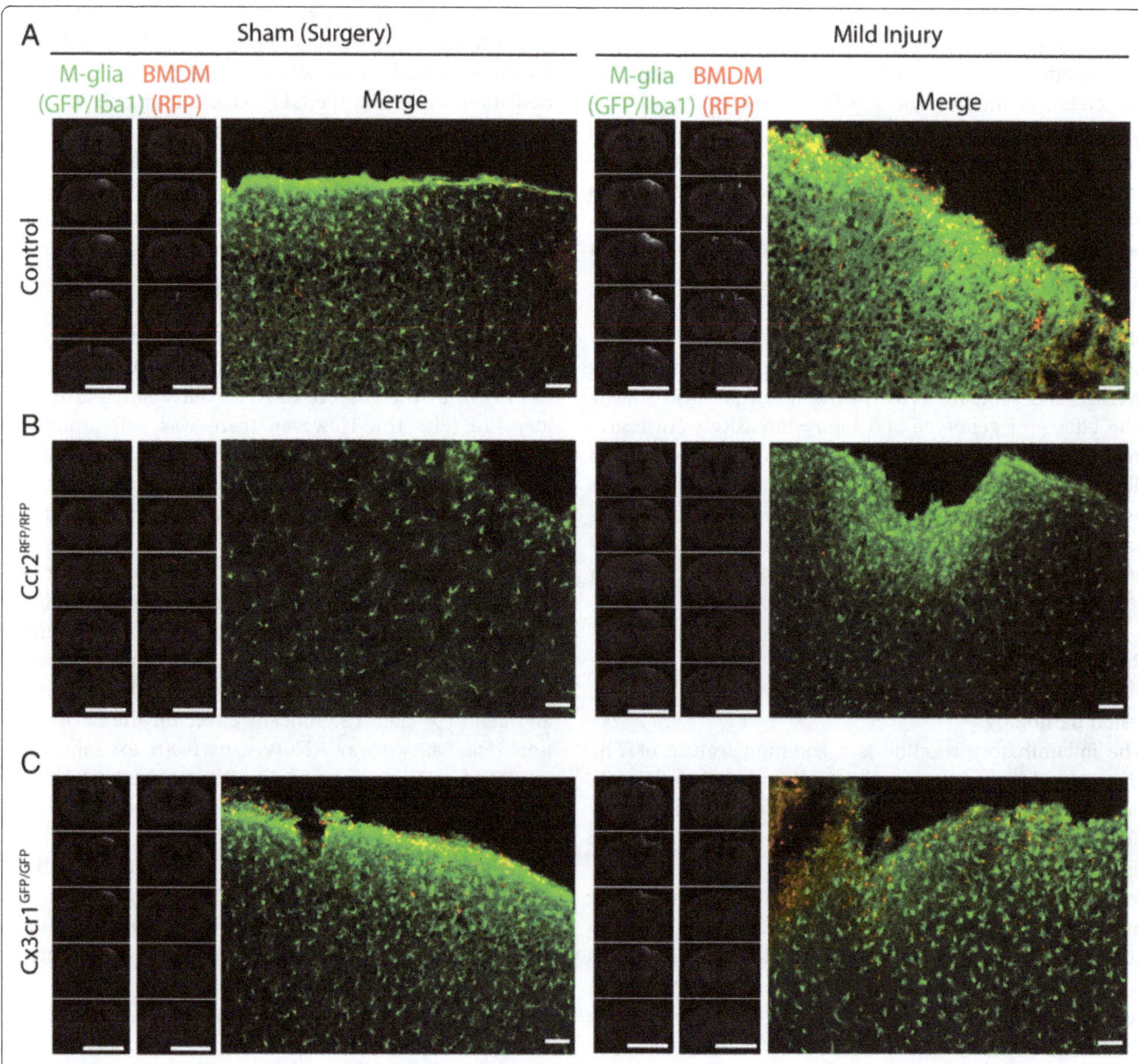

Fig. 1 Modulation of the inflammatory reaction at 3 days after LFPI in CCR2 and CX3CR1 transgenic mice. Control $Ccr2^{RFP/+}$;$Cx3cr1^{GFP/+}$ (**a**), $Ccr2^{RFP/RFP}$ (**b**), and $Cx3cr1^{GFP/GFP}$ (**c**) mice were subjected to surgery (craniotomy; Sham mice) or mild injury, and brains were collected 3 days later. Serial sections were stained for GFP (**a**, **b** (Mild), and **c**) or Iba1 (**b** (Surgery)) to visualize microglia or RFP to visualize infiltrating bone marrow-derived monocytes (BMDM). Inflammatory cells are mostly restricted to the site of injury. *Scale bar* on images with whole slices, 1 cm. The brightness on the images was adjusted to allow an easier distinction of the brain sections from the background; all sections in a series were adjusted to the same brightness level. Magnified images show a close up view of microglial and monocyte distribution around the cavity size. Note the reduced number of RFP^+ cells in $Ccr2^{RFP/RFP}$ mice. *Scale bar* for magnified images, 100 μm

indicating axotomy at sites remote to the injury [28]. In the present study, we detected increased APP immunoreactivity, especially in the corpus callosum underlying the injury site at 3 dpi (Fig. 3a). Examining the corpus callosum at higher magnification showed that many of the APP-positive structures seemed to align with the direction of axonal tracts (Fig. 3b). Deletion of *Ccr2* appeared to reduce APP immunoreactivity after TBI. Quantifying axonal pathology as the percentage of the corpus callosum with APP immunoreactivity confirmed reduced axonal pathology in $Ccr2^{RFP/RFP}$ mice at 3 dpi compared to controls (Fig. 3c; two-way ANOVA and Tukey's *post hoc* test, $p < 0.05$).

Ccr2 deletion alters tau phosphorylation and localization

Because inflammation has been shown to modulate tau pathology and *Ccr2* deletion reduces monocyte-mediated inflammation after TBI [10–12, 23, 30], we examined the effect of TBI on tau phosphorylation in $Ccr2^{RFP/RFP}$ mice. We initially analyzed changes in tau phosphorylation by

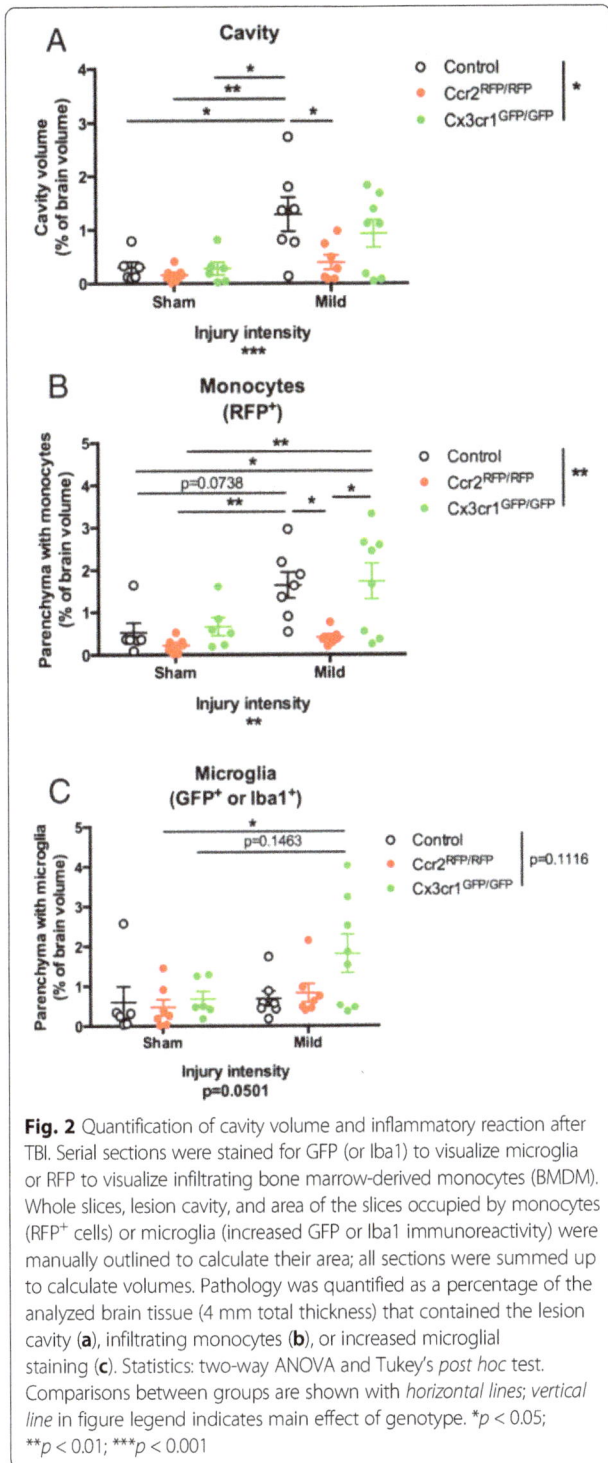

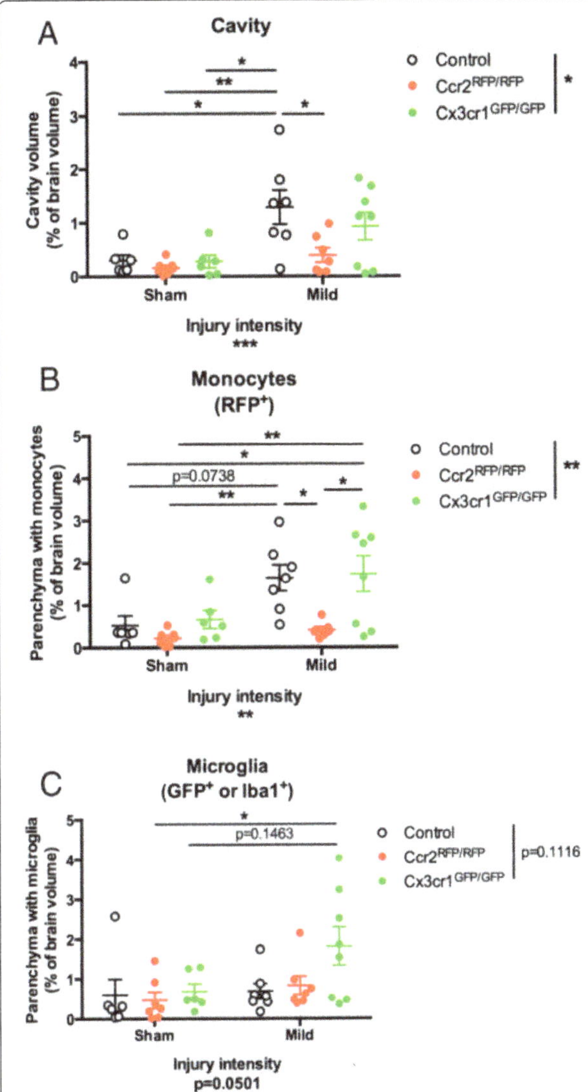

Fig. 2 Quantification of cavity volume and inflammatory reaction after TBI. Serial sections were stained for GFP (or Iba1) to visualize microglia or RFP to visualize infiltrating bone marrow-derived monocytes (BMDM). Whole slices, lesion cavity, and area of the slices occupied by monocytes (RFP^+ cells) or microglia (increased GFP or Iba1 immunoreactivity) were manually outlined to calculate their area; all sections were summed up to calculate volumes. Pathology was quantified as a percentage of the analyzed brain tissue (4 mm total thickness) that contained the lesion cavity (**a**), infiltrating monocytes (**b**), or increased microglial staining (**c**). Statistics: two-way ANOVA and Tukey's *post hoc* test. Comparisons between groups are shown with *horizontal lines*; *vertical line* in figure legend indicates main effect of genotype. *$p < 0.05$; **$p < 0.01$; ***$p < 0.001$

fluorescent immunohistochemistry to determine the localization of pTau (Fig. 4). Tissue staining for the AT8 pTau epitope showed increased staining at the site of injury in the cortex of both control heterozygous and $Ccr2^{RFP/RFP}$ mice (Fig. 4a). While the pTau immunoreactivity at the lesion site appeared rather diffuse in heterozygous mice, pTau signal was mostly perinuclear in $Ccr2^{RFP/RFP}$ mice (Fig. 4c). It should be noted that the physiological location of tau is in the axon; hence, both increased phosphorylation and mislocalization to the cell soma after TBI are abnormal.

Increased tau phosphorylation was also detected remote to the injury at 3 dpi, in the underlying hippocampus in both control and $Ccr2^{RFP/RFP}$ mice (Fig. 4b). However, the pattern of pTau immunoreactivity appeared different in the two genotypes. As in the cortex, AT8 immunoreactivity in the hippocampus of heterozygous $Ccr2^{RFP/+}$ TBI mice was mostly diffuse and located in the hilus of the dentate gyrus, outside the granule cell layer. In contrast, AT8 signal in the hippocampus of $Ccr2^{RFP/RFP}$ mice was the highest around cell bodies in the granule cell layer of the dentate gyrus and hilus (Fig. 4b, c). Thus, TBI increases tau phosphorylation in both control and $Ccr2^{RFP/RFP}$ mice, but only $Ccr2^{RFP/RFP}$ mice show clear pTau translocation to the cell soma.

Both injury and *Ccr2* genotype affect pTau levels by Western blot

In order to quantify the changes in pTau after TBI, we performed Western blot analysis for the AT8 pTau epitope in microdissected cortical or hippocampal lysates. Because the hub-placement surgery itself influenced the inflammatory reaction (Fig. 1) and pTau immunoreactivity (Fig. 4a, compare sham ipsilateral and contralateral staining), we also included treatment-naïve mice that did not undergo surgery but received ketamine/xylazine anesthesia. Interestingly, there was not an injury- and side-dependent increase in pTau levels in the cortex at 3 dpi (Fig. 5a). Yet, mice with both sham surgery and mild LFPI exhibited higher AT8 pTau levels than naïve mice in a side-independent manner (Fig. 5a). The levels of pTau were also modulated differentially in the hippocampus. While hub-placement surgery did not affect pTau in control mice, they increased pTau in $Ccr2^{RFP/RFP}$ mice in a "dose"- and side-dependent manner. That is, even surgery itself led to higher pTau on the ipsilateral side compared to naïve mice, and the higher "dose"—mild injury—led to an even larger increase in pTau (Fig. 5b).

We quantified pTau levels on the ipsilateral and contralateral sides separately in order to evaluate the effects of injury intensity and genotype (Fig. 6). In the ipsilateral cortex, both injury and genotype had a significant effect on pTau levels (Fig. 6a; two-way ANOVA, $p < 0.01$ for Injury and $p < 0.001$ for Genotype). Overall, *Ccr2* deletion resulted in higher pTau levels after experimental manipulation of the mice. There was a significant increase in pTau in $Ccr2^{RFP/RFP}$ mice in sham (surgery) mice compared to naïve mice (two-way ANOVA and Tukey's *post hoc* test, $p < 0.01$) but not an additional

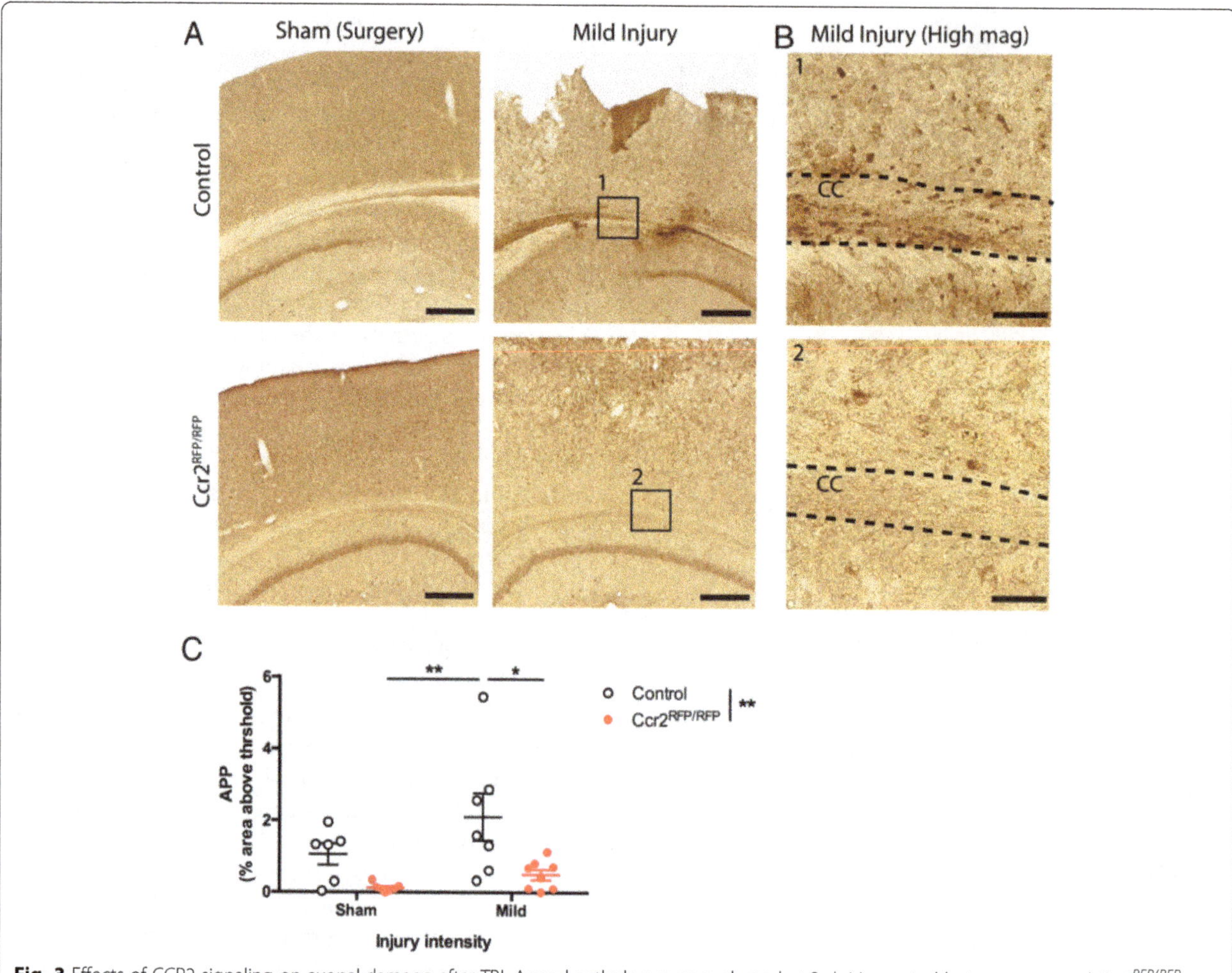

Fig. 3 Effects of CCR2 signaling on axonal damage after TBI. Axonal pathology was evaluated at 3 dpi in control heterozygous and *Ccr2^{RFP/RFP}* mice by APP staining. **a** The injury induces APP accumulation in axons of the ipsilateral side to the injury, particularly in the corpus callosum. *Ccr2* deletion decreases APP accumulation in axons. *Scale bar*, 500 μm. **b** Higher magnification images of the indicated regions (*boxes*) show that APP immunoreactivity aligns with axonal tracks in the corpus callosum (CC). *Scale bar*, 100 μm. **c** Quantification of axonal pathology as percent area of the corpus callosum with APP immunoreactivity above threshold. Statistics: two-way ANOVA and Tukey's *post hoc* test. Comparisons between groups are shown with *horizontal lines*; *vertical line* in figure legend indicates main effect of genotype. *$p < 0.05$; **$p < 0.01$

increase after mild injury (Fig. 6a). There was a significant difference between control and $Ccr2^{RFP/RFP}$ mice only for the sham surgery groups (Fig. 6a; two-way ANOVA and Tukey's *post hoc* test, $p < 0.01$). Despite the change in pTau immunoreactivity in tissue staining (Fig. 4), there was not a significant difference after injury in pTau levels in control heterozygous mice (Fig. 6a). $Ccr2^{RFP/RFP}$ mice were also significantly different from control mice on the contralateral side of the cortex (two-way ANOVA, $p < 0.05$), but there were no significant inter-group changes (Fig. 6b).

Consistent with tissue staining (Fig. 4b), we detected robust changes in pTau levels in the hippocampus on both the ipsilateral and contralateral sides (Fig. 6c, d), with both injury and genotype having significant effects (two-way ANOVA, $p < 0.0001$ for Genotype for both the ipsilateral and contralateral sides, $p < 0.01$ and $p < 0.05$ for Injury intensity for the ipsilateral and contralateral sides, respectively). There was a significant difference in pTau levels after mild injury between control heterozygous and $Ccr2^{RFP/RFP}$ mice (two-way ANOVA and Tukey's *post hoc* test, $p < 0.0001$ for both sides). As in the cortex, the sham surgery induced an increase in pTau in $Ccr2^{RFP/RFP}$ mice compared to naïve mice that was not subsequently increased by mild injury (Fig. 6c, d; two-way ANOVA and Tukey's *post hoc* test, $p < 0.0001$ and $p < 0.01$ comparing naïve and mild injured $Ccr2^{RFP/RFP}$ mice on the ipsilateral and contralateral sides, respectively). Experimental manipulation or surgery did not significantly affect pTau levels in control heterozygous mice. Thus, *Ccr2* deletion resulted in increased pTau levels on both the ipsilateral and contralateral sides at 3 days after injury or sham surgery.

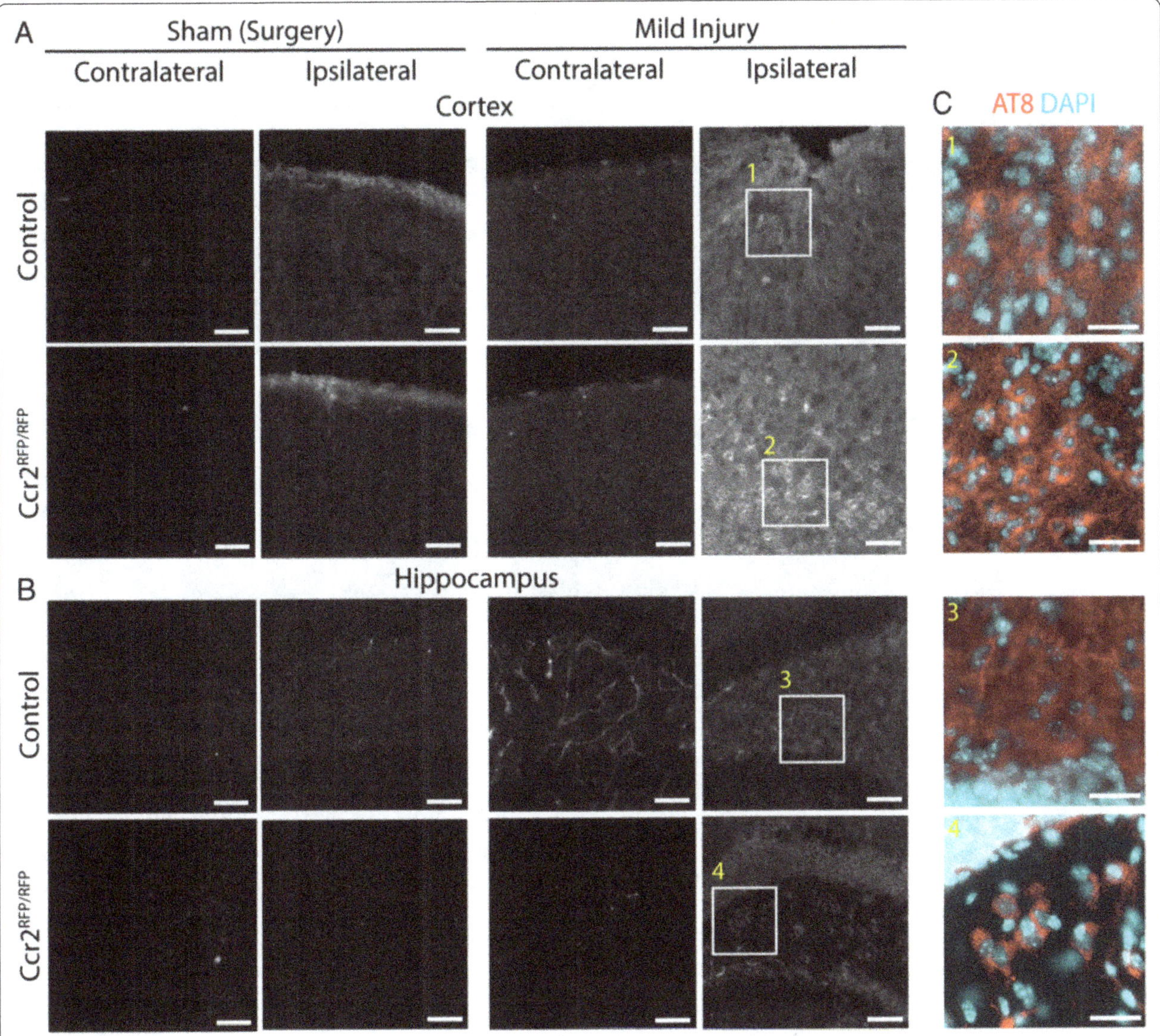

Fig. 4 Assessment of tau phosphorylation and localization by tissue staining. Sections from control heterozygous and *Ccr2*$^{RFP/RFP}$ mice after surgery (Sham) or mild injury were stained with the AT8 pTau antibody. Images were taken from the cortex near the lesion cavity (**a**) and the underlying hippocampus (**b**) and the corresponding contralateral side. Injury induces increased pTau immunoreactivity as background neuropil staining in control mice and mislocalization to the cell body in *Ccr2*$^{RFP/RFP}$ mice. *Scale bar,* 100 μm. **c** *Insets* show pTau staining (AT8, *red*) in relation to DAPI-positive nuclei (*cyan*) for the indicated ipsilateral regions (*boxes*). *Scale bar,* 50 μm

Discussion

The inflammation that develops after TBI has the potential to influence subsequent neuronal pathology [14, 18]; preventing or mitigating aspects of inflammation could help prevent secondary tissue damage and promote recovery [17]. Because inflammation is also a feature of many neurodegenerative conditions, we wanted to examine if modulating inflammation will also affect aspects of neurodegeneration such as altered Tau phosphorylation. We initially examined two models of altered inflammation: deletion of the chemokine receptor CX3CR1, which primarily affects microglia in the brain, and deletion of the chemokine receptor CCR2, which primarily affects bone marrow-derived monocytes and their extravasation to sites of damage [25, 29]. Only reduced monocyte infiltration through *Ccr2* deletion reduced cavity volume and axonal pathology (Figs. 1, 2, and 3), which led us to examine its effects on tau phosphorylation. Surprisingly, despite the reduced accumulation of monocytes at 3 dpi, *Ccr2*$^{RFP/RFP}$ mice showed increased pTau levels by both tissue staining and Western blot analyses (Figs. 4, 5, and 6). Moreover, pTau was translocated from the axon to the cell body in both the cortex and hippocampus of *Ccr2*$^{RFP/RFP}$ mice (Fig. 4). The pathology

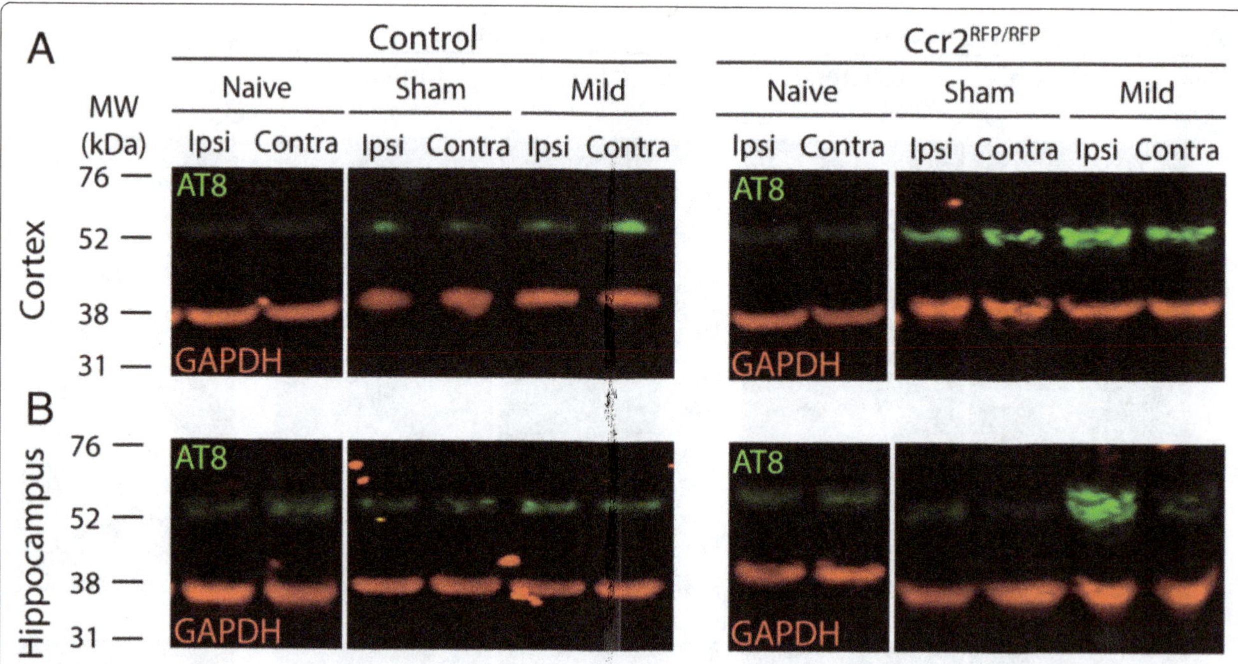

Fig. 5 Assessment of tau phosphorylation by Western blot. Protein lysates from the cortex (**a**) or hippocampus (**b**) of treatment-naïve, sham (surgery only), or mild injured control or *Ccr2*$^{RFP/RFP}$ mice were probed for pTau (AT8 antibody, *green*). GAPDH was used as loading control (*red*). Mild injury induced a visible increase on the ipsilateral side of the cortex and hippocampus in *Ccr2*$^{RFP/RFP}$ mice

seen in TBI mice here is reminiscent to the neurofibrillary tangles seen in human tauopathies [31] and in patients with CTE or after a single TBI event [3, 32, 33].

Modulation of inflammation in *Cx3cr1*$^{GFP/GFP}$ and *Ccr2*$^{RFP/RFP}$ mice

The *Cx3cr1*$^{GFP/GFP}$ mice that we employed here are commonly used to study and visualize microglia in the brain [29, 34]. Indeed, parenchymal microglia are the predominant cell type expressing CX3CR1—and GFP—in the brain as peripheral CX3CR1-positive cells do not cross the intact blood–brain barrier (BBB) in physiological conditions. However, disruption of the BBB in TBI will allow peripheral CX3CR1^{+} cells to enter the brain. In a dorsal column crush model of spinal cord injury, CX3CR1^{+} "patrolling" monocytes mediate axonal pathology [35]. In our studies, the great majority of GFP^{+} cells after TBI had ramified or bushy morphology (Fig. 1), suggesting that they are microglia. Yet, additional studies are necessary to establish the ontology of all GFP^{+} cells after TBI.

Delivery of mild TBI to *Cx3cr1*$^{GFP/GFP}$ mice did not significantly affect any of the pathological signs we examined: microglial activation, recruitment of CCR2^{+} cells, or lesion cavity, which was in contrast to the clear effect of *Ccr2* deletion (Figs. 1 and 2). Thus, we focused on CCR2 signaling rather than CX3CR1 signaling in subsequent analyses. It should be noted that microglial CX3CR1 signaling has been shown to affect tau phosphorylation in models of tauopathy. Specifically, deletion of *Cx3cr1* or its ligand *Cx3cl1* results in increased tau phosphorylation in mice overexpressing human tau or the APPPS1 model of AD [11, 36, 37]. Hence, it is plausible that *Cx3cr1* deletion might lead to changes in tau phosphorylation in our mild TBI model, but this question remains to be addressed.

As with *Cx3cr1*$^{GFP/GFP}$ mice, *Ccr2*$^{RFP/RFP}$ mice are simplistically used to study responses by inflammatory CD45^{hi}Ly6C^{hi} monocytes [25, 26]. However, subsets of T cells, NK cells, and Ly6C^{lo} monocytes express CCR2 or the RFP reporter in some conditions [26]. Although the frequency of these other CCR2/RFP^{+} cells is significantly lower than the frequency of CCR2^{+} inflammatory monocytes after TBI [24], we cannot rule out that these cell types contribute to the pathology. Thus, additional studies will be necessary to carefully phenotype the different lymphoid populations that respond to TBI and their role in TBI outcomes.

Tau phosphorylation after TBI

There is ample evidence that phosphorylated, aggregated tau is present in the brain of humans that had suffered from various tauopathies, including CTE, AD, frontotemporal dementia, Pick's disease, and others [31]. In the context of TBI, pTau has been observed in numerous individuals who had experienced traumatic events ranging from repetitive sports-related injuries to isolated head traumas (for examples, see 32, 3). Yet, there are only a handful of studies that have examined tau phosphorylation

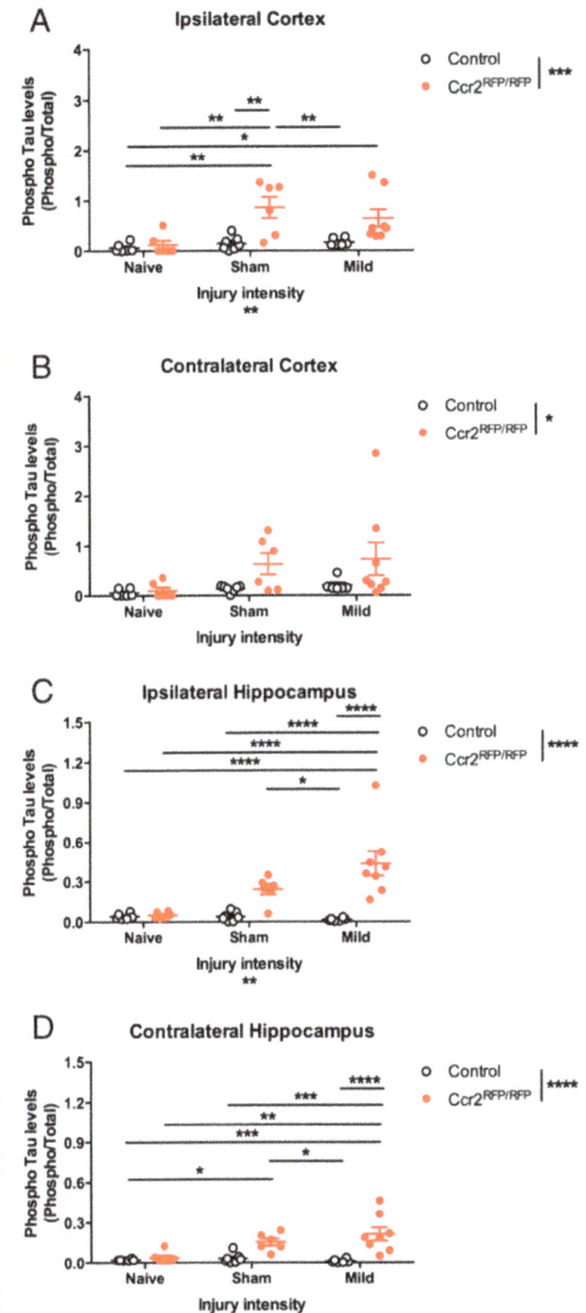

Fig. 6 Quantification of pTau Western blots. The levels of pTau (AT8 antibody) were normalized to the levels of total tau (Tau5 antibody). **a**, **b** *Ccr2* genotype significantly affects pTau levels in both the ipsilateral (**a**) and contralateral (**b**) cortex, but pTau levels are elevated after experimental manipulation (surgery or mild injury) only on the ipsilateral side. **c**, **d** pTau levels in the hippocampus are increased on both the ipsilateral (**c**) and contralateral (**d**) side in injury- and genotype-dependent manner. As in the cortex, sham surgery itself elevates pTau levels in the hippocampus. Statistics: two-way ANOVA and Tukey's *post hoc* test. Comparisons between groups are shown with *horizontal lines*; *vertical line* in figure legend indicates main effect of genotype. *$p < 0.05$; **$p < 0.01$; ***$p < 0.001$; ****$p < 0.0001$

in animal models of TBI. In two different transgenic tau-overexpressing animals, TBI accelerates tau pathology [38, 39]. Using wild type mice, Genis et al. [40] and Iliff et al. [41] show that TBI can cause tau hyperphosphorylation in the absence of mutated transgene expression. However, although Genis et al. [40] suggest that tau phosphorylation is transient, peaking at 4 h, Iliff et al. [41] demonstrate increased levels of pTau in the brain even at 28 days after injury. Similar to our study, they found that increased tau phosphorylation is not restricted to the injured ipsilateral side, but is also detectable to the contralateral side.

Another noteworthy observation from our study is that the surgery that is required to prepare mice for fluid percussion injury is sufficient to increase pTau levels when compared to treatment-naïve mice. Furthermore, certain types of anesthetics quickly increase the levels of pTau in the brain [42–44]. In our study, all groups received anesthesia, including the treatment-naïve mice. Thus, the effects of anesthesia alone are not sufficient to explain the increase of pTau after surgery and injury. Yet, these findings suggest that tau phosphorylation may represent an immediate physiological response to brain disturbances or a biomarker of altered brain homeostasis. It is worth investigating if tau becomes phosphorylated in other conditions in which brain function is impaired, such as stroke, epilepsy, etc. Moreover, although pTau is more prone to aggregation [9], it remains to be determined if it serves physiological functions that may be aimed at returning the brain to homeostasis in the acute time scales.

We were not able to detect a significant increase in pTau levels after mild injury compared to the surgery itself. One possibility for this is that the surgery and *Ccr2*$^{RFP/RFP}$ genotype synergized to produce a strong pTau signal, and the deletion of *Ccr2* itself sensitizes the mice to anesthesia- or surgery-mediated effects on pTau. Then, the delivery of an additional injury with mild intensity may not be sufficient to substantially increase pTau levels (Fig. 6). However, despite the lack of protein increase by Western blot, the injury does induce pTau translocation from the axon to the cell body (Fig. 4). As a result, surgery (or other brain disturbances) and traumatic injury may play distinct, sequential roles to lead to frank tau pathology.

Ccr2 modulation in TBI

Preventing monocyte accumulation in the brain has become a promising therapeutic approach to treat TBI and prevent the development of secondary pathologies. Deletion of *Ccl2*, a ligand for CCR2, *Ccr2* itself or antagonism of CCR2 with small molecules have all been shown to be beneficial after TBI [23, 30, 45–47]. Importantly, interfering with CCR2 signaling results in improved cognitive function for up to 4 weeks after the injury.

Yet, here we show that *Ccr2* deletion also leads to increased phosphorylation of tau protein—an event that is commonly associated with loss of physiological function and gain of pathological function by tau in a variety of neurodegenerative diseases [31]. In many of these conditions, tau is found in hyperphosphorylated form in the cell body of neurons, similar to what we observed here after TBI in $Ccr2^{RFP/RFP}$ mice. This raises the question whether interfering with CCR2 signaling might have unexpected consequences of promoting the development of pathologies.

There are still important questions that need to be addressed about the role of CCR2 signaling in tau pathology after TBI. First, are the effects of *Ccr2* deletion on tau phosphorylation long lasting or transient? Second, are other disease-associated epitopes of pTau, such as AT180, PHF-1, or CP13, affected? The work by Iliff et al. [41] suggests that tau phosphorylation could persist for at least 28 days after TBI and affect a variety of pTau epitopes. Finally, how can the absence of a peripheral cell type, which is normally not found in the brain, lead to increased tau phosphorylation? One possible answer to this last question is that the infiltrating monocytes modulate the function of resident brain cells such as neurons, astrocytes, and microglia in the context of TBI; in the absence of infiltrating monocytes, the resident cells may release factors that in turn regulate tau phosphorylation. Indeed, we did not detect a reduction in the brain parenchyma occupied by activated microglia in $Ccr2^{RFP/RFP}$ mice (Figs. 1 and 2). Whether these microglia are functionally and molecularly different from microglia in control mice after TBI remains to be determined. Similarly, whether the function of other brain-resident cell types is affected by the absence of $CCR2^+$ cells in TBI still needs to be examined.

Conclusions

Here we show an unexpected outcome of inhibiting monocyte infiltration into the brain after TBI in $Ccr2^{RFP/RFP}$ mice. Although *Ccr2* deletion is protective in terms of lesion volume, axonal pathology, and subsequent behavioral outcomes, it leads to increased phosphorylation and mislocalization of tau protein. The latter has been associated with neurodegenerative diseases and should be carefully considered if strategies aimed at CCR2 signaling continue to be pursued for therapeutic purposes in TBI and other conditions.

Abbreviations

AD: Alzheimer's disease; ANOVA: analysis of variance; APP: amyloid precursor protein; BBB: blood–brain barrier; CCL2: chemokine (C-C motif) ligand 2; CCR2: chemokine (C-C motif) receptor 2; CNS: central nervous system; CX3CR1: chemokine (C-X3-C motif) receptor 1; CTE: chronic traumatic encephalopathy; dpi: days post injury; GFP: green fluorescent protein; LFPI: lateral fluid percussion injury; MAPT: microtubule-associated protein tau; NGS: normal goat serum; PBS: phosphate-buffered saline; PFA: paraformaldehyde; pTau: (hyper)phosphorylated tau; RFP: red fluorescent protein; RT: room temperature; TBI: traumatic brain injury.

Competing interests

The authors declare that they have no competing interests.

Authors' contributions

SG performed surgeries and injuries, immunofluorescence tissue staining, Western blot, and statistical analysis. DK carried out APP tissue staining and quantification. AK was involved in imaging pTau-stained tissue sections. ONKC participated in design of the study. BTL and RMR participated in design of the study and data interpretation. All authors read and approved the final manuscript.

Acknowledgements

This work was supported by a grant from the National Institutes of Health (R21 NS082798) to BTL and RMR. We thank Anna Rietsch for technical assistance.

Author details

[1]Department of Neurosciences, Lerner Research Institute, Cleveland Clinic Foundation, Cleveland, OH, USA. [2]Department of Chemistry, Case Western Reserve University, Cleveland, OH, USA. [3]Neuroinflammation Research Center, Cleveland Clinic Foundation, Cleveland, OH, USA. [4]Neuroimmunology, Biogen, 225 Binney St, Cambridge, MA 02142, USA.

References

1. Faul M, Xu L, Wald MM, Coronado VG. Traumatic brain injury in the United States: emergency department visits, hospitalizations and deaths 2002–2006. Centers for Disease Control and Prevention National Centers for Injury Prevention and Control. 2010.
2. Kiraly MA, Kiraly SJ. Traumatic brain injury and delayed sequelae: a review—traumatic brain injury and mild traumatic brain injury (concussion) are precursors to later-onset brain disorders, including early-onset dementia. Sci World J. 2007;7:1768–76.
3. McKee AC, Cantu RC, Nowinski CJ, Hedley-Whyte ET, Gavett BE, Budson AE, et al. Chronic traumatic encephalopathy in athletes: progressive taupathy after repetitive head injury. J Neuropathol Exp Neurol. 2009;68(7):709–35.
4. Schofield P, Tang M, Marder K, Bell K, Dooneief G, Chun M, et al. Alzheimer's disease after remote head injury: an incidence study. J Neurol Neurosurg Psychiatry. 1997;62:119–24.
5. Stern RA, Riley DO, Daneshvar DH, Nowinski CJ, Cantu RC, McKee AC. Long-term consequences of repetitive brain trauma: chronic traumatic encephalopathy. PM&R. 2011;3(10S2):S460–7.
6. Yi J, Padalino DJ, Chin L, Montenegro P, Cantu RC. Chronic traumatic encephalopathy. Curr Sports Med Rep. 2013;12(1):28–32.
7. Nemetz PN, Leibson C, Naessens JN, Beard M, Kokmen E, Annegers JF, et al. Traumatic brain injury and time to onset of Alzheimer's disease: a population-based study. Am J Epidemiol. 1999;149(1):32–40.
8. Guo Z, Cupples L, Kurz A, Auerbach S, Volicer L, Chui H, et al. Head injury and the risk of AD in the MIRAGE study. Neurology. 2000;54:1316–23.
9. Mazanetz MP, Fischer PM. Untangling tau hyperphosphorylation in drug design for neurodegenerative diseases. Nat Rev Drug Discov. 2007;6:464–79.
10. Kitazawa M, Oddo S, Yamasaki TR, Green KN, LaFerla FM. Lipopolysaccharide-induced inflammation exacerbates tau pathology by a cyclin-dependent kinase 5-mediated pathway in a transgenic model of Alzheimer's disease. J Neurosci. 2005;25(39):8843–53.
11. Bhaskar K, Konerth M, Kokiko-Cochran ON, Cardona A, Ransohoff RM, Lamb BT. Regulation of tau pathology by the microglial fractalkine receptor. Neuron. 2010;68:19–31.
12. Ghosh S, Wu MD, Shaftel SS, Kyrkanides S, LaFerla FM, Oschowka JA, et al. Sustained interleukin-1β overexpression exacerbates tau pathology despite reduced amyloid burden in an Alzheimer's mouse model. J Neurosci. 2013;33(11):5053–64.

13. Das M, Mohapatra S, Mohapatra SS. New perspectives on central and peripheral immune responses to acute traumatic brain injury. J Neuroinflammation. 2012;9:236.
14. Rhodes J. Peripheral immune cells in the pathology of traumatic brain injury? Curr Opin Crit Care. 2011;17:122–30.
15. Kelley BJ, Lifshitz J, Povlishock JT. Neuroinflammatory responses after experimental diffuse traumatic brain injury. J Neuropathol Exp Neurol. 2007;66(11):989–1001.
16. Morganti-Kossmann MC, Rancan M, Otto VI, Stahel PF, Kossmann T. Role of cerebral inflammation after traumatic brain injury: a revisited concept. Shock. 2001;16(3):165–77.
17. Gyoneva S, Ransohoff RM. Inflammatory reaction after traumatic brain injury: therapeutic potential of targeting cell-cell communication by chemokines. Trends Pharmacol Sci. 2015;36(7):471–80.
18. Giunta B, Obregon D, Velisetty R, Sanberg PR, Borlongan CV, Tan J. The immunology of traumatic brain injury: a prime target for Alzheimer's disease prevention. J Neuroinflammation. 2012;9:185.
19. Dixon CE, Lyeth BG, Povlishock JT, Findling RL, Hamm RJ, Marmarou A, et al. A fluid percussion model of experimental brain injury in the rat. J Neurosurg. 1987;67:110–9.
20. Xiong Y, Mahmood A, Chopp M. Animal models of traumatic brain injury. Nat Rev Neurosci. 2013;14:128–42.
21. Prinz M, Priller J, Sisodia SS, Ransohoff RM. Heterogeneity of CNS myeloid cells and their roles in neurodegeneration. Nat Neurosci. 2011;14(10):1–9.
22. Shi C, Pamer EG. Monocyte recruitment during infection and inflammation. Nat Rev Immunol. 2011;11:762–74.
23. Morganti JM, Jopson TD, Liu S, Riparip L-K, Guandique CK, Gupta N, et al. CCR2 antagonism alters brain macrophage polarization and ameliorates cognitive dysfunction induced by traumatic brain injury. J Neurosci. 2015;35(2):748–60.
24. Holmin S, Mathiesen T, Shetye J, Biberfeld P. Intracerebral inflammatory response to experimental brain contusion. Acta Neurochir (Wien). 1995;132:110–9.
25. Chu HX, Arumugam TV, Gelderblom M, Magnus T, Drummond GR, Sobey CG. Role of CCR2 in inflammatory conditions of the central nervous system. J Cereb Blood Flow Metab. 2014;34:1425–9.
26. Saederup N, Cardona AE, Croft K, Mizutani M, Cotleur AC, Tsou C-L, et al. Selective chemokine receptor usage by central nervous system myeloid cells in CCR2-red fluorescent protein knock-in mice. PLoS One. 2010;5(10), e13693.
27. Ajami B, Bennett JL, Krieger C, McNagny KM, Rossi FMV. Infiltrating monocytes trigger EAE progresson, but do not contribute to the resident microglia pool. Nat Neurosci. 2011;14(9):1142–9.
28. Greer JE, McGinn MJ, Povlishock JT. Diffuse traumatic axonal injury in the mouse induces atrophy, c-Jun activation, and axonal outgrowth in the axotomized neuronal population. J Neurosci. 2011;31(13):5089–105.
29. Cardona AE, Pioro EP, Sasse ME, Kostenko V, Cardona SM, Dijkstra IM, et al. Control of microglial neurotoxicity by the fractalkine receptor. Nat Neurosci. 2006;9:917–24.
30. Hsieh CL, Niemi EC, Wang SH, Lee CC, Bingham D, Zhang J, et al. CCR2 deficiency impairs macrophage infiltration and improves cognitive function after traumatic brain injury. J Neurotrauma. 2014;31:1677–88.
31. Clavaguera F, Akatsu H, Fraser G, Crowther RA, Frank S, Hench J, et al. Brain homogenates from human taupathies induce tau inclusions in mouse brain. Proc Natl Acad Sci U S A. 2013;110(23):9535–40.
32. Johnson VE, Stewart W, Smith DH. Widespread tau and amyloid-beta pathology many years after a single traumatic brain injury in humans. Brain Pathol. 2012;22:142–9.
33. Omalu BI, DeKosky ST, Minster RL, Kamboh MI, Hamilton RL, Wecht CH. Chronic traumatic encephalopathy in a National Football Leage Player. Neurosurgery. 2005;57:128–34.
34. Jung S, Aliberti J, Graemmel P, Sunshine MJ, Keutzberg GW, Sher A, et al. Analysis of fractalkine receptor CX_3CR1 funstion by targeted deletion and green fluorescent protein reporter gene insertion. Mol Cell Biol. 2000;20(11):4106–14.
35. Evans TA, Barkauskas DS, Myers J, Hare EG, You J, Ransohoff RM, et al. High-resolution intravital imaging reveals that blood-derived macrophages but not resident microglia facilitate secondary axonal dieback in traumatic spinal cord injury. Exp Neurol. 2014;254:109–20.
36. Maphis N, Xu G, Kokiko-Cochran ON, Jiang S, Cardona A, Ransohoff RM, et al. Reactive microglia drive tau pathology and contribute to the spreading of tau in the brain. Brain. 2015;138(Pt 6):1738–55.
37. Lee S, Xu G, Jay TR, Bhatta S, Kim K-W, Jung S, et al. Opposing effects of membrane-anchored CX3CL1 on amyloid and tau pathologies via the p38 MAPK pathway. J Neurosci. 2014;34(37):12538–46.
38. Tran HT, Sanchez L, Esparza TJ, Brody DL. Distinct temporal and anatomical distributions of amyloid-β and tau abnormalities following controlled cortical impact in transgenic mice. PLoS One. 2011;6(9):e25475.
39. Ojo J-O, Mouzon B, Greenberg MB, Bachmeier C, Mullan M, Crawford F. Repetitive mild traumatic brain injury augments tau pathology and glial activation in aged hTau mice. J Neuropathol Exp Neurol. 2013;72(2):137–51.
40. Genis L, Chen Y, Shohami E, Michaelson D. Tau hyperphosphorylation in apolipoprotein E-deficient and control mice after closed head injury. J Neurosci Res. 2000;60:559–64.
41. Iliff JJ, Chen MJ, Plog BA, Zeppenfeld DM, Soltero M, Yang L, et al. Impairment of glymphatic pathway function promotes tau pathology after traumatic brain injury. J Neurosci. 2014;34(49):16180–93.
42. Holscher C, van Aalten L, Sutherland C. Anaesthesia generates neuronal insulin resistance by inducing hypothermia. BMC Neurosci. 2008;9:100.
43. Planel E, Richter KEG, BNolan CE, Finley JE, Liu L, Wen Y, et al. Anesthesia leads to tau hyperphosphorylation through inhibition of phosphatase activity by hypothermia. J Neurosci. 2007;27(12):3090–7.
44. Run X, Liang Z, Zhang L, Iqbal K, Grundke-Iqbal I, Gong C-X. Anesthesia induces phosphorylation of tau. J Alzheimers Dis. 2009;16(3):619–26.
45. Semple BD, Bye N, Rancan M, Ziebell JM, Morganti-Kossmann MC. Role of CCL2 (MCP-1) in traumatic brain injury (TBI): evidence from severe TBI patients and CCL2–/– mice. J Cereb Blood Flow Metab. 2010;30:769–82.
46. Liu S, Zhang L, Wu Q, Wu Q, Wang T. Chemokine CCL2 induces apoptosis in cortex following traumatic brain injury. J Mol Neurosci. 2013;51:1021–9.
47. Israelsson C, Kylberg A, Bengtsson H, Hillered L, Ebendal T. Interacting chemokine signals regulate dendritic cells in acute brain injury. PLoS One. 2014;9(8):e104754.

Permissions

All chapters in this book were first published in JN, by BioMed Central; hereby published with permission under the Creative Commons Attribution License or equivalent. Every chapter published in this book has been scrutinized by our experts. Their significance has been extensively debated. The topics covered herein carry significant findings which will fuel the growth of the discipline. They may even be implemented as practical applications or may be referred to as a beginning point for another development.

The contributors of this book come from diverse backgrounds, making this book a truly international effort. This book will bring forth new frontiers with its revolutionizing research information and detailed analysis of the nascent developments around the world.

We would like to thank all the contributing authors for lending their expertise to make the book truly unique. They have played a crucial role in the development of this book. Without their invaluable contributions this book wouldn't have been possible. They have made vital efforts to compile up to date information on the varied aspects of this subject to make this book a valuable addition to the collection of many professionals and students.

This book was conceptualized with the vision of imparting up-to-date information and advanced data in this field. To ensure the same, a matchless editorial board was set up. Every individual on the board went through rigorous rounds of assessment to prove their worth. After which they invested a large part of their time researching and compiling the most relevant data for our readers.

The editorial board has been involved in producing this book since its inception. They have spent rigorous hours researching and exploring the diverse topics which have resulted in the successful publishing of this book. They have passed on their knowledge of decades through this book. To expedite this challenging task, the publisher supported the team at every step. A small team of assistant editors was also appointed to further simplify the editing procedure and attain best results for the readers.

Apart from the editorial board, the designing team has also invested a significant amount of their time in understanding the subject and creating the most relevant covers. They scrutinized every image to scout for the most suitable representation of the subject and create an appropriate cover for the book.

The publishing team has been an ardent support to the editorial, designing and production team. Their endless efforts to recruit the best for this project, has resulted in the accomplishment of this book. They are a veteran in the field of academics and their pool of knowledge is as vast as their experience in printing. Their expertise and guidance has proved useful at every step. Their uncompromising quality standards have made this book an exceptional effort. Their encouragement from time to time has been an inspiration for everyone.

The publisher and the editorial board hope that this book will prove to be a valuable piece of knowledge for researchers, students, practitioners and scholars across the globe.

List of Contributors

Renana Baratz, Chaim G Pick and Vardit Rubovitch
Department of Anatomy and Anthropology, Sackler School of Medicine, Tel-Aviv University, Tel-Aviv, Israel

David Tweedie, Weiming Luo and Nigel H Greig
Drug Design and Development Section, Translational Gerontology Branch, Intramural Research Program, National Institute on Aging, National Institutes of Health, BRC Room 05C220, 251 Bayview Blvd., Baltimore, MD 21224, USA

Jia-Yi Wang
Graduate Institute of Medical Sciences, College of Medicine, Taipei Medical University, Taipei, Taiwan

Barry J Hoffer
Department of Neurosurgery, Case Western Reserve University School of Medicine, Cleveland, OH, USA

Xiangrong Chen, Chunnuan Chen, Sining Fan, Shukai Wu, Fuxing Yang, Zhongning Fang and Yasong Li
The Second clinical medical college, The Second Affiliated Hospital, Fujian Medical University, Quanzhou 362000, Fujian Province, China

Huangde Fu
Department of Neurosurgery, Affiliated Hospital of YouJiang Medical University for Nationalities, Baise 533000, Guangxi Province, China

Anna Teresa Mazzeo, Vito Fanelli, Barbara Assenzio and Ilaria Mastromauro
Anesthesia and Intensive Care Unit, Department of Surgical Sciences, University of Torino, Torino, Italy

Claudia Filippini
Department of Surgical Sciences, University of Torino, Torino, Italy

Rosalba Rosato
Department of Psychology, University of Torino, Torino, Italy

Ian Piper
Department of Clinical Physics, Southern General Hospital, Glasgow, UK

Timothy Howells
Section of Neurosurgery, Department of Neuroscience, Uppsala University, Uppsala, Sweden

Maurizio Berardino
Anesthesia and Intensive Care Unit, AOU Citta' della Salute e della Scienza di Torino, Presidio CTO, Torino, Italy

Alessandro Ducati
Neurosurgery Unit, Department of Neuroscience, University of Torino, Torino, Italy

Luciana Mascia
Dipartimento di Scienze e Biotecnologie Medico Chirurgiche, Sapienza University of Rome, Rome, Italy

Junfang Wu, Jessica J. Matyas, Alok Kumar, Marie Hanscom, Shruti V. Kabadi and Alan I. Faden
Department of Anesthesiology and Center for Shock, Trauma and Anesthesiology Research (STAR), University of Maryland School of Medicine, Baltimore, MD 21201, USA

Jacob W. Skovira
Department of Anesthesiology and Center for Shock, Trauma and Anesthesiology Research (STAR), University of Maryland School of Medicine, Baltimore, MD 21201, USA
Research Division Pharmacology Branch, United States Army Medical Research Institute of Chemical Defense, Aberdeen Proving Ground, Aberdeen, MD 21010, USA

Raymond Fang
Program in Trauma, Center for the Sustainment of Trauma and Readiness Skills (C-STARS), University of Maryland School of Medicine, Baltimore, MD 21201, USA

Alok Kumar, Bogdan A. Stoica, David J. Loane, Gelareh Abulwerdi, Niaz Khan, Asit Kumar and Alan I. Faden
Department of Anesthesiology, University of Maryland School of Medicine, Baltimore, MD, USA
Shock, Trauma and Anesthesiology Research (STAR) Center, University of Maryland School of Medicine, Health Sciences Facility II (HSFII), #S247 20 Penn Street, Baltimore, MD 21201, USA

Ming Yang and Stephen R. Thom
Department of Emergency Medicine, University of Maryland School of Medicine, Baltimore, MD, USA

Audrey D. Lafrenaye, Susan A. Walker and John T. Povlishock
Department of Anatomy and Neurobiology, Virginia Commonwealth University Medical Center, Richmond, VA 23298, USA

Masaki Todani
Department of Anatomy and Neurobiology, Virginia Commonwealth
University Medical Center, Richmond, VA 23298, USA
Advanced Medical Emergency and Critical Care Center, Yamaguchi University Hospital, Yamaguchi, Japan

Jin Yu, Hong Zhu, Saeid Taheri and William Mondy
Department of Pharmaceutical Sciences, College of Pharmacy, University of South Florida, 12901 Bruce B. Downs Blvd., MDC 30, Tampa, FL 33612, USA

Stephen Perry
NutriFusion, LLC, 10641 Airport Pulling Rd., Suite 31, Naples, FL 34109, USA

Mark S. Kindy
Department of Pharmaceutical Sciences, College of Pharmacy, University of South Florida, 12901 Bruce B. Downs Blvd., MDC 30, Tampa, FL 33612, USA
Departments of Molecular Medicine, Molecular Pharmacology, Physiology and Pathology and Cell Biology, and Neurology, College of Medicine, University of South Florida, Tampa, FL, USA
James A. Haley VA Medical Center, Tampa, FL, USA
Shriners Hospital for Children, Tampa, FL, USA

Kyria M. Webster, Mujun Sun, Terence J. O'Brien, Sandy R. Shultz and Bridgette D. Semple
Department of Medicine (The Royal Melbourne Hospital), The University of Melbourne, Kenneth Myer Building, Melbourne Brain Centre, Royal Parade, Parkville, VIC 3050, Australia

Peter Crack
Department of Pharmacology and Therapeutics, The University of Melbourne, Parkville, VIC 3050, Australia

Fengchen Zhang, Tao Lv, Ke Jin, Yichao Jin, Xiaohua Zhang and Jiyao Jiang
Department of Neurosurgery, Ren-Ji Hospital, School of Medicine, Shanghai Jiao Tong University, No. 160 Pujian Road, Shanghai 200127, People's Republic of China

Haiping Dong
Department of Anesthesiology, Ren-Ji Hospital, School of Medicine, Shanghai Jiao Tong University, No. 160 Pujian Road, Shanghai 200127, People's Republic of China

Tingting Dong, Liang Zhi, Brijesh Bhayana and Mei X. Wu
Wellman Center for Photomedicine, Massachusetts General Hospital, Department of Dermatology, Harvard Medical School, 50 Blossom Street, Boston, MA 02114, USA

Edwin B. Yan
Department of Physiology, Monash University, Clayton, VIC 3800, Australia

Tony Frugier
Department of Pharmacology and Therapeutics, The University of Melbourne, Melbourne, Australia

Chai K. Lim, Benjamin Heng and Gilles J. Guillemin
Neuroinflammation group, Faculty of Medicine and Health Sciences, Macquarie University, Sydney, Australia

Gayathri Sundaram
Applied Neurosciences Program, Peter Duncan Neurosciences Research Unit, St Vincent's Centre for Applied Medical Research, Sydney, Australia

May Tan
Hospital Queen Elizabeth, Karung Berkunci No. 2029, 88586 Kota Kinabalu, Sabah, Malaysia

Jeffrey V. Rosenfeld
Department of Neurosurgery, The Alfred Hospital, Melbourne, Australia
Department of Surgery, Central Clinical School and Monash Institute of Medical Engineering, Monash University, Melbourne, Australia

David W. Walker
The Ritchie Centre, Hudson Institute of Medical Research, Monash Medical Centre, Melbourne, Australia

Maria Cristina Morganti-Kossmann
Australian New Zealand Intensive Care Research Centre, Department of Epidemiology and Preventive Medicine, Monash University, Melbourne, Australia
Department of Child Health, Barrow Neurological Institute, University of Arizona, Phoenix, AZ, USA

Amar Abdullah, Moses Zhang, Tony Frugier, Juliet M. Taylor and Peter J. Crack
Neuropharmacology Laboratory, Department of Pharmacology and Therapeutics, University of Melbourne, Parkville, Melbourne 3010, Australia

Sammy Bedoui
Department of Microbiology and Immunology, Peter Doherty Institute, Melbourne 3010, Australia

Frances Corrigan, Kimberley A. Mander and Anna V. Leonard
Adelaide Centre for Neuroscience Research, School of Medicine, The University of Adelaide, Adelaide, South Australia, Australia

Robert Vink
Sansom Institute for Health Research, The University of South Australia, Adelaide, South Australia, Australia

Atsuko Katsumoto, O. Nicole Kokiko-Cochran and Bruce T. Lamb
Department of Neurosciences, Lerner Research Institute, Cleveland Clinic Foundation, Cleveland, OH, USA
Neuroinflammation Research Center, Cleveland Clinic Foundation, Cleveland, OH, USA

Stefka Gyoneva and Richard M. Ransohoff
Department of Neurosciences, Lerner Research Institute, Cleveland Clinic Foundation, Cleveland, OH, USA
Neuroinflammation Research Center, Cleveland Clinic Foundation, Cleveland, OH, USA
Neuroimmunology, Biogen, 225 Binney St, Cambridge, MA 02142, USA

Daniel Kim
Department of Chemistry, Case Western Reserve University, Cleveland, OH, USA
Neuroinflammation Research Center, Cleveland Clinic Foundation, Cleveland, OH, USA

Index

www.ingramcontent.com/pod-product-compliance
Lightning Source LLC
Chambersburg PA
CBHW082036190326
41458CB00010B/3385

* 9 7 8 1 6 3 9 2 7 3 3 3 1 *